AF886227

Kidney Transplantation: Challenging the Future

Editor

Massimiliano Veroux

Vascular Surgery and Organ Transplantation Unit
University Hospital of Catania
Italy

Co- Editor

Pierfrancesco Veroux

Vascular Surgery and Organ Transplantation Unit
University Hospital of Catania
Italy

DEDICATION

This book is dedicated to my family.

CONTENTS

CHAPTERS

FOREWORD

During the last 30 years the progress in transplantation has been impressive. Advances in surgery and medicine and the development of new immunosuppressive drugs have allowed that thousands of patients could be transplanted successfully.

Over 1 million people worldwide have received an organ and some of them have already survived more than 25 years.

However the shortage of organ donors remains the major obstacle preventing the full development of transplant services and imposes a severe limit to the number of patients who benefit from this form of therapy. The shortage of organs increases the gap between the number of available organs and the patients on waiting lists; that's the reason why, patients who respond to a specific profile have more chances to be recorded on waiting list.

As such, multidirectional efforts are required to expand donor pool. Nowadays one more therapeutic option is represented by transplantation of organs from living donors; living donation is demonstrated to be associated with superior results for the recipient, and relatively benign long-term outcomes for donors.

It is important to remember that organ donation, both from living and dead donor, is an expression of self-giving to another person, the recipient, characterizing every voluntary transplantation primarily as an interpersonal action. The act of organ donation can be seen as offering a gift; the reason is that the giver wants to benefit the recipient, acting freely, and nothing being expected in return for the donation.

"Challenging the future" is a "must" for every worker in transplant field and for every citizen: research on immunology, improvement on surgical techniques, enhancement on procurement and allocation of organs, spread communication to create a culture of donation represent the main way to imagine a future where more people can be transplanted and can rely on a better quality of life.

Dr. Alessandro Nanni Costa
Director
Italian National Transplant Centre
Rome
Italy

PREFACE

Kidney transplantation is worldwide considered the best replacement therapy in patients with end-stage renal disease. However, although impressive improvements in surgical techniques and in the management of immunosuppression, long-term results have not significantly changed over the last decades.

The purpose of this book is not to be a comprehensive review on kidney transplantation, but it would overview the recent acquisitions in the field of kidney transplantation, by offering to clinicians the future directions and the possible fields of research to improve the long term outcome.

The book is divided into 27 chapters. The first part of the book is devoted to the basic principles of immunity and organ transplantation and the clinical evaluation of potential recipient. Moreover, in this section are discussed the most recent strategies to increase the donor pool trying to offer a kidney transplantation to a growing number of patients. The second part of the book is devoted to the immunosuppression. In these two chapters, the authors present an overview on the immunosuppressive management of kidney transplant recipients, with particular emphasis on the minimization of immunosuppression. The third part of the book is devoted to the complications of immunosuppression and to the psychological aspects of transplantation. This section is particularly detailed, and offers a complete point of view on the consequences and benefits of kidney transplantation. Last section is devoted to the future. The clinical tolerance and xenotransplantation are not still the present, but the authors illustrate the fields of application of these fundamental aspects of organ transplantation.

The authors and editors have tried to select an appropriate mix of citations, but it has not been possible to cite all the relevant articles. Apologies are due to those authors whose works we have failed to cite.

Our goal was to provide the most recent acquisitions in a practical manner. We hope that we have succeeded.

Special thanks to all the authors for their excellent and enthusiastic collaboration and special thanks to our patients to whom are dedicated all our efforts.

Massimiliano Veroux, MD, PhD

University Hospital of Catania

Catania

Italy

List of Contributors

Susan Ackerman Medical University of South Carolina, Charleston, South Carolina, USA

Vincent T. Armenti Department of Surgery, Thomas Jefferson University, Philadelphia, USA

Joshua Augustine Department of Medicine, University Hospitals Case Medical Center and Case Western Reserve University, Cleveland, Ohio, USA

Ugo Boggi Operative Unit Chirurgia Generale e Trapianti nell'Uremico e nel Diabetico, University Hospital of Pisa, Italy

Pietro Castellino Department of Medicine, University Hospital of Catania, University of Catania, Italy

Claudia Cimaglia Department of Epidemiology, National Institute for Infectious Diseases "L. Spallanzani", Rome, Italy

Daniela Corona Vascular Surgery and Organ Transplant, Department of Surgery, Transplantation and Advanced Technologies, University Hospital of Catania, Italy

Lisa A. Coscia Department of Surgery, Thomas Jefferson University, Philadelphia, USA

Benedict Cosimi Massachusetts General Hospital, Transplant Center, Harvard Medical School, Boston, USA

Chiara Croce Operative Unit Chirurgia Generale e Trapianti nell'Uremico e nel Diabetico, University Hospital of Pisa, Italy

Daniela Dalla Gasperina Department of Clinical Medicine, Section of Infectious Diseases, University of Insubria, Varese, Italy

Sabina De Geest Institute of Nursing Science, University of Basel, Basel, Switzerland and Center for Health Services and Nursing Research, Katholieke Universiteit Leuven, Leuven, Belgium

Nelide De Lio Operative Unit Chirurgia Generale e Trapianti nell'Uremico e nel Diabetico, University Hospital of Pisa, Italy

Marco Del Chiaro Operative Unit Chirurgia Generale e Trapianti nell'Uremico e nel Diabetico, University Hospital of Pisa, Italy

Kris Denhaerynck Institute of Nursing Science, University of Basel, Basel, Switzerland

Fabienne Dobbels Center for Health Services and Nursing Research, Katholieke Universiteit Leuven, Leuven, Belgium

Dejan Dobi Department of Pathology, University of Szeged, Szeged, Hungary

Adrian Egli Transplantation Virology, Institute for Medical Microbiology, Department of Biomedicine, University of Basel, Switzerland and Department of Medicine, University Hospital Basel, Switzerland

Burcin Ekser Kidney and Pancreas Transplantation Unit, Department of Surgery and Organ Transplantation, University of Padua, Padua, Italy

Miran Epstein Barts and The London School of Medicine and Dentistry, Queen Mary University of London, United Kingdom

Bengt Fellström Department of Nephrology, University of Uppsala, Sweden

Enrico Girardi Department of Epidemiology, National Institute for Infectious Diseases "L. Spallanzani", Rome, Italy

Giuseppe Giuffrida Vascular Surgery and Organ Transplant, Department of Surgery, Transplantation and Advanced Technologies, University Hospital of Catania, Italy

Giuseppe Grandaliano Nephrology, Dialysis and Transplantation Unit, Department of Emergency and Organ Transplantation, University of Bari, Italy

Paolo Antonio Grossi Department of Clinical Medicine, Section of Infectious Diseases, University of Insubria, Varese, Italy

Ilkka Helantera Transplant Unit Research Laboratory, Transplantation and Liver Surgery Clinic; Helsinki University Hospital, and University of Helsinki, Meilahti, Helsinki, Finland and Department of Medicine, Division of Nephrology; Helsinki University Hospital, and University of Helsinki, Finland

Kevin Herman Medical University of South Carolina, Charleston, South Carolina, USA

Hans Hirsch Transplantation Virology, Institute for Medical Microbiology, Department of Biomedicine, University of Basel, Switzerland and Infectious diseases & Hospital Epidemiology, Department of Internal Medicine, University Hospital Basel, Switzerland

Hallvard Holdaas Department of Nephrology, University of Oslo, Norway

Donald Hricik Department of Medicine, University Hospitals Case Medical Center and Case Western Reserve University, Cleveland, Ohio, USA

Giuseppe Ippolito Department of Epidemiology, National Institute for Infectious Diseases "L. Spallanzani", Rome, Italy

Abid Irshrad Medical University of South Carolina, Charleston, South Carolina, USA

Bela Ivanyi Department of Pathology, University of Szeged, Szeged, Hungary

Alan Jardine Department of Nephrology, University of Glasgow, UK

Tatsuo Kawai Massachusetts General Hospital, Transplant Center, Harvard Medical School, Boston, USA

Eva Kemeny Department of Pathology, University of Szeged, Szeged, Hungary

Andrea Laudani, Anaesthesia and Intensive Care, University Hospital of Catania, Italy

Petri Koskinen Department of Medicine, Division of Nephrology; Helsinki University Hospital, Helsinki, Finland

Irmeli Lautenschlager Transplant Unit Research Laboratory, Transplantation and Liver Surgery Clinic; Helsinki University Hospital, Finland and Department of Virology, Helsinki University Hospital, Helsinki, Finland

Vincenzo Losappio Nephrology, Dialysis and Transplantation Unit, Department of Emergency and Organ Transplantation, University of Bari, Italy

Annamaria Maiorano Nephrology, Dialysis and Transplantation Unit, Department of Emergency and Organ Transplantation, University of Bari, Italy

Roberto Marcen Department of Nephrology. Ramon y Cajal Hospital. University of Alcalá de Henares, Spain

Jessica Maugeri Anaesthesia and Intensive Care, University Hospital of Catania, Italy

Carolyn H McGrory Department of Surgery, Thomas Jefferson University, Philadelphia, USA

Emily McQuarrie Department of Nephrology, University of Glasgow, UK

Gianluigi Morello Vittorio Emanuele Hospital, Gela, Italy

Carlo Moretto Operative Unit Chirurgia Generale e Trapianti nell'Uremico e nel Diabetico, University Hospital of Pisa, Italy

Kar-Hui Ng Department of Pediatrics, Yong Loo Lin School of Medicine, National University of Singapore and University Children's Medical Institute, National University Health System, Singapore

Laura Parrinello Anaesthesia and Intensive Care, University Hospital of Catania, Italy

Neha Patel Northwestern Memorial Hospital, USA

Vittorio Perrone Operative Unit Chirurgia Generale e Trapianti nell'Uremico e nel Diabetico, University Hospital of Pisa, Italy

Pierluca Piselli Department of Epidemiology, National Institute for Infectious Diseases "L. Spallanzani", Rome, Italy

Vincenzo Puro Department of Epidemiology, National Institute for Infectious Diseases "L. Spallanzani", Rome, Italy

Lidia Puzzo Histopathology Unit, Department GF Ingrassia, University Hospital of Catania, Italy

David Rush Transplant Manitoba Adult Kidney Program, University of Manitoba, Winnipeg, MB, Canada

Diego Serraino Unità di Epidemiologia e Biostatistica, IRCCS Centro di Riferimento Oncologico, Aviano, Italy

Mirko Sidoti Anaesthesia and Intensive Care, University Hospital of Catania, Italy

Guido Sireci Dipartimento di Biopatologia e Metodologie Biomediche, University of Palermo, Italy

Massimiliano Sorbello Anaesthesia and Intensive Care, University Hospital of Catania, Italy

Mehwish Shazly Medical University of South Carolina, Charleston, South Carolina, USA

Stefano Signori Operative Unit Chirurgia Generale e Trapianti nell'Uremico e nel Diabetico, University Hospital of Pisa, Italy

Jurg Steiger Department of Transplant Immunology and Nephrology, University Hospital Basel, Basel, Switzerland

Edit Szederkenyi Renal Transplantation Unit, Clinics of Surgery, University of Szeged, Szeged, Hungary

Kazunari Tanabe Department of Urology, Tokyo Women's Medical University, Tokyo, Japan

Enrico Vasquez Histopathology Unit, Department GF Ingrassia, University Hospital of Catania, Italy

Massimiliano Veroux Vascular Surgery and Organ Transplant, Department of Surgery, Transplantation and Advanced Technologies, University Hospital of Catania, Italy

Pierfrancesco Veroux Vascular Surgery and Organ Transplant, Department of Surgery, Transplantation and Advanced Technologies, University Hospital of Catania, Italy

Fabio Vistoli Operative Unit Chirurgia Generale e Trapianti nell'Uremico e nel Diabetico, University Hospital of Pisa, Italy

Nicole Weimert Medical University of South Carolina, USA

Hui-Kim Yap Department of Pediatrics, Yong Loo Lin School of Medicine, National University of Singapore and University Children's Medical Institute, National University Health System, Singapore

Wee-Song Yeo Department of Pediatrics, Yong Loo Lin School of Medicine, National University of Singapore and University Children's Medical Institute, National University Health System, Singapore

Luca Zanoli Department of Medicine, University Hospital of Catania, University of Catania, Italy

Annamaria Zoccolo Department of Medicine, University Hospital of Catania, University of Catania, Italy

CHAPTER 1

Immunological Basis of Acute and Chronic Kidney Rejection

Guido Sireci*

Dipartimento di Biopatologia Biotecnologie Mediche e Forensi, Università di Palermo, Italia

Abstract: For the vast majority of the 54 years since the first kidney transplant, T cell–mediated inflammation was believed to be the central process in allograft rejection. The therapies to prevent and treat allograft rejection consequently have been directed primarily against T cells. The improvements in these drugs have led to greatly improve rates of acute cellular rejection and 1-yr graft survival; however, acute rejection does still occur, as does long-term chronic rejection. It was the development of the immunohistochemical process for visualization of complement split product C4d in graft tissue that provides concrete evidence linking antibody binding and complement activation in renal allografts to the mechanism by which damage occurs in this setting. We now recognize that alloantibodies play a role in rejections that do not respond to T cell therapies and, indeed, require targeted therapies that address the various mechanisms by which they exert their effects. Newer, more sensitive technologies for serum antibody screening are allowing for clearer delineation of the relationship between antibodies and acute and/or chronic allograft pathologies and their attendant clinical outcomes. This chapter tries to clarify the antigenic targets of the humoral alloimmune response, the mechanism of antibody generation, the pathophysiology of antibody-mediated cell damage, the phenomenon of accommodation, the mechanisms of allorecognition, the T cell-mediated rejection and overview of the current understanding and classification of antibody-mediated syndromes. In addition two new aspects of allograft rejection are discussed: the roles of chemokines and Toll-Like Receptors pathway involvement in allograft rejections.

Keywords: Allografts, Antibodies, T cells, Chemokines, Antibody-Mediated Rejection, Acute Rejection, Co-stimulation, Immunosuppression, Immunoodulation.

ANTIGEN TARGETS

Alloantibodies that are of key interest in transplantation are those that principally are directed against the MHC molecules (also known as Human Leukocyte Antigens), which are "classically" responsible for presentation of foreign antigens to T cells. Donor MHC may act as a direct antigenic target (direct allorecognition) or processed by recipient antigen-presenting cells (APC) for subsequent presentation to recipient T cells (indirect allorecognition). In addition, autoantibodies and antibodies to minor histocompatibility antigens are acknowledged increasingly as potential targets of the humoral alloimmune response. The most ubiquitous antigens to which the population is sensitized are the ABO blood group antigens [1]; on the basis of population frequencies in the United States and Europe, the chance that any two individuals will be ABO incompatible is 35%. MHC class I molecules (known as A, B, and C antigens) are found on the surface of all nucleated cells in the body, of which endothelial cells are of particular significance in transplantation. MHC class II molecules (DR and DQ antigens) expression is limited to the surface of B cells, APC, and microvascular endothelial cells. MHC molecules are extremely polymorphic, with more than 1600 different alleles presently documented in humans. This property increases the chances of sensitization (development of alloantibodies or activation of alloreactive T cells), which can happen upon exposure to nonself MHC or other nonself antigens (commonly through blood transfusion, pregnancy, or previous transplantations) [2, 3].

In addition to these major histocompatibility antigens, a large number of minor histocompatibility antigens have been recognized. These minor histocompatibility antigens were defined as significant during rejection

***Address correspondence to Guido Sireci:** Dipartimento di Biopatologia e Metodologie Biomediche, Università degli Studi di Palermo, Corso Tukory 211, 90134 Palermo. Phone: +39 091 6555939; Fax: +39 091 6555924; E-mail: sireci@unipa.it

Massimiliano Veroux and Pierfrancesco Veroux (Eds)

in mouse skin graft models and have been shown further to cause endothelial cell apoptosis [4]. However, a significant effect was reported of HA-1 mismatch in Chronic Allograft Nephropathy (CAN) in renal transplantation, as evidenced by increase in the number of failed grafts [5].

Allo-antibodies against nonclassical MHC molecules, such as MHC class I polypeptide-related sequences A (MICA) and B (MICB) have been implicated with acute renal allograft rejection and loss [6-8].

Autoantibodies also may be important but are similarly incompletely described at this time. An intriguing recent study demonstrated an association between autoantibodies specific for angiotensin II type 1 receptor and hypertension, fibrinoid necrosis, and acute renal allograft dysfunction [9]. Antivimentin and antimyosin antibodies have been shown in cardiac transplantation to relate to long-term allograft survival [10, 11], and antibodies against collagen and percalan are associated with chronic renal rejection in animal studies [12].

Exposure to inherited paternal human leukocyte antigens (IPA) and the noninherited maternal HLA antigens (NIMA) can lead to either immunization or tolerance. Exposure to IPA seems to have a more immunizing effect as the mature immune system of a mother can form anti-HLA antibodies against the foreign paternal HLA molecules. On the other hand, exposure of a child to the NIMA antigens during pregnancy may lead to NIMA-specific tolerance [13]. A study by Smits *et al.* in deceased donor kidney transplant recipients compared the survival rate of grafts with a single mismatched antigen identical to the NIMA with the survival rate of grafts in which the mismatched antigen was not identical to the NIMA [14]. They showed that recipients from donors mismatched for an HLA-A antigen that were identical to the NIMA had a significantly better survival rate when compared to recipients of grafts with no mismatches. This evidence suggests that an active process of immune regulation is involved in the NIMA effect and that HLA class I plays a role in the NIMA-specific tolerance, as it is also suggested by an earlier study that showed an unresponsive state at both the cellular and the humoral level towards maternal HLA class I antigens, even during late rejection [15].

T–B CELL INTERACTIONS AND ANTIBODY PRODUCTION

High-affinity antibody production by B cells to a particular target is dependent on sufficient help from antigen specific T cells. Furthermore, the T and B cells that respond to a new antigen must be in close proximity to each other within the lymphoid organs and must be activated from their naïve state before they can interact to produce an effector response. When an APC (usually a dendritic cell) moves to the lymph node (or spleen) to interact with the effector cells, a series of events ensue to meet this geographic requirement. Upon antigen presentation to a T cell, a change in the T cell shape occurs, consistent with impending diapedesis [16], and the chemokine receptor CXCR5 is upregulated [17]. Subsequently, in response to the chemokine CXC13, located in the primary follicles where B cells reside, the T cells migrate toward the B cell location [18]. Reciprocal activity occurs with the B cell [19], which upon its activation acquires chemokine receptor CCR7 that responds to chemokines CCL19 and CCL21, ensuring interaction of T and B cells at the junction of their respective locations. Once activated, B cells then process antigen in a similar manner to the dendritic cells, displaying the peptide in the groove of class II MHC [20]. In the case of transplantation, this antigen is either donor MHC itself or donor MHC processed and subsequently presented by recipient B cells. Upon B cell antigen presentation to T cell receptor, several hours of interaction occur. Both cells change shape and maximize their contact surface area, permitting efficient and sustained interaction between their respective surface receptors and counter receptors [21]. In this way, soluble factors also may exchange between these cells.

The molecular mechanism that triggers the ultimate antibody response is the recognition by T cell receptors of the specific peptide in the MHC class II groove on the B cell. This initial bridging is augmented quickly by a series of additional links to facilitate the first signal. First, CD4 on the T cell binds a nonpolymorphic (ubiquitous) region on the MHC class II molecule, and then the adhesion molecule CD11a/CD18 (also called LFA-1) T cell integrin expresses high affinity for its intracellular adhesion molecule (ICAM; CD54) ligand upon B cell activation, mechanically stabilizing the bridge. At this time, the CD4–class II links that are located at the peripheral part of the synapse with LFA-1–ICAM adhesion complexes locate centrally

[22]. As the binding is stabilized, the antigen bridge moves centrally to initiate signalling in both cells [23]. The activation of T cells forms an independent complex discussion and is not considered further here.

Additional molecular interactions (or accessory signals) between T and B cells work in concert, leading to their successive induction and recruitment. Four distinct pathways must be functional to mediate the second signal, which facilitates class switching and formation of the germinal center [24-27]. The T and B cell molecules involved are, respectively: 1) CD100 to CD72, enhancing B cell survival and class II molecule upregulation [24]; 2) CD154 to CD40, increasing CD80 and CD86, class II and CD95 expression, isotype switching, germinal center formation, and formation of B memory cells, as well as inducing IL-6, IL-10, IL-12, Lymphotoxin, TNF and chemokines [25]; 3) CD28 to CD86 transducing activation signals in the T cell, with the subsequent indirect effect on B cells [25]; 4) Icos to B7 resulting in B cell proliferation, differentiation and germinal center formation [24-27]. The prolongation of activation is achieved by accessory signals, including CD134/CD134L, which assists in proliferation (likely *via* its effect on T cell activation [28, 29]), isotype switching and CD70/CD27, which stimulates production of memory B cells and plasma cells [30]. Negative accessory signals also exist to modulate the T–B cell response. CTLA-4 expression is upregulated on activated T cells, and this in turn interacts with CD80/CD86 and then downregulates T cell activity after a few days [31]. T cell CD153 and B cell CD30 interact late in activation to prevent isotype switching and additional B cell maturation. Finally, to distinguish an immune response, the CD95-CD95L (Fas-FasL) modulators induce apoptosis in activated T and B cells [32]. The result of initial T and B cell interaction is class-switch recombination [33], with B cells then making all Ig types in addition to their constitutive expression of IgM. Initially, short-lived plasma cells and memory B cells locate in the T zone, and a small percentage produce the first peak of specific (IgM) antibodies [34], which display low-medium affinity for the antigen. Subsequently, B cells form the germinal center, where they proliferate with numerous mutations in the variable regions of the antibodies. Each "new and different" B cell's receptor is tested by dendritic-like cells in the follicle, and those with insufficient affinity for the antigen are deleted by apoptosis [32, 35, 36]. Multiple generations of mutation occur, and, eventually, only a small number remains, forming long-term memory B cells and plasma cells that produce high-affinity antibody of all isotypes [37]. These long-term memory B cells can survive for many years and upon re-exposure to the same or similar antigens can be almost immediately reactivated to produce copious highly specific antibody. The analysis of B cells producing antibodies specific for donor antigens may be an useful tool for identifying and monitoring the humoral immune response in organ transplant recipients [38].

ANTIBODY-MEDIATED DAMAGE

Complement Activation

Complement fixing IgG or IgM antibodies (irrespective of target) on the vascular endothelium are the predominant ways by which antibodies exert their effects on the target organ, classically characterized as hyperacute or acute rejection. The two major pathways of complement activation are the classical pathway, in which certain isotypes of antibodies bind to antigens, initiating the complement cascade, and the alternative pathway, which is activated on microbial cell surfaces in the absence of antibody. We discuss only the former antibody-dependent pathway here [39]. IgG or IgM antibody bound to antigen on the allograft endothelium activates C1 (composed of C1q, C1r, and C1s components) *via* direct interaction with the C1q globular domain. A conformational change in C1q follows, with subsequent cleavage of C1r, which in turn cleaves and activates C1s, which then activates C2 and C4.

When C1s cleaves C4, C4a (small) and C4b (large) fragments are formed, exposing a sulfhydryl group on C4b that rapidly inactivates by binding to nearby molecules as esters or amides and after inactivation by factor I to C4d remains covalently bound in tissue, thereby easily detectable as a marker of complement activation and, by interference, previous recent antibody–antigen interaction [40-42]. There is no evidence that C4d has any functional activity; however, it contributes with type IV collagen along the capillary basement membrane and along endothelium [43] and is cleared from tissue after antibody activity has ceased. The presence of C4d does not guarantee that the final common pathway and attendant tissue damage will occur. If activation stops at the C4 level (where C4d would be present in the graft) but activation of C3 did not occur (and no C3d would be detectable in the graft), then graft injury may not occur.

For graft injury to occur, C4b combines with the enzymatically active fragment C2a to form a C4b/C2a complex known as C3-convertase. After C3-convertase has formed, C3 cleaves into C3a and C3b. When the C3b product is present along with C3-convertase, it covalently binds to form C4b/C2a/C3b (the C5-convertase).

This cleaves C5, forming C5a and C5b, with the latter initiation formation of the membrane attack complex (MAC) composed of membrane-bound C5b and subsequent complement proteins C6, 7, 8, and 9. The MAC causes lysis of endothelial cells and graft rejection, dependent on C6. Furthermore, C3a and C5a are chemoattractant to neutrophils and macrophages, which express surface receptors for these fragments. C3a also releases prostaglandin E2 from macrophages, and C5a results in edema *via* histamine release from mast cells [44].

Activation of endothelial cells also is an effect of complement; C3a and C5a activity on their receptors results in increased adhesion molecule expression from endothelial cells [45, 46]. Exposure to soluble (as opposed to membrane bound) C5b-C9 also increases expression of endothelial adhesion molecules (E-selectin, ICAM-1, and vascular cellular adhesion molecule-1) *via* IL-1a [47]. The MAC can trigger proliferation of endothelial cells *via* release of growth factors (platelet-derived growth factor, -FGF) [48] and chemokines (CCL2, CCL5, and CXCL8) *via* IL-1a. Similarly, soluble C5b-C9 promotes secretion of CCL2 and CXCL8 *via* NF-B pathways [49]. Both C5a and C5b-C9 also can trigger synthesis of tissue factor [50], which may be responsible in part for the thrombotic injury that dominates severe humoral rejection. The complement system also is involved in maintaining the normal immune response. Both B and dendritic cells express complement receptor 1 (which binds C3b-C4b) and complement receptor 2 (which binds C3d). CR2 activation lowers the threshold for B cell activation, and complement deficiencies in animal models have been associated with prolonged graft survival and reduced chronic rejection [51, 52].

Antibody Action without Complement

The action of antibody on endothelial cells in the absence of complement activation also may have a role in allograft rejection, particularly chronic allograft rejection [53]. Even in the absence of complement, endothelial cells demonstrate activation and proliferation in the presence of MHC class I antibodies *in vitro* [54-57].This activation may be at least partly causative of arterial intimal proliferation that is characteristic of chronic humoral rejection. Noncomplement mechanisms also may stem from direct antibody cell lysis through an Fc receptor on the surface of natural killer cells and macrophages; however, there is only limited evidence that this mechanism is related to acute rejection [56].

DETECTION OF ANTIBODIES IN SERUM

Lymphocytotoxicity assays, as first described in 1969 by Patel and Terasaki [58], have formed the basis of antibody detection through the present. More recently, high-throughput methods of increasing sensitivity (for low-level antibodies) and specificity (for anti-HLA antibodies) have been developed, which has greatly facilitated the increased interest in antibody-mediated processes. The differences in sensitivity of these tests can be dramatic, with luminex tests being more sensitive than flow cytometric tests that are more sensitive than either ELISA or cytotoxic methods. This difference in sensitivity must be considered when interpreting studies of antibodies and subsequent clinicopathologic outcomes.

Complement-Dependent Cytotoxicity Methods

Lymphocytes from a single donor (in the case of a crossmatch) or a panel of donors (selected to represent the most common HLA antigens in a particular population) are mixed with sera from a potential recipient. Donor-specific antibodies, if present, will bind to their appropriate antigen. When complement is added, complement-activating antibodies that are present in sufficient amount will activate it, the membrane attack complex will be formed, and the cells to which the antibody was bound will be killed. A vital dye is added to the reaction well and is taken up by the dead cells, which subsequently appear red on microscopy.

In the case of panel reactive antibody (PRA) testing, the fraction of wells that contain a majority of dead cells compared with the total number of wells examined forms the percentage of PRA.

Depending on the nature of the cells used in the panel, it also may be possible to determine the specificity of the antibody (*i.e.* to which antigen[s] it is binding). For cross-matching, the donor lymphocytes are B and T cells from a single potential donor, such that any antibodies detected are, by definition, donor specific. A positive T cell cross-match suggests class I donor-specific antibodies and is a contraindication to transplantation. Positive B cell cross-matches with negative T cell reactions may indicate low titer class I antibody, class II antibody, or autoantibody/non-HLA antibody, and their effect on subsequent transplantation is determined on an individual basis.

The antibodies that are detected by cytotoxicity are usually against HLA antigen but occasionally may be against non-HLA antigen also. They may be IgG or IgM, the latter of which is not usually of concern in transplantation unless the recipient has experienced a sensitizing event (*e.g.*, blood transfusion) in the preceeding few weeks. Heat treatment of the serum or treatment with DTT breaks the IgM pentamer, rendering them nonreactive, such that IgG antibodies may be reliably identified.

Anti-Human Globulin–Enhanced Complement-Dependent Cytotoxicity

If antibodies are of lower titer, then they may not be present in sufficient amount to activate the complement cascade. When anti-human globulin (AHG) is added to the reaction well of a cytotoxicity assay, it binds to antidonor antibody that is already present and bound to the lymphocytes. Unbound antibody along with AHG will be removed in the wash step. The remainder of the assay is performed as described above, but lower titer antibody than standard complement-dependent cytotoxicity (CDC) methods is detectable. AHG enhancement of the T cell CDC cross-match is routine.

Flow Cytometry

Cells. Even lower titer antibodies and those that do not bind complement may be detected using the most sensitive method of flow cytometry. Donor cells (either panel for PRA or single specific donor for a cross-match) are mixed with recipient serum and washed to remove unbound antibody. Instead of addition of complement, however, antibody to human Ig that has been conjugated with a fluorescent dye is added. This secondary antibody will bind to lymphocyte-bound antibody. When passed through a flow cytometer, cells with primary (antidonor) and secondary (fluorochrome-labelled) antibody are counted as having higher fluorescence, when the flow cytometer laser excites the colour tag. If a threshold of fluorescence is reached, then the test is considered to be positive for the detection of antibody. Neither complement activation nor high-titer antibody is required to render this test positive. As such, it is possible that a donor–recipient pair may have a negative CDC cross-match but a positive flow cytometry cross-match. Although not a cause of hyperacute rejection *per se*, these antibodies do have important clinical consequences, with higher rates of acute rejection, worse rejections, and higher rates of graft loss than in patients without these low-level antibodies [58-68]. Furthermore, because the secondary antibody is usually specific to IgG, there is no false positivity from IgM antibody. The decision to transplant across a positive flow cross-match is currently center-specific.

Solid Phase

In these assays, which are used for antibody screening before transplantation and confirmation of antibody specificity both before and after transplantation, recipient serum is mixed with inert beads (or an ELISA platform) that bear purified recombinant HLA antigen. As such, only anti-HLA antibody, if present, will bind. Addition of a secondary fluorescence antibody permits for quantification of how many beads have anti-HLA antibody bound. The degree of fluorescence measured represents the amount of anti-HLA antibody present in the original serum sample. The ELISA solid-phase platform has similar sensitivity. This particular method can be used for screening and also to determine reliably specificity of any antibodies found; however, clinical interpretation is necessary to determine the significance of these results . The assay is specific for IgG, and non-HLA antibodies are not detected.

ANTIBODY-MEDIATED SYNDROMES

The first clinically recognized antibody-mediated syndrome in the modern era of transplantation was described in 1968 in the landmark paper of Terasaki and Patel [58]. In a study of 225 renal transplant patients, in which

32 had primary nonfunction of the graft, 24 of 32 had evidence of a circulating factor in recipient serum that caused CDC of donor lymphocytes, compared with only six of 193 with primary graft function who had this factor demonstrable. The primary nonfunction in this case now is recognized as hyperacute rejection in which catastrophic intravascular thrombosis and necrosis are almost immediate after graft reperfusion. The circulating factor described now is known to be antidonor antibody, in most cases, anti-HLA antibody. The CDC assay used in this study, with relatively little modification in the past 41 yr, has formed the basis for the T cell cross-match. Recognition of this antibody-mediated syndrome and the ability of the T cell cross-match to predict its occurrence if positive have virtually eliminated the entity of hyperacute rejection in modern transplantation. Rejection refers to the activation of the recipient immune system against the allograft and, depending on the time course and clinical presentation, can be classified as subclinical, acute, or chronic. Subclinical rejection occurs when renal biopsy shows the presence of histologic findings of acute rejection without accompanying clinical deterioration [69]. Acute rejection develops over days and results in a sudden decline in renal function in association with specific pathologic findings that demonstrate acute inflammation. Chronic rejection, however, is characterized by tubular atrophy and interstitial fibrosis in the clinical setting of a slow decline in renal function over months to years [70]. Despite awareness of the importance of antibodies at the time of transplantation, there remained for many years considerable scepticism regarding any role of antibodies in any of these other clinical presentations after transplantation. The breakthrough came with the use of immunoperoxidase staining for C4d as "proof" of antibody activity in a graft. This technique has allowed for renewed interest and definition of more specific antibody-mediated syndromes in both the early and late posttransplantation periods. We discuss the evidence supporting the role of antibodies in these clinical syndromes next.

Role of Antibodies in Acute Rejection

Strong suggestion that circulating antibodies may be present and exerting a role in the pathogenesis of acute rejection in addition to the cellular cytotoxicity that was already well described and recognized was reported in 1990 by Halloran *et al.* [71]. In a series of 64 patients, anti-HLA class I antibodies were present in the sera of 100% of patients with acute rejection, demonstrating peritubular capillaritis and vascular lesions, compared with only 41% of patients without similar histology. Subsequent reporting of C4d deposits in peritubular capillaries in patients who demonstrated cellular rejection allowed for further definition and refinement of the histologic findings that are associated with acute antibody-mediated rejection (AAMR). C4d staining as indicative of AAMR is present in up to 50% of patients who undergo biopsy because of renal dysfunction and up to 32% of biopsies that demonstrate acute rejection [72-79]. Furthermore, C4d staining can be present subclinically, as can cellular rejection, in up to 25% of protocol biopsies, without [80] or with subclinical cellular rejection [69]. The presence of C4d in AAMR is highly correlated with circulating donor-specific antibody detected in recipient serum, with sensitivity and specificity of 95%, and is superior to histology alone, with sensitivity and specificity of 68 and 96%, respectively [72]. The presence of C4d as a footprint of the activity of the corresponding alloantibodies is not merely academic. Rather, C4d staining portends a worse prognosis for acute rejection, independent of other known predictors of rejection outcome. Herzenberg *et al.* [73] showed that, independent of the severity of cellular rejection, C4d positivity was associated with approximately 70% 1-yr graft survival compared with 90% survival in the C4d negative group, with similar results being reported by other groups [81]. Given the evidence linking more adverse clinical outcomes with histologic findings suggestive of antibody-dependent activity and with C4d staining sustaining the mechanistic connection between circulating antibody and observed tissue damage, the entity of acute humoral rejection was formally defined, separate from cellular rejection, in an update of the 1997 Banff criteria in 2003 [82].

Role of Antibodies in Chronic Rejection and Transplant Glomerulopathy

Newer evidence supports the hypothesis that the action of antibodies on allografts also may play a role in the pathogenesis of transplant glomerulopathy as well as classically defined chronic rejection. Chronic rejection remains a significant problem after transplantation, despite improvement in the diagnosis and the treatment of acute (clinical and subclinical) cellular rejection.

Chronic rejection should be considered distinct from other causes of chronic allograft dysfunction (including drugs, ischemia, aging *etc.*), and recent studies confirm that both circulating and intragraft alloantibodies indeed are strongly associated with the histologic processes that are consistent with chronic rejection. Just as peritubular capillary C4d staining is associated with circulating alloantibodies in biopsies that demonstrate acute rejection histology, it is similarly associated with circulating alloantibodies in up to 21 to 85% of biopsies that show chronic rejection changes, in comparison with 0 to 22% of biopsies that demonstrate nonimmune chronic injury [83-89]. Furthermore, acute rejections with C4d positive staining are more likely to lead to chronic rejection (32 to 44%) compared with those that are C4d negative (8 to 14%) [90, 91].

Transplant glomerulopathy is a late post-transplantation complication in approximately 3 to 8% of recipients, characterized clinically by nephrotic-range proteinuria and pathologically by duplication of the glomerular basement membrane and peritubular capillary basement membrane multilayering (PTCBMML), possibly indicative of repetitive waves of injury. In biopsy series of allografts that demonstrate different glomerular diseases, C4d deposits may be seen in up to 25% with transplant glomerulopathy and PTCBMML, whereas the C4d is negative in other allograft glomerulopathies [87]. C4d positivity not only is associated with chronic rejection and transplant glomerulopathy but also predicts it. Regele *et al.* [77] demonstrated that in first-year biopsies, C4d staining was a strong predictor of subsequent glomerulopathy after 12 mo (46% *versus* only 6% in the control group). Anti-HLA antibodies also have been eluted from needle biopsies of functional grafts with chronic allograft nephropathy [84], and a significant correlation between their presence and the presence of C4d staining and plasma cell infiltrate was found [92]. Furthermore, anti-HLA antibodies were not found in the biopsy eluates of well-tolerated transplants, strongly supporting a pathogenic role of donor-specific anti-HLA antibody in chronic rejection and chronic allograft nephropathy. Therefore, analogous to the new criteria approved for acute humoral rejection, chronic antibody-mediated damage is increasingly recognized as a distinct entity [93] and is currently pending addition to the Banff Criteria. Considerable research has established an association between HLA antibodies and chronic rejection. Two new major developments now provide evidence that this relationship is in fact causative. First, recent studies of serial serum samples of 346 kidney transplant patients from four transplant centers show that *de novo* antibodies can be detected before rejection. Moreover, serial testing revealed that when antibodies were not present, good function was demonstrable in 149 patients. Second, among 90 patients whose grafts chronically failed, 86% developed antibodies before failure. To assess the likelihood of a causal link, it was applied the nine widely accepted Bradford Hill criteria and concluded that the evidence supports a causal connection between HLA antibodies and chronic rejection [94].

Importance of Circulating Antidonor Antibodies

Multiple mechanisms of antibody action that results in eventual graft loss are suggested by both this unpredictability of antibody duration before loss [95, 96] and the variation in clinical syndromes that precede that loss. At a recent National Institutes of Health consensus conference, criteria that begin to address this paradigm mechanistically were established and outlined four theoretical stages of antibody action, each of which is a requirement for the next, with the final common pathway being that of chronic graft dysfunction and loss. In this model, the first evidence of antibody activation is detection of circulating antidonor alloantibody. Post-transplantation alloantibodies are more likely to be present in women, patients with a significant transfusion history, patients with pre-transplantation alloantibodies, and patients with graft dysfunction [93]. Their detection may be underestimated by the sensitivity of the assay being used, that solid-phase assays may not detect non-HLA antibodies that may have clinical relevance, and because antibody may in fact be significantly adsorbed to the graft. This last hypothesis is suggested by examination of intragraft eluates of transplant nephrectomies in which 70.6% had antidonor antibodies present within the graft. Furthermore, at the time of transplant nephrectomy, 31.6% of patients had circulating antibodies, but 4 wk after, 74% had alloantibodies demonstrated [97]. Although this latter observation may be explained, in part, by the withdrawal of immunosuppression, the intragraft eluates with high-titer antibodies suggest that the rise in alloantibody after nephrectomy may be attributed at least partly to release of antibody from the graft. This presence of antibody within the graft is the basis of stage 2 of the proposed model in which C4d is detectable in the microvasculature of the graft but no evidence of graft dysfunction is present. By stage 3, in addition to the C4d staining, there are pathologic changes consistent with antibody-mediated damage, and by stage 4, graft dysfunction is present. Although each stage is a prerequisite for the next, the progression through all stages is not known to be inevitable. Nonetheless, it is an important model that facilitates more precise definitions of antibody-mediated processes and allow for the development of stage-specific interventions and treatment strategies.

Role of Non-HLA Antibodies

A plethora of non-HLA antibodies have been shown in a variety of small studies to be associated with acute and chronic humoral rejections. The extent to which these have been explored is related to the lack of commercially available and reproducibly validated assays for the infinite number of potential antibodies to a myriad of targets in the renal allograft. Certainly, the observation that 10% of cases with C4d positivity fail to show circulating anti-HLA antibody is suggestive that non-HLA antibodies also are to be considered. Correlations between anti-endothelial antibodies and chronic allograft rejection have been documented [98-100]. Antivimentin (a cytosolic protein derived from endothelial cells and expressed in the intima and media of arteries) antibodies are associated with early transplantation coronary artery disease (chronic rejection) in cardiac allografts [10]. It has been shown that posttransplantation development of alloantibody specific to MICA is correlated with chronic rejection and poor allograft survival [101].

T CELL RESPONSE TO ALLOANTIGENS

Until recently, alloimmune responses against foreign MHC antigens were thought to be induced by either intact allogenic MHC molecules (direct pathway of allorecognition) or by peptides derived from polymorphic sequences of allogenic MHC molecules presented by self-MHC molecules (indirect pathway of allorecognition). The uniquely high frequency of T cells with direct allospecificity and the relatively low frequency of T cells with indirect allospecificity in the normal T cell repertoire has led to the suggestion that the direct alloresponse dominates the early phase after transplantation, and the indirect pathway plays a major role in the later forms of alloresponses. It is conceivable that the strength of the direct anti-donor alloresponse diminishes with time as donor DCs are eliminated after transplantation. It was reported that, in renal and cardiac transplant patients, the frequency of T cells with direct, anti-donor allospecificity declines with time [102]. In one short-term study [103] this decline was most pronounced in the $CD4^+CD45RO^+$ (memory) subset, consistent with the proposal that it is an encounter with graft parenchymal cells that leads to the fall in frequency. Importantly, the decline in the direct response was as pronounced in patients with classical features of chronic rejection as in those with stable good graft function. These findings suggest that the direct pathway of anti-donor allospecificity is not an important driver of chronic rejection. The data also imply that alloantigen presentation by the non-immunogenic parenchymal cells of the transplanted tissue could result in transplantation tolerance instead of alloimmunity. Indeed, co-culture of $CD4^+CD45RO^+$ T cells with HLA- mismatched, IFN-γ-treated primary epithelial cells derived from human thyroid or kidney have been reported to induce allospecific hyporesponsiveness [104, 105].

Clinical studies have demonstrated an increased frequency of $CD4^+$ T cells with indirect anti-donor allospecificity in patients with established chronic graft rejection [106-110]. Furthermore, the development of chronic allograft dysfunction in numerous experimental models has been associated with the increased numbers of alloreactive $CD4^+$ T cells with indirect anti-donor allospecificity [111-114]. The indirect pathway was thought to involve recipient DCs presenting exogenous antigens derived from an allograft to recipient $CD4^+$ T cells. Indirect recognition by $CD8^+$ T cells has received little attention. Activation of cytotoxic $CD8^+$ T cells generally requires endogenous antigen presentation by self-MHC class I molecules. DCs, nonetheless, have been shown to be capable of 'cross-priming' self MHC-restricted $CD8^+$ T cells to exogenous antigens [115].

Any studies, however, have blurred the boundary between the two pathways of allorecognition. A third pathway, which may serve to link the direct and indirect pathways, has been proposed. Recipient dendritic cells (DCs) can acquire intact MHC molecules from donor cells or tissues and stimulate direct anti-donor alloimmune responses. It was coined the term 'semi-direct' to describe this third pathway of allorecognition. The transfer of intact MHC molecules between cells was first noted by immunoelectron microscopy of murine thymocytes more than two decades ago [116]. Subsequently, Huang *et al.* [117] and our laboratory [118] have observed MHC acquisition by mature $CD8^+$ and $CD4^+$ T cells from APCs.

Furthermore, the DCs were then able to present these acquired MHC complexes efficiently to antigen-specific and alloreactive T cells. DCs can also acquire intact MHC class I and II molecules from exosomes secreted by other DCs, and prime naïve $CD8^+$ and $CD4^+$ T cell responses [119, 120]. Together with previous reports by Knight's group in human studies [121], it was proposed that this represents a third mode of allorecognition, the 'semi-direct' pathway. If this occurs to a significant extent *in vivo*, as recipient DCs constantly traffic through a transplanted tissue, it could provide a link between T cells with direct and indirect allospecificity, thereby solving the four-cell conundrum. Recipient DCs could acquire and present intact donor MHC class I molecules to direct pathway $CD8^+$ T cells, and simultaneously could present internalized and processed donor MHC molecules as peptides to $CD4^+$ T cells with indirect anti-donor allospecificity.

A growing body of evidence has pointed to the conclusion that alloreactive $CD4^+$ and $CD8^+$ T cells with both direct and indirect specificity contribute to graft rejection, whereas $CD4^+CD25^+$ regulatory T cells with indirect anti-donor specificity maintain transplantation tolerance. Over the past decade, several subpopulations of regulatory cells have been identified both in mice and in man, including naturally occurring innate regulatory NKT, adaptive $CD4^+CD25^+$ cells, and several *in vitro*-generated regulatory cells, such as IL-10-producing type 1 regulatory T cells (Tr1), TGF-β-producing T helper 3 (Th3) cells, $CD8^+CD28^-$ cells, $CD3^+CD4^-CD8^-$ cells and anergic $CD4^+$ T cells [122]. A large body of evidence derived from models of adoptive transferable tolerance suggests that $CD4^+CD25^+$ regulatory T cells play an important role in maintaining dominant transplantation tolerance [123-126]. It is believed that $CD4^+CD25^+$ cells have antigen specificity for a variety of self-peptides, the substrate that leads to their selection in the thymus, and that facilitates their role in the prevention of autoimmunity in the periphery [127, 128]. Given the fact that these cells have a diverse TCR repertoire, it is reasonable to argue that they are capable of cross-reactivity on alloantigens, similar to conventional T cells. Indeed, many groups have shown that the cells that maintain experimental transplantation tolerance have indirect anti-donor allospecificity [129-132]. In a clinical transplantation setting, it was observed that $CD4^+CD25^+$ regulatory cells did not significantly contribute to direct pathway hyporesponsiveness in stable renal transplant patients [133]. However, depletion of $CD4^+CD25^+$ T cells revealed significant indirect pathway anti-donor alloresponses in a fraction of stable transplant patients [134]. Furthermore, data from *ex vivo* studies showed that it was possible to raise and expand $CD4^+CD25^+$ T cell lines with indirect allospecificity against a defined allopeptide from human peripheral blood $CD4^+CD25^+$ T cells [135].

TOLL LIKE RECEPTORS (TLR) INVOLVEMENT IN KIDNEY REJECTION

The innate immunity is considered the first line of defense of the host against the growth and the proliferation of bacteria in the first phase of the infection. The identification of Toll-like receptors (TLRs) revealed that the innate immunity can recognize conserved molecular patterns associated to pathogens. The TLR are expressed on effector cells including T and B lymphocytes, dendritic cells, macrophages and epithelial cells [136]. TLR activations induce the cytokine production and increase in the expression of costimulatory molecules in macrophages, favouring the activation of T lymphocytes [137]. Classically, the TLR activation by LPS begins the cascade of intracellular signalling that involves the adapting protein MYD88, IL-1 (interleukin-1), IkB (inhibitor of the NFkB) and TRAF6 (tumor necrosis factor receptor-associated factor 6), all favouring the transmigration of NFkB for the nucleus. With the activation of NFkB, several inflammatory genes are transcripted including genes for adhesion molecules, cytokines and inducible NO synthase.

TLR4 can also recognize endogenous ligands, including heat shock proteins [138]. Surgical trauma and ischemia–reperfusion injury are likely to provide exposure to endogenous ligands for TLR4 in virtually all kidney transplant recipients [139]. Some works demonstrated in animal models that the TLR are involved not only in the immune response to bacterial infections but also in graft rejection of solid organ transplants [140-144]. 5 candidate genes were identified [145] that were differentially expressed in nephrectomy with vascular and nonvascular AR and CAN. It was hypothesized that TLR2 and TLR4 on tubular epithelial cells would be activated by endogenous ligands, but in all groups studied, the expression of these genes, TLR2 and TLR4, were not enhanced. This result corroborated other study where the expression of TLR4 was not related to kidney function or AR. However, expression of TLR2 in proximal and distal tubules was related with protection of allograft [146]. IL-6 and IRAK-3 were increased in vascular AR in relation to nonvascular AR. Several studies have shown that serum IL-6 levels can identify individuals who are at greater risk for AR [147]. Between CAN and vascular AR, other genes were also expressed (Pellino 2, IL-8 and Ubiquitin-conjugating enzyme E2). Pellino protein seems to function as evolutionary conserved scaffold protein in TLR/IL-1R signalling and as novel ubiquitin ligases for IL-1R associated kinase 1 (IRAK-1) [148]. There are no studies about E2-UBE2V1 and transplantation. IL-8 is an important acute-phase response chemokine. In one study about ischemia/reperfusion injury in kidney transplant, the expression of IL-8 was at low in ischemic biopsies from living and cadaveric donor graft, but during reperfusion increased 1.5 fold when compared to levels in the ischemic biopsy in living donor grafts and 13.3-fold over the ischemic sample during reperfusion of cadaveric donor grafts [149]. In lung transplantation, IL-8 correlated closely with TLR4 gene expression before and after reperfusion [150]. The analysis of nephrectomy showed that TLR pathway is indeed activated in the presence of graft dysfunction.

CHEMOKINES AND ALLOGRAFT REJECTION

Chemokines and Chemokine Receptors

Chemokines are a large family of low molecular weight (8–11 kDa), heparin-binding protcins with chemoattractant activity for leukocytes. Approximately 60 chemokines are grouped into C, CC, CXC and CX3C subfamilies based on cysteine motifs near the amino-terminal end of the molecule [151]. Structural similarities within subfamilies, however, do not imply common function. Chemokines within the same structural subgroup (*e.g.,* CXC chemokines) can have varied biological targets and/or functions. To better represent these aspects of chemokine biology, chemokines have been grouped with respect to their inflammatory *versus* homeostatic functions. Inflammatory chemokines are expressed in areas of tissue damage, infection or other inflammatory processes. For example, IL-8, MIP-2, Gro-α/KC and MCP-1 recruit innate immune cells, such as neutrophils and macrophages, to inflammatory sites whereas MIG, IP-10, and I-TAC recruit antigen-primed T cells to such sites. The homeostatic chemokines such as PARC, TECK and SDF-1α/β direct cell trafficking and positioning during tissue development and homeostasis. Such chemokines have been shown to be critical elements in the organization of secondary lymphoid tissues and thymic microenvironment structure [152, 153]. Chemokines mediate their activities through seven transmembrane-spanning, G-protein-coupled receptors differentially expressed on leukocyte populations and somatic tissues. Currently, 18 chemokine receptors have been identified, with some receptors binding multiple chemokines and some chemokines binding multiple receptors. Although this suggests a high degree of redundancy in the chemokine system, as discussed below, antagonism of specific chemokines or chemokine receptors has a profound effect in attenuating leukocyte infiltration into allografts.

Chemokines in Transplantation

A key event in allograft rejection is the infiltration of alloantigen-primed T cells into the graft. Recent work from many laboratories has demonstrated the presence of specific chemokines during the progression of the rejection process and the ability to inhibit rejection by targeting the chemokines. Collectively, these studies demonstrate that chemokines are important factors directing T cells and other leukocytes into transplanted organs. It was reported that the expression of chemokine genes and their production in murine skin and heart allograft models have indicated two general cascades of chemokine production during acute rejection [154]. The early chemokine cascade is primarily directed at the recruitment of cellular components of the innate immune system including neutrophils, macrophages and NK cells to the graft. Animal models of skin and heart transplantation have demonstrated that early chemokines are quickly produced in allografts and isografts; in either allografts or isografts, early chemokines are produced with similar kinetics and to an equal degree. As this early inflammation subsides, a later chemokine cascade appears in allografts, not in isografts, that directs the recruitment of alloantigen-primed T cells into the grafts. The early chemokine cascade directly influences the appearance and intensity of the later cascade, although mechanistic links between the two remain poorly understood. In renal transplants, upregulated expression of several chemokines has been documented during rejection episodes. Among the chemokines detected at elevated levels during acute rejection were RANTES, MIP-1α, IP-10, fractalkine and lymphotactin [155, 156]. In addition, MCP-1 and MIP-1β expression correlated with the histological grade of rejection in renal biopsies and the respective receptors CCR2, CCR3 and CCR5 were expressed on the graft-infiltrating leukocytes [157, 158]. This correlation suggests a direct relationship between the type and level of chemokine expression and the particular pattern of allograft-infiltrating leukocytes. Important evidence for the role of chemokines in renal allograft rejection has been provided by observations that allografts in recipients with a mutation negating the function of CCR5 have fewer acute rejection episodes and better survival [159]. Recently, urinary CXCL9 and CXCL10 were detected in adults and children during acute kidney rejection providing a role for the chemokines as non invasive markers for transplant rejection [160].

CONCLUSIONS

In the past few years, there has been an increasing interest in immune-mediated injury in renal transplant recipients. This tissue damage could be due to antibody-, T cell- and/or NK-dependent mode of action in allografts. This interest has been spurred by the improved ability to detect antibody activity through C4d staining as well as the development of increasingly sensitive methods for detecting circulating antibodies. Antibody-associated injury has been found to be associated with both acute and chronic types of injury, although it is unclear whether some of the humorally mediated injury that is currently being reported has always been present but undetected or it represents a heightened humoral response that is brought on by changes in immunosuppressive medications. T-cell-mediated tissue damage is also of interest as T cells could act directly *versus* alloantigens or inducing the generation of alloantibodies. The role of chemokines and the involvement of TLR-pathway provide intriguing evidences to better understand the immune mechanisms able to induce kidney rejection. In conclusion, many factors, any of these probably cohoperating among them, could damage transplanted kidney (Fig. **1**).

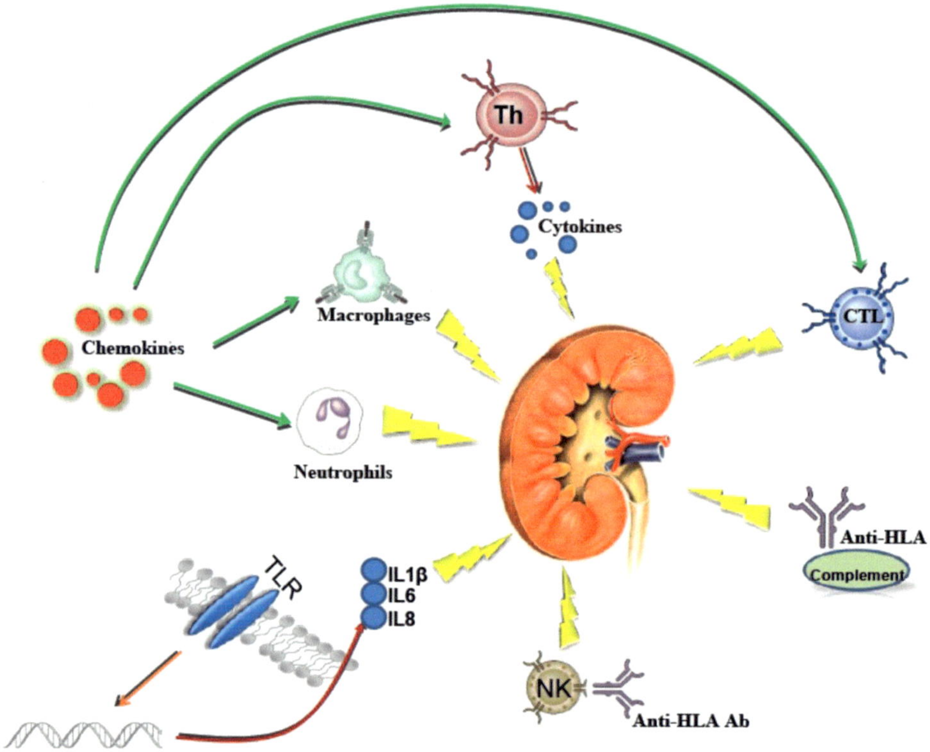

Figure 1: Here a scenario of transplanted kidney damage due to many factors is shown. Anti-HLA antibodies, T cells, Chemokines and Toll Like Receptors could cooperate each other, as depicted in the Figure, affecting allografts.

Undoubtedly, this will continue to be an area of great interest in terms of fully understanding the immune-mediated injury as well as the potential for clinical intervention to prevent kidney rejection.

REFERENCES

[1] Race RR, Sanger R. Blood groups in man. Blackwell Sci(Oxford) 1958.

[2] Erlich HA, Opelz G, Hansen J. HLA DNA typing and transplantation. Immunity 2001, 14: 347–356.

[3] Derhaag JG, Duijvestijn AM, Damoiseaux JG, van BredaVriesman PJ. Effects of antibody reactivity to major histocompatibilitycomplex (MHC) and non-MHC alloantigens on graft endothelial cells in heart allograft rejection. Transplantation 2000; 69: 1899–1806.

[4] Wu GD, Jin YS, Salazar R, Dai WD, *et al.* Vascular endothelial cell apoptosis induced by anti-donor non-MHC antibodies: A possible injury pathway contributing to chronic allograft rejection. J Heart Lung Transplant 2002; 21: 1174–1187.

[5] Krishnan NS, Higgins RM, Lam FT, *et al.* HA-1 Mismatch Has Significant Effect in Chronic Allograft Nephropathy in Clinical Renal Transplantation. Transplant Proc 2007; 39: 1439–1445.

[6] Sumitran-Holgersson S, Wilczek HE, Holgersson J, Soderstrom K. Identification of the nonclassical HLA molecules, MICA, as targets for humoral immunity associated with irreversible rejection of kidney allografts. Transplantation 2002;74: 268–277.

[7] Zou Y, Heinemann FM, Grosse-Wilde H, *et al.* Detection of anti-MICA antibodies in patients awaiting kidney transplantation, during the post-transplant course, and in eluates from rejected kidney allografts by Luminex flow cytometry. Hum Immunol. 2006; 67: 230-237.

[8] Mizutani K, Terasaki P, Rosen A, Esquenazi V, *et al.* Serial ten-year follow-up of HLA and MICA antibody production prior to kidney graft failure. Am J Transplant 2005; 5: 2265–2272.

[9] Dragun D, Muller DN, Brasen JH, *et al.* Angiotensin II type 1-receptor activating antibodies in renal-allograft rejection. N Engl J Med 2005; 352: 558–569.

[10] Jurcevic S, Ainsworth ME, Pomerance A, *et al.* Antivimentin antibodies are an independent predictor of transplant-associated coronary artery disease after cardiac transplantation. Transplantation 2001; 71: 886–892.

[11] Morgun A, Shulzhenko N, Unterkircher CS, *et al.* Pre- and post-transplant anti-myosin and anti-heat shock protein antibodies and cardiac transplant outcome. J Heart Lung Transplant 2004; 23: 204–209.

[12] Joosten SA, van Dixhoorn MG, Borrias MC, *et al.* Antibody response against perlecan and collagen types IV and VI in chronic renal allograft rejection in the rat. Am J Pathol 2002; 160:1301–1310.

[13] van den Boogaardt DEM, van Rood JJ, Roelen DL, Claas FHJ. The influence of inherited and noninherited parental antigens on outcome after transplantation. Transplant Int 2006; 19:360-371.

[14] Smits JMA, Claas FHJ, van Houwelingen HC, Persijn GG. Do noninherited maternal antigens (NIMA) enhance renal graft survival? Transplant Int 1998; 11: 82-88.

[15] Burlingham WJ, Grailer AP, Fechner JH, *et al.* Microchimerism linked to cytotoxic T lymphocyte functional unresponsiveness (clonal anergy) in a tolerant renal-transplant recipient. Transplantation 1995; 59: 1147-1155.

[16] von Andrian UH, Mackay CR. T-cell function and migration. Two sides of the same coin. N Engl J Med 2000; 343: 1020–1034.

[17] Ono SJ, Nakamura T, Miyazaki D, *et al.* Chemokines: Roles in leukocyte development, trafficking, and effector function. J Allergy Clin Immunol 2003; 111:1185–1199.

[18] von Andrian UH, Mempel TR. Homing and cellular traffic in lymph nodes. Nat Rev Immunol 2003; 3: 867–878.

[19] Cyster JG. Homing of antibody secreting cells. Immunol Rev 2003; 194: 48–60.

[20] Zinkernagel RM, Doherty PC. The discovery of MHC restriction. Immunol Today 1997; 18: 14–17.

[21] Huppa JB, Davis MM. T-cell-antigen recognition and the immunological synapse. Nat Rev Immunol 2003; 3: 973–983.

[22] Jacobelli J, Andres PG, Boisvert J, Krummel MF. New views of the immunological synapse: Variations in assembly and function. Curr Opin Immunol 2004; 16: 345–352.

[23] Scholl PR, Geha RS. MHC class II signaling in B-cell activation.Immunol Today 1994; 15: 418–422.

[24] Kumanogoh A, Watanabe C, Lee I, *et al.* Identification of CD72 as a lymphocyte receptor for the class IV semaphorin CD100: A novel mechanism for regulating B cell signaling. Immunity 2000; 13: 621–631.

[25] Sharpe AH, Freeman GJ. The B7-CD28 superfamily. Nat Rev Immunol 2002; 2: 116–26.

[26] Bishop GA, Hostager BS. The CD40-CD154 interaction in B cell-T cell liaisons. Cytokine Growth Factor Rev 2003; 14: 297–209.

[27] Coyle AJ, Lehar S, Lloyd C, *et al.* The CD28-related molecule ICOS is required for effective T cell-dependent immune responses. Immunity 2000; 13: 95–105.

[28] Kato H, Kojima H, Ishii N, *et al.* Essential role of OX40L on B cells in persistent alloantibody production following repeated alloimmunizations. J Clin Immunol 2004; 24: 237–248.

[29] DeBenedette MA, Wen T, Bachmann MF, *et al.* Analysis of 4–1BB ligand (4 –1BBL)-deficient mice and of mice lacking both 4–1BBL and CD28 reveals a role for 4–1BBL in skin allograft rejection and in the cytotoxic T cell response to influenza virus. J Immunol 1999; 163: 4833–4841.

[30] Raman VS, Akondy RS, Rath S, *et al.* Ligation of CD27 on B cells *in vivo* during primary immunization enhances commitment to memory B cell responses. J Immunol 2003; 171: 5876–5881.

[31] Cerutti A, Schaffer A, Shah S, *et al.* CD30 is a CD40-inducible molecule that negatively regulates CD40-mediated immunoglobulin class switching in non-antigen-selected human B cells. Immunity 1998; 9: 247–256.

[32] Krammer PH. CD95's deadly mission in the immune system. Nature 2000; 407: 789–795.

[33] Posey JE, Brandt VL, Roth DB. Paradigm switching in the germinal center. Nat Immunol 2004; 5: 476–477.

[34] McHeyzer-Williams MG. B cells as effectors. Curr Opin Immunol 2003; 15: 354–361.

[35] Manser T. Textbook germinal centers? J Immunol 2004; 172:3369–3375.

[36] Tarlinton D. Germinal centers: Form and function. Curr Opin Immunol 1998; 10: 245–251.

[37] Slifka MK, Ahmed R. Long-lived plasma cells: A mechanism for maintaining persistent antibody production. Curr Opin Immunol 1998; 10: 252–258.

[38] Han M, Rogers JA, Lavingia B, Stastny P. Peripheral blood B cells producing donor-specific HLA antibodies *in vitro*. Hum Immunol. 2009;70 :29-34.

[39] Prodinger WM, Wurzner R, Stoiber H, Dierich MP. Complement. In: Fundamentals in Immunology, edited by Paul WE, Philadelphia, Lippincott Williams & Wilkins, 2003, pp1077–103.

[40] van den Elsen JM, Martin A, Wong V, *et al.* X-ray crystal structure of the C4d fragment of human complement component C4. J Mol Biol 2002; 322:1103–1115.

[41] Collins AB, Schneeberger EE, Pascual MA, *et al.* Complement activation in acute humoral renal allograft rejection: Diagnostic significance of C4d deposits in peritubular capillaries. J Am Soc Nephrol 1999; 10: 2208–2214.

[42] Bohmig GA, Exner M, Habicht A, *et al.* Capillary C4d deposition in kidney allografts. A specific marker of alloantibody-dependent graft injury. J Am Soc Nephrol 2002; 13: 1091–1099.

[43] Nakashima S, Qian Z, Rahimi S, *et al.* Membrane attack complex contributes to destruction of vascular integrity in acute lung allograft rejection. J Immunol 2002; 169: 4620–4627.

[44] Saadi S, Platt JL. Humoral rejection and endothelial cell activation. Xenotransplantation 2002; 9: 239–241.

[45] Albrecht EA, Chinnaiyan AM, Varambally S, *et al.* C5a-induced gene expression in human umbilical vein endothelial cells. Am J Pathol 2004; 164: 849–859.

[46] Monsinjon T, Gasque P, Chan P, *et al.* Regulation by complement C3a and C5a anaphylatoxins of cytokine production in human umbilical vein endothelial cells. FASEB J 2003; 17: 1003–1014.

[47] Saadi S, Holzknecht RA, Patte CP, Platt JL. Endothelial cell activation by pore-forming structures: Pivotal role for interleukin-1alpha. Circulation 2000; 101: 1867–1873.

[48] Benzaquen LR, Nicholson-Weller A, Halperin JA. Terminal complement proteins C5b-9 release basic fibroblast growth factor and platelet-derived growth factor from endothelial cells. J Exp Med 1994; 179: 985–992.

[49] Kilgore KS, Schmid E, Shanley TP, *et al.* Sublytic concentrations of the membrane attack complex of complement induce endothelial interleukin-8 and monocyte chemoattractant protein-1 through nuclear factor-kappa B activation. Am J Pathol 1997; 150: 2019–2031.

[50] Ikeda K, Nagasawa K, Horiuchi T, *et al.* C5a induces tissue factor activity on endothelial cells. Thromb Haemost 1997; 77: 394–398.

[51] Saadi S, Holzknecht RA, Patte CP, *et al.* Complement-mediated regulation of tissue factor activity in endothelium. J Exp Med 1995; 182: 1807–1814.

[52] Qian Z, Wasowska BA, Behrens E, *et al.* C6 produced by macrophages contributes to cardiac allograft rejection. Am J Pathol 1999; 155: 1293–1302.

[53] Ota H, Fox-Talbot K, Hu W, *et al.* Terminal complement components mediate release of von Willebrand factor and adhesion of platelets in arteries of allografts. Transplantation 2005; 79: 276–281.

[54] Pratt JR, Basheer SA, Sacks SH. Local synthesis of complement component C3 regulates acute renal transplant rejection. Nat Med 2002; 8: 582–587.

[55] Rahimi A, Sepehri H, Pakravesh J, Bahar K.Quantification of C3 and C4 in infertile men with antisperm antibody in their seminal plasma. Am J Reprod Immunol 1999; 41: 330–336.

[56] Smith JD, Lawson C, Yacoub MH, Rose ML. Activation of NF-kappa B in human endothelial cells induced by monoclonal and allospecific HLA antibodies. Int Immunol 2000; 12: 563–571.

[57] Jin YP, Singh RP, Du ZY, *et al.* Ligation of HLA class I molecules on endothelial cells induces phosphorylation of Src, paxillin, and focal adhesion kinase in an actin-dependent manner. J Immunol 2002; 168: 5415–5423.

[58] Patel R, Terasaki PI. Significance of the positive crossmatch test in kidney transplantation. N Engl J Med 1969; 280: 735–739.

[59] Yuan FF, Watson N, Sullivan JS, *et al.* Association of Fc gamma receptor IIA polymorphisms with acute renal-allograft rejection. Transplantation 2004; 78: 766–769.

[60] Gebel HM, Bray RA. Sensitization and sensitivity. Defining the unsensitized patient. Transplantation 2000; 69: 1370–1374.

[61] Iwaki Y, Lau M, Cook DJ, *et al.* Crossmatching with B and T cells and flow cytometry. Clin Transpl 1986; 277–284.

[62] Cook DJ, Fettouh HI, Gjertson DW, Cecka JM. Flow cytometry crossmatching (FCXM) in the UNOS Kidney Transplant Registry. Clin Transpl 1998; 413–419.

[63] Mahoney RJ, Ault KA, Given SR, *et al.* The flow cytometric crossmatch and early renal transplant loss. Transplantation 1990; 49: 527–535.

[64] Ogura K, Terasaki PI, Johnson C, *et al.* The significance of a positive flow cytometry crossmatch test in primary kidney transplantation. Transplantation 1993; 56: 294–298.

[65] Karpinski M, Rush D, Jeffery J, *et al.* Flow cytometric crossmatching in primary renal transplant recipients with a negative anti-human globulin enhanced cytotoxicity crossmatch. J Am Soc Nephrol 2001; 12: 2807–2814.

[66] Kimball P, Rhodes C, King A, *et al.* Flow cross-matching identifies patients at risk for postoperative elaboration of cytotoxic antibodies. Transplantation 1998; 65: 444–446.

[67] El Fettouh HA, Cook DJ, Bishay E, *et al.* Association between a positive flow cytometry crossmatch and the development of chronic rejection in primary renal transplantation. Urology 2000; 56: 369–372.

[68] Gebel HM, Harris SB, Zibari G, Bray RA. Conundrums with FlowPRA beads. Clin Transplant 2002; 16: 24–29.

[69] Rush D, Somorjai R, Deslauriers R, *et al.* Subclinical rejection—a potential surrogate marker for chronic rejection—may be diagnosed by protocol biopsy or urine spectroscopy. Ann Transplant 2000; 5: 44–49.

[70] Racusen LC, Solez K, Colvin RB, *et al.* The Banff 97 working classification of renal allograft pathology. Kidney Int 1999; 55: 713–723.

[71] Halloran PF, Wadgymar A, Ritchie S, *et al.* The significance of the anti-class I antibody response. I. Clinical and pathologic features of anti-class I-mediated rejection. Transplantation 1990; 49: 85–91.

[72] Mauiyyedi S, Crespo M, Collins AB, *et al.* Acute humoral rejection in kidney transplantation: II. Morphology, immunopathology, and pathologic classification. J Am Soc Nephrol 2002; 13: 779–787.

[73] Herzenberg AM, Gill JS, Djurdjev O, Magil AB. C4d deposition in acute rejection: An independent long-term prognostic factor. J Am Soc Nephrol 2002; 13: 234–241.

[74] Nickeleit V, Zeiler M, Gudat F, *et al.* Detection of the complement degradation product C4d in renal allografts: Diagnostic and therapeutic implications. J Am Soc Nephrol 2002; 13: 242–251.

[75] Lederer SR, Kluth-Pepper B, Schneeberger H, *et al.* Impact of humoral alloreactivity early after transplantation on the long-term survival of renal allografts. Kidney Int 2001; 59: 334–341.

[76] Regele H, Exner M, Watschinger B, *et al.* Endothelial C4d deposition is associated with inferior kidney allograft outcome independently of cellular rejection. Nephrol Dial Transplant 2001; 16: 2058–2066.

[77] Regele H, Bohmig GA, Habicht A, *et al.* Capillary deposition of complement split product C4d in renal allografts is associated with basement membrane injury in peritubular and glomerular capillaries: A contribution of humoral immunity to chronic allograft rejection. J Am Soc Nephrol 2002 ; 13: 2371–2380.

[78] Sund S, Hovig T, Reisaeter AV, *et al.* Complement activation in early protocol kidney graft biopsies after living-donor transplantation. Transplantation 2003; 75: 1204–1213.

[79] Koo DD, Roberts IS, Quiroga I, *et al.* C4d deposition in early renal allograft protocol biopsies. Transplantation 2004; 78: 398–403.

[80] Bolmig G, Regele H. Diagnosis and treatment of antibody mediated kidney allograft rejection. Transpl Int 2003; 16: 773–787.

[81] Fidler ME, Gloor JM, Lager DJ, *et al.* Histologic findings of antibody-mediated rejection in ABO blood-group-incompatible living-donor kidney transplantation. Am J Transplant 2004; 4: 101–107.

[82] Racusen LC, Colvin RB, Solez K, *et al.* Antibody- mediated rejection criteria: An addition to the Banff 97 classification of renal allograft rejection. Am J Transplant 2003; 3: 708–714.

[83] Mauiyyedi S, Pelle PD, Saidman S, *et al.* Chronic humoral rejection: Identification of antibody-mediated chronic renal allograft rejection by C4d deposits in peritubular capillaries. J Am Soc Nephrol 2001; 12: 574–582.

[84] Cardarelli F, Pascual M, Tolkoff-Rubin N, *et al.* Prevalence and significance of anti-HLA and donorspecific antibodies long-term after renal transplantation. Transpl Int 2005; 18: 532–540.

[85] Herman J, Lerut E, Van Damme-Lombaerts R, *et al.* Capillary deposition of complement C4d and C3d in pediatric renal allograft biopsies. Transplantation 2005; 79: 1435–1440.

[86] Mroz A, Durlik M, Cieciura T, *et al.* C4d complement split product expression in chronic rejection of renal allograft. Transplant Proc 2003; 35: 2190–2192.

[87] Vongwiwatana A, Tasanarong A, Hidalgo LG, Halloran PF. The role of B cells and alloantibody in the host response to human organ allografts. Immunol Rev 2003; 196: 197–218.

[88] Sijpkens YW, Doxiadis, II, van Kemenade FJ, *et al.* Chronic rejection with or without transplant vasculopathy. Clin Transplant 2003; 17: 163–170.

[89] Jeong HJ, Kim SH, Kim YS, *et al.* Peritubular capillary C4d deposition in chronic allograft dysfunction. Yonsei Med J 2004; 45: 859–864.

[90] Rotman S, Collins AB, Colvin RB. C4d deposition in allografts: Current concepts and interpretation. Transplantation Reviews 2005;19: 65–77.

[91] Piazza A, Poggi E, Borrelli L, *et al.* Impact of donor-specific antibodies on chronic rejection occurrence and graft loss in renal transplantation: Posttransplant analysis using flow cytometric techniques. Transplantation 2001; 71: 1106–1112.

[92] Rifle G, Mousson C, Martin L, *et al.* Donorspecific antibodies in allograft rejection: Clinical and experimental data. Transplantation 2005; 79: S14–18.

[93] Takemoto SK, Zeevi A, Feng S, *et al.* National conference to assess antibody mediated rejection in solid organ transplantation. Am J Transplant 2004; 4: 1033–1041.

[94] Terasaki PI, Cai J. Human leukocyte antigen antibodies and chronic rejection: from association to causation.Transplantation 2008; 86: 377-383.

[95] Lee PC, Terasaki PI, Takemoto SK, *et al.* All chronic rejection failures of kidney transplants were preceded by the development of HLA antibodies. Transplantation 2002 ; 74: 1192–1194.

[96] Worthington JE, Martin S, Al-Husseini DM, *et al.* Posttransplantation production of donor HLA specific antibodies as a predictor of renal transplant outcome. Transplantation 2003; 75: 1034–1040.

[97] Hourmant M, Cesbron-Gautier A, Terasaki PI, *et al.* Frequency and clinical implications of development of donor-specific and non-donor-specific HLA antibodies after kidney transplantation. J Am Soc Nephrol 2005; 16: 2804–2812.

[98] Martin L, Guignier F, Mousson C, *et al.* Detection of donor-specific anti-HLA antibodies with flow cytometry in eluates and sera from renal transplant recipients with chronic allograft nephropathy. Transplantation 2003;76: 395–400.

[99] Ferry BL, Welsh KI, Dunn MJ, *et al.* Anti-cell surface endothelial antibodies in sera from cardiac and kidney transplant recipients: Association with chronic rejection. Transpl Immunol 1997; 5: 17–24.

[100] Ball B, Mousson C, Ratignier C, *et al.* Antibodies to vascular endothelial cells in chronic rejection of renal allografts. Transplant Proc 2000; 32: 353–354.

[101] Mizutani K, Terasaki PI, Rosen A, *et al.* Serial ten-year followup of HLA and MICA antibody production prior to kidney graft failure. Am J Transplant 2005; 5: 2265-2272.

[102] Hornick PI,Mason PD, Yacoub MH, *et al.* Assessment of the contribution that direct allorecognition makes to the progression of chronic cardiac transplant rejection in humans. Circulation 1998; 97:1257-1263.

[103] Baker RJ, Hernandez-Fuentes MP, Brookes PA, *et al.* Loss of direct and maintenance of indirect alloresponses in renal allograft recipients: implications for the pathogenesis of chronic allograft nephropathy. J Immunol 2001; 167:7199-7206.

[104] Marelli-Berg FM, Weetman A, Frasca L, *et al.* Antigen presentation by epithelial cells induces anergic immunoregulatory CD45RO+ T cells and deletion of CD45RA+ T cells. J Immunol 1997; 159: 5853-5861.

[105] Marelli-Berg FM, Scott D, Bartok I, *et al.* Activated murine endothelial cells have reduced immunogenicity for CD8+ T cells: a mechanism of immunoregulation? J Immunol 2000; 165:4182-4189.

[106] Hornick PI, Mason PD, Baker RJ, *et al.* Significant frequencies of T cells with indirect anti-donor specificity in heart graft recipients with chronic rejection. Circulation 2000; 101: 2405-2410.

[107] Vella JP, Spadafora-Ferreira M, Murphy B, *et al.* Indirect allorecognition of major histocompatibility complex allopeptides in human renal transplant recipients with chronic graft dysfunction. Transplantation 1997; 64:795-800.

[108] Ciubotariu R, Liu Z, Colovai AI, *et al.* Persistent allopeptide reactivity and epitope spreading in chronic rejection of organ allografts. J Clin Invest 1998; 101:398-405.

[109] Liu Z, Colovai AI, Tugulea S, *et al.* Indirect recognition of donor HLA-DR peptides in organ allograft rejection. J Clin Invest 1996; 98: 1150-1157.
[110] Preston EH, Light JA, Kampen RL, Kirk AD. Human renal allograft rejection despite the absence of allogeneic passenger leukocytes. Am J Transplant 2004; 4: 283-285.
[111] Benichou G, Valujskikh A, Heeger PS. Contributions of direct and indirect T cell alloreactivity during allograft rejection in mice. J Immunol 1999; 162: 352-358.
[112] Lee RS, Yamada K, Houser SL,*et al.* Indirect recognition of allopeptides promotes the development of cardiac allograft vasculopathy. Proc Natl Acad Sci USA 2001; 98:3276-3281.
[113] Ensminger SM, Spriewald BM, Witzke O, *et al.* Indirect allorecognition can play an important role in the development of transplant arteriosclerosis. Transplantation 2002; 73:279-286.
[114] Richards DM, Dalheimer SL, Ehst BD, *et al.* Indirect minor histocompatibility antigen presentation by allograft recipient cells in the draining lymph node leads to the activation and clonal expansion of $CD4^+$ T cells that cause obliterative airways disease. J Immunol 2004; 172: 3469-3479.
[115] Albert ML, Sauter B, Bhardwaj N. Dendritic cells acquire antigen from apoptotic cells and induce class I-restricted CTLs. Nature 1998; 392: 86-89.
[116] Sharrow SO, Mathieson BJ, Singer A. Cell surface appearance of unexpected host MHC determinants on thymocytes from radiation bone marrow chimeras. J Immunol 1981; 126:1327-1335.
[117] Huang JF, Yang Y, Sepulveda H, Shi W, *et al.* TCR-Mediated internalization of peptide-MHC complexes acquired by T cells. Science 1999; 286: 952-954.
[118] Tsang JY, Chai JG, Lechler R. Antigen presentation by mouse CD4+ T cells involving acquired MHC class II:peptide complexes: another mechanism to limit clonal expansion? Blood 2003; 101: 2704-2710.
[119] Andre F, Chaput N, Schartz NE, Flament C, *et al.* Exosomes as potent cell-free peptide-based vaccine. I. Dendritic cell-derived exosomes transfer functional MHC class I/peptide complexes to dendritic cells. J Immunol 2004;172: 2126-2136.
[120] Thery C, Duban L, Segura E, Veron P, *et al.* Indirect activation of naive CD4+ T cells by dendritic cell-derived exosomes. Nat Immunol 2002; 3: 1156-1162.
[121] Bedford P, Garner K, Knight SC. MHC class II molecules transferred between allogeneic dendritic cells stimulate primary mixed leukocyte reactions. Int Immunol 1999; 11: 1739-1744.
[122] Jiang S, Lechler RI. Regulatory T cells in the control of transplantation tolerance and autoimmunity. Am J Transplant 2003; 3: 516-524.
[123] Hall BM, Pearce NW, Gurley KE, Dorsch SE. Specific unresponsiveness in rats with prolonged cardiac allograft survival after treatment with cyclosporine. III. Further characterization of the CD4+ suppressor cell and its mechanisms of action. J Exp Med 1990; 171: 141-157.
[124] Gregori S, Casorati M, Amuchastegui S, *et al.* Regulatory T cells induced by 1 alpha, 25-dihydroxyvitamin D3 and mycophenolate mofetil treatment mediate transplantation tolerance. J Immunol 2001; 167: 1945-1953.
[125] Zhai Y, Shen XD, Lehmann M, Busuttil R, *et al.* T cell subsets and *in vitro* immune regulation in 'infectious' transplantation tolerance. J Immunol 2001; 167: 4814-4820.
[126] Graca L, Cobbold SP, Waldmann H. Identification of regulatory T cells in tolerated allografts. J Exp Med 2002; 195: 1641-1646.
[127] Wood KJ, Sakaguchi S. Regulatory T cells in transplantation tolerance. Nat Rev Immunol 2003; 3: 199-210.
[128] Sakaguchi S. Naturally arising $CD4^+$ regulatory T cells for immunologic self-tolerance and negative control of immune responses. Annu Rev Immunol 2004; 22:531-562.
[129] Hara M, Kingsley CI, Niimi M, Read S, *et al.*IL-10 is required for regulatory T cells to mediate tolerance to alloantigens *in vivo*. J Immunol 2001, 166: 3789-3796.
[130] van Maurik A, Herber M, Wood KJ, Jones ND. $CD4^+CD25^+$ alloantigen-specific immunoregulatory cells that can prevent $CD8^+$ T cell-mediated graft rejection: implications for anti- CD154 immunotherapy. J Immunol 2002; 169: 5401-5404.
[131] Quezada SA, Fuller B, Jarvinen LZ, Gonzalez M, *et al.* Mechanisms of donorspecific transfusion tolerance: preemptive induction of clonal T-cell exhaustion *via* indirect presentation. Blood 2003; 102: 1920-1926.
[132] Mirenda V, Berton I, Read J, Cook T, *et al.* Modified dendritic cells coexpressing self and allogeneic major histocompatability complex molecules: an efficient way to induce indirect pathway regulation. J Am Soc Nephrol 2004; 15: 987-997.
[133] Game DS, Hernandez-Fuentes MP, Chaudhry AN, Lechler RI. $CD4^+CD25^+$ regulatory T cells do not significantly contribute to direct pathway hyporesponsiveness in stable renal transplant patients. J Am Soc Nephrol 2003; 14: 1652-1661.

[134] Salama AD, Najafian N, Clarkson MR, *et al.* Regulatory CD25$^+$ T cells in human kidney transplant recipients. J Am Soc Nephrol 2003; 14: 1643-1651.

[135] Jiang S, Camara N, Lombardi G, Lechler RI. Induction of allopeptide-specific human CD4$^+$CD25$^+$ regulatory T cells *ex vivo*. Blood 2003; 102: 2180-2186.

[136] Schaefer TM, Desouza K, Fahey JV, Beagley KW, *et al.* Toll-like receptor (TLR) expression and TLR-mediated cytokine/chemokine production by human uterine epithelial cells. Immunology 2004; 112: 428–436.

[137] Akira S, Sato S. Toll-like receptors and their signaling mechanisms. Scand J Infect Dis 2003; 35: 555–562.

[138] Vabulas RM, Ahmad-Nejad P, da Costa C, Miethke T, *et al.* Endocytosed HSP60s use toll-like receptor 2 (TLR2) and TLR4 to activate the toll/ interleukin-1 receptor signaling pathway in innate immune cells. J Biol Chem 17; 276: 31332–31339.

[139] Lin T, Zhou W, Sacks SH. The role of complement and Toll-like receptors in organ transplantation. Transplant Int 2007; 20: 481–489.

[140] Wolfs TGA, BuurmanWA, van Schadewijk A, Vries B, *et al. In vivo* expression of toll-like receptor 2 and 4 by renal epithelial cells: IFN- and TNF-mediated up-regulation during inflammation. J Immunol 2002; 168: 1286–1293.

[141] Supajatura V, Ushio H, Nakao A, Okumura K, *et al.* Protective roles of mast cells against enterobacterial infection are mediated by Toll-like receptor 4. J Immunol 2001; 167: 2250–2256.

[142] Goldstein DR, Tesar BM, Akira S, Lakkis FG. Critical role of the Toll-like receptor signal adaptor protein MyD88 in acute allograft rejection. J Clin Invest 2003;111: 1571–1578.

[143] Ducloux D, Deschamps M, Yannaraki M, *et al.* Relevance of Toll-like recpetor-4 polymorphisms in renal transplantation. Kidney Int 2005; 67: 2454–2461.

[144] Deng JF, Geng L, Qian YG, *et al.* The role of toll-like receptors 2 and 4 in acute allograft rejection after liver transplantation. Transplant Proc 2007 ; 39: 3222–3224.

[145] Nogueira E, Campos Conciano V, Naka EL, *et al.* Toll-like receptors-related genes in kidney transplant patients with chronic allograft nephropathy and acute rejection. Int Immunopharmacol 2009; 9: 673–676.

[146] De Groot K, Kuklik K, Brocker V, *et al.* Toll-like receptor 2 and renal allograft function. Am J Nephrol 2008; 28: 583–588.

[147] Ioannidou E, Kao D, Chang N, *et al.* Elevated serum interleukin-6 (IL-6) in solid-organ transplant recipients is positively associated with tissue destruction and IL-6 gene expression in the periodontium. J Periodontol 2006; 77: 1871–1878.

[148] Schauvliege R, Janssens S, Beyaert R. Pellino proteins: novel players in TLR and IL-1R signalling. J Cell Mol Med 2007; 11: 453–461.

[149] Araki M, Fahmy N, Zhou L,*et al.* Expression of IL-8 during reperfusion of renal allografts is dependent on ischemic time. Transplantation 2006; 81: 783–788.

[150] Andrade CF, Kaneda H, Der S, *et al.* Toll-like receptor and cytokine gene expression in the early phase of human lung transplantation. Heart Lung Transplant 2006; 25: 1317–1323.

[151] Murphy PM, Baggiolini M, Charo IF, *et al.* International union of pharmacology. XXII. Nomenclature for chemokine receptors. Pharmacol Rev 2000; 52: 145-176.

[152] Rossi D, Zlotnik A. The biology of chemokines and their receptors. Annu Rev Immunol 2000; 18: 217-242.

[153] Campbell JJ, Butcher EC. Chemokines in tissue-specific and microenvironment-specific lymphocyte homing. Curr Opin Immunol 2000; 12: 336-341.

[154] Morita K, Miura M, Paolone DR, Engeman TM, *et al.* Early chemokine cascades in murine cardiac grafts regulate T cell recruitment and progression of acute allograft rejection. J Immunol 2001; 167: 2979-2984.

[155] Cockwell P, Chakravorty SJ, Girdlestone J, Savage CO. Fractalkine expression in human renal inflammation. J Pathol 2002, 196:85-90.

[156] Segerer S, Cui Y, Eitner F, *et al.* Expression of chemokines and chemokine receptors during human renal transplant rejection. Am J Kidney Dis 2001, 37: 518-531.

[157] Robertson H, Morley AR, Talbot D, *et al.* Renal allograft rejection: β-chemokine involvement in the development of tubulitis. Transplantation 2000, 69: 684-687.

[158] Chakravorty SJ, Howie AJ, Girdlestone J, *et al.* Potential role for monocyte chemotactic protein-4 (MCP-4) in monocyte/macrophage recruitment in acute renal inflammation. J Pathol 2001; 194: 239-246.

[159] Fischereder M, Luckow B, Hocher B, *et al.* CC chemokine receptor 5 and renal-transplant survival. Lancet 2001; 357:1758-1761.

[160] Jackson JA, Kim EJ, Begley B, *et al.* Urinary chemokines CXCL9 and CXCL10 are noninvasive markers of renal allograft rejection and BK viral infection. Am J Transplant 2011; doi: 10.1111/j. 1600-6143.2011.03680.x.

CHAPTER 2

The Clinical Evaluation of the Renal Transplant Candidate

Pietro Castellino*, Luca Zanoli and Annamaria Zoccolo

Department of Medicine, University Hospital of Catania, University of Catania, Italy

Abstract: The clinical evaluation of the renal transplant candidate is a complex medical procedure. Its final goal is to select the patients in whom renal transplantation is likely to improve the clinical outcome. Potential candidate should be referred to the transplant center within six months from the onset of dialysis. The first step of the evaluation is to identify those conditions such as active alcohol or drug abuse, cancer, infections which may represent a major barrier to a successful transplant. If present, they should be removed before any further step in the evaluation process. Special attention should be focused on the detection of any active neoplastic disease and an adequate disease free interval, generally between 2 and 5 years, should be allowed prior to transplant. Similarly, careful evaluation and treatment of any active infectious disease should be undertaken prior to transplant. Cardiovascular diseases represent the major cause of death in patients with renal failure as well as in transplant recipients. Their detection and treatment in the evaluation process greatly improve the clinical outcome of the transplant recipients.

Keywords: Neoplastic Disease, Infections, Glomerular Disease, Gastrointestinal Disease, Cardiovascular Disease, Hepatitis C, Chronic Hepatitis, Waiting List, End-Stage Renal Disease, Kidney Disease.

INTRODUCTION

Renal transplantation is a complex procedure which is not devoided of medical risks and various social implications. Therefore, the ultimate goal of the evaluation process is to provide a correct assessment of the risks *vs.* benefits ratio of transplantation in the potential candidate. In fact, the transplant procedure should be undertaken only in patients in whom the clinical outcome is likely to be more favourable with transplantation than with other forms of renal replacement therapy.

The evaluation starts when a potential candidate is referred to the transplant center. The first step is to schedule an initial interview, or information session [1]. The patient may be encouraged to participate with family members and/or friends. During this session the patient should be informed about the various therapeutic options and about the risks and benefits of transplantation. The patient may either decide to proceed or, alternatively, he/she may not be interested in any further evaluation process. At this time it is often possible to identify one or more clinical problems which represent an obvious barrier to a successful transplantation. In this case the patient should be referred to the appropriate specialist to evaluate and eventually remove the barrier before any additional test is performed. Common examples of these limiting clinical conditions are drug addictions, active cardiovascular diseases, recent or active neoplastic or infectious diseases (Fig. **1**).

Once it is clear than the potential candidate is truly interested and that there is no obvious barrier to transplantation, the remainder of the evaluation can be performed. Timing of evaluation is also important, ideally, it should represent the best balance between the risks of medical and/or dialysis treatment of uraemia and the risks of transplantation. In clinical practice, the patient should be referred to the transplant center within six months prior the expected start of a renal replacement therapy, when GFR is between 10 and 15 ml/ min, or at least not later than six months after the onset of dialysis. This policy allows making the best choice between the various options available for uraemia therapy. The clinical evaluation of the transplant candidate also provide important information on the overall clinical status of the patients which,

***Address correspondence to Pietro Castellino:** Department of Medicine, University Hospital of Catania, *Via* S. Sofia, 86 95123, Catania, Italy; Tel: +39 095 3782736; E-mail: pcastell@unict.it

Massimiliano Veroux and Pierfrancesco Veroux (Eds)

in turn, represents one of the major determinants of the outcome both in dialysis and after transplantation (Table **1**). This evaluation may influence significantly the choice between the various therapeutic option such as the use of marginal deceased donor kidney or the exclusion from a living kidney donor program.

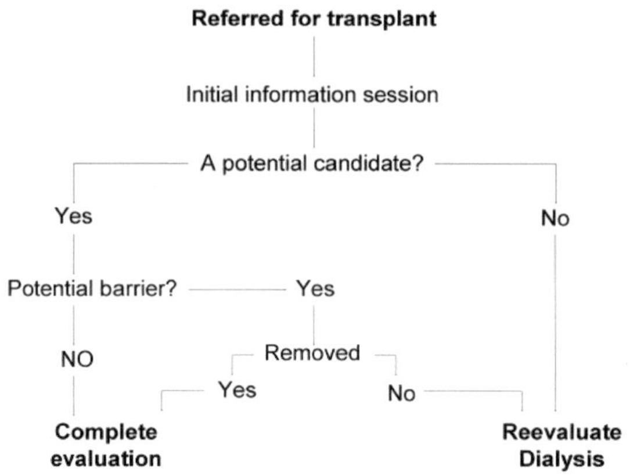

Figure 1: The renal transplant candidate evaluation process.

Table 1: The clinical outcome of renal transplantation based upon the clinical fitness of the recipients [1]

Fitness	Survival at 5 years	Survival
Good	51%	12.7 yrs
Moderate	31%	9.8 yrs
Poor	13%	8.7 yrs
Inacceptable	6%	

CANCER

Cancer is responsible of 1-5% of all deaths in the dialysis population [2]. Although the incidence varies significantly by the various tumours, the overall incidence of cancer in the dialysis population is higher than in the general population [3]. This is particularly evident in younger patients on dialysis. Albeit no specific screening program for cancer is routinely implemented in the dialysis population, younger patients and transplant candidates may gain the maximal benefit from an accurate screening. Cancer is responsible of 10-12% of deaths after transplantation [2] and the effect of intense pre transplant screening is still unclear. Post transplant immunosuppression is likely to offset the surveillance mechanism that counteracts the development of malignancies. Minor malignancies are extremely common in transplant recipients. Thus, it is more than likely that eliminating premalignant lesions or overt malignancies prior to transplantation may contribute to a lower rate of post transplant malignancies. Active cancer is most often an absolute barrier to transplantation. However, dialysis patients who have been successfully treated for cancer are generally suitable for transplantation. It is unanimously suggested waiting an appropriate time between successful treatment of cancer and renal transplantation. To this regard, it has been observed that more than 50% of cancer recurrence occur in patients who had their malignancy treated within two years from transplantation, 33% of recurrence occurs in patients treated between 2 and 5 years prior to transplantation and only 13% of cases recurred after more than 5 years [4]. With these data in mind, it has been suggested that all patients treated for cancer should have a waiting period prior to transplantation. Duration of the waiting period is still a matter of debate, however it appears prudent to avoid transplantation prior of 2 year after cancer eradication. In many cases a disease free period of 5 years is recommended. For some specific tumours the risk of recurrence remains too high even after 5 years from successful treatment. For each specific tumour it has been proposed clinical practice guidelines to approach both the screening and the treatment phases of transplantation. The detailed discussion of the single cancers and their screening and treatment options goes beyond the scope of the present chapter and the reader is referred to the specific guidelines for an in depth evaluation. In general, the overall approach for cancer screening can be outlined as follows [1, 4]:

Screening procedures – Tests of choices which are suggested in the screening procedure of the potential candidate.

Incidence and rationale – Incidence of specific cancer in the general population and in the dialysis population, rate and time of recurrence, mortality rate in case of recurrence, effect of therapy.

Recommendations – Exclusion criteria, specific therapy, protocol for screening and follow up, disease free intervals prior to transplantation.

It should be pointed out that the various transplant centers may follow their own screening program for malignancies with tests and schedules which may differ even significantly from one center to another. A list of the most frequently performed screening and procedures is summarized in Table **2**.

Table 2: Screening procedures for cancer in potential transplant recipients

Cancer	Screening
Kidney	Ultrasound imaging
Bladder	Urinalysis and urine cytology
Uterus	Cervical cytology and pelvic examination
Thyroid	Ultrasound imaging, Fine Needle Biopsy
Kaposi's sarcomas	Human herpes virus-8 infection's test
Breast	Mammography
Colorectal	Fecal occult blood, colonscopy, double contrast barium enema X-ray
Prostate	Prostate specific antigen, digital rectal examination
Liver	Alpha-fetoprotein, ultrasound imaging
Multiple myeloma	Serum and urine immunoelectropheresis
Linphoma and posttransplant lymphoproliferative disorders	Antibodies to the Epstein-Barr Virus
Leukemias	Complete blood count
Malignant melanoma	Medical history and physical examination
Lung	Chest X-ray

INFECTIONS

Because of the concomitant immunosuppression, infections represent a significant medical risk in the transplanted patient. The clinical course and the outcome of viral, bacterial or fungal diseases are almost invariably more severe in the transplant recipients than in the general population. Therefore all efforts should be made to eradicate all treatable infections prior to transplantation. A relevant part of the evaluation process is focused to identify and to eliminate infections that may become life threatening after transplantation or may lead to a worsening in kidney function and even to a loss of the transplanted organ. In specific cases viral infections associated with immunosuppression may lead to development of coetaneous or generalized tumoral diseases, as for Kaposi's sarcoma. The list of potential infections is indeed quite large and there are significant differences between the various countries in the prevalence of specific infective agents and diseases. Patients who have not been immunized prior to or early in the course of renal insufficiency should receive immunization prior to transplantation as a part of the evaluation protocol, if this has not been possible the transplant candidate should receive immunization after renal transplantation.

The most common infections which may be encountered in transplant candidates will be briefly evaluated.

HIV

Testing for HIV antibody is mandatory in order to be included in the active waiting list. For many years, the large majority of transplant centers have been reluctant to transplant asymptomatic HIV – positive patients. Early reports described the rapid onset of serious infection in HIV positive patients or through an inadverted HIV infected organ. HIV infected organs are excluded from transplant. After the advent of more potent anti retroviral agents, the issue of transplant in asymptomatic HIV positive patients has been reconsidered. In recent years more favourable outcomes have been reported [5]. The procedure is still considered experimental and is limited to centers with a large experience both in transplantation and HIV management. The potential candidate should have and undetectable HIV viral load with a CD4 count > 300/ml, adherence to the antiviral regimen and no signs of opportunistic infections.

Tuberculosis

The prevalence of exposure to tuberculosis ranges between 10 and 20% [6] but it varies significantly between countries. The rate of false negative test is higher in ESRD than in the general population. Protocols for prophylaxis and treatment are reported in Table **3**.

Table 3: Tuberculosis - Prophylaxis and treatment protocols in transplant candidates

PPD skin test Positive Rx Suggestive	→	- Prophilaxis for 6 months with isoniazide
Active disease Positive sputum colture	→	- Pyridoxine + Isoniazide + Rifampin
Post trasplant exposure to Mycobacterium	→	- Prophilaxis for 6 months with isoniazide

Cytomegalovirus (CMV)

The proposed screening is to test the presence of CMV antibody both in the recipient and in the donor. The proportion of antibody positive patients varies with age and geography but is in general > 50%. The risk of active CMV infection after transplantation is < 5% if both donor and recipients are CMV negative but it increases to 20-40% if the recipient is positive and up to 50-70% if the recipient is negative and the donor is positive [7]. In the last two cases post transplant prophylaxis is indicated.

RECURRENT DISEASES

With the exception of Alport syndrome, Fabry disease and polycystic kidney disease, all other renal diseases can recur in the transplanted kidney. Percentage of recurrence varies significantly according to the original disease as shown in Table **4** [8]; however the percentage of graft loss that can be attributed to recurrent disease is less than 9% [9].

Frequency of recurrence and outcome are significantly influenced by the length of follow-up, the longer the more frequent the recurrence, and the type of diagnostic approach, clinical *vs.* histological, with an higher rate of recurrence if the latter criteria is used for the diagnosis. The potential transplant recipient should be informed about the risk of recurrence and, in order to do so, all efforts should be made to reach an accurate diagnosis of the original cause of renal failure. To this regard, it should be pointed out that in many countries including Italy, at time of starting the renal replacement therapy, a large percentage of patients do not have a clear diagnosis of the cause of renal insufficiency. This limits the correct prognosis of disease recurrence.

Table 4: Post Transplant recurrence of primary renal diseases [8]

Glomerular disease	Recurrence rate
Focal Segmental GN	**20-30%**
Ig A GN	**20-60%**
HENOCH-SCHOENLEIN Purpura	**10-20%**
Membranous GN	**10-30%**
Membrano proliferative GN Type I	**20-30%**
Membrano proliferative Type II	**50-100%**
Hemolitic uremic Sindrome	**10-25%**
GOODPASTURE Syndrome	**10-25%**
WEGENER granulomatosis	**15-50%**
LES	**2-10 %**
Diabetic Nephropaty	**100%**

GASTROINTESTINAL DISEASES

Prevalence of diverticulitis is increased in uraemic patients, in particular in ADPKDs with an increased risk of post transplant intestinal perforation; at present no specific screening is suggested, however, in patients with advanced disease selective resection may be indicated prior to transplantation [10].

Peptic ulcer was a common and potentially lethal complication of transplantation and of long term steroids administration. The generalized use of H2 blockers and proton pump inhibitors has drastically reduced the incidence of the disease. The recognition and treatment of Helicobacter Pylori has reduced even further the morbidity associated with gastric diseases. No unanimous recommendations are available on the need of GI endoscopy or HP screening in pretransplant evaluation. Similarly, the approach to patients with cholelithiasis is not univocal, the disease is present in approximately 10% [11] of renal transplant recipients and morbidity and mortality post transplant, including pancreatitis are increased. All transplant candidates should be screened for stones and gall bladder diseases; however the need for routine pretransplant cholecystectomy in patients with asymptomatic cholelithiasis is still a matter of debate.

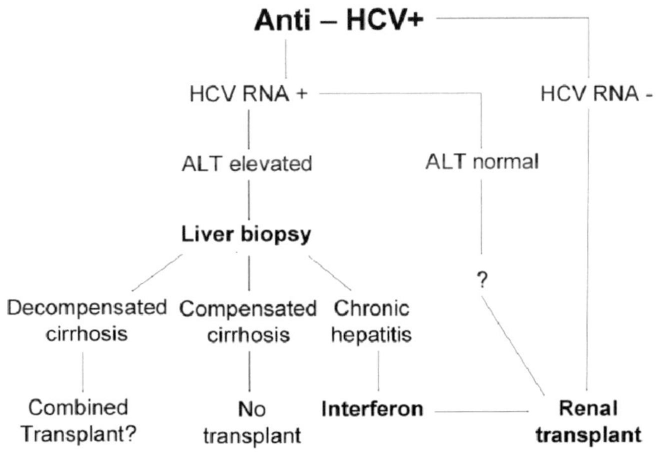

Figure 2: Management HCV+ in hemodialysis pre transplant.

The prevalence of Hepatitis B virus in the dialysis population is rather low in western countries but it remains elevated in developing countries. Vaccination is recommended prior to transplantation, but the rate of conversion is lower than in the general population. Pretransplant screening should include HBsAg and HbeAg evaluations and HBV DNA determination. Patients with active viral replication or HBeAg positive are at an increased risk for liver disease progression. The use of antiviral drugs pre and post transplant and pretransplant liver biopsy are strongly recommended. Hepatitis C Virus infection is more common among dialysis patients and its prevalence is 3-23% [12]. Pre-transplant screening should include HCV Ab evaluation and HCV RNA determinations. The flow chart for the pretransplant management of HCV positive patients is rather complex and it is shown in Fig. **2**.

Pretransplant interferon with ribavirine treatments and liver biopsy are strongly recommended; however compliance and rate of response are often poor. Patients with cirrhosis, both HBV and HCV related, have an elevated risk of liver failure and may be advised to forgo isolated renal transplantation.

CARDIOVASCULAR DISEASES

Cardiovascular diseases represent the leading cause of death among the dialysis population with more than 50% of the total events and a relative risk of death that is increased up to 100 fold among younger patients in comparison to the general aged matched population. The prevalence of cardiovascular diseases is also increased in transplant patients. More than 50% of deaths within the first 30 days from transplantation are related to ischemic heart diseases [13]. Therefore, cardiovascular evaluation represents a critical aspect of the pretransplant screening procedures. A prior history of ischemic heart diseases and an elevated cardiac risk index are both predictive of post transplant cardiac events. All patients with a positive history of myocardial infarction, angina or congestive heart failure should undergo cardiac stress testing and coronary angiography. Because of the high prevalence of critical coronary lesions, patients with diabetes may be suggested to undergo angiography even in absence of symptoms. In the near future, electron beam tomography and multi slice CT scan may represent a valid and non invasive alternative to angiography in the screening procedures. Patients who appear to have critical lesions should probably undergo revascularization prior to transplantation. In patients who have undergone to successful revascularization and are asymptomatic may proceed to renal transplantation. Aggressive treatment of smoking and hypertension are recommended, in contrast the role of dislipidemia is currently a matter of debate with no clear advantages of treatment in the dialysis population.

Congestive heart failure is a common condition in renal insufficiency, while a history of heart failure is reported in approximately 50% of dialysis patients [14]. Left ventricular hypertrophy and some degree of diastolic dysfunction are even more common. Medical history, electrocardiogram and echocardiogram should often be performed. Reversible form of heart failure should be treated; in particular anaemia, fluid overload and hypertension may contribute to cardiac dysfunction. In patients with systolic dysfunction may also be important to screen for ischemic heart disease, even if asymptomatic. Heart failure *per se* is not a contraindication to transplantation. Patients with mild to moderate cardiac dysfunction may improve after transplantation. In contrast, severe and irreversible heart failure may preclude surgery unless combined renal and heart transplant can be considered. Atrial fibrillation, if ventricular function is preserved, is not a contraindication to transplantation; anticoagulant therapy can be managed in most cases with no increased risk of bleeding or thrombosis. Both carotid and peripheral vascular diseases are rather common in the dialysis population also because of the high prevalence of diabetics. Management of vascular disease does not differ significantly from what is suggested for moderate to high risk patients who are evaluated for surgery.

ENDOCRINE

In the general population, the prevalence of obesity is continuously increasing; the incident rate of obese patients who are started on dialysis is even higher. It is estimated that in the next five to ten years approximately 50% of patients starting dialysis will be either obese, diabetics or both, 10-20% of transplant recipients has a BMI >30 [15]. In the dialysis population moderate overweight and low grade obesity are associated with a good survival, probably because of the strong role of malnutrition in mortality. In contrast, obesity is a significant risk factor in transplant recipient, with reported delayed graft function, surgical complications and infections. In obese individuals long term outcome and rate of complications after transplant are also worsen with an increased incidence of hypertension, diabetes and cardiovascular diseases. As a result, severe obesity may be considered an exclusion criterion from transplant programs and a weight reduction to a BMI < 30 is often requested prior to transplant.

Diabetes mellitus is the leading cause of renal failure in western countries, the US renal data System reports that approximately 50% of new cases of renal failure are attributed to diabetes [16]. Clinical outcome of diabetics after transplantation is better than on dialysis; however their outcome is always worse than in the non diabetic population. In spite of the high incidence of complications, diabetes *per se* in not a barrier to transplantation but because of the high rate of cardiovascular complications a careful screening is requested even in apparently asymptomatic patients.

REFERENCES

[1] Kasiske BL, Cangro CB, Hariharan S, *et al.* American Society of Transplantation. The evaluation of renal transplantation candidates: clinical practice guidelines. Am J Transplant 2001;1 Suppl 2:3-95.

[2] U.S. Renal Data System. Causes of death. USRDS 1999 Annual Data Report. Bethesda, MD: National Institutes of Health, National Institute of Diabetes, Digestive and Kidney Diseases; 1999. p. 89-100.

[3] Maisonneuve P, Agodoa L, Gellert R, *et al.* Cancer in patients on dialysis for end-stage renal disease: an international collaborative study. Lancet. 1999;354:93-99.

[4] Penn I. Evaluation of transplant candidates with pre-existing malignancies. Ann Transplant 1997; 2: 14-17.

[5] Hogg RS, Heath KV, Yip B, *et al.* Improved survival among HIV infected individuals following initiation of antiretroviral therapy. JAMA 1998;11:450-454.

[6] Woeltje KF, Mathew A, Rothstein M, *et al.* Tuberculosis infection and anergy in hemodialysis patients. Am J Kidney Dis 1998;31:848-852.

[7] Jassal SV, Roscoe JM, Zaltzman JS, *et al.* Clinical practice guidelines: prevention of cytomegalovirus disease after renal transplantation. J Am Soc Nephrol 1998;9:1697-1708.

[8] Golgert WA, Appel GB, Hariharan S. Recurrent glomerulonephritis after renal transplantation: an unsolved problem. Clin J Am Soc Nephrol 2008;3:800-807.

[9] Briganti EM, Russ GR, McNeil JJ, Atkins RC, Chadban SJ. Risk of renal allograft loss from recurrent glomerulonephritis. N Engl J Med 2002;347:103-109.

[10] Lederman ED, Conti DJ, Lempert N, *et al.* Complicated diverticulitis following renal transplantation. Dis Colon Rectum 1998;;4:613-618.

[11] Graham SM, Flowers JL, Schweitzer E, *et al.* The utility of prophylactic laparoscopic cholecystectomy in transplant candidates. Am J Surg 1995;169:44-48.

[12] Fissell RB, Bragg-Gresham JI, Woods JD, *et al.* Patterns of hepatitis C prevalence and seroconversion in hemodialysis units from three continents: the DOOPS. Kidney Int 2004;65:2335–2342.

[13] Ojo AO, Hanson JA, Wolfe RA, *et al.* Long-term survival in renal transplant recipients with graft function. Kidney Int 2000;57:307-313.

[14] Rahman M, Fu P, Sehgal AR, Smith MC. Interdialytic weight gain, compliance with dialysis regimen, and age are independent predictors of blood pressure in hemodialysis patients. Am J Kidney Dis 2000;35:257-265.

[15] Drafts HH, Anjum MR, Wynn JJ, *et al.* The impact of pre-transplant obesity on renal transplant outcomes. Clin Transplant 1997;11(5 Pt 2):493-496.

[16] U.S. Renal Data System. USRDS 2000 Annual Data Report. Bethesda, MD: National Institutes of Health, National Institute of Diabetes, Digestive and Kidney Disease; 2001.

CHAPTER 3

High-Risk Recipients in Kidney Transplantation

Neha Patel[1,*] and Nicole A. Weimert[2]

[1]PharmD, BCPS- Northwestern Memorial Hospital and [2]PharmD, MSCR, BCPS-Medical University of South Carolina, USA

Abstract: Renal transplantation among high-risk transplant recipients is becoming more and more common. As the incidence of end-stage renal disease is increasing the need for organ donors is also increasing, and with the shortage of organs the use of marginal donors has increased. All these factors impact patient and graft survival. As time has progressed the incidence of acute rejection has decreased significantly due to improvements in immunosuppressive medications. However, even though rates of acute rejection have decreased significantly overall patient and graft survival has not changed much over the years. In order to fully understand the stratification of "high-risk" renal transplantation many donor, recipient and allograft variables need to be considered.

Keywords: High-Risk, Desensitization, Rejection, Immunologic Risk, Immunosuppression, Kidney Transplantation, Antibody-Mediated Rrejection, Crossmatch.

INTRODUCTION

Solid organ transplant has evolved substantially over the past two decades. More and more patients are receiving the gift of life through historical obstacles. These obstacles include immunologic, medical, as well as socioeconomic. For example, many cultures preclude transplantation of deceased donor organs, and with the scarcity of kidney donors, for example, end stage renal disease was essentially a death sentence. Now under modern immunosuppression and immune monitoring transplantation can be performed across immunologic barriers giving patients options. However, doing so places a patient at "high risk" for infection, malignancy and perhaps rejection depending on the presence of an immunologic barrier. Today, there are many definitions of "high risk" in solid organ transplantation, but for purposes of this chapter we will focus on immunologic high risk.

Initially the definition of high risk was limited to patients that were highly sensitized after exposure to non-self human leukocyte antigens (HLA) during pregnancy, blood transfusions, previous organ transplants or other immunosensitizing events. Patients with pre-formed antibodies against HLA are at increased risk for early antibody mediated rejection, and in most cases the presence of these antibodies will delay or preclude transplantation. With current immunologic testing we are able to define and monitor the presence of donor specific antibodies and their potential impact post-transplant. Therefore, the definition of "high-risk" transplantation has broadened and now variables beyond the immunologic characteristics must be considered. These include donor and recipient age, donor cause of death, time to transplant and pre- and post procurement variables [1]. Throughout the next several paragraphs we will attempt to define these variables and describe their impact of allograft rejection and graft loss.

REJECTION

Rejection will occur when the recipient's immune system recognizes the allograft as foreign tissue and attempts to destroy it. We mitigate the recipient's immune system with immunosuppressants in an attempt to prevent this recognition. However, administration of a high level of immunosuppression may lead to infection and malignancy while a low level will lead to rejection. This constant balance requires intense surveillance for overimmunosuppression and underimmunosuppression.

***Address correspondence to Neha Patel:** PharmD, BCPS,Northwestern Memorial Hospital, Dept of Pharmacy and Transplant Surgery,251 E. Huron St. LC-700,Chicago, IL 60611; Fax: 312-926-5891; Phone: 312-926-8814; E-mail: neha727@gmail.com

Massimiliano Veroux and Pierfrancesco Veroux (Eds)

Before we discuss "high-risk" kidney transplantation it is essential to understand the types of rejection that can exist and their etiology post-transplant. These types of rejections include: hyperacute rejection, acute cellular rejection, antibody-mediated/humoral rejection, and chronic allograft nephropathy [1].

Hyperacute Rejection

Hyperacute rejection occurs when the recipient has pre-formed circulating antibodies against HLA or other antigens in the allograft. These antibodies are present prior to transplant and will bind to the vascular endothelium, then activate the complement cascade causing an immediate immune response against the allograft. A common clinical scenario associated with hyperacute rejection is following implantation of the organ, causing an immediate thrombosis of graft due to the rapid immunologic response and clot formation, shutting down blood supply to the graft. Risks factor for hyperacute rejection are high panel-reactive antibody (PRA) level, a positive crossmatch prior to transplant, or an ABO-incompatible kidney transplantation[1,2].

Acute Cellular Rejection

Acute cellular rejection occurs typically within the first 30 days after transplant. This is the most common type of acute rejection encountered. Acute cellular rejection involves the development of naïve and memory lymphocytes. The immune response is elicited by antigen presenting cells (APCs) [3]. Donor APCs can activate the recipient's immune system through either the direct or indirect pathway. In the direct pathway the donor allograft "passively" expresses donor alloantigens through the excursion of donor APCs out of the allograft into the recipients lymphatic system. The donor alloantigens can be directly recognized by the recipient's T-lymphocytes. The indirect pathway requires the shedding of donor alloantigens from the graft, which are then taken up by the recipient's APCs and presented to the T-lymphocytes [1-3]. Both pathways will lead to an immune response. Once the antigen is engulfed by an APC it is processed into multiple peptides and presented on the surface of the APC to the CD-4 (helper) T-cells on the major histocompatibilty complex II (MHC II). The MCH II receptor then binds to the T-cell receptor (TCR) initiating the cellular immune response. However, for the T-cell to become fully activated it needs a co-stimulatory signal such as activation of the cluster of differentiation (CD) 86 and CD 80, on the surface of APC which stimulates CD 28 on the recipient's T-cells. The co-stimulation leads to the initiation of several intracellular pathways within the T-cell, including: calcium calcineurin, renin-angiotensin aldosterone system (RAAS)-mitogen activated protein (MAP) kinase and nuclear factors causing cytokine release, T-cell receptor expression and clonal expansion of T-cells, B-cells, activated macrophages, and various other inflammatory events. This leads to rapid and aggressive infiltration of the graft causing cellular rejection [1-3].

Kidney transplant recipients are at higher risk for acute cellular rejection if their PRA prior to transplant is elevated, had a previous transplant, exhibit poor compliance with medications, have received low levels of immunosuppression, are African-American, or their kidney has delayed graft function (DGF) [1].

Biopsy findings include infiltration of tubular epithelium by lymphocytes (tubulitis) and in the intima of small arteries (arteritis). Other findings may include interstitial edema, or endothelialitis [1,3]. The severity of graft injury is graded *via* the Banff 97 criteria, which will also help determine treatment of acute cellular rejection [4].

Antibody-Mediated/Humoral Rejection

Antibody-mediated rejection accounts for 5-10% of rejection [5]. It typically occurs within weeks of transplant. However, recently there has been evidence to suggest that there is a late form of antibody-mediated rejection which can occur >1 year post-transplant as a result of circulating HLA-specific antibodies [5]. Antibody-mediated rejection is similar to hyperacute rejection in that is it characterized by the presence of pre-formed antibodies against the donor graft. However, in this case the antibodies develop in magnitude and specificity overtime, likely to the common practice of decreasing immunosuppression overtime to prevent side effects and sequelae associated to prolonged exposure to these agents. These antibodies initiate a cascade of events leading to activation of the complement system, which ultimately leads to thrombosis of arteries, arterioles and glomeruli [1,3-8]

Recipients are at higher risk for antibody mediated rejection if they have had a previous transplant, pregnancy, female sex, a positive crossmatch prior to transplant, and increased PRA, especially in the presence of low levels of immunosuppression [3,8]. Biopsy findings include acute glomerulonephritis, infiltration of the glomerulus with mononuclear cells, peritubular capillary C4d staining, severe vasculitis, fibrin thrombi, fibrinoid necrosis, infarction and neutrophils in the peritubular capillaries [3,5,8].

Finally, another interesting issue associated with humoral rejection is a condition termed accommodation. This is the rare circumstance that the allograft will acquire resistance to humoral injury. In the case of accommodation early complement fragments such as C4d may be present on biopsies with the absence of histologic evidence of tissue injury [5-7].

Chronic Allograft Nephropathy

Chronic allograft nephropathy (CAN) occurs months to years post-transplant. It occurs due to a combination of an immune response against the allograft and medication toxicity [1]. Many donor characteristics may contribute to the development of CAN, including donor size, age, ischemia-reperfusion injury, and procurement factors [9,10]. Other factors may include obesity, hypertension, diabetes, and calcineurin inhibitors (CNI) based immunosuppression [9,10].

Transplant-associated risk factors for the development of CAN include multiple acute rejections, deceased donor graft, acute tubular necrosis, delayed graft function, HLA mismatch, increased PRA at time of transplant, noncompliance, and calcineurin inhibitor toxicity [1]. Biopsy findings include glomerulosc--lerosis, tubular atrophy, interstitial fibrosis, and vascular fibrointimal proliferation [1].

PRE-TRANSPLANT IMMUNOLOGIC RISK DETERMINATION

Blood Group

Erythrocyte blood group antigens are structures located of the surface of the red blood cell (RBC) membrane. They are carbohydrate or protein structures. There are over 250 associated blood groups within 29 different blood group systems [11]. When an individual whose RBCs lack an antigen is exposed to RBCs that possess the antigen, an immune response occurs and produces antibodies that will react to the antigen [11]. Depending on the characteristics of the antibody the interaction between the antibody and the antigen can result in sensitization, agglutination or hemolysis when complement is activated [11].

Historically transplantation across ABO incompatible blood groups has lead to hyperacute rejection and has been previously considered a contraindication to kidney transplantation. Based on the distribution of blood groups in the United States there is a 35% chance that any two individuals will be ABO incompatible, therefore about one-third of living donors are excluded due to ABO incompatibility with the potential recipient [12]. Since then, there have been many strategies to transplant across ABO incompatibility since there is a limited number of deceased donor organs for the demand. Warren and colleagues [12] report the first successful renal transplantation of 3 patients that had ABO incompatible living donors and a positive crossmatch. Each of these patients received a preconditioning regimen of plasmapheresis, Cytomegalovirus (CMV) hyperimmune globulin, and standard immunosuppressive medications. In addition, all 3 patients underwent a splenectomy at time of transplant. All 3 patients did experience rejection within the first year of transplant, however, they were successfully treated with additional doses of plasmapheresis and CMV hyperimmune globulin [12]. Although some alternatives have been created to successfully transplant across blood groups that are still some risks of developing antibody-mediated rejection.

Toki and colleagues [13] studied the risk of antibody-mediated rejection in ABO incompatible kidney transplantation and the long-term effects on graft function. The study included 57 patients that underwent living ABO incompatible kidney transplants. To remove anti-blood group antibodies, all patients underwent 3-4 rounds of double-filtration plasmapheresis and a splenectomy at time of transplant. After performing univariate analyses, acute antibody-mediated rejection was associated with lack of pre-transplant MMF administration, anti-blood group antibody IgG titers of 1:32 at transplant, and donor-specific anti-HLA antibodies (DSHA). A multivariate logistic regression analysis was used to identify independent risk factors for acute antibody-mediated rejection, which included anti-blood group antibody titers of 1:32 and pre-transplant DSHA [13].

The practice of transplantation across ABO blood groups remains controversial but continues to be explored as a way to increase the donor pool. Because of the substantial immunologic and infectious risk to the recipient, patients must be thoroughly informed of the risks and benefits associated with this type of transplant. In addition, they must be willing and able to be compliant with immunosuppression and immunologic testing to ensure the best possible outcome.

Human Leukocyte Antigen Tissue Testing (HLA)

HLA-tissue typing is done during the initial transplant evaluation to determine the presence of anti-donor HLA antibodies in the recipient's serum. HLA tissue typing is an important factor in deceased organ allocation. HLA class I (HLA-A, -B) are present on all nucleated cell surfaces and recognized by CD8+ T-cells (cytotoxic T-cells). HLA class II (HLA-DR) are found on B-cells, dendritic cells, and macrophages, and they are recognized by CD4+ helper T-cells [1]. The tissue typing is performed from the lymph nodes, spleen and blood [1].

Renal transplants in recipients with high levels of antibodies to donor HLA antigens may have various degree of graft damage, ranging from hyperacute rejection to increased numbers of rejection episodes and overall poorer graft survival. HLA typing involves identification of 6 major histocompatibility complexes of the donor and recipient. HLA typing and the recipient's time on waiting list are the most important key factors in deceased donor allocation. However, this policy contributes to a higher transplantation rate among whites than non-whites.

A 6-antigen match or zero-antigen mismatch have been shown to have better overall outcomes. In 1994 Heid and colleagues [14] examined 30564 kidney transplant recipients from the United States Renal Data System (USRDS), to estimate the effects of HLA mismatches on graft survival. Overall the adjusted 1-year graft survival was 84.3% in recipients that received a kidney from a zero HLA mismatch compared to 77% of grafts with 4 mismatches.

Ting and colleagues [15] reviewed the effects of HLA matching and mismatching on graft outcomes and access to transplant for minority patients. Unsensitized recipients (PRA 0-9%) of transplants with zero -B and -DR mismatches did not have an increase in the risk of graft loss when compared with transplants with zero -A, -B, and -DR mismatches. However, transplants with more than two -B and -DR mismatches were significantly different than those with zero or one -B and -DR mismatches in terms of long-term graft survival ($p<0.0001$).

If recipients had one or two mismatches at the HLA-A or -B locus as compared with zero mismatches had no statistically significant effect after adjustment for mismatches at the other two loci. However, mismatches at HLA-DR did increase the risk of graft failure (relative risk with 1 mismatch, 1.15; $p<0.001$; relative risk with 2 mismatches, 1.26; $p<0.001$)[16-18].

Many authors hypothesized that changing the allocation policy would affect graft survival and would lead to a racial balance among transplant recipients [15,16].

Detection of Donor-Specific Antibodies

The presence of donor-specific antibodies in a transplant recipient has been widely accepted as an indirect index of T-cell sensitization [19]. This occurs because of IgG production by alloantigen stimulated B-cells, and this requires alloantigen stimulated T-cells. The presence of anti-HLA IgG is then detected in the recipient serum [19].

All transplant candidates are submitted to pre-transplant blood tests to determine the presence of circulating antibodies to class I and class II HLA antigens. The most frequent HLA antigens in the potential donor pool are collated into a panel. The percentage of antigens in the panel that the potential recipient reacts to is known as their PRA percent. The higher the percentage the more likely the potential recipient has preformed antibodies against potential donors in their donor pool. The presence of preformed complement-fixing alloantibodies is well established to be associated with increased risk for rejection and overall poor graft outcomes [20]. There are two methods used to assess PRA: flow cytometry PRA, and complement-dependent cytotoxicity (CDC) PRA.

The CDC PRA entails the inoculation of the potential recipient's serum with a panel of donor cells which have the most common HLA antigens. The donor cells are placed in several wells and combined with the potential recipient's blood along with complement. Then the wells are observed for cytolysis. There are a few things to consider when interpreting this data and it is very difficult to obtain a test that could represent all the human leukocyte antigens specificities [3,20]. Another potential disadvantage of this test is the high rate of false-positive results caused by IgM or IgG lymphocytotoxic autoantibodies reacting with non-HLA lymphocyte surface antigens [3,20]. False-positive results can also occur because of the use of antilymphocyte antibody for induction or treatment of rejection [20].

In contrast, flowPRA can detect antibodies at a more sensitive level. Flow cytometry has also been used to differentiate between IgG and IgM antibodies by using anti-IgG secondary antibodies [20]. Flow cytometry screens for both class I and class II anti-bodies using a panel of microbeads. These beads are known as flowPRA beads that are coated with either purified HLA class I or purified HLA class II antigens [3,20,21].These beads react specifically with HLA antibodies in the serum decreasing the chance of false reactions. A pool of 30 different class I and class II beads can be used and the percentage is determined by the percent of microbeads that react positively to the serum [3,20]. Overall, flow cytometry is a more sensitive and specific test compared to CDC PRA [20,21]. However, using FlowPRA it is difficult to distinguish between complement-fixing alloantibodies and less harmful non-complement-fixing reactivities [20,21].

The current practice of transplantation involves the use of both CDC PRA and FlowPRA to determine the presence of preformed antibodies (Fig. **1**).

Crossmatch result: IgG HLA-specific antibodies	Contraindicated	High-risk	Intermediate risk	Low risk
Current Positive Cytotoxicity Flow Cytometry	*	*		
Historical Positive Cytotoxicity Flow Cytometry		*	*	
Current and historical negative Cytotoxicity Flow Cytometry			*	*

Figure 1: Risk assessment for antibody-mediated rejection [23] (with permission).

Crossmatching

A crossmatch is performed prior to transplant to determine the presence of anti-donor HLA antibodies in the recipient's blood [1,3]. The presence of preformed antibodies or a positive cross-match, specifically against HLA class I antigens will contraindicate kidney transplantation. B-cell positive cross-matches are considered acceptable at some centers as long as the appropriate monitoring and immunosuppression is used. Traditionally, the CDC crossmatch was performed. The CDC or standard crossmatch, which is similar to the CDC PRA, involves inoculating the potential recipient's serum with cells from the potential donor. Complement is added to the mixture and direct cell cytotoxicity is observed to determine the presence of preformed antibodies to the donor tissue [13,22]. Since then, a more sensitive method has evolved which uses anti-human globulin (AHG). This was developed in 1972 to detect low titer and/or noncomplement fixing antibodies [22]. The AHG/complement-dependent T and B-cell crossmatch is more sensitive due to the addition of anti-human light chain antibody, which increases the crosslinking of antibodies on the surface of the cell leading to increased complement fixation and cell death [1,22].

A more recently developed technique is the flow crossmatch, which detects donor-specific antibodies without the use of complement. In this case the recipient's serum is inoculated with the donor lymphocytes that are stained with fluorochrome-conjugated anti-IgG antibodies [3,22]. One particular advantage with this method is that the detection of antibody reactivity can be independently evaluated on donor T and B lymphocytes. However, just like the CDC crossmatch there is still the possibility for false positives or false negative results [1,22].

DESENSITIZATION

Over the last decade a growing number of highly sensitized patients are awaiting renal transplantation. In 2006, 33% of patients in the United States had an elevated PRA, and approximately 40% of them were considered highly sensitized with a PRA of >80% [24]. Due to the current shortage of allografts and the growing number of patients on the waiting list transplantation across previously incompatible immunologic barriers is occurring. Transplantation across a positive T or B-cell crossmatch or across ABO blood groups puts the patient at risk for hyperacute rejection. Therefore the goal of desensitization is the remove circulating anti-HLA antibodies and prevent the formation of new anti-HLA antibodies [3,17].

Intravenous Immune Globulin (IVIg)

Intravenous Immune Globulin (IVIg) has been shown to reduce the presence of circulating anti-HLA antibodies. IVIg is a commercially prepared product from IgG derived from pooled human plasma. Therefore, it is likely that IVIg contains the entire compilation of antibodies found in normal human serum [23]. The product itself contains >90% intact IgG and traces of IgM and IgA. It contains antibodies against: T-cell receptor idiotypes, CD4, CD5, CD40, CD95, HLA class I, HLA class II-DR, RhD antigen, IL-1α, IL-4, IL-6, TNF-α, GM-CSF, and IL-1β [24,25]. Although the exact mechanism of IVIg in desensitization is not fully understood there are many theorized mechanisms. It is postulate to exert its effects on B-cells by causing selective down-regulation and up-regulation of antibody production and neutralizes circulating autoantibodies by anti-idiotypes [24,25]. IVIg also works on T-cells by regulating the production of helper T-cell cytokines [24,25]. IVIg can also inhibit lymphocyte proliferation and regulate apoptosis. IVIg molecules also bind their Fc region to Fcγ receptors on macrophages, neutrophils, eosinophils, platelets, mast cells, natural killer cells, and B-cells.The Fc region of the antibody interacts with the cells to diable or up-regulate cellular activities depending of the Fcγ region [24].

There have been various protocols and dosing strategies used in the literature for desensitization. They are summarized in Table **1**. Currently there is no consensus on the exact dose or dosing strategy. Some institutions have used cytomegalovirus hyperimmune IgG, in an attempt to maximize IgG concentrations [3,25]. There are currently many commercial preparations

The incidence of adverse events related to IVIg administration ranges from 12-23%. The most common adverse events include headache, fever, fatigue, chills, myalgias, dizziness, hypotension, nasal congestions, chest tightness, wheezing, and nausea. These adverse effects are usually self-limiting and usually respond to slowing the infusion or treatment with nonsteroidal anti-inflammatory drugs (NSAIDs). Severe anaphylactic transfusion reactions may occur in patients with complete IgA deficiency that has developed anti-IgA antibodies [25]. Treatment of infusion-related adverse events include slowing or stopping the infusion, treatment with diphenhydramine, NSAIDs, and/or corticosteroids, administration of intravenous fluids, epinephrine, and benzodiazepines [25].

Plasmapheresis

Plasmapheresis removes and reduces the level of circulating antibody to the donor and removes other factors that induce or sustain inflammation as well as effector molecules such a complement [18]. As shown in Table **1** most plasmapheresis sessions are followed by IVIg infusions to replenish IgG and to prevent rebound antibody production. Albumin is typically used to help maintain oncotic pressure during the plasmapheresis session.

Table 1: High risk recipients. Clinical studies

Study	Indication	Plasmapheresis (PP)	Rituximab	CMV IgG	IVIg Dose	IVIg Interval	Preoperative Immunosuppression	Endpoint
Schweitzer *et al.* (n=15) [69]	Positive CM, LD	Yes 3 times weekly for 6 treatments	No	No	500 mg/kg total dose	Divided over 7 days	MMF + tacrolimus + prednisone started on initiation of desensitization OKT3 at time of transplant	CM at 2 and 3 weeks and pre-operative, if negative then received a transplant
Montgomery *et al.* (n=14) [70]	AHR (n=10) or positive CM (n=4)	Yes alternative day for AHR until clinical improvement and/or DSA no longer detectable Yes alternative day for CM positive group until CM negative and then 2 additional doses post-transplant	No	No	100 mg/kg	Alternative day following PP	No	Serial CM and DSA
Sonnenday *et al.* (n=18) [71]	Positive CM, LD	Yes alternative day	No	Yes 100 mg/kg	No	N/A	MMF + tacrolimus on initiation of desensitization Dacluzimab before reperfusion	Serial CM until negative
Glotz *et al.* (n=15) [72]	Class I PRA >50% or positive T-cell CM	No	No	No	2 g/kg	Day 0 or 1 Day 20 or 21 Day 40 of 41 All doses administered over 48 hrs	No	PRA and CM repeated 3 wks following last dose of IVIg, considered successful is PRA fell ≥50% from baseline or negative CM
Sonnenday *et al.* (n=6) [73]	ABO blood group incompatible	Yes alternative day and 3 days post-transplant (days 1,3,5)	Yes 375 mg/m^2 1-2 days prior to transplant	Yes 100 mg/kg following each PP	No	N/A	MMF + tacrolimus on initiation of desensitization Daclizumab before reperfusion	ABO antibody titer ≤16
Jordan *et al.* (n=98) [17]	PRA ≥ 50%	No	No	No	2 g/kg	Month x 4 months with additional infusions at 12, 24, and 30 months	No	Serial PRA
Thielke *et al.* (n=16) [74]	Positive CM by flow cytometry, CM positive for T-cell for number of channel shifts >20 and for B-cell >40	Every other day starting 1 wk prior to transplant	No	No	100 mg/kg	Every other day following PP	Induction with thymoglobulin 1.5 mg/kg x 5 doses at time of transplant, PP/IVIg every other day x 1 wk post-transplant	Negative CM by the third treatment

Table 1: cont….

Stegall *et al.* (n=61) [75]	Positive CM, 3 protocols compared	Protocol 1 (n=32): PP daily Protocol 2 (n=13): No Protocol 3 (n=16): daily	Yes 375 mg/m^2 4-7 days prior to transplant No Yes 375 mg/m^2 4-7 days prior to transplant	No No No	100 mg/kg 2.1-3 g/kgg 100 mg/kg	Daily after PP 1-3 days prior to transplant, if positive CM received another dose on following day Daily after PP	18/32 splenectomy and 2-3 days post-transplant PP/IVIg on days 1-3 If positive CM then used protocol 1 without splenectomy Thymoglobulin 1.5 mg/kg	Serial CM and AHR in the first 6 wks of transplant	Negative 5/13, grou 11/30, grc patient an respective
Vo *et al.* (n=20) [76]	Highly HLA-sensitized (PRA 77±19%) or DSA present	No	Yes 1 gm day 7 and 22	No	2 g/kg	Day 0 and 30	Induction with alemtuzumab	Serial DSA and PRA	16/20 rece 10 still ha transplant. 100% and rejection r antibody- antibody- DSA

CM =crossmatch; LD = living donor; CMV = cytomegalovirus; IVIg = intravenous immunoglobulin; MMF = mycophenolate mofetil; AHR = acute humoral rej
DSA= donor-specific antibodies; PRA = panel reactive antibody.

Rituximab

Rituximab is a chimeric murine/human antibody directed against the CD20 molecule on pre-B and mature B-cells, but not on plasma cells. It directly inhibits B-cell proliferation by antibody-dependent, cell-mediated, and complement-mediated cytotoxicity [26,27]. It is currently used as single dose of 375 mg/m^2 for the treatment of humoral rejection. The use of rituximab has recently been studied in highly sensitive recipients. Munoz and colleagues [27] describe a case series of highly sensitized patients who received rituximab as part of induction therapy. Patients received one or two doses of rituximab 375 mg/m^2 1 day prior to transplant along with an IL-2 receptor antagonist or alemtuzumab as an induction agent at time of transplant. This combination has displayed favorable graft outcomes [27]. The average PRA of the 7 patients included in the analysis was 35.7%. Except for 2 patients, all others showed immediate graft function. The other 2 patients had an average serum creatinine of 1.8-2 mg/dL a week after transplant with decreasing urine output. Biopsy on these 2 patients revealed acute humoral rejection with positive C4d at 1-week and 1-month post-transplant. However, the other 5 patients were rejection free for the mean follow up time of 3 months (range 1.5-5 months) [27].

Bortezomib

As time has progressed more and more centers have gained experience with the use of plasmapheresis, IVIg, rATG, and rituximab for treating antibody-mediated rejection and in desensitization. Currently these methods are effective but unreliable and provide suboptimal results. Some of the limitations the current therapies include the gradual reversal of antibody-mediated rejection compared to a prompt result, expense, rejection reversal rates <80%, and long-term detection of donor-specific antibodies [28].Therefore, Bortezomib, the first proteosomal inhibitor that has been FDA approved for the treatment of multiple myeloma has been evaluated in the treatment of antibody mediated rejection. Bortezomib is considered a proteosomal inhibitor which will suppress T-cell function and therefore it has the potential for the treatment or prevention of antibody-mediated rejection. Everly and colleagues [29] describe their initial experience with the use of Bortezomib as an antihumoral agent. This case series described 6 patients that experienced humoral rejection that was refractory to plasmapheresis, IVIg, rATG, or rituximab. All 6 patients were treated wit Bortezomib (1.3 mg/m2 in 4 doses) and the allograft was salvageable. The 6 patients also had a sustained reduction in both immunodominant DSA and nonimmunodominant DSA. It is thought that the effects of Bortezomib on T-cell function including apoptosis induction in activated T-cells, T-cell depletion, decrease in major histocompatibility class I expression, and decrease in Th1 responses. It also effects the B-lymphocytes by inhibiting IL-6 production by bone marrow stromal cells leading to apoptosis of B-cell maturation. The current role of Bortezomib is still unclear [28,29].

OTHER FACTORS THAT MAKE PATIENTS "HIGH-RISK"

African-Americans

African-American race has also correlated with suboptimal allograft outcomes and therefore they are considered "high risk" transplant recipients. Since the 1970s, African-Americans have been recognized to have a significantly higher risk of developing end-stage renal disease compared to Caucasians [30]. African-Americans tend to have lower rates of transplantation secondary to a variety of immunologic, genealogic, socio/economic factors placing them at higher risk for transplantation. African-Americans tend to also have a higher incidence of hypertension, diabetes which limits their number of familial living donors [30]. African-Americans tend to be on the waiting list longer than other ethnicities, therefore, receiving deceased donor allografts bearing a greater number of mismatched donor-recipient HLA blood group antigens [30]. Compared to Caucasians, African-Americans require higher doses of immunosuppressive drugs to achieve similar drug concentrations. They display more rapid drug clearance rates of cyclosporine and tacrolimus [30]. African-Americans exhibit a smaller volume of distribution and lower clearance rates, which result in higher cortisol levels, therefore, displaying a pharmacodynamic resistance to methylprednisolone. Furthermore, African-Americans rapidly methylate, therefore, inactivate azathioprine. Lastly, African-Americans have a greater rate of noncompliance to medications [30].

Pregnancy

Pregnancy also makes a patient highly sensitized for transplant. Sautner and colleagues [31] evaluated the impact of potential risk factors for the development of PRA in 1,078 deceased donor transplant recipients. After performing a multivariate analysis, multiple transplants, transfusions of great than 5 units of blood and more than two pregnancies were factors that significantly impacted the formation of high levels of PRA. Soosay and colleagues also tried to define the causes of sensitization in potential renal allograft recipients and they found similar results [32].

Pediatric Recipients

Pediatric patients tend to have significantly decreased long-term patient and allograft survival for several reasons [33]. Hwang and colleagues [34] evaluated UNOS data for early and late risk factors for deceased donor graft loss in pediatric kidney transplantation from January 1, 1994 to December 31, 2002. Overall graft survival at both 1 (95%) and 3-years (79%) significantly improved during 1999-2002 compared with those between 1994-1998 (88% and 76% at 1 and 3-years respectively, long rank p=0.02). Overall when the 2 groups were compared, factors that significantly affected early transplant outcomes adversely within 3 months post-transplant included prolonged cold ischemia time (>36 hours, OR = 3.38 *vs.* 0-36 hours) and young recipient age (2-5 years old, OR = 2.02 *vs.* 6-12 years). After 3 months, significant risk factors included African-American recipients, teenage recipients (13-20 years old), and patients with focal glomerulosclerosis as the cause of their renal failure [34].

Variables which may contribute to these observations, include anatomy, pharmacokinetics and adherence. Vascular thrombosis is still a major cause of graft failure. Singh and colleagues [35] conducted a study to identify risk factors for vascular thrombosis. As total of 4,394 transplants were evaluated. After performing a univariate analysis it showed that the rate of thrombosis leading to graft loss was significantly higher in younger children (<2 years of age) as compared with older age groups (2-5 year, 6-12 years, and >12 years of age). Recipients of kidneys from deceased donors <5 years of age had a significantly higher rate of thrombosis (8.3%) than did recipients from older donor age (5-10 year, 4.5%; >10 years of age, 3.2%) [35].

The pharmacokinetics of immunosuppressants have been extensively studied in adults, however, these parameters are generally not applicable to children. Developmental changes in physiology contribute to significantly altered absorption, distribution, metabolism and excretion of immunosuppressive agents, therefore, higher doses may be needed in younger recipients.

Adolescents have the best 1-year graft survival compared to any other age group [36], however, non-adherence with immunosuppressive medications is one of the most important factors that contribute to graft rejection and loss in teenagers. One theory is that a typical adolescent likes to establish autonomy and freedom from parents, however, at the same time with a transplant they need the support and guidance of parents [37]. It is difficult for teenagers to understand the long term consequences of their immediate actions. There are some patient characteristics that correlate with pediatric and adolescent non-adherence, including: low self-esteem, depression of anxiety, poor communication and socialization skills, single parent families, family instability, insufficient family support, low income and poor intra-family communication [36]. There are many approaches to the issue of non-adherence: using pill boxes, education and group discussions with other transplant recipients and lastly psychiatric consultation. Most importantly early identification of medication non-adherence with the appropriate interventions will lead to significant improvement in adolescent graft survival.

Older Patients

Older recipients are also at high-risk. Patients aged 60 years and older represent the fastest growing population with chronic kidney disease and ESRD. In 2002 about 137,000 patients over the age of 65 were on dialysis and the number of older patients registered on the kidney transplant list is also increasing [37]. Between 1994 and 2003 the number of patients listed on the kidney transplant wait list aged between 54-64 doubled and the number of patients older than 64 tripled [37]. Only a small minority of patients over the age of 65 on dialysis are placed on the list. Therefore, the majority of the elderly population is not being referred to the waiting list because of other co-morbid conditions and lower life expectancy [37]. Patients with ESRD who receive a transplant have greater survival then those who remain on dialysis [37]. Due to the improvement in quality of life, there are greater number of patients being placed on the waiting list for deceased donor kidney transplants which leads to increased wait times. This increase in wait time impacts older patients (>60 years of age) more than younger patients who may be in better health and have fewer co-morbidities. Because risk for death increases with patient age and length of time on the waiting list, older patients are more likely to die on the waiting list [37]. Of these older patients who do get a transplant, the risks for immunosuppression induced complications are increased [37].

Donor age also plays an important role in long-term patient and graft survival. There have been many studies that have evaluated donor risk factors for graft survival. Pessione and colleagues [38] presented data on the impact of donor risk factors that might influence 3-year graft outcomes along with recipient and transplantation factors between 1996 and 2000. After performing a multivariate analysis they determined that cerebrovascular cause of death, history of hypertension, and elevated creatinine were all significant independent donor risk factors for graft survival [38].

As previously discussed there is an increasingly critical shortage of kidneys for transplantation, therefore, there has been increasing use of kidneys that were at one point deemed unsuitable. Currently there is no universal definition of what is considered an ideal or "marginal" transplantable kidney. There are many factors that characterize an organ as being marginal: advanced donor age, long standing hypertension, diabetes, prolonged cold ischemia time and non-heartbeating cadaver donor. Ojo and colleagues [39] evaluated the survival of recipients of marginal cadaveric donor kidneys compared with other recipients. Overall, they found that 5-year graft and patient survival was 53% and 74% for marginal donor kidney recipients compared with 67% ($p<0.001$) and 80% ($p<0.001$) for ideal donor kidneys.

Recurrent Diseases

There are numerous reasons for renal failure that can lead to dialysis. The most concerning etiologies are those that can reoccur, which include glomerulonephritis. Glomerulonephritis includes a variety of diseases that are characterized by inflammation of the glomeruli, or small blood vessels in the kidneys. They are categorized into several pathological patterns, which include non-proliferative (FSGS, membranous glomerulonephritis) or proliferative types (IgA nephropathy, membranoproliferative/mesangiocapillary GN) [40].

Overall, glomerulonephritis is the primary cause of end-stage renal disease in up to 50% of patients [40]. Recurrence rates range between 6% and 19.4% in renal allograft recipients and increases with longer follow-up [40]. Recipients that have a recurrence, have a higher rate of graft loss. Briganti and colleagues [40] evaluated the incidence and timing of risk factors for allograft loss due to biopsy-proven glomerulonephritis and compared this data with those patients that had graft loss due to acute rejection, chronic rejection or death with a functioning graft. A total of 1505 patients with biopsy-proven glomerulonephritis were transplanted between 1988 and 1997. The most common glomerulonephropathy was IgA nephropathy (n=532). Allograft loss due to recurrence of glomerulonephritis occurred in 52 patients, with a 10-year incidence of 8.4% (CI 5.9-12). Multiple characteristics of the donors and recipients were examined as potential predictors of 10-year actuarial incidence if allograft loss due to recurrence. The characteristics included: age, sex, peak PRA, duration of dialysis prior to transplant, and type of glomerulonephritis. Overall, the type of glomerulonephritis, sex of recipient, and peak PRA were independent predictors of recurrence. Recurrence was the third leading cause of graft loss after chronic rejection and death from a functioning graft. Despite glomerulonephritis graft loss was similar between both groups (45.4% CI 40.9-50.2 glomerulonephritis *vs.* 45.8% CI 42.3-49.3 other, $p=0.09$). Overall, recurrence is an important cause of allograft loss in patients with glomerulonephritis as the etiology of their renal failure [40].

Human Immunodeficiency Virus (HIV)

The natural history of HIV has been dramatically impacted by the availability of highly active antiretroviral therapies (HAART), therefore, leading to reductions in mortality, hospitalizations, and opportunistic infections.

Since patients are now living longer, kidney disease has become an important complication of HIV infection. Up to 30% of patients with HIV have chronic kidney disease and are at risk for end-stage renal disease as a result of HIV-associated nephropathy and other diseases such as immune complex glomerulonephropathy, hepatitis B and C related membranous nephropathy. In the pre-HAART era HIV infection was an absolute contraindication to kidney transplantation largely due to the concerns of a more rapid progression of HIV due to the heightened immunosuppression. Interestingly, many commonly used immunosuppressive agents have anti-retroviral qualities. For example, cyclosporine may suppress HIV replication that is associated with the inhibition of IL-2 dependent T-cell proliferation [41,42] Mycophenolate mofetil acts synergistically with some nucleoside analogues [41,42]. In pilot studies of renal transplants in HIV positive recipients have shown an excellent 100% 1-year survival [41,42]. Progression of HIV was not an issues however, rates of acute rejection were double than that seen in HIV-negative recipients [41,42]. Most cases of rejection were classified as moderate to severe requiring aggressive treatment with thymoglobulin. This may be a result of immune dysregulation [41,42]. Overall, transplantation in HIV positive patients is now a viable option. Some things to keep in mind include the drug interactions that can occur between immunosuppressants and highly active antiretroviral therapies, additional prophylaxis may be indicated for those recipients that have a CD4 count <200, and co-infections with hepatitis B or C [41,42].

Socioeconomic and Patient Support

It has been shown that economic hardship predicts poorer transplantation outcomes [30]. Kahil and colleagues [43] evaluated the impact of socioeconomic factors on long-term outcomes after renal transplantation. They evaluated the effects of family income of 202 kidney transplanted patients between 1976-1982. When low income patients were compared to patients with adequate income at time of transplantation low income recipients were more likely to return to dialysis after 1 year (36% *vs.* 17%, p <0.01) [43]. Patients that complied with fewer than 85% of visits during the first 2 years were also most likely to return to dialysis after 1 year (35% *vs.* 16%, p<0.01). The relative risk for returning to dialysis after 5 years was 2.4 (p<0.05) for low income and 3.0 (p<0.05) for less than 85% compliance for visits. These effects were independent of prior transplantation, HLA mismatches, elevated PRA, delayed graft function (DGF), age, sex, diabetes, or race. A more recent analysis of transplantation outcomes according to ZIP code documented a significantly greater risk of graft loss in lower income areas. Also of note patients without private insurance at the time of transplantation who were African-Americans, were at increased risk of graft loss [43]. As we know noncompliance with medications and office visits were a significant predictor of graft loss and it occurred more frequently among African-Americans, however, after correction of socioeconomic factors, there was no difference between races. Overall, there is a strong correlation among socioeconomic status, educations background, and medication compliance [30,44,45].

Procurement Issues

With the growing number of patients on the waiting list there has been a need to expand the donor pool beyond those from brain-dead donors with a heart-beat. Alternative sources of organs include the elderly, living donors and non-heart beating donors. Non-heart beating donors are defined as donors with irreversible cessation of circulatory and respiratory function, whereas brain dead donors are classified according to neurologic criteria [46,47]. Therefore, non-heart beating donors have a prolonged phase of hypotension followed by cardiac arrest before organ procurement [46].This seems to be an alternative to transplanting the "ideal" organ, however, there are some risks with using non-heart beating donors. Graft loss from non-heart beating donors depends on multiple factors: age, donor co-morbidity's such as hypertension, peripheral vascular disease or diabetes can all cause nephron loss [3].Therefore, donor disease can lead to ischemia/reperfusion injury.

Sanchez-Fructuoso and colleagues [48] evaluated survival and renal function of kidneys from non-heart beating donors with those of heart-beating donors. 144 kidneys were evaluated. There was not significant difference in renal function and the number of rejections between either groups. The non-heart beating donors had a 5.73-fold increase in the incidence if delayed graft function (adjusted relative risk 95% CI, 2.82 to 11.62). One- and five-year survival rates were similar between both groups. With the increasing number of patients on the wait last and the lack of adequate donors, non-heart beating donors may be an option for some patients [48].

Overall, ischemia to the graft is associated with procurement, preservation and storage of the kidney. Reperfusion is critical to the viability of the organ and can amplify ischemic injury. Increases in cold ischemia time (CIT) or warm ischemia time (WIT) increases the incidence of DGF (the need for hemodialysis within 7 days of transplant) [49,50]. For every 6-hour increase in CIT the risk of DGF increases by 23%, and DGF has been associated with acute rejection and early graft loss [49,50]. Ischemia/reperfusion injury increases the organs expression of HLA class I and II, interferon, transforming growth factors, granulocyte monocyte-colony stimulating factors, interleukin-2 and 10 that may cause the kidney to be more immunogenic [49]. Bryan and colleagues [49] determined if CIT influenced the production of HLA class I-directed antibodies in 90 unsensitized recipients (PRA <10%) undergoing their first renal transplant who lost their graft function after transplant. After performing a multivariate analysis a CIT >15 hours independently increased the risk of antihuman globulin class I panel reactive antibody level being >20% after unsensitized patients rejected their first kidneys (RR- 3.57, CI 1.26-10.14; p =0.01). The overall mean PRA was significantly lower in the recipients with a CIT <15 hours (25.9%+/-33.9 *vs.* 46.3%+/-36.5, p<0.0010). Overall, a longer CIT adversely effects graft outcomes and increases immunologic risk [49].

IMMUNOSUPPRESSIVE STRATEGIES TO MITIGATE FACTORS

Induction

Antithymocyte Globulins (ATG)

Antithymocyte globulins are considered polyclonal antibodies and therefore, have activity on a variety of T-cell receptors. They are among the most potent induction agents used in transplantation. ATG is produced by immunizing horses or rabbits with human lymphoid cells, harvesting the IgG and removing toxic antibodies [51-54]. ATG will bind to T-cell surface receptors, opsonising lymphocytes for complement-mediated lysis or reticuloendothelial cell mediated phagocytosis [51-54].

Early trials compared the efficacy, safety, and potency of rabbit *versus* horse derived antithymocyte globulins. Brennen and colleagues [51] conducted a study to evaluate the safety and efficacy of thymoglobulin (rabbit derived) versus ATGAM (horse derived) in high-risk renal transplant patients. All patients received quadruple immunosuppressive therapy consisting of induction therapy with rabbit ATG or horse ATG for 7 days followed with triple maintenance therapy. Patients that were randomized to rabbit ATG received 1.5 mg/kg/day intravenously with the first dose intraoperatively and then continued for 7 days, and patients that were randomized to horse ATG received 15 mg/kg/day also for 7 days. Both induction agents were adjusted based on platelet count and white blood cell count. Maintenance immunosuppression consisted of azathioprine, cyclosporine and corticosteroids. High-risk recipients received mycophenolate mofetil in place of azathioprine. Both 1 and 5-year results revealed greater patient and graft survival for recipients that received rabbit ATG [51,52]. Patients that received rabbit ATG experienced a lower rate of acute rejection at 1 and 5 years compared to those that received horse ATG (4 *vs.* 25%, p=0.014) [51,52]. Just recently Hardinger and colleagues [53] published the 10-year results from the Brennen and colleagues initial study. At 10 years after transplantation, the composite endpoint of freedom from death, graft loss, and rejection, "event-free survival" was higher with thymoglobulin (48%) compared with ATGAM (29%, p=0.011). In regards to rejection there were 6 episodes in the thymoglobulin group compared with 8 episodes in the ATGAM group (11% *vs.* 42% respectively, p=0.004). The incidence of CMV disease remained less with thymoglobulin then ATGAM at 10 years, with no additional cases after the first year (13% *vs.* 33%, p=0.056) [53]. Historically rabbit ATG has been the drug of choice for induction for "high-risk" kidney transplant recipients, however, the exact dose and duration of therapy still remains controversial.

Common adverse effects include an infusion like syndrome due to profound cytokine release. These effects can be mitigated by pre-medicating with an anti-histamine, acetaminophen, and corticosteroids. Other adverse effects include hypotension, malaise, chest tightness, and fever/chills/rigors. The initial infusion should be run over 6 hours and if tolerated subsequent doses can be infused over 4 hours. If patients experience extreme fluid overload or are intolerant to the cytokine release the infusion can be extended up to 24 hours [54].

IL-Receptor Antagonists (IL-2RA)

Daclizumab and basiliximab are humanized and chimeric IgG monoclonal antibodies. They have a high affinity for the α subunit of the lymphocyte IL-2 receptor (CD25) on the surface of activated T-cells [24]. These agents inhibit binding of IL-2 to the IL-2 receptor; competitively inhibiting IL-2 mediated activation and proliferation of T-cells. Since these agents only affect activated T-cells they are considered nondepleting antibodies, and therefore can not be used in the treatment of allograft rejection. The biological half-life of these agents correlates with receptor saturation. IL-2 receptor antagonists have been used with aggressive maintenance regimens for high immunological risk patients that may not be able to tolerate the hematological and infectious complications of antilymphocyte globulins [40,55-59].

Webster and colleagues [60] systematically identified and summarized the effects of IL-2 receptor antagonists as induction agents, as an addition to standard therapy or in comparison to antibody therapies. After exclusion criteria, 38 trials were included in the meta-analysis. 16 trials compared IL-2 receptor antagonists with placebo or no treatment; 14 trials compared IL-2 receptor antagonists to another mono- or polyclonal antibody (monomurab-CD3 or antithymocyte globulin); 1 trial had 3 arms which compared an IL-2 receptor antagonist with no treatment and with a polyclonal antibody; 2 trials compared basiliximab with daclizumab and the remaining involved comparisons with calcineurin-inhibitor free regimens and steroid-free regimens. The majority of the trials were restricted to unsensitized recipients. However, 11 trials included recipients with a PRA >50% and 8 trials included a proportion of recipients with previously failed renal transplants. The incidence of clinically diagnosed acute rejection was reduced by 34% compared to that of a placebo (RR 0.66; CI 0.59-0.74). There was no difference in graft or patient survival. When IL-2 receptor antagonists were compared with other antibody therapy, there were no significant differences in adverse effects, but IL-2 receptor antagonists had fewer adverse events. Since this meta-analysis only included a small number of trials with "high-risk" patients it is difficult to determine the role of IL-2 receptor antagonists as induction agents in this particular patient population [60].

Haririan and colleagues [44] evaluated the use of basiliximab compared with thymoglobulin in 88 African-American kidney transplant recipients. Baseline characteristics were similar between both groups except for recipients that received thymoglobulin had more patients with a PRA >50%. At the end of study follow-up patient and graft survival were similar between both groups. Although the overall incidence of acute rejection was lower in patients that received thymoglobulin the difference did not reach statistical significance (14% *vs.* 29%; p=0.10). Although the incidence the rejection tended to be higher in patients that received basiliximab , the patients that received thymoglobulin had more risk factors for rejection, but the type of induction was not found to be an independent risk factor for acute rejection when adjusting the effect of all other variables. There was also no significant difference in the severity of the acute rejection episodes between groups (p=0.16 for grade I; 0.17 for grade II; and 0.3 for humoral rejection). Further analysis showed that the number of HLA mismatches, presence of delayed graft function, and acute rejection were significantly associated with decreased graft survival. Overall, IL-2 receptor antagonists may be used in African-Americans that are at low immunologic risk at time of transplant [44].

Compared to other induction agents the adverse event profile for the IL-2 receptor antagonist is fairly benign. An acute hypersensitivity reaction including anaphylaxis is rare but mostly related to basiliximab. Neither agent appeared to increase the risk of post-transplant lymphoproliferative disorders, and the incidence of infectious episodes including CMV are similar to that of a placebo [55-59].

IL-2 receptor antagonists have been shown to be more beneficial then placebo, however, the current evidence indicates that they may not provide the protection that antilymphocyte globulins can in "high-risk" renal transplant recipients [44,60].

Alemtuzumab

Alemtuzumab (Campath-1H), is a humanized, monoclonal antibody directed against glycoprotein CD52, which is found on B-cells, T-cells, macrophages, monocytes, granulocytes, and natural killer cells. It is currently FDA approved for B-cell chronic lymphocytic leukemia but recent studies have investigated its use in solid-organ transplantation [40,61]. It was first used in solid-organ transplantation in 1998 to prevent rejection and is being used with increased frequency [61].

Thomas and colleagues [62] studied the use of alemtuzumab as induction in high-risk kidney transplantation. They defined high-risk as those recipients with a PRA >20% or were a re-transplant. Twenty-one patients between January 2005-May 2006 underwent randomization to either receive thymoglobulin (control group) or alemtuzumab. The control group received the first dose of thymoglobulin 1.5 mg/kg preoperatively along with mycophenolate mofetil. Tacrolimus was started when the creatinine decreased to <3 mg/dL or on post-operative day 3, with a target trough of 10 ng/mL. The recipients that received alemtuzumab received a 30 mg dose before reperfusion and monotherapy with tacrolimus was started on post-operative day 1. The only difference in baseline characteristics was the peak PRA was significantly higher among recipients in the control group (81.8%±6.5% *vs*. 38.5%±9.5%). Graft survival at 1-year was similar between both groups with 85.7% survival in the alemtuzumab group and 87.5% in the thymoglobulin group. Three patients in the thymoglobulin group and two in the alemtuzumab group suffered acute cellular rejection. Overall, rates of infections and malignancies were small and there was no difference between groups. Although this study was small and underpowered the results are encouraging and the study is still continuing to recruit patients [62].

Kaufman and colleagues [63] evaluated the use of alemtuzumab and basiliximab as induction immunosuppression in kidney transplantation. This was a single-center, retrospective, nonrandomized, sequential study design that evaluated the outcomes of alemtuzumab (n=123) or basiliximab (n=155) induction with a prednisone free maintenance protocol. Baseline characteristics were similar between both groups, the basiliximab group included 19% African- Americans and the alemtuzumab had 23% of recipients African-Americans. Overall 1-year patient and graft survival were similar between both the basiliximab and alemtuzumab group. When patient and graft survival was analyzed based on donor type there was also no difference between groups. The 12-month actual rejection rates for recipients that received alemtuzumab and basiliximab were 14.9% and 13.5% respectively. The mean days to rejection in the alemtuzumab group was 153 days compared with 10 days in the basiliximab group. Within 90 days of transplant only 5 recipients that received alemtuzumab had a rejection episode compared with 18 recipients in the basiliximab group. Infection rates were also similar between both groups. Overall, some things to note are that although maintenance agents were the same in both groups there was a difference in the exposure of agents. Patients that were treated with alemtuzumab had an overall lower dose of mycophenolate mofetil. However, alemtuzumab does offer some benefits in contrast to other induction agents. First, its a one time dose given in the operating room. Second, unlike the IL-2 receptor antagonist, alemtuzumab may be more effective in prophylaxing against rejection. Lastly, in the immediate/early transplant period alemtuzumab may allow for less exposure to maintenance immunosuppression [63].

Overall, alemtuzumab may be an option for induction in "high-risk" patients, however, to determine its full role in therapy trials with longer follow-up need to be done, along with a larger population, especially those that are considered "high-risk."

Maintenance Immunosuppression

The goals of maintenance immunosuppression are very similar in all transplant recipients including those that are considered "high-risk." It is important to maintain a fine balance between efficacy and toxicity. There are a variety of agents that can be used in a variety of combinations. Some things to consider when creating the "ideal" cocktail of medications is the recipients risk for: malignancy, adverse effects, delayed graft function, acute rejection, and infection.

Calcineurin Inhibitors

Calcineurin inhibitors have been a key component in maintenance immunosuppression regimens. They have significantly decreased rates of acute rejection which at one time were greater >70% to most recently <15%

[24]. Currently two calcineurin inhibitors are available: tacrolimus and cyclosporine. They inhibit the secretion of IL-2 and other cytokines and inhibit both humoral and cellular-mediated immunity. Although calcineurin inhibitors have decreased the rates of acute rejection, one the main reasons long-term patient or graft survival has not improved is due to chronic allograft nephropathy. Chronic toxicity of the calcineurin inhibitors may contribute to the etiology of chronic allograft nephropathy leading to long-term allograft dysfunction.

Similarly to corticosteroids the long-term effects of calcineurin inhibitors are detrimental. They can cause hypertension, hyperlipidemia, or even glucose intolerance. Calcineurin inhibitors can also cause direct nephrotoxicty. Acutely calcineurin inhibitors cause afferent arteriolar vasoconstriction resulting in decreased renal blood flow and glomerular filtration. There changes occur because of an imbalance in prostaglandin E2 and thromboxane A2, increase systemic vascular resistance, and endothelin-1 release [9]. Several strategies have been used to minimize the long-term use of calcineurin inhibitors. These strategies include converting patients to sirolimus in place of the anti-metabolite and continuing the calcineurin inhibitor at a lower dose (calcineurin minimization) or converting to sirolimus and continuing the anti-metabolite. However, there is limited data comparing the effectiveness of these strategies especially in the "high-risk" population.

Anti-Metabolites

Anti-metabolite agents includes azathioprine and mycophenolate mofetil. Since mycophenolate mofetil has been on the market, azathioprine has fallen out of favor. Mycophenolate mofetil is an ester of mycophenolic aicd (MPA), which is rapidly and extensively absorbed. Mycophenolic acid is a potent and specific inhibitor of *de novo* purine synthesis and blocks the proliferation of both T and B cells. There have been a couple of studies that have evaluated the use of mycophenolate mofetil in African-American recipients, which are considered "high-risk" [64-70].African-Americans have a higher rate of acute rejection despite donor age, patient age, gender, weight, CIT, noncompliance, and socioeconomic factors. African-Americans tend to benefit from 3 grams/day of mycophenolate mofetil in comparison to Caucasians that only need 2 grams/day, in the setting of cyclosporine [64]. Pescovitz and colleagues [65] evaluated the pharmacokinetics of twice daily mycophenolate mofetil in African-Americans and Caucasians. Overall, it seems that the exposure of MPA is unrelated to the risk of rejection, however the risk of rejection is more dependent on additional risk factors for rejection [65].

Corticosteroids

Corticosteroids have been the cornerstone to immunosuppression regimens for more than 40 years. The mechanism at which they inhibit the immune system is not fully understood. Corticosteroids alter the distribution of circulating lymphocytes and cause sequestering of the CD4+cells in the reticuloendothelial system [66,67] Steroids also inhibit the proliferation and function of lymphocytes by blocking various lymphokines and cytokines [66,67]. Current evidence shows that steroids also inhibit the action of transcription factors such as activating protein-1 and various nuclear factors [66, 67]. Steroids also inhibit expression of other pro-inflammatory cytokines. Finally corticosteroids inhibit the expression of IL-2 impeding the effects of DNA binding proteins that normally stimulate IL-2 gene transcription [66, 67]. Unfortunately many trials of steroid avoidance have been shown to increase the risk of acute or chronic rejection. However, the long-term adverse effects of long-term steroid use can lead to hypertension, hyperlipidemia, and glucose intolerance and in that case new comorbidities. One of the key questions that arises is when is it safe to withdraw steroids. In 2002 Hricik [64] published an editorial of steroid-free immunosuppression proposed criteria for late and early steroid withdrawal. Recipients that should be considered for later withdrawal are those that are: high-risk for rejection, African-Americans, pediatrics, highly sensitized, and re-transplants Recipients that may qualify for early withdrawal include those that are at: low-risk for rejection, Asian or Caucasian decent, primary transplant, living donors, family history of diabetes, or osteoporosis [64].

There is minimal data on steroid withdrawal in "high-risk" transplant patients. Woodle and colleagues [68] evaluated the risk factors for acute rejection with early steroid withdrawal (within 7 days of transplant). Data from 4 prospective trials were analyzed. A total of 308 patients were included and of that 27% were

African-American and 11% had a current PRA >25%. Overall rate of acute rejection was 17.1% which occurred prior to steroid withdrawal. The overall acute rejection rate after withdrawal was 14.3% [68]. The highest acute rejection rates occurred in re-transplants and sensitized patients. Overall, based on a logistic regression analysis the recipients at highest risk of rejection are re-transplants and type I diabetics [68]. Intermediate risk patients are those with a PRA >25%, DGF, and HLA DR mismatches >0. Recipients at the lowest risk are those that received thymoglobulin induction, type 2 diabetics, living donor transplant, and Caucasian recipient race and male gender. Overall, more studies need to be done on a larger population of highly sensitized recipients to determine the safety and efficacy of steroid withdrawal [64].

CONCLUSION

The definition of "high-risk" has changed significantly over time. It is important to perform the appropriate testing prior to transplant to minimize the risk of rejection. Overall, there are no concrete guidelines in transplanting the "high-risk" population. Most importantly recipient risk factors should aid in the ideal immunosuppressive regimen for the patient.

REFERENCES

[1] Davis, CL. Transplant: immunology and treatment of rejection. Am J Kidney Dis 2004; 6: 1116-1134.

[2] Michaels PJ, Fishbein MC, Colvin RB. Humoral rejection of human organ transplants. Semin Immunopathol 2003; 25: 119-140.

[3] Weimert NA, Alloway RR. Renal transplantation in high-risk patients. Drugs 2007; 67: 1603-1627.

[4] McCarthy GP, Roberts IS. Diagnosis of acute renal allograft rejection. Transplant 2002; 73: 1518-1526.

[5] Colvin RB, Smith RN. Antibody-mediated organ-allograft rejection. Immunology 2005; 5: 807-817.

[6] Takemoto SK, Zeevi A, Feng S, *et al.* National conference to assess antibody-mediated rejection in solid organ transplantation. Am J Transplant 2004; 4: 1033-1041.

[7] Moll S, Pascual M. Humoral rejection of organ allografts. Am J Transplant 2005; 5: 2611-2618.

[8] Racusen LC, Colvin RB, Solez K, *et al.* Antibody-mediated rejection criteria – an addition to Banff '97 classification of renal allograft rejection. Am J Transplant 2003; 3: 708-714.

[9] Flechner SM, Kobashingawa J, Klintmalm G, *et al.* Calcineurin inhibitor-sparing regimens in solid organ transplantation: focus on improving renal function and nephrotoxicity. Clin Transplant 2008: 22: 1-15.

[10] Montgomery RA, Hardy MA, Jordan SC, *et al.* Consensus opinion from the antibody working group of the diagnosis, reporting, and risk assessment for antibody-mediated rejection and desensitization protocols. Transplantation 2004; 78: 181-185.

[11] Reid ME, Olsson ML. Human blood group antigens and antibodies in: Hoffman R, Benz EJ, editors. Hematology: basic principles and practice. 4th ed. Philadelphia (PA): WB Saunders, 2005;2370-74.

[12] Warren DS, Zachary AA, Sonnenday CJ, *et al.* Successful renal transplantation across simultaneous ABO incompatible and positive crossmatch barriers. Am J Transplant 2004; 4: 561-568.

[13] Toki D, Ishida H, Setoguchi K, *et al.* Acute antibody-mediated rejection in living ABO-incompatible kidney transplantation: long-term impact and risk factors. Am J Transplant 2009; 9: 567-577.

[14] Held PJ, Kahan BD, Hunsicker LG. *et al.* The impact of HLA mismatches on the survival of 1st cadaveric kidney transplants. New Engl J Med 1994; 331: 765-770.

[15] Ting A, Edwards LB. Human leukoctye antigen in the allocation of kidney from cadaveric donorjs in the United States. Transplant 2004; 77: 610-633.

[16] Roberts JP, Wolfe RA, Bragg-Gresham JL, *et al.* Effect of changing the priority for HLA matching on rates and outcomes of kidney transplantation in minority groups. New Engl J Med 2004; 350: 545-551.

[17] Jordan SC, Tyan D, Stablein D, *et al.* Evaluation of intravenous immunoglobulin as an agent to lower allosensitization and improve transplantation in highly sensitized adult patients with end-stage renal disease: a report of the NIH IG02 trial. J Am Soc Nephrol 2004; 15: 3256-3262.

[18] Peng A, Vo A, Jordan SC. Transplantation of the highly human leukocyte antigen-sensitized patient: long-term outcomes and future directions. Transplant Rev 2006; 20: 146-156.

[19] Pelletier RP, Hennessy PK, Adams PW *et al.* High incidence of donor-reactive delayed-type hypersensitivity reactivity in transplant patients. Am J Transplant 2002; 2: 926-933.

[20] Wahrmann M, Exner M, Haidbauer B, *et al.* {C4d} FlowPRA screening - a specific assay for selective detection of complement-activating anti-HLA alloantibodies. Hum Immunol 2005; 66: 526-534.

[21] Pei R, Wang G, Tarsitani C, *et al.* Simultaneous HLA class I and class II antibodies screening with flow cytometry. Hum Immunol 1998; 59: 313-322.

[22] Gebel HM, Bray RA, Nickerson P. Pre-transplant assessment of donor-reactive, HLA-specific antibodies in renal transplantation: contraindication *vs.* risk. Am J Transplant 2003; 3: 1488-1500.

[23] Fuggle SV, Martin S. Toward performing transplantation in highly sensitized patients. Transplant 2004; 78: 186-189.

[24] Beimler JHM, Susal C, Zeier M. Desensitization strategies enabling successful renal transplantation in highly sensitized patients. Clin Transplant 2006; 20: 7-12.

[25] Jordan S, Cunningham-Rundles C, McEwan R. Utility of intravenous immune globulin in kidney transplantation: efficacy, safety, and cost implications. Am J Transplant 2003; 3: 653-664.

[26] Becker YT, Becker BN, Pirsch JD, *et al.* Rituximab as treatment for refractory kidney transplant rejection. Am J Transplant 2004; 4: 996-1001.

[27] Munoz AS, Rioveros AA, Cabanayan-Casasola CB, Danguilan RA, *et al.*Rituximab in highly sensitized kidney transplant recipients. Transplant Proc 2008; 40: 2218-2221.

[28] Everly JJ, Walse RC, Alloway RR *et al.* Protease inhibition for antibody-mediated rejection. Curr Opin Organ Transplant 2009; 14: 1-5.

[29] Everly MJ, Everly JJ, Susskind B, *et al.* Bortezomib provides effective therapy for antibody- and cell-mediated acute rejection. Transplant 2008; 86: 1754-1761.

[30] Young CJ, Gaston RS. Renal transplantation in black Americans. N Engl J Med 2000; 343: 1545-1552.

[31] Sautner T, Gnant M, Banhegyi C, *et al.* Risk factors for development of panel reactive antibodies and their impact on kidney transplantation outcomes. Tranplant Int 1992; 5: 5116-5120.

[32] Soosay A, O'Neill D, Counihan A, *et al.* Causes of sensitization in patients awaiting renal transplantation in Ireland. Ir Med J 2003; 96: 109-112.

[33] Montini G, Ujka F, Varagnolo C, *et al.* The pharmacokinetics and immunosuppressive response of tacrolimus in pediatric renal transplant recipients. Pediatr Nephrol 2006; 21: 719-724.

[34] Hwang AH, Cho YW, Cicciarelli J, *et al.* Risk factors for short- and long-term survival of primary cadaveric renal allografts in pediatric recipients: a UNOS analysis. Transplant 2005; 80: 466-470.

[35] Singh A, Stablein D, Tejani A, *et al.* Risk factors for vascular thrombosis in pediatric renal transplantation: a special report of the North American Pediatric Renal Transplant Cooperative Study. Transplant 1997; 63: 1263-1267.

[36] Rianthavorn P, Ettengr RB. Medication non-adherence in the adolescent renal transplant recipient: clinicians viewpoint. Pediatr Transplant 2005; 9: 398-407.

[37] Danovitch G, Savransky E. Challenges in the counseling and management of older kidney transplant candidates. Am J Kidney Dis 2006; 47: S86-97.

[38] Pessione F, Cohen S, Durand D, *et al.* Multivariate analysis of donor risk factors for graft survival in kidney transplantation. Transplantation 2003; 75: 361-367.

[39] Ojo AO, Wolfe RA, Agadoa LY, *et al.* Prognosis after primary renal transplant failure and the beneficial effect of repeat transplantation: multivariate analysis from the United States Renal Data System. Trasplantation 1998; 66: 1651-1659.

[40] Briganti EM, Epi MC, Russ GR, *et al.* Risk of renal allograft loss from recurrent glomerulonephritis. N Eng J Med 2002; 347: 103-109.

[41] Stock PG, Roland ME. Evolving clinical strategies for transplantation in the HIV-positive recipient. Transplant 2007; 84: 563-571.

[42] Ciuffreda D, Pantaleo G, Pascual M. Effects of immunosuppressive drugs on HIV infection: implications for solid-organ transplantation. Transplant International 2007; 20: 649-658.

[43] Kalil RSN, Heim-Duthoy KL, Kasiske BL, *et al.* Patients with low income have reduced renal allograft survival. Am J Kidney Dis 1992; 20: 63-69.

[44] Haririan A, Morawski K, Sillix DH, *et al.* Induction therapy with basiliximab versus thymoglobulin in African-American kidney transplant recipients. Transplantation 2005; 79: 716-721.

[45] Epstein AM, Ayanian JZ, Keogh JH *et al.* Racial disparities in access to renal transplantation. New Eng J Med 2000; 343: 1537-1544.

[46] Weber M, Dindo D, Detartines N *et al.* Kidney transplantation from donors without a heartbeat. N Eng J Med 2002; 347: 248-255.

[47] Recommendations for nonheartbeating organ donation. Crit Care Med 2001; 29: 1826-1831.

[48] Sanchez-Fructuso AL, Prats D, Torrent K, *et al.* Renal transplantation from non-heart beating donors: a promising alternative to enlarge the donor pool. J Am Soc Nephrol 2000; 11: 350-358.

[49] Bryan CF, Luger AM, Martinez J, *et al.* Cold ischemia time: an independent predictor of increased HLA class I antibody production after rejection or a primary cadaeric renal allograft. Transplant 2001; 71: 875-879.

[50] Loverre A, Difonno P, Crovace A *et al.* Ischemia-reperfusion injury induces glomerular and tubular activation of proinflammatory and antiapoptotic pathways, differential modulation by rapamycin. J Am Soc Nephrol 2204; 15: 2675-2686.

[51] Brennen DC, Agha I, Bohl DL, *et al.* A randomized, double-blinded comparison of thymoglobulin versus ATGAM for induction immunosuppressive therapy in adult renal transplant recipients. Transplantation 1999; 67: 1011-1018.

[52] Hardinger KL, Schnitzler MA, Miller B, *et al.* Five-year follow up of thymoglobulin versus ATGAM induction in adult renal transplant. Transplantation 2004; 78: 136-141.

[53] Hardinger KL, Rhee S, Buchanan P, *et al.* A prospective, randomized, double-blinded comparison of thymoglobulin versus ATGAM for induction immunosuppressive therapy: 10-year results. Transplantation 2008; 86: 947-952.

[54] Thymoglobulin (Anti-thymocyte globulin [rabbit]) [package insert]. Genzyme Polyclonals SAS Lyons, France. Revision 6. 2005

[55] Wiseman LR, Faulds D. Daclizumab. Drugs. 1999;58(6):1029-1042.

[56] Chapman TM, Keating GM. Basiliximab. Drugs. 2003;63(24):2804-2835.

[57] Cibrik DM, Kaplan B, Meier-Kriesche H. Role of anti-interleukin-2 receptor antibodies in kidney transplantation. Biodrugs. 2001;15(10):655-666.

[58] Roche Pharmaceuticals: Daclizumab (Zenapax) Package Insert. (2003). Nutley, NJ: Roche Pharmaceuticals Corporation.

[59] Novartis Pharmaceuticals: Basiliximab (Simulect) Package Insert. (2005). East Hanover, NJ: Novartis Pharmaceuticals Corporation

[60] Webster AC, Playford EG, Higgins G, *et al.* Interleukin 2 receptor antagonists for renal transplant recipients: a meta-analysis of randomized trials. Transplantation 2005; 77: 166-176.

[61] Morris PJ, Russell NK. Alemtuzumab (Campath-1H): a systemic review in organ transplantation. Transplantation 2006; 81: 1361-1367.

[62] Thomas PG, Woodside KJ, Lappin JA, *et al.* Alemtuzumab (Campath 1H) induction with tacrolimus monotherapy is safe for high immunological risk renal transplantation. Transplant 2007; 83: 1509-1512.

[63] Kaufman DB, Leventhal JR, Axelrod D, *et al.* Alemtuzumab induction and prednisone-free maintenance immunotherapy in kidney transplantation: comparison with basiliximab induction-long-term results. Am J Transplant 2005; 5: 2539-2548.

[64] Neylan JF. Immunosuppressive therapy in high-risk transplant patients: dose-dependent efficacy of mycophenolate mofeti in African-American renal allograft recipients. Transplant 1997; 64: 1277-1282.

[65] Pescovitz MD, Guasch A, Gaston R, *et al.* Equivalent pharmacokinetics of mycophenolate mofetil in African-American and Caucasian male and female stable renal allograft recipients. Am J Transplant 2003; 3: 1581.

[66] Hricik DE. Steroid-free immunosuppression in kidney transplantation: an editorial review. Am J Transplant 2002; 2: 19-24.

[67] Alawi WY, Itardo ET, Strom TB. Evidence that glucocorticosteroid mediated immunosuppressive effects do not involve altering second messenger function. Transplant 1991; 52: 133-140.

[68] Woodle ES, Alloway RR, Buell JF, *et al.* Multivariate analysis of risk factors for acute rejection in early corticosteroid cessation regimens under modern immunosuppression. Am J Transplant 2005; 5: 2740-2744.

[69] Schweiter EJ, Wilson JS, Fernandez-Vina M, *et al.* A high panel-reactive antibody rescue protocol for cross-match positive live donor kidney transplants. Transplantation 2000; 70: 1531-1536.

[70] Montgomery RA, Zachary AA, Racusen LC, *et al.* Plasmapheresis and intravenous immune globulin provides effective rescue therapy for refractory humoral rejection and allows kidneys to be successfully transplanted into cross-match positive recipients. Transplantation 2000; 70: 887-895.

[71] Sonnenday CJ, Ratner LE, Zachary AA, *et al.* Preemptive therapy with plasmapheresis/intravenous immunoglobulin allows successful live donor renal transplantation in patients with a positive cross-match. Transplant Proc 2002; 34: 1614-1616.

[72] Glotz D, Antoine C, Suberbielle-Boissel PJC, Boudjeltia S, *et al.* Desensitization and subsequent kidney transplantation of patients using intravenous immunoglobulins (IVIg). Am J Transplant 2002; 2: 758-760.

[73] Sonnenday CJ, Warren DS, Cooper M, *et al.* Plasmapheresis, CMV hyperimmune globulin, and anti-CD20 allow ABO-incompatible renal transplantation without splenectomy. Am J Transplant 2004; 4: 1315-1322.

[74] Thielke J, DeChristopher PJ, Sankary H, *et al.* Highly successful living donor kidney transplantation after conversion to negative of a previously positive flow-cytometry cross-match by pretransplant plasmapheresis. Transplant Proc 2005; 37: 643-644.

[75] Stegall MD, Gloor J, Winters JL, *et al.* A comparison of plasmapheresis versus high-dose IVIg desensitization in renal allograft recipients with high levels of donor specific alloantibody. Am J Transplant 2006; 6: 346-351.

[76] Vo AA, Lukosky M, Toyoda M, *et al.* Rituximab and intravenous immune globulin for desensitization during renal transplantation. N Engl J Med 2008; 359: 242-251.

CHAPTER 4

ABO-Incompatible Renal Transplantation

Kazunari Tanabe*

Department of Urology, Tokyo Women's Medical University, Tokyo, Japan

Abstract: In an effort to overcome the severe organ shortage, ABO-incompatible kidney transplantation has been carried out in many transplant centers worldwide over the last decade. In the 1980s, ABO-incompatible kidney transplantation was electively performed in Europe and Japan and the early results were acceptable though short-term results were significantly poorer than those of ABO-compatible kidney transplantation (80% *vs.* 95% at one year, 79% *vs.* 92% at three years in ABO-incompatible *vs.* ABO-compatible transplantations, respectively). The original preconditioning regimens included splenectomy, plasmapheresis, and immunosuppression with ciclosporin, azathioprine and steroids.

Early in this century, many potent immunosuppressive agents, such as tacrolimus, mycophenolate mofetil, rituximab, basiliximab, thymoglobulin and daclizimab were introduced in the field of clinical kidney transplantation. With these potent immunosuppressive agents, the outcomes of ABO-incompatible kidney transplantation improved significantly. Currently, in most transplant programs, preconditioning and immunosuppressive regimens typically include a rituximab injection, plasmapheresis or immunoadsorption and immunosuppression with tacrolimus, mycophenolate mofetil and steroids. The latter is a mild regimen comparable to those for ABO-compatible kidney transplantation. Recently, one year graft survival in most ABO-incompatible programs has exceeded 90-95%. Furthermore, the incidence of rejection is less than 10% in most reports of ABO-incompatible kidney transplantation.

ABO-incompatible kidney transplantation has become a safe, excellent treatment option for renal failure patients.

Keywords: ABO Incompatible Kidney Transplantation, Rituximab, Plasmapheresis, C4d, Acute Rejection, Living Donor, Organ Shortage, Desensitization.

INTRODUCTION

The supply of cadaver donor kidneys is not sufficient to meet the demand of an increasing number of patients requiring renal transplantation worldwide. To resolve this serious problem, expansion of the donor pool employing various options, such as transplantation using ECD, DCD and ABO-incompatible donors, donor exchange programs, or cross-match-positive donors, has been carried out over the last decade.

ABO-incompatible kidney transplantation (ABO-IKT) began in the early 1970s [1, 2]. In the early experience, the outcomes of ABO-IKT were not sufficient to make this a routine procedure in kidney transplantation. However, in the 1990s, Japanese groups accumulated major experience with ABO-IKT because there were not enough cadaver kidneys available. Their early experience, while not excellent, was acceptable given the extreme shortage of kidney donors in Japan [3, 4].

Since 2000, even in countries with well organized deceased donor systems, the number of renal failure patients has been rapidly increasing and the gap between the number of cadaver organs available and potential recipients has been increasing rapidly. Under these circumstances, ABO-IKT programs were launched in some European and US centers since as many as 20% of potential living donors had been excluded because of ABO-incompatibility [5-7].

In this chapter, we will review the clinical outcomes of ABO-IKT obtained to date.

***Address correspondence to Kazunari Tanabe:** Department of Urology, Tokyo Women's Medical University, 8-1 Kawada-cho, Shinjuku-ku, Tokyo, 162-8666, Japan; Phone +81-3-3353-8111 ext: 37414; Fax: +81-3-5269-7353; E-mail:tanabe@kc.twmu.ac.jp

Massimiliano Veroux and Pierfrancesco Veroux (Eds)

BLOOD GROUP ANTIGEN EXPRESSIONS IN THE KIDNEY

Blood group A is characterized by the terminal trisaccharide GalNA alfa-3[Fuc alfa 1-2] Gal BETA-, blood group B by the terminal trisaccharide Gal alfa 1-3[Fuc alfa 1-2] Gal BETA -, and blood group O by the disaccharide Fuc alfa 1-2 Gal BETA- [8, 9]. Blood group A can be further divided into A1 and A2 subgroups. The A2 subgroup constitutes about 20% of the European blood group A population, but only 0.15% of the Japanese population [3].

In the kidney, ABH antigens are expressed on the vascular endothelium and in the distal convoluted tubules and collecting tubules, whereas Lewis blood group antigens are expressed on epithelial cells of the distal convoluted and collecting tubules, but not the vascular endothelium. The gycosyltransferase activity necessary for the synthesis of ABH and Lewis antigens is found in the cortex, medulla and glomeruli of the kidney. All vascular endothelia have ethanol-soluble ABH antigens in both secretors and non-secretors, but the blood group antigens on epithelial cells of the collecting tubules and the calyceal epithelium are water-soluble and are expressed only in secretors [3, 10-13].

HISTORY OF ABO-INCOMPATIBLE KIDNEY TRANSPLANTATION

In the 1960s, some very important phenomena in the field of blood group antigen expression and tissue compatibility were reported by two research groups. Economidou *et al.* [14] showed that the expression of A2 antigens on erythrocytes was much weaker than that of A1 antigens. Also, Ceppellini *et al.* [15] reported that skin grafts from blood group A2 to O individuals survived for almost the same period as skin grafts from blood group O to O whereas skin grafts from A1 or B to O individuals were rejected immediately. They speculated that solid organ transplantation from blood group A2 to O might be possible [15].

In the 1970s, Rydberg *et al.* started A2-incompatible renal transplantation using azathioprine and steroids without pre-transplant conditioning. Among 20 A2-incompatible renal transplant recipients, eight lost their graft within one month of transplantation, whereas the remaining 12 grafts functioned long term [1, 2].

Since blood group B or O transplant candidates usually have difficulty finding compatible donors, some US and European transplant centers have established programs to preferentially allocate blood group A2 or A2B cadaver kidneys to blood type O or B recipients [16-18]. Nelson *et al.* [19] reported that they performed A2-incompatible renal transplantation in 41 cases between 1994 and 2000 with neither pre-transplant treatment nor splenectomy. The 1- and 5-year graft survival rates were 91% and 85%, respectively. These data did not differ from those of compatible kidney transplantation. The authors concluded that blood group B recipients could successfully receive kidneys from blood group A2 or A2B donors and thereby, eventually, expand the donor pool.

During the same period, several immunomodulating techniques such as plasmapheresis and immunoadsorption contributed to donor pool expansion. These techniques played an important role in successful renal transplantation from ABO-incompatible or anti-HLA antibody positive donors.

In 1981, Slapak *et al.* [20] reported a favorable effect of plasmapheresis on hyper-acute rejection in a patient who accidentally received a kidney from an ABO-incompatible donor. After transplantation, plasmapheresis was performed to remove anti-ABO antibodies and the graft was successfully rescued. In 1984, they also reported three cases of successful A1 to O renal transplantation with pre-transplant immunoadsorption and plasmapheresis treatment [21]. Subsequently, they reported their updated data from 16 cases receiving ABO-incompatible renal transplantation in 1990, with a one-year graft survival rate of 87%. Splenectomy was performed in five of the 16 patients, but had no impact on graft survival [22].

Alexander *et al.* reported their first experience with ABO-incompatible renal transplantation in 26 patients [23]. Their preconditioning and immunosuppressive regimen included ciclosporin, azathioprine, steroids, anti-lymphocyte globulin, donor specific platelet transfusion and splenectomy, in most cases. Their one-year graft survival was 85% and they reported splenectomy to be essential for successful ABO-incompatible renal transplantation.

In 1989, Japanese transplant centers started to perform ABO-incompatible renal transplantation to resolve the severe organ donor shortage in this country. In the early 1990s, the Tokyo Women's Medical University (TWMU) team reported their single center result for ABO-incompatible living kidney transplantation (ABO-ILKT) [24-27]. Toma *et al.* [28] reported their experience with 141 ABO-incompatible renal transplantations and showed short-term graft survivals up to 4 years after transplantation to be significantly poorer than those of ABO-compatible cases. However, interestingly, long-term graft survival did not differ between ABO-incompatible and ABO-compatible cases.

In 2004, the same group reported that one week of pre-transplant immunosuppression using potent immunosuppressive drugs, such as tacrolimus (TAC), mycophenolate mofetil (MMF) and steroids (ST), produced excellent graft survival and a significantly lower incidence of AMR as compared to those who did not receive one week of pre-transplantation immunosuppression [29]. Forty-five patients were enrolled in this study and 25 were given the pre-transplantation immunosuppression regimen (group 1) while 13 were not (group 2). Two-year graft survival rates were 97% and 92% in groups 1 and 2, respectively. The incidences of rejection were 56% and 19% in groups 1 and 2, respectively.

The Mayo Clinic team reported their experience with 18 ABO-ILKT using A2 and non-A2 living donors [30]. Their preconditioning regimen included plasmapheresis followed by IVIG and post-transplant immunosuppressive medications included thymoglobulin induction, TAC, MMF and steroids. They also performed splenectomy at the time of transplantation. Their outcomes were excellent. The 1-year graft survival rate was 89% and antibody-mediated rejection (AMR) occurred in 28% of recipients.

Table 1: Current outcome of ABO-ILKT

Current outcome of ABO-ILKT

	TWMU	Stocholm	Johns Hopkins	Mayo Clinic
Pre-transplant management				
TAC	Y	Y	Y	Y
MMF	Y	Y	Y	Y
ST	Y	Y	N	Y
splenectomy	N	N	N	N
rituximab	Y	Y	N	Y
Post-transplant				
prophylactic PEX/Id	N	Y	Y	Y
Rejection	5-10%	5%>	6%	30%
IYgraft suwuival	97%	100%	100%	93%

Y: yes、N: no、PEX: plasma pheresis, Id: immuno-adsorption

TAC: tacrolimus、MMF: mycophenolate mofetil、ST: steroids

CURRENT SITUATION OF ABO-INCOMPATIBLE KIDNEY TRANSPLANTATION

The TWMU team has the largest number of ABO-ILKT in worldwide in a single center. In TWMU, immunosuppression, including TAC (0.1 mg/kg, with a target trough level of 10 ng/ml), MMF (1-2 g/day) and ST (20 mg/day, increased to 500 mfg on the day of transplantation) is usually started 7 days prior to renal transplantation. This is accompanied by four sessions of concomitant double filtration plasmapheresis (DFPP) to remove anti-A and/or anti-B antibodies. Whereas till 2004 all recipients underwent splenectomy at the time of renal transplantation, rituximab has been injected instead of performing splenectomy since 2005 (Fig. **1**) (Table **1**).

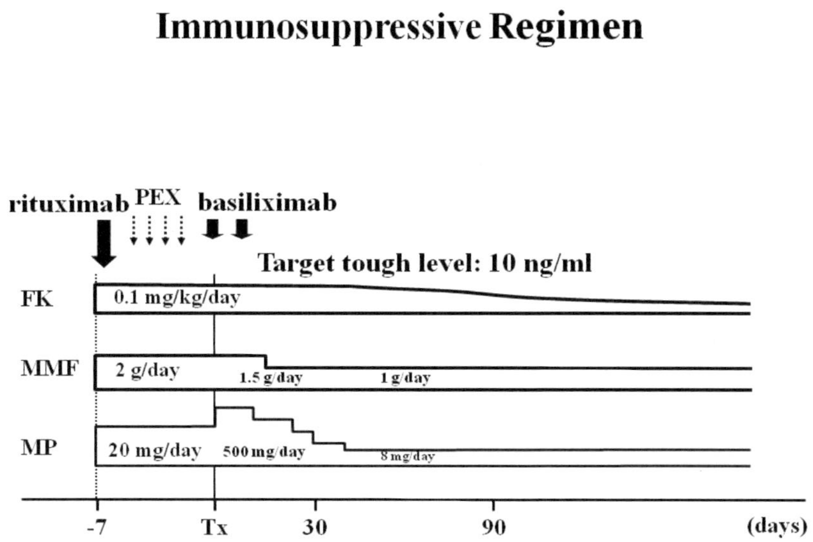

Figure 1: Preconditioning and immunosuppressive regimen in TWMU. FK, MMF and MP were used as basic immunosuppressive agents. We administered FK(0.1 mg/kg/day)/MMF(1-2g/day)/MP(20-125 mg/day) concomitantly with PEX starting 7 days before transplantation. FK was reduced according to the target trough level, which was around 10ng/ml in the induction phase. MMF was reduced to 1,500 mg/day 2 weeks after surgery, and to 1,000 mg/day 1 month after ABO-ILKT. MP wad reduced to 8 mg/day 1 month after transplantation. In the maintenance phase (6 months after transplantation), all patients were placed on low-dose immunosuppression with FK/MMF/MP. The average doses of FK, MMF and MP were 0.07 mg/kg, 1,000 mg/day and 5 mg/day, respectively. The target trough level of FK was 5 ng/ml during the maintenance phase. Neither ALG nor DSG were used. Local irradiation of the graft was not performed. Anti-IL-2 receptor blocker (basiliximab) was used in the induction phase. Rituximab at a dose of 200 mg/person was administered 7 days prior to renal transplantation in place of splenectomy. In this study, pre- or posttransplant prophylactic administration of intravenous immunoglobulin (IVIG) was not performed in all patients.

The effects of immunosuppression on outcomes of ABO-ILKT at TWMU were recently evaluated. In total, 222 ABO-ILK performed between 1989 and 2004 at TWMU were assessed. All patients were divided into group 1 (105 patients who underwent ABO-LKT between 1989 and 1999) or group 2 (117 patients who underwent ABO-LKT between 2001 and 2004). There were significant differences in the 1- and 5-year graft survival rates between groups 1 and 2 (1-year: 78% in group 1 *vs.* 94% in group 2; 5-year: 73% in group 1 *vs.* 90% in group 2). Also, a significantly higher incidence of rejection was observed in group 1 (48%) than in group 2 (15%) [31].

Toki *et al.* reported that acute AMR has a strong impact on the long-term outcome of ABO-ILKT [32]. They evaluated 57 consecutive ABO-ILKT performed at TWMU between 1999 and 2004. Out of 57 patients, 19 experienced acute AMR (AMR group) and 38 did not (non-AMR group). The graft survival rate of the AMR group was significantly poorer than that of the non-AMR group (AMR *vs.* non-AMR, respectively; 5 years: 84% *vs.* 95%; 8 years: 45% *vs.* 95%; $p=0.009$). The prevalence of transplant glomerulopathy at 1 year post-transplantation was significantly higher in the AMR group (AMR 64% *vs.* non-AMR 3%, $p<0.001$). Also, they reported that donor-specific anti-HLA antibody (DSA) detected by the Luminex single bead method was an independent risk factor for acute AMR regardless of the baseline anti-blood group IgG antibody titers. They concluded that DSA had a more significant association with poor graft outcomes than anti-blood group antibodies in ABO-ILKT.

Setoguchi *et al.* reviewed 89 protocol biopsy specimens of ABO-ILKT performed between 2000 and 2004 at TWMU [33]. They reported that subclinical rejection was found in 10-30% of ABO-ILKT patients by protocol biopsy. Furthermore, they showed positive PRA and a prior history of AMR to be strong risk factors for transplant glomerulopathy.

Tanabe *et al.* reported up-dated data on ABO-ILKT in 2009 [34]. They evaluated two different preconditioning regimens for ABO-ILKT, namely splenectomy *vs.* rituximab-treatment non-splenectomy preconditioning regimens. Seventy recipients underwent ABO-ILKT between 2001 and 2006 and were enrolled in this study. Forty-six patients were treated with splenectomy (SPX group) and 24 were given rituximab injections without splenectomy (RIT group). Fifty-five ABO-compatible renal transplant recipients were employed as a matched control group (Control group). The three-year graft survival rates did not differ among the three groups; 98.2%, 93.5% and 95.8% in the ABO-C, SPX and RIT groups, respectively. The RIT group showed significantly lower incidences of acute AMR and chronic AMR than the other two groups. The RIT group had an 8.3% AMR and a 4.2% chronic AMR incidence, whereas the SPX and Control groups had significantly higher incidences of acute AMR (acute AMR; 9.1%, 19.6% and 8.3% in the Control, SPX and RIT groups, respectively) and chronic AMR (chronic AMR; 25.5%, 2.2% and 4.2% in the Control, SPX and RIT groups, respectively). Their conclusion was that the RIT group showed the best outcome in terms of the incidences of both acute and chronic AMR and graft survival.

SPLENECTOMY *VS.* NON-SPLENECTOMY

In the early ABO-ILKT experience, most immunosuppressive regimens included splenectomy as a standard protocol.

Tyden *et al.* [5] performed the first ABO-ILKT with a new preconditioning regimen including rituximab injection instead of splenectomy with antigen specific immunoadsorption in 2001 and reported their experience in 2003. They described the first successful ABO-ILKT with a non-splenectomy regimen, using rituximab. This new non-splenectomy regimen has rapidly spread to many transplant centers performing ABO-ILKT. Their preconditioning regimen included injection of one dose of rituximab, followed by full doses of TAC, MMF and prednisolone. Antigen-specific immunoadsorption was performed on days -6, -5, -2 and -1, and 0.5 g/kg of IVIG was given on day -1. They also added three sessions of prophylactic immunoadsorption after transplantation. Genberg *et al.* reported their 3-year data. The graft survival rate was 86.7% and rejection occurred in only one patient [35] (Fig. **2**) (Table **1**).

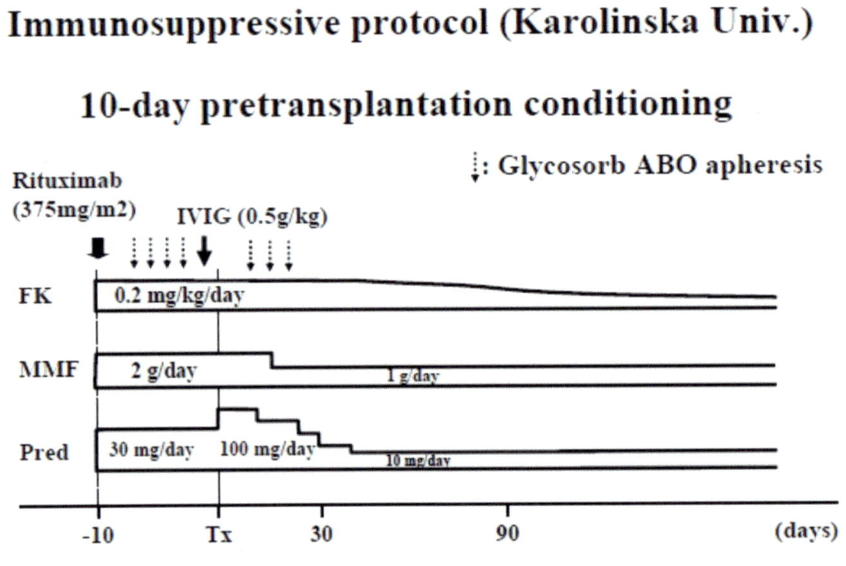

Figure 2: Preconditioning and immunosuppressive regimen in Stockholm. Removal of A/B antibody was achieved by repeated antigen-specific immunoadsorption (GlycosorbABO; Glycorex, Lund, Sweden) preoperatively on day -6, -5, -2, and -1. In addition, a single dose of rituximab 375mg/m^2 body surface area was given on day -30 and oral immunosuppression (tacrolimus, mycophenolate mofetil, and prednisolone) instituted on day -10. On day -1, intravenous immunoglobulin, 0.5 g/kg body weight (b.w.), was administered. Postoperatively, immunoadsorption was performed on days 2, 5, and 8. Additional immunoadsorptions were performed preoperatively If A/B antibody titers exceeded 1:4 after the last preoperative session and postoperatively if there was a rise in A/B antibody titers with a concomitant impairment of the kidney function.

Since that time, in most ABO-ILKT programs, rituximab injection was adopted as a part of the standard preconditioning regimens. The Johns Hopkins group reported their experience with ABO-ILKT in 2004 [7]. Their preconditioning regimen included plasmapheresis followed by Cytomegalovirus immune globulin (CMVIg) at a dose of 100 mg/kg and concomitant immunosuppression with TAC (0.1 mg/kg) and MMF (2g/day). One to 2 days prior to transplantation, a single dose of rituximab (375 mg/m2) was given. On the day of surgery, methylprednisolone 500 mg plus daclizmab 2 mg/kg was initiated and post-transplant plasmapheresis/CMVIg treatments were typically performed on days 1, 3 and 5 (Fig. **3**) (Table **1**).

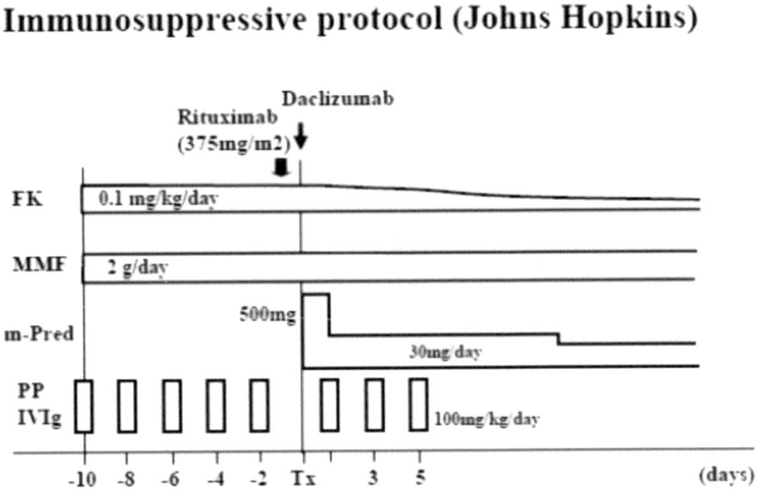

Figure 3: Preconditioning and immunosuppressive regimen in Johns Hopkins. Plasmapheresis was delivered using a COBE Spectra (Gambro BCT, Lakewood, CO, USA). In brief, 1-1.5 plasma volumes were removed per treatment with 100% volume replacement using either 5% albumin solution or fresh frozen plasma. CMVIg (Cytogam^{TM}, Medlmmune Inc., Gaithersburg, MD, USA) was administered at 100 mg/kg following each PP treatment. Pre-transplant treatments were given every other day on an outpatient basis until ABO antibody titer $\leq$16 was achieved. One to 2d prior to the anticipated transplant date, after the last pre-transplant PP treatment wad delivered , a single dose of rituximab was given (375 mg/m^2). Tacrolimus (0.1 mg/kg/day) and mycophenolate mofetil (2 g/day in 2-4 divided doses) were started at the initiation of preoperative PP/CMVIg treatments. Daclizumab 2 mg/kg prior to reperfusion then 1 mg/kg every other week for four doses, and steroids (methylprednisolone 500 mg intra-operative then 125 mg every 6h for six doses; followed by prednisone 30 mg/day) were begun at the time of transplantation. When tacrolimus reached target levels (10-12 ng/mL) post-transplant, the prednisone dose wad decreased to 20 mg/day. After transplantation, protocol PP/CMVIg treatments were given on postoperative days 1, 3 and 5.

They recently reported their up-dated data from 53 cases of ABO-ILKT and the 3-year graft survival rate was 93.4% with excellent graft function (the median creatinine concentration was 1.2 mg/dl at 3 years after surgery) [36, 37]. More recently, they reported that even without rituximab injection, successful desensitization could be achieved by plasmapheresis alone as a preconditioning regimen. They concluded that neither splenectomy nor rituximab injection is necessary for successful ABO-ILKT [38].

Recently, they reported up-dated data on 28 ABO-ILKT without splenectomy or rituximab injection. In total, 8 patients had acute clinical or subclinical rejection but with 100% graft survival. They concluded that the use of routine splenectomy or rituximab injection is not essential for engraftment of ABO-incompatible kidneys [39].

PATHOLOGICAL ANALYSIS OF ABO-ILKT

The significance of C4d staining in peritubular capillaries after ABO-ILKT remains controversial [34, 40-42]. In 2003, a Japanese group, Kato and colleagues [41], showed diffuse/bright C4d deposition in PTC to be valuable as a specific and sensitive indicator of AAMR in ABO-ILKT. However, recent accumulated data pertaining to this issue indicate that C4d deposition is not a good indicator of AMR.

The clinical relevance of C4d deposition in peritubular capillaries in ABO-ILKT has been widely reported. At present, the author recognizes that there is a consensus that C4d deposition in PTC is a non-specific finding of AMR in the majority of published articles [43-45]. The Johns Hopkins team found that PTC C4d staining did not correlate significantly with histologic changes of AAMR in biopsies from ABO-I renal transplants. The extent of PTC C4d staining is divided into diffuse, focal and negative categories. The incidences of PTC neutrophil margination are nearly the same among different grades of C4d staining.

Moreover, the Johns Hopkins group has shown that diffuse and bright C4d deposition, without morphological features of AMR and renal dysfunction, results in better chronic pathological findings in ABO-ILKT [46].

We also found C4d deposition to have no relevance in ABO-ILKT. In our protocol biopsy study using 250 ABO-compatible and 89 ABO-incompatible specimens, 89% of ABOC grafts showed no PTC C4d deposition, while 94% of ABOI specimens showed focal and diffuse C4d deposition in the PTC [33].

Most previous studies have examined C4d deposition during the early period after ABOI kidney transplantation. However, the details of C4d deposition in late biopsies are not well understood. The incidence of C4d deposition in ABO-C grafts was about 20% over the long-term. C4d deposition was, however, observed in over 80% of specimens even in late biopsies in ABO-ILKT (unpublished data).

Since, in the ABO-ILKT setting, C4d staining is not a reliable criterion for the diagnosis of AMR, we need to define new diagnostic criteria for AMR in ABO-ILKT.

CONCLUSION

The outcomes of ABO-ILKT have recently improved dramatically thanks to potent immunosuppression and one-year graft survival rates of 90-95% are now being achieved in most transplant programs.

REFERENCES

[1] Rydberg L, Breimer ME, Samuelsson Be, Brynger H. Blood group ABO-incompatible(A2 to O) kidney transplantation in human subjects: a clinical, serologic, and biochemical approach. Transplant Proc 1987; 19: 4528-4537.

[2] Rydberg L. ABO-incompatibility in solid organ transplantation. Transfus Med 2001: 11: 325-342.

[3] Toma H. ABO-incompatible renal transplantation. Urol Clin North Am 1994; 21: 299-310.

[4] Tanabe K, Takahashi K, Sonda K, *et al.* Long-term results of ABO-incompatible living kidney transplantation. Transplantation 1998; 65: 224-248.

[5] Tyden G, Kumlien G, Fehrman I. Successful ABO-incompatible kidney transplantations without splenectomy using antigen-specific immunoadsorption and rituximab. Transplantation 2003; 76: 730-743.

[6] Gloor JM, Lager DJ, Moore SB at al. ABO-incompatible kidney transplantation using both A2 and non-A2 living donors. Transplantation 2003; 75(7): 971.

[7] Sonnenday CJ, Warren DS, Cooper M, *et al.* Plasmapheresis, CMV hyperimmune globulin, and anti-CD20 allow ABO-incompatible renal transplantation without splenectomy. Am J Transplant 2004; 4: 1315.

[8] Clausen H, Levery SB, Nudelman E, *et al.* Repetitive A epitope(type 3 chain A) defined by blood group A1 specific monoclonal anti-body TH-1: Chemical basis of a qualitative A1 and A2 distinction. Proc Nat Acad Sci 1985; 82: 1199-1203.

[9] Clausen H, Levery SB, Dabelsteen E, Hakomori S. Blood group ABH antigens: a new series of blood group A-associated structures(genetic regulation and tissue distribution). Transplant Proc 1987; 19: 4408-4412.

[10] Tanabe K, Tyden G. Overcoming ABO incompatibility. Living Donor Kidney Transplantation 2005; 119-129.

[11] Samuelsson BE, Breimer ME. ABH antigens: some basic aspects. Transplant Proc 1987; 19: 4401-4404.

[12] Bariety J, Oriol R, Hinglais N, *et al.* Distribution of blood group antigen A in normal and pathologic human kidneys. Kidney Int 1980; 17: 820-826.

[13] Oriol R, Cartron JP, Cartron J, *et al.* Biosynthesis of ABH and Lewis antigens in normal and transplanted kidneys. Transplantation 1980; 29: 184-188.

[14] Economidou J, Hugh-Jones N, Gardner B. Quantitative measurements concerning A and B antigen sites. Vox Sang 1967; 12: 321-328.

[15] Ceppellini R, Bigliani S, Curtoni ES, Leigheb G. Experimental allotransplantation in man: The role A1, A2 and B antigens. Enhancement by circulating antibody. Transplant Proc 1969; 1: 390-384.

[16] Alkhunaizi AM, de Mattos AM, Barry JM, *et al.* Renal transplantation across the ABO barrier using A2 kidneys. Transplantation 1999; 67: 1319-1324.

[17] Bryan CF, Shield CF, Nelson PW, *et al.* Transplantation rate of the blood group B waiting list is increased by using A2 and A2B kidneys. Transplantation 1998; 66: 1714-1717.

[18] Schnuelle P, van der Woude FJ. Should A2 kidneys be transplanted into B or O recipients? Lancet 1998; 351: 1675-1676.

[19] Nelson PW, Shield CF, Muruve NA, *et al.* Increased access to transplantation for blood group B cadaveric waiting list candidates by using A2 kidneys: time for a new nation system. Am J Transplant 2002; 2: 94-99.

[20] Slapak M, Naik RM, Lee HA. Renal transplant in a patient with major donor-recipient blod group incompatibility. Transplantation 1981; 31: 4-7.

[21] Slapak M, Evans P, Trickett L, *et al.* Can ABO-incompatible donors be used in renal transplantation? Transplant Proc 1984; 16:75-79.

[22] Slapak M, Digard N, Ahmed M, *et al.* Renal transplantation across the ABO-barrier. A 9-year experience. Transplant Proc 1990; 22: 1425-1428.

[23] Alexandre GPJ, Squifflet JP, De Bruyere M, *et al.* Present experiences in a series of 26 ABO-incompatible living donor renal allografts. Transplant Proc 1987; 19: 4538-4542.

[24] Takahashi K, Yagisawa T, Sonda K, *et al.* ABO-incompatible kidney transplantation in a single-center trial. Transplant Proc 1993; 25: 271-273.

[25] Tanabe K, Takahashi K, Sonda K, *et al.* ABO-incompatible living kidney donor transplantation: results and immunological aspects. Transplant Proc 1995; 27: 1020-1023.

[26] Tanabe K, Takahashi K, Sonda K, *et al.* Long-term results of ABO-incompatible living kidney transplantation: a single-center experience. Transplantation 1998; 65: 224-228.

[27] Toma H, Tanabe K, Tokumoto T. Long-term outcome of ABO-incompatible renal transplantation. Urol Clin North Am 2001; 28: 769-780.

[28] Toma H, Tanabe K, Tokumoto T, *et al.* Excellent long-term outcome of ABO-incompatible renal transplantation. A single center experience[abstract]. Am J Trasnplant 2004; 4: 402.

[29] Tanabe K, Tokumoto T, Ishida H, *et al.* Excellent outcome of ABO-incompatible living kidney transplantation under pretransplant immunosuppression with tacrolimus, mycophenolate mofetil, and steroids. Transplant Proc 2004; 36: 2175-2177.

[30] Gloor JM, Lager DJ, Moor SB, *et al.* ABO-incompatible kidney transplantation using both A2 and non-A2 living donors. Transplantation 2003; 7: 971-977.

[31] Ishida H, Miyamoto N, Tanabe K *et al.* Evaluation of immunosuppressive regimens in ABO-incompatible living kidney transplantation single center analysis. Am J Transplant 2007; 7: 825-831.

[32] Toki D, Ishida H, Tanabe K, *et al.* Acute antibody-mediated rejection in living ABO-incompatible kidney transplantation: long-term impact and risk factors. Am J Transplant 2009; 9: 567-577.

[33] Setoguchi K, Ishida H, Tanabe K, *et al.* Analysis of renal transplant protocol biopsies in ABO-incompatible kidney transplantation. Am J Transplant 2008; 8: 86-94.

[34] Tanabe K, Ishida H, Shimizu T, *et al.* Evaluation of two different preconditioning regimens for ABO-incompatible living kidney donor transplantation. Humoral Immunity in Kidney Transplantation 2009; 162: 61-74.

[35] Genberg H, Kumlien G, Wennberg L, *et al.* ABO-incompatible kidney transplantation using antigen-specific immunoadsorption and rituximab: A 3-year follow-up. Transplantation 2008; 85(12): 1745-1754.

[36] Montgomery RA, Locke JS. ABO-incompatible transplantation: less may be more. Transplantation 2007; 84(12S): S8-S9.

[37] Tobian AAR, Shirey RS, Montgomery RA, Ness PM, King KE. The critical role of plasmapheresis in ABO-incompatible renal transplantation. Transfusion 2008; 48: 2453-2460.

[38] Segev DL, Simpkins CE, Warren DS, *et al.* ABO incompatible high-titer renal transplantation without splenectomy or anti-CD20 treatment. Am J Transplant 2005; 5: 2570.

[39] Montgomery RA, Locke JE, King KE, *et al.* ABO incompatible renal transplantation: A paradigm ready for broad implementation. Transplantation 2009; 87: 1246-1255.

[40] Onitsuka S, Yamaguchi Y, Tanabe K, *et al.* Peritubular capillary deposition of C4d complement fragment in ABO-incompatible renal transplantation with humoral rejection. Clin Transplant 1999; 3(suppl1): 33-37.

[41] Kato M, Morozumi K, Takeuchi O, *et al.* Complement fragment C4d deposition in peritubular capillaries in acute humoral rejection after A BO blood group-incompatible human kidney transplantation. Transplantation 2003; 75: 663-665.

[42] Fidler ME, Gloor JM, Lager DJ, *et al.* Histologic findings of antibody-mediated rejection in ABO blood-group-incompatible living-donor kidney transplantation. Am J Transplant 2004; 4: 101-107.

[43] Kanetsuna Y, Yamaguchi Y, Toma H, Tanabe K. Histological evalution of renal allograft protocol biopsies in the early period and 1 year after transplantation. Clin Transplant 2003; 17(suppl10): 25-29.

[44] Haas M, Rahman MH, Racusen LC, *et al.* C4d and c3d stainig in biopsies of ABO- and HLA-incompatible renal allografts: Correlation with histologic findings. Am J Transplant 2006; 6: 1829-1840.

[45] Oettl T, Halter J, Bachmann A, *et al.* ABO blood group-incompatible living donor kidney transplantation: a prospective, single-centre analysis including serial protocol biopsies. Nephrol Dial Transplant 2009; 24: 298-303.

[46] Hass M, Segev DL, Racusen LC, *et al.* C4d deposition without rejection correlates with reduced early scarring in ABO-incompatible renal allografts. J Am Soc Nephrol 2009; 20: 197-204.

CHAPTER 5

Pre-Transplant Histological Evaluation in Kidney Transplantation

Lidia Puzzo* **and Enrico Vasquez**

Histopathology Unit, Department G. F. Ingrassia, University Hospital of Catania, Italy

Abstract: The increased discrepancy between the number of patients on the waiting list and the kidney graft availability has prompted most of the transplant centers to expand their suitability criteria for deceased donor kidneys. However, these grafts have a potential lower graft functionality and must be properly allocated to ensure the best outcome. Histopathological pre-transplant evaluation has progressively assumed as the best prognostic factor for graft function in kidney transplantation from older donors. However, there is not consensus about the best strategy of scoring the bioptic samples and there are no clinical trials comparing the best allocation strategy of these kidneys. In this chapter will be reviewed the recent acquisition on pre-transplant histopathologic examination with a brief overview on the role of kidney biopsy in living kidney donors.

Keywords: Expanded Criteria Donor, Dual Kidney Transplantation, Biopsy, Histological Evaluation, Glomerulosclerosis, Tubular Necrosis, Interstitial Fibrosis, Vascular, Marginal Donor, Dual Kidney Transplantation.

INTRODUCTION

Kidney transplantation is the preferred treatment for all end-stage renal diseases (ESRD). Although younger deceased donors renal function is assessed only by terminal serum creatinine, older donors must be better evaluated, including the clinical characteristics, such as the presence of long-standing diabetes, hypertension, atherosclerotic vascular disease together with an analysis of the pathological features [1-3].

In the last few years, the popularity of living donor renal transplantation has risen dramatically, for the increasing disparity between organ availability and patients on the transplant waiting list. Organ availability, preservation quality, lack of reperfusion injury and favourable outcomes are the most obvious advantages of living donation [4, 5].

Kidney transplant from living donor has been often linked with a better outcome for the recipients and a low risk of adverse outcome for the donors. In a small number of donors, increased risk of chronic kidney disease, end stage kidney disease or other complications have been shown; in any case, acute rejection must be considered the most important risk factor of graft and patient failure both in living and deceased donors [4-6].

A kidney biopsy could be performed either before the transplantation, as pretransplant biopsy or before graft implantation [7-9], or after the transplantation; in all cases, the grade of inflammatory activity and the stage of interstitial and vascular fibrosis must be evaluated. Therefore, the aims of renal biopsy in kidney transplant are:

- The functional pretransplant assessment of suitability in kidneys from deceased or living donors.
- The evaluation of post transplant outcomes.
- The evaluation of recurrent glomerulonephritis.

***Address correspondence to Lidia Puzzo:** Histopathology Unit, Department G. F. Ingrassia, University Hospital of Catania, Italy; Phone: + 39 095 378 2026; E-mail lipuzzo@unict.it

Massimiliano Veroux and Pierfrancesco Veroux (Eds)

PRETRANSPLANT ASSESSMENT OF SUITABILITY

The kidney suitability represents a checkpoint of clinical outcome for the recipient: clinical criteria (donor age, estimated glomerular filtration rate (eGFR) and mainly pre existing chronic kidney disease) and histopathological assessment of the kidneys provide the most useful information about organ quality and short and long term graft survival.

In a recent review, Mueller *et al.* [10] showed more favourable outcomes in transplant from living donors than from deceased donors and donor's age has been evaluated as the most useful clinical parameter for a long term outcome.

Nowadays, in the evaluation of kidney suitability we should consider:

1. Intrinsic donor factors: age, gender, hypertensive disease, but also stress factors related with transplantation, as brain death, anaesthesia, ischemia-reperfusion injury;

2. Recipient factors: age, hypotension and poor cardiac output.

There is an increased need for kidney transplant among older adults: while the number of younger patients in the waiting list is constant, due to its increasing success, kidney transplantation has been now offered to an increasing number of older recipients: moreover, the median age of deceased donors has progressively increased, so that more than 50% of deceased kidney donors are 50 years or older [11-13].

Recently, the Scientific Registry of Transplant Recipients expanded the criteria of kidney suitability, reassessing mainly the clinical criteria: age, gender, related or unrelated donor, blood pressure, hypertension or family history of hypertension in unrelated donor, body mass index (BMI) >30, other comorbidities, as diabetes, last serum creatinine, 24-hour creatinine clearance [14].

Despite these clinical data, both the donor and recipient age is still considered the most important risk factor for chronic kidney allograft failure; the kidneys from elderly donors are more susceptible to the ischemia-reperfusion injury and to a higher incidence of delayed graft function (DGF), and their preferred allocation is into an older recipient [15].

The Expanded Criteria Donor (ECD) concerns both donors older than 60 years without co-morbidities and donors older than 50 years with at least two co-morbidities, among hypertension, death from cerebro-vascular accident, terminal serum creatinine levels >1.5 mg/dl; often pre-transplant assessment of renal quality and function has been related mainly to the serum creatinine measurements, despite their known limitations [16-21].

Nowadays, perhaps we can only have general criteria to assess what age is really a risk factor and what is the advantage/disadvantage ratio between expanded criteria donor (ECD) kidneys and standard criteria donor (SCD) kidneys [18, 20, 22].

Considering only the age, recipients older than 60 years have a lower rate of acute cellular rejection (ACR) but a worse overall survival than younger recipients, while there was no significant difference in the onset of DGF.

Lastly, kidneys from a young donor with a known history of cerebral malignant tumour or intravenous drug abuse can not be transplanted in a young recipient, but may be offered to an old recipient, with a lower life expectancy.

Nowadays, ECD kidney outcome is considered generally favourable, provided that kidneys from elderly donors are allocated to older recipients. In fact, the age-related changes of the immune system may have an impact both on the elderly recipient and on the aged graft.

Age related immunologic changes in elderly donors include [23]:

- increased number of T-cells subset (CD3+, CD4+, CD8+).
- chronic activation of the immune system.
- increased production of pro-inflammatory cytokines.

These immunological changes may be responsible of a higher risk of chronic rejection and chronic allograft injury.

Age related non immunologic changes in elderly include:

- atherosclerosis and hypertension with vascular smooth cell proliferation.
- impaired anti-oxidative and repair/remodeling capacity.
- associated co-morbidity (dislipidemic diseases, diabetes, cardiovascular disease, chronic infections).

These changes may also contribute to chronic allograft dysfunction.

Lastly, all the aging processes may produce structural and functional changes in the graft, as reduction of renal function for atrophy and fibrosis.

Since 1999, to provide an adequate nephron mass, the transplant of two marginal kidneys from an ECD in a single recipient may be performed [14]; dual kidney transplant from an elderly donor shows a significantly lower incidence of DGF and an excellent short-term outcome, when compared to a single kidney transplant from the same age group [24, 25].

The kidney availability from donors older than 60 years could be improved by the histological evaluation of pre-transplant biopsy; therefore, the clinical data of graft dysfunction (serum creatinine and creatinine clearance) should be related to the donor factors (age and cause of death in case of deceased donors) and mainly to the morphology of zero-time biopsy.

In fact, ESRD of the graft could develop in a very small fraction of living donors with hypertensive nephrosclerosis, mainly in case of unknown baseline clinical and histopathological renal findings; the unknown baseline graft morphology could lead to a misdiagnosis of chronic rejection or drug toxicity instead of native chronic disease, as arteriosclerosis or arteriolar hyalinisation. The age-linked arteriolar hyalinisation may predispose to acute kidney disease and also donor related vasculopathy could have a significant impact on the subsequent graft function [26].

There is universal consensus about the role of zero-time biopsy in the evaluation of kidney suitability and many scores have been proposed: in his report, Anglicheau *et al.* [27] performed pre-transplant biopsies from donors older than 50 years and concluded that a simple clinical/pathological composite score, including donor serum creatinine, hypertension and global glomerulosclerosis, was able to predict graft survival at 1 year; while Munivenkatappa *et al.* [28] proposed a histopathological composite score, the Maryland aggregate pathology index (MAPI), including arteriolar hyalinosis, periglomerular fibrosis, global interstitial sclerosis, glomerulosclerosis and wall-to-lumen ratio of interlobular arteries.

Histological Evaluation of Kidney Biopsy

There are two bioptic techniques to perform a renal sample: wedge biopsy and core needle biopsy [29, 30]; both are still used and evaluated and a full agreement has not yet been reached to choose the wedge or the needle biopsy and the histopathological criteria to discharge the donor kidneys.

Open wedge biopsy is more frequently performed from a deceased donor to assess pretransplant suitability at time of transplant (zero-time biopsy); the criteria of suitability have been assessed by frozen surgical sections, using the score system of Remuzzi [31] (Table **1**).

Table 1: Pre-transplant histological assessment of kidney from a deceased donor [31]

Glomerular Global Sclerosis	0: absent	1+: <20%	2+: 20-50%	3+: >50%
Tubular Atrophy	0: absent	1+: <20%	2+: 20-50%	3+: >50%
Interstitial Fibrosis	0: absent	1+: <20%	2+: 20-50%	3+: >50%
Arterial/Arteriolar Narrowing	0: absent	1+: <20%	2+: 20-50%	3+: >50%

The total score specifies the suitability for single transplant (score 0-3), double transplant (score 4-6) or the unsuitability for the transplant (score 7-12).

Since 1998, Sund *et al.* [29], showed poor correlation between Banff '97 criteria and graft function at 1 and 3 years after transplantation: thus, a needle core biopsy has been performed from living donors and showed at least mild arteriosclerosis also in normotensive and young donors . It is certain that both techniques have their advantages and limitations.

The standard wedge biopsy is the preferred technique in cases of deceased donor, providing more tissue and greater glomerular area; the examination of histological frozen sections at multiple levels allows, in few minutes, to assess the suitability for transplantation. However, the sample size of wedge biopsy is operator dependent [32] and therefore highly variable; moreover, a too superficial sample includes mainly the subcapsular cortical area and shows an higher percentage of globally sclerosed glomeruli and, often, only the distal portions of interlobular arteries. Considering the frozen sections and the same sections routinely processed, the final score of frozen sections is usually at least one grade higher than in routinely sections, due to the freezing artefacts (Fig. **1**).

The needle biopsy sizes are operator independent [32], depending on the technique, and include always cortico-medullary area with the proximal portions of interlobular arteries or arciform arteries; however, needle biopsy could show only few glomeruli and be considered inadequate to evaluate global glomerulosclerosis.

Moreover, needle biopsy may be routinely processed and stained with ematoxilin-eosin (EE), periodic acid's Schiff (PAS), silver methenamine, Masson trichrome stains; multiple sections may be used for eventual immunofluorescence and immunohistochemical stains. On the other hand, the needle biopsy could lead to a higher risk of complications, as arteriovenous fistulas, perirenal and intraparenchymal hematomas and bleeding in the urinary tract.

Regardless to the wedge or the needle biopsy, perhaps the issue is the agreement among the histopathological criteria and the interobserver variability: nowadays, an almost universal consensus has been reached about the criteria, considering globally sclerosed glomeruli, vascular narrowing, tubular atrophy and interstitial fibrosis, while the interobserver disagreement still remains [33-35].

About glomerular scores, concerning both the number of glomeruli and the number of globally sclerosed glomeruli, only a moderate agreement has been reached; a wedge biopsy could overestimate the percentage of globally sclerosed glomeruli, more frequently found in the subcortical area, while a needle biopsy could underestimate this parameter; considering that in needle biopsy the number of glomeruli increases with the sample size, the ratio between global sclerotic glomeruli and the sample size could provide an accurate evaluation. In summary, both the wedge and the core specimens with at least seven glomeruli could be considered adequate samples, but glomerular score should be considered with more caution [35].

There is statistically significant disagreement in the evaluation of interstitial scarring and tubular atrophy, but a higher agreement between pathologists could improve combining interstitial fibrosis and tubular atrophy into a single parameter [35].

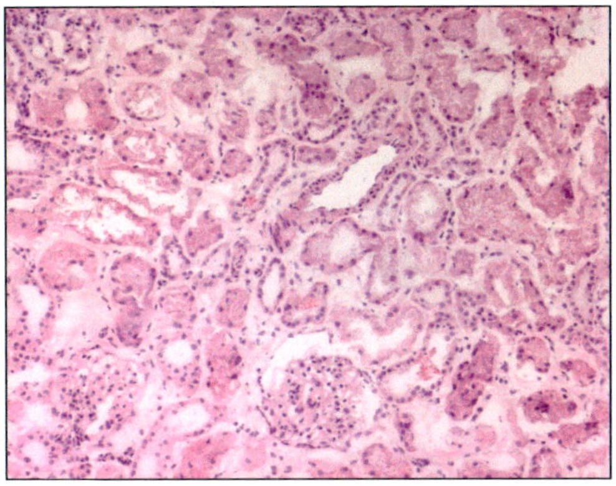

A. Frozen section (score 2)

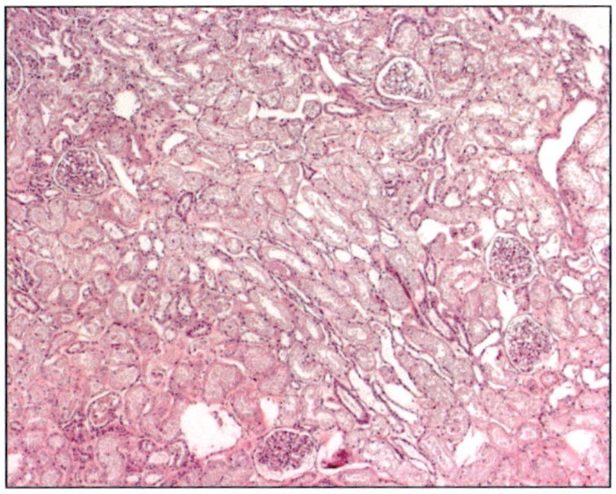

a. Frozen section control (score 1)

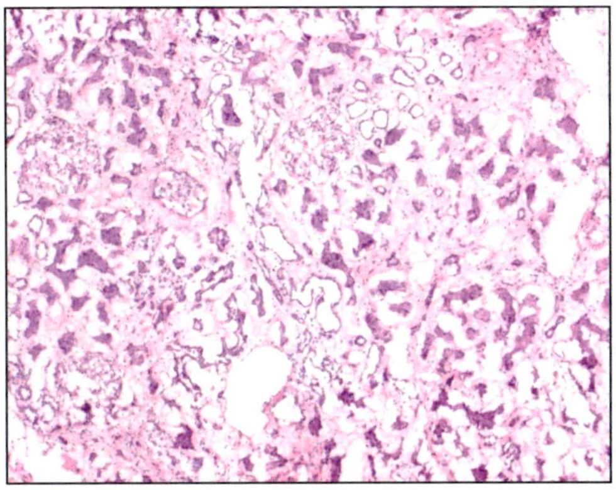

B. Frozen section (score 4)

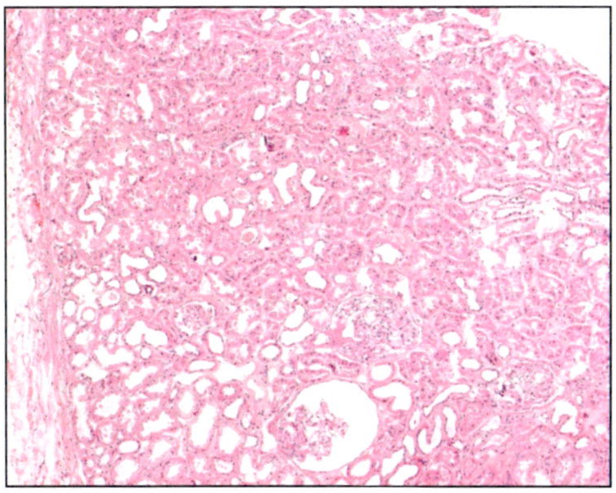

b. Frozen section control (score 3)

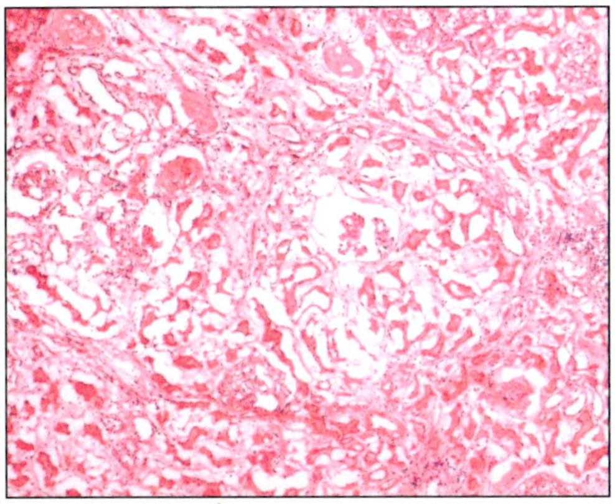

C. Frozen section (score 6)

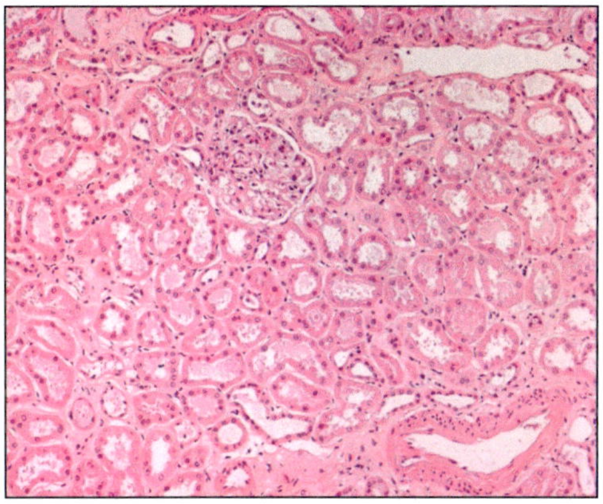

c. Frozen section control (score 5)

Figure 1: Frozen sections show more severe arteriolar, tubular, glomerular and interstitial score, E.E. 10X; A, a: mild tubular atrophy and arteriolar narrowing in frozen section (score 2), only mild arteriolar narrowing in frozen section control (score 1); B, b: moderate interstitial scarring and arteriolar narrowing in frozen section (score 4), moderate arteriolar narrowing and mild interstitial scarring (score 3); C, c: global glomerular sclerosis, moderate tubular atrophy, interstitial scarring and arteriolar narrowing in frozen section (score 6), moderate interstitial scarring, arteriolar narrowing and mild tubular atrophy in frozen section control (score 5).

Regarding the vascular changes, considered the most predictive factor for short and long term outcome, the disagreement is mainly related to the method of sampling; in fact, the earliest arteriosclerotic changes, like sub intimal fibroplasia, have been seen mainly in the proximal portions of interlobular and arciform arteries, also in individuals of an age between 25 and 45 years, without overt systemic hypertension, while fibrointimal thickening in more periferical portions of interlobular arteries has been found only in hypertensive or individuals more than 55 years old [30, 32-35].

For all these reasons the needle biopsy could be preferred to wedge biopsy.

Molecular Profile

To evaluate the donor renal quality at time zero, molecular profile seems to go beyond histopathological and clinical scores [36, 37]. Molecular profile correlates with acute tissue injury, not necessarily seen by pathological examination and clinical markers. Thus a histological normal biopsy could also show an abnormal molecular profile. Naesens *et al.* [37] showed that complement activation and related complement gene expression were associated with early and late graft function and could be more sensitive than clinical or histologic markers. However, description of molecular profile should consider that the inflammatory response reflect the tissue injury, but is also necessary for repair.

In 2009, Perco *et al.* [36] has selected 80 genes in kidneys with or without histological damage, demonstrating that only three genes were sufficient to predict medium-term graft function; also polymerase chain reaction-based study showed that a combination of few selected genes and clinical markers could be associated with kidney outcome. Ischemia-reperfusion injury has a great impact on early and medium-term graft function and perhaps a panel of markers of acute kidney failure, (as IL18, LCN2) and senescence (as p21 or p16INK4a) could identify subjects at risk for ischemia-reperfusion injury, delayed graft function and poor long term function.

In conclusion, nowadays almost all scoring systems include clinical and histological criteria, but in the future the molecular profile may provide better information about quality and long term function of the kidney transplant.

REFERENCES

[1] Saxena R, Yu X, Giraldo M, *et al.* Renal transplantation in the elderly. Int Urol Nephrol 2009; 41: 195–210.

[2] Naderi GH, Mehraban D, Kazemeyni SM, *et al.* Living or deceased donor kidney transplantation: a comparison of results and survival rates among iranian patients. Transplant Proc 2009; 41: 2772–2774.

[3] Grassi G, Abdelkawy H, Barsotti M, *et al.* Living kidney transplantation: evaluation of renal function and morphology of potential donors. Transplant Proc 2009; 41: 1121–1124.

[4] Gaston RS, Danovitch GM, Adams PL, *et al.* The report of a National Conference on the Wait List for Kidney Transplantation. Am J Transplant 2003; 3: 775-785.

[5] Neipp M, Jackobs S, Jaeger M, *et al.* Living kidney donors >60 years of age: is it acceptable for the donor and the recipient? Transplant Int 2006; 19: 213–217.

[6] Wu C, Shapiro R, Tan H, *et al.* Kidney transplantation in elderly people: the influence of recipient comorbidity and living kidney donors. J Am Geriatr Soc 2008; 56: 231–238.

[7] Mengel M, Sis B. An Appeal for Zero-Time Biopsies in Renal Transplantation. Am J Transplant 2008;8:2181-2182.

[8] Lin NC, Yang AH, King KL, *et al.* Results of kidney transplantation from high–terminal creatinine donors and the role of time-zero biopsy. Transplant Proc 2010; 42: 3382–3386.

[9] Okamoto M, Koshino K, Nobori S, *et al.* Analysis of preexisting baseline kidney lesions revealed by biopsy in living kidney donors: relationship with clinical parameters at the time of donation, Clin Transplant 2010; 24: 27–30.

[10] Mueller TF, Solez K, Mas V. Assessment of kidney organ quality and prediction of outcome at time of transplantation, Semin Immunopathol 2011;33:185-199.

[11] Lee S, Kim J, Shin M, *et al.* Comparison of outcomes of living and deceased donor kidney grafts surviving longer than 5 years in Korea. Transplant Proc 2010; 42: 775–777.

[12] Sharma AK, Tolani SL, Rathi GL, *et al.* Evaluation of factors causing delayed graft function in live related donor renal transplantation. Saudi J Kidney Dis Transpl 2010; 21: 242-245.

[13] Wolfe RA, Merion RM, Roys EC, *et al.* Trends in organ donation and transplantation in the United States. Am J Transplant 2009; 9: 869-878.

[14] Remuzzi G, Grinyò J, Ruggenenti P, *et al.* Early experience with dual kidney transplantation in adults using expanded donor criteria. J Am Soc Nephrol 1999; 10: 2591–2598.

[15] Cabello M, Cobelo C, Gonzalez-Molina M, *et al.* Renal transplantation in old recipients from expanded criteria donors selected by kidney biopsy. Transplant Proc 2010; 42: 2845– 2847.

[16] Textor S, Taler S. Expanding criteria for living kidney donors: what are the limits?, Transplant Rev 2008; 22: 187–191.

[17] Sung RS, Christensen LL, Leichtman AB, *et al.* Determinants of discard of expanded criteria donor kidneys: impact of biopsy and machine perfusion. Am J Transplant 2008; 8: 783–792.

[18] Iordanous Y, Seymour N, Young A, *et al.* Recipient outcomes for expanded criteria living kidney donors: the disconnect between current evidence and practice. Am J Transplant 2009; 9: 1558–1573.

[19] Domagala P, Kwiatkowski A, Perkowska-Ptasinska A, *et al.* Assessment of kidneys procured from expanded criteria donors before transplantation. Transplant Proc 2009;41: 2966-2969.

[20] Goplani KR, Kute VB, Vanikar AV, *et al.* Expanded criteria donor kidneys for younger recipients: acceptable outcomes. Transplant Proc 2010; 42: 3931–3934.

[21] Goplani KR, Firoz A, Ramakrishana P, *et al.* Deceased donor organ transplantation with expanded criteria donors: a single-center experience from india. Transplant Proc 2010; 42: 171-174.

[22] Lucarelli G, Bettocchi C, Battaglia M, *et al.* Extended criteria donor kidney transplantation: comparative outcome analysis between single versus double kidney transplantation at 5 years. Transplant Proc, 2010; 42: 1104-1107.

[23] Weinstein JR, Anderson S. The aging kidney: physiological changes; Adv Chronic Kidney Dis 2010; 17: 302-307.

[24] Kayler LK, Mohanka R, Basu A, *et al.* Single versus dual renal transplantation from donors with significant arteriosclerosis on pre-implant biopsy. Clin Transplant 2009; 23: 525–531.

[25] Ekser B, Furian L, Broggiato A, *et al.* Technical aspects of unilateral dual kidney transplantation from expanded criteria donors: experience of 100 patients. Am J Transplant 2010;10:2000-2007.

[26] Woestenburg AT, Verpooten GA, Ysebaert DK, *et al.* Fibrous intimal thickening at implantation adversely affects long-term kidney allograft function. Transplantation 2009; 87: 72-78.

[27] Anglicheau D, Loupy A, Lefaucheur C, *et al.* A simple clinico-histopathological composite scoring system is highly predictive of graft outcomes in marginal donors. Am J Transplant 2008; 8: 2325-2334.

[28] Munivenkatappa RB, Schweitzer EJ, Papadimitriou JC, *et al.* The Maryland Aggregate Pathology Index: a deceased donor kidney biopsy scoring system for predicting graft failure. Am J Transplant 2008; 8: 2316–2324.

[29] Sund S, Reisaeter AV, Scott H, *et al.* Morphological studies of baseline needle biopsies from living donor kidneys: light microscopic, immunohistochemical and ultrastructural findings, APMIS 1998;106: 1017-1034.

[30] Haas M, Segev DL, Racusen LC, *et al.* Arteriosclerosis in kidneys from healthy live donors comparison of wedge and needle core perioperative biopsies. Arch Pathol Lab Med 2008; 132:37–42.

[31] Remuzzi G, Cravedi P, Perna A, *et al.* Long-term outcome of renal transplantation from older donors. N Engl J Med 2006; 354: 343-352.

[32] Yushkov Y, Dikman S, Alvarez-Casas J, *et al.* Optimized technique in needle biopsy protocol shown to be of greater sensitivity and accuracy compared to wedge biopsy. Transplant Proc 2010; 42: 2493–2497.

[33] Mazzucco G, Magnani C, Fortunato M, *et al.* The reliability of pre-transplant donor renal biopsies (PTDB) in predicting the kidney state. A comparative single-centre study on 154 untransplanted kidneys. Nephrol Dial Transplant 2010; 25: 3401–3408.

[34] Sulikowski T, Tejchman K, Ziętek Z, *et al.* Histopathologic evaluation of pretransplantation biopsy as a factor influencing graft function after kidney transplantation in 3-year observation. Transplant Proc 2010; 42: 3375–3381.

[35] Snoeijs MG, Boonstra LA, Buurman WA, *et al.* Histological assessment of pre-transplant kidney biopsies reproducible and representative. Histopathology 2010; 56:198-202.

[36] Perco P, Kainz A, Wilflingseder J, *et al.* Histogenomics: association of gene expression patterns with histological parameters in kidney biopsies. Transplantation 2009; 87: 290-295.

[37] Naesens M, Sarwal MM. Molecular diagnostics in transplantation. Nat Rev Nephrol 2010; 6:614-628.

CHAPTER 6

Renal Transplantation from Expanded Criteria "Marginal" Donors

Burcin Ekser*

Kidney and Pancreas Transplantation Unit, Department of Surgery and Organ Transplantation, University of Padua, Padua, Italy

Abstract: Due to the increased demand in transplantable organs, the gap between kidney graft and supply grows. The organ shortage continues despite the fact that surgeons have liberalized their acceptance criteria for suitable deceased donor organs, have exploited the use of ABO-incompatible and marginal 'expanded criteria donors (ECD)'. However, kidneys from ECD donors come with their relative risk of graft failure of 1.7 compared with a reference group. Therefore, selection of kidneys from ECD donors remains extremely important to guarantee an adequate kidney function and graft survival for long-term. Some ECD donor kidneys are not accepted by many centers due to their extreme age and additional risk factors such as hypertension, diabetes mellitus of the donor. A comprehensive assessment of the ECD kidney is mandatory and long-term graft survival and kidney function need to be assured.

Keywords: Donor Selection, Expanded Criteria Donors, Marginal, Old, Old-to-old, Renal transplantation, Single Transplant, Dual Transplant, Organ shortage, Kidney Biopsy, Renal Function.

INTRODUCTION

Kidney transplantation has been accepted to be the best choice of treatment for end-stage renal disease more than 50 years ago [1]. Because of its benefits such as free of dialysis, longer patient survival, and increased quality of life, many patients with end-stage renal disease become candidates for a renal transplant being a member of the waiting list. However, demand for a renal transplant and supply for all patients remain to be a big problem. By October 2009, in the United Network for Organ Sharing of the United States there are more than 82, 000 patients waiting to be transplanted by a kidney graft [2]. Despite increased transplants numbers - in the United States, the number of kidneys transplanted increased from 16, 076 in 2005 to 16, 646 in 2006 (a 3.5% increase) [3], the gap between demand and supply grows. The shortage continues despite the fact that surgeons have liberalized their acceptance criteria for suitable deceased donor organs, have exploited the use of ABO-incompatible and marginal 'expanded criteria donors (ECD)', and have also used living related kidney grafts.

Expanded criteria donor (ECD) kidneys (marginal, old) became a reality more than a decade ago with the term of 'kidneys nobody wanted' [4] to expand the donor pool. Despite controversies on shorter graft survival, ECD kidneys are utilized in the USA and more commonly in Europe especially in old-for-old allocation [5].

DEFINITION OF ECD KIDNEYS

On October 31, 2002, the Organ Procurement and Transplantation Network/United Network for Organ Sharing (OPTN/UNOS) Board of Directors adopted a new ECD allocation policy, establishing an ECD definition based on age and 3 statistically significant risk factors determined by a previous SRTR (The Scientific Registry of Transplant Recipients) analysis: arterial hypertension history, terminal serum creatinine level greater than 1.5 mg/dL (serum creatinine in mg/dL may be converted to μmol/L by multiplying by 88.4), or cause of death from cerebrovascular accident [2, 3]. Consequently, ECDs were defined as any deceased donor 60 years or older or older than 50 years with at least 2 of the cited risk factors. Each of these criteria was defined by a relative risk of graft failure that exceeded a relative risk of

***Address correspondence to Burcin Ekser:** Kidney and Pancreas Transplantation Unit, Department of Surgery and Organ Transplantation, University of Padua, *Via* Giustiniani, 2 35128 Padua, Italy; Tel: +1-412-624-1402; Fax: +1-412-624-1172; E-mail: burcinexer@yahoo.com

Massimiliano Veroux and Pierfrancesco Veroux (Eds)

graft loss of 1.7 compared with a reference group of “ideal donors”: those aged 10 to 39 years, without hyper-tension, who did not die of cerebrovascular accident, and with a pre-donation serum creatinine level less than 1.5 mg/dL [3] (Table **1**).

Table 1: Definition of expanded criteria donors by UNOS

a) Brain-dead donor ≥ 60 years
b) Brain-dead donor < 60 years with 2 of the following:
- history of hypertension
- terminal serum creatinine level > 1.5 mg/dL
- death resulting from a cerebvascular accident

The number of donated kidneys that met the definition of ECD (including the small numbers of ECD-DCD [donation after cardiac death]) has increased by 36.3% from 1, 235 in 1999 to 1, 683 in 2005. Despite these differences, ECDs still represent only about 17% of all deceased donors in the United States, a small increase from 15% in 1999. These kidneys are allocated to those listed as ECD candidates by using an algorithm based on wait time rather than HLA matching. Donation service areas have their own ECD list, and there is marked variation among the 58 areas in the United States regarding the proportion of candidates listed for an ECD kidney (range, 1.9% to 94.9%) [6]. More than 50% of candidates are listed for an ECD kidney in 23 of 58 areas [7] (Table **2**).

Table 2: Kidney transplants by donor type in the United States

Donor Type	**1996**	**1999**	**2002**	**2005**
All deceased donors	7, 729 (100%)	8, 042 (100%)	8, 538 (100%)	9, 914 (100%)
SCD	6, 558 (84.8)	6, 680 (83.1)	7, 018 (88.2)	7, 554 (76.2)
ECD	1, 076 (13.9)	1, 218 (15.1)	1, 230 (14.4)	1, 609 (16.2)
DCD non-ECD	82 (1.1)	127 (1.6)	264 (3.1)	677 (6.8)
DCD, ECD	13 (0.2)	17 (0.2)	26 (0.3)	74 (0.7)

SCD: standard criteria donors.

It was hoped that ECD policy would reduce waiting times for older patients, diabetics and those with limited vascular access in exchange for their willingness to accept a kidney with an increased risk of failure [9] and would encourage recovery and transplantation of these kidneys. Although the number of ECD kidneys procured and transplanted increased following the implementation of this policy, the proportion of discarded kidneys did not change [10]. Similarly, the goals of reduced waiting times and more rapid placement appear only to have been achieved at centers with fewer than 20% of their renal candidates listed for an ECD kidney [11].

Cecka *et al.* have shown that, in the United States, 54% of kidneys procured from donors >65 years and 12% of those in the Eurotransplant region are discarded [12].

In Europe, ECD donors are often called marginal donors and different countries apply different selection criteria which are mainly based on age limit. Some countries accept older donors more than 60 years others define marginal more than 65 years.

CONTROVERSIES ON ECD ‘ MARGINAL’ KIDNEYS

Deterioration of kidney function with age is well-known. Nephron mass decreases with age in a normal population and so does glomerular filtration rate [13]. Therefore, controversies on accepting an aged kidney to guarantee an adequate renal function after kidney transplant continue. In most cases, cold ischemia time, one or more acute rejections, and toxicity of medications—particularly cyclosporin A and tacrolimus—

further reduce the already limited number of nephrons that a single suboptimal kidney provides [14]. This remnant kidney—now containing 20 to 30% of viable parenchyma or less compared to that in two optimal kidneys—initiates a self-perpetuating program of progressive deterioration, as commonly seen in animals undergoing renal mass ablation [15]. That nephron mass is a determinant of chronic allograft failure has been formally tested in animal experiments showing that increasing the number of viable nephron mass by simultaneous transplantation of two kidneys into the same recipient effectively prevented the progressive deterioration in renal function that occurs in control subjects given a single kidney [16]. Shorter graft survival has been shown using ECD kidneys [8] and also lower glomerular filtration rate (GFR) is now added to the discussion of worse outcome from ECD donors. An adequate GFR is even more important to the recipient of ECD kidneys since these kidneys are usually transplanted to older recipients in the United States and also in Europe with old-for-old allocation. GFR 50 to 60 mL/min should be offered to the older recipient after transplantation, especially in the first year post-transplant, to assure a non-increased cardiac risk for increased stage of a chronic kidney disease (Table **3**).

Table 3: Stages of chronic kidney disease

Stage	**Description**	**GFR, ml/min per 1.73m^2**
1	Kidney damage with normal or increased GFR	>90
2	Kidney damage with mildly decreased GFR	60 to 89
3	Moderately decreased GFR	30 to 59
4	Severely decreased GFR	15 to 29
5	Kidney failure	<15or dialysis

Upper stages of chronic kidney disease will reflect on increased cardiovascular disease risk on recipients who are already in a high risk due to their age. Cardiovascular disease risk status according to chronic kidney disease is shown in Table **4**.

Table 4: Cardiovascular risk according to stages of chronic kidney disease

Stage	**Cardiovascular Risk (Odds Ratio)**
1	Depending on degree of proteinuria
2	1.5
3	2 to 4
4	4 to 10
5	10 to 50
ESRD	20 to 1000

ESRD: end-stage renal disease.

ALLOCATION OF ECD KIDNEYS

The 'transplantability' of ECD kidneys is an important issue of debate since the use of ECD kidneys is associated with shorter graft survival. However, not all ECD kidneys are the same and can be transplanted. Therefore, they require an accurate assessment to evaluate their '*transplantability*'. It has been proposed to transplant 2 ECD kidneys into a single recipient (dual kidney transplantation, DKT) with the aim of increased number of viable nephrons which is essential for better GFR and subsequently longer graft survival.

Until today, there is no established criteria to allocate older kidneys. Some centers decide ECD kidneys' destiny with pre-transplant biopsy after a generalized macroscopic evaluation [17] some centers apply donor scoring using donor age, donor race, donor history of hypertension, donor history of diabetes, donor death due to cerebrovascular accident, cold ischemic time, HLA mismatch, donor/recipient cytomegalovirus match [18].

In the literature, there are several donor scoring system to study deceased donors, especially ECD donors. These criteria recently reviewed by Moore *et al.* [19]. Of donor scoring systems, Donor Risk Score studied by Schold *et al.* [18] was best associated with subsequent allograft function.

In Europe many centers are based on biopsy assessment of marginal kidneys. Of several biopsy scoring, Remuzzi histology score is commonly used [17]. However, the decision of which kidneys are undergone a pre-transplant biopsy is crucial to not increase the cold ischemia time.

In Italy, the assessment and allocation of old kidneys are commonly used as showed in Fig. **1**. Low risk and high risk marginal donors are defined. In the basis of risk stratification, grafts are undergone a pre-transplant biopsy and according to biopsy score kidneys are allocated as single kidney transplant (SKT), or DKT, or discarded.

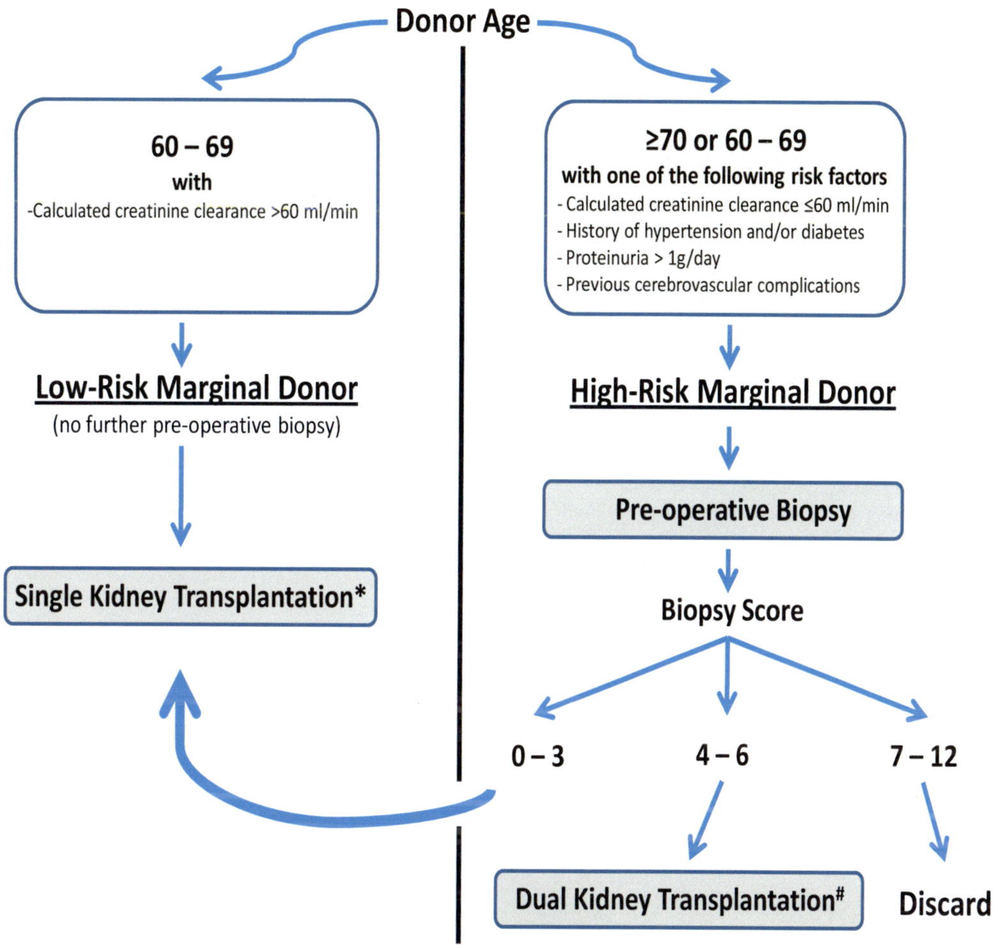

Figure 1: Assessment and allocation algorithm of aged kidneys in Italy.

Table 5: Hurdles in dual kidney transplantation

Donor selection
Recipient selection (often old recipients with pre-existing cardio-vascular disease)
Increased surgical trauma due to bilateral access
Increased risk of surgical complications due to 2 Gibson incisions, including urological complications
Monolateral technique could be offered but the technique comes with its own surgical risks
Choice of immunosuppression (ECD kidneys are more susceptible to CNI nephrotoxicity)
Long-term results (>5 years) ?

DUAL KIDNEY TRANSPLANTATION

The introduction of DKT approach has rendered the selection of ECD kidneys more difficult than before because the decision, now, should include not only the '*transplantability*' of these kidneys but how to transplant them, *i.e.* SKT or DKT.

Remuzzi *et al.* reported early results of DKT using ECD kidneys in 1999 [17]. In a prospective, case-control study they compared adverse events and graft outcome in 24 recipients of two marginal kidneys from donors who were >60 year old or who had diabetes, hypertension, or non-nephrotic proteinuria (cases), with that of 48 age- and gender-matched control subjects who received single ideal grafts at the same center and were given the same immunosuppressive therapy. Marginal kidneys with no macroscopic abnormalities were selected for the double transplant on the basis of a predefined score of histologic damage. Six-month patient and kidney survival was 100% with both of the procedures. They concluded that dual transplants of marginal kidneys were as safe and tolerated as single transplants, and possibly offer an improved filtration power without exposing the recipient to enhanced risk of delayed renal function recovery, acute allograft rejection, or major surgical complications [15]. However, 6-month follow-up was too short to evaluate the renal function of DKT if they would ever offer an adequate long-term outcome.

DKT has created more hurdles in transplantation field (Table **5**). A comprehensive evaluation of marginal donors and their recipients are required to offer a better outcome in long-term follow up.

Since the first DKT was reported in 1996 [20], many centers now perform DKT using different organ selection criteria and surgical techniques [21-25], including the bilateral placement of both kidneys, intra- or extra-peritoneally [20], through two separate Gibson incisions or one midline incision [20], and the monolateral placement of both kidneys extraperitoneally through a single Gibson incision [26].

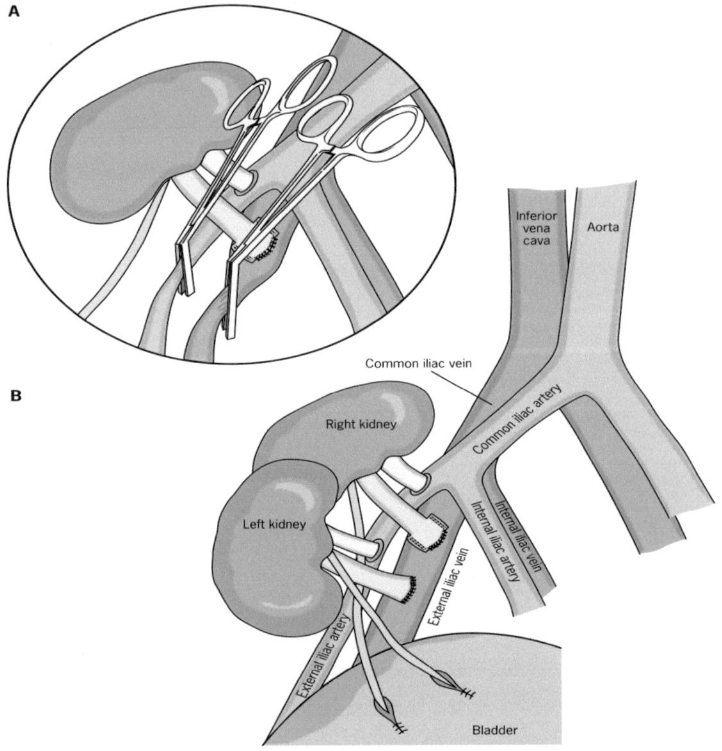

Figure 2: Monolateral placement of both kidneys using 2 ECD grafts.

The issue of which surgical technique to use for this procedure is very relevant because the potential disadvantages of DKT include a longer operating time and greater surgical risk.

Monolateral placement of both kidneys in DKT (Figs. **2** and **3**) offers the advantage of a single incision with less surgical trauma and a shorter operating time, keeping the contralateral iliac fossa available for further transplantation procedures, with no increase in the surgical complication rate [27-29].

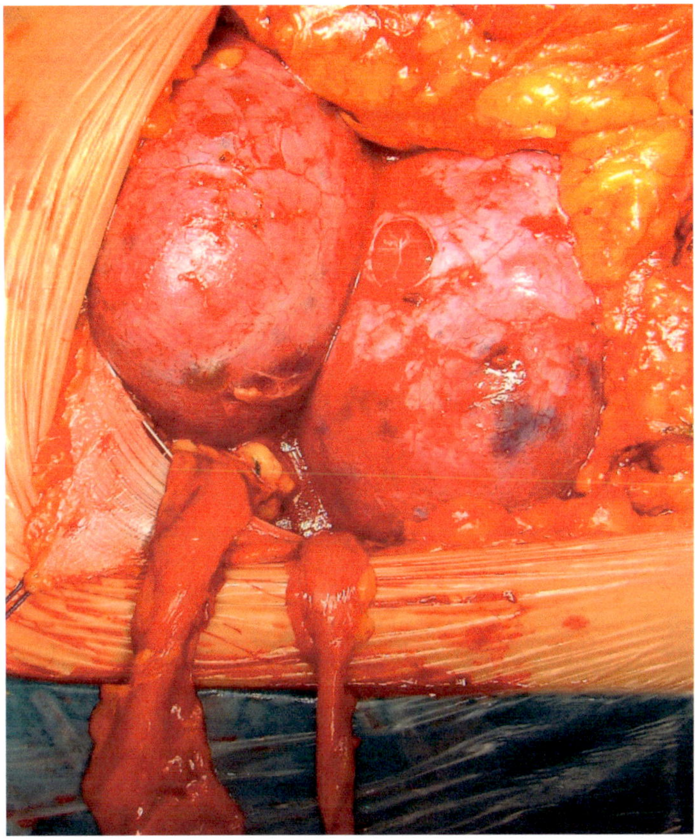

Figure 3: Operating picture of monolateral positioning of 2 ECD kidneys.

SELECTED RECENT STUDIES USING ECD KIDNEYS

Snanoudj R *et al.* have recently proposed donor-estimated GFR to allocate ECD kidneys in a prospective study comparing SKT or DKT allocation [30]. They suggest a simple criterion – donor estimated GFR (eGFR) – to decide ECD kidneys' destiny, studying deceased donors over 65 years with one of the following risk factors: history of hypertension, diabetes mellitus, atherosclerotic disease or death from a cardiovascular cause. According to their study, grafts from donors with eGFR >60 mL/min were allocated to SKT, those with eGFR of 30-60 mL/min were allocated to DKT, and those with eGFR<30 mL/min were discarded.

Snanoudj *et al.* have simulated three different selection criteria to their ECD donors and they did not see any difference in one year eGFR. A unique clinical parameter to evaluate ECD kidneys would be an optimal and desirable assessment tool if it could give an optimistic outcome for long-term follow up. There would be enough space to increase DKT activity using older ECD kidneys, however several hurdles as shown in Table **5**, and the transplantation team policy make DKT non-preferable choice in front of SKT. An advance in surgical technique such as monolateral placement [27, 28] and expertise in DKT would reduce surgical complication rate which was extraordinarily high in Snanoudj and colleagues' study [30] (13 of 81 DKT recipients, 16% experienced one graft loss).

With an alternative selection criteria , in 2006, Remuzzi *et al.* have reported in a prospective, multicenter, matched-cohort study, the long-term graft survival of 62 kidney recipients who received a transplant (either SKT or DKT) from a donor of >60 years of age (mean donor age, 69±8) after preimplantation histologic evaluation of the donor kidneys [31]. Histologic changes in the vessels (i), glomeruli (ii), tubules (iii), and connective tissue (iv) in biopsy specimens obtained from the donor kidneys before transplantation were scored on a scale from 0 (no changes) to 3 (severe changes) for each variable. When both donor kidneys had a total score from 0 to 3, the two kidneys were used for two SKTs, while a total score from 4 to 6, the two kidneys were transplanted as DKT. Kidneys were discarded when a total score of 7 or more was obtained (Fig. **1**). The outcome was compared with long-term graft survival in two cohorts of matched recipients of SKT from donors 60 years of age or younger or older than 60 years of age without a preimplantation biopsy. The results were unexpectingly interesting, though the allocation after a pre-transplant biopsy permitted to obtain equal graft survival of >90% at 3-year with donors >60 years and donors <60 years (mean donor age, 49±9). Moreover, a comparison of graft survival between donors >60 years allocated with or without pre-transplant biopsy showed an important difference (93% *vs.* 72%, respectively) [31].

Using the same biopsy criteria like Remuzzi *et al.* [31], in 2009, Rigotti *et al.* have shown that donors >70 years (mean donor age, 73.8±3.0) and donors between 60-69 years (mean donor age, 65.2±2.8) have same graft survival of >90% at 2-year follow up [32]. When we study these donors according to their allocation for DKT and SKT (DKT, n=74, mean age, 72.2±4.4 *vs.* SKT, n=64, mean age, 66.7±4.4), the graft survival resulted equal, however, eGFR resulted >50mL/min at 2 years in DKT group (*Ekser et al., unpublished data*).

Being aware the mean donor age for DKT and SKT was 75 .1±5.8 and 71.4±4.1 years, respectively, 1-year GFR in Snanoudj *et al*'s study was reported 44.8 and 39 mL/min, respectively. It is well known that DKT recipients, who are constantly older than single transplant recipient population, have increased risk of cardiovascular (CV) events and often die with functioning graft mainly due to a CV disorder. Bearing in mind of this knowledge, it could be dangerous to offer kidneys to senior recipients who will become a member of stage 4 (GFR= 15-29 mL/min) chronic kidney disease within 2-3 years after transplantation which has a 4 to 10-fold increased risk of CV event (Tables **3** and **4**) [34].

There are several factors needed to consider for ECD risk evaluation if we will ever offer these kidneys to a two different recipients (SKT), or to a single recipient as a DKT, or discard both of them due to expected worse short and long-term outcome. Pre-transplant evaluation should consist of clinical evaluation of donor, macroscopic assessment of ECD kidneys during harvesting (vasculopathy, anatomical variations and feasibility, important renal cysts, *etc.*) and ultimately histological evaluation to make the final arbitration before allocation. A comprehensive assessment would imply a better GFR and longer graft survival. The choice of immunosuppression in these recipients is more likely important to avoid CNI toxicity post-transplant [7, 33].

Therefore, a better selection of ECD kidneys to offer a longer survival to recipients is mandatory considering that recipient demographics in dialysis would not be ameliorated easily. It may be better to perform less transplants, but instead should be offered longer and better graft survival.

REFERENCES

[1] Morris, Peter and Knechtle Stuart J. Kidney Transplantation: principles and practice. Saunders, 6th Edition, 2008.

[2] UNOS – United Network for organ Sharing. http://www.unos.org (last accessed on October 1st, 2009).

[3] Port FK, Merion RM, Roys EC, *et al.* Trends in organ donation and transplantation in the United States., 1997-2006. Am J Transplant 2008; 8: 911-921.

[4] Lee CM, Scandling JD, Shen GK, *et al.* The kidneys that nobody wanted: support for the utilization of expanded criteria donors. Transplantation 1996; 62: 1832-1841.

[5] Moers C, Kornmann NS, Leuvenink HG, Ploeg RJ. The influence of deceased donor age and old-for-old allocation on kidney transplant outcome. Transplantation 2009; 88: 542-552.

[6] Sung RS, Guidinger MK, Leichtman AB, *et al.* Impact of the expanded criteria donor allocation system on candidates for and recipients of expanded criteria donor kidneys. Transplantation 2007; 84:1138-1144.

[7] Pascual J, Zamora J, Pirsch JD. A systematic review of kidney transplantation from expanded criteria donors. Am J Kidney Dis 2008; 52: 553-586.

[8] Port FK, Bragg-Gresham JL, Metzger RA, *et al.* Donor characteristics associated with reduced graft survival: an approach to expanding the pool of kidney donors. Transplantation 2002; 74: 1281-1286.

[9] Gaston RS, Danovitch GM, Adams PL, *et al.* The report of a national conference on the waitlist for kidney transplantation. Am J Transplant 2003; 3: 775–785.

[10] Sung RS, Guidinger MK, Lake CD, *et al.* Impact of the expanded criteria donor allocation system on the use of expanded criteria donor kidneys. Transplantation 2005; 79: 1257–1261.

[11] Schold JD, Howard RJ, Scicchitano MJ, Meier-Kriesche H-U. The expanded criteria donor policy: An evaluation of program objectives and indirect ramifications. Am J Transplant 2006; 6: 1689–1695.

[12] Cecka JM, Cohen B, Rosendale J, *et al.* Could more effective use of kidneys recovered from older deceased donors result in more kidney transplants for older patients? Transplantation 2006; 81: 966-970.

[13] Stevens LA, Coresh J, Greene T, *et al.* Assessing kidney function – measured and estimated glomerular filtration rate. N Engl J Med 2006; 354: 2476-2483.

[14] Brenner BM, Cohen RA, Milford EL. In renal transplantation, one size may not fit all. J Am Soc Nephrol 1992; 3 : 162-169.

[15] Rennke HG: Pathology of glomerular hyperfiltration. In: The Progressive Nature of Renal Disease: Contemporary Issues in Nephrology, Vol. 14, edited by Mitch WE, Brenner BM, Stein JH, New York, Churchill-Livingstone, 1986, pp111 -113.

[16] MacKenzie HS, Azuma H, Rennke HG, Tilney NL, Brenner BM: Renal mass as a determinant of late allograft outcome: Insights from experimental studies in rats. Kidney Int 1995; 52: S38 -S42.

[17] Remuzzi G, Grinyo J, Ruggenenti P, *et al.* Early xxperience with dual kidney transplantation in adults using expanded donor criteria. J Am Soc Nephrol 1999; 10: 2591-2598.

[18] Schold JD, Kaplan B, Baliga RS, Meier-Kriesche HU. The broad spectrum of quality in deceased donor kidneys. Am J Transplant 2005; 5(4 Pt 1): 757-765.

[19] Moore J, Ramakrishna S, Tan K, *et al.* Identification of the optimal donor quality scoring system and measure of early renal function in kidney transplantation. Transplantation 2009; 87: 578-586.

[20] Johnson LB, Kuo PC, Dafoe DC, *et al.* Double adult renal allografts: a technique for expansion of the cadaveric kidney donor pool. Surgery 1996; 120: 580-583.

[21] Dafoe DC, Alfrey EJ. Dual renal grafts: expansion of the donor pool from an overlooked source. Transplant Int 1998; 11: 164-168.

[22] Alfrey EJ, Lee CM, Scandling JD, *et al.* When should expanded criteria donor kidneys be used for single *versus* dual kidney transplants? Transplantation 1997; 64: 1142-1146.

[23] Jerius JT, Taylor RJ, Murillo D, *et al.* Double renal transplants from marginal donors: 2-year results. J Urol 2000; 163: 423-425.

[24] Rigotti P, Baldan N, Valente ML, *et al.* Evaluation of 84 elderly donors in renal transplantation. Clin Transplant 2004; 18: 440-445.

[25] Wolters HH, Palmes D, Heidenreich S, *et al.* Long-term follow-up of double kidney transplantation using a score for evaluation of marginal donors. Transplant Int 2005; 18:453-457.

[26] Masson D, Hefty T. A technique for the transplantation of 2 adult cadaver kidney grafts into 1 recipient. J Urol 1998; 160: 1779-1780.

[27] Ekser B, Baldan N, Margani G, *et al.* Monolateral placement of both kidneys in dual kidney transplantation: low surgical complication rate and short operating time. Transplant Int 2006; 19: 485-491.

[28] Veroux M, Corona D, Gagliano M, *et al.* Monolateral dual kidney transplantation from marginal donors. Transplant Proc 2007; 39: 1800-1802.

[29] Ekser B, Furian L, Baldan N, *et al.* Dual kidney transplantation after liver transplantation: a good option to rescue a patient from dialysis. Clin Transplant 2009; 23: 124-128.

[30] Snanoudj R, Rabant M, Timsit MO, *et al.* Donor-estimated GFR as an appropriate criterion for allocation of ECD kidneys into single or dual kidney transplantation. Am J Transplant 2009; 9: 2542-2551.

[31] Remuzzi G, Cravedi P, Perna A, *et al.* Long-term outcome of renal transplantation from old donors. N Engl J Med 2006; 354: 343-352.

[32] Rigotti P, Ekser B, Furian L, *et al.* Outcome of renal transplantation from very old donors. N Engl J Med 2009; 360: 464-465.

[33] Furian L, Baldan N, Margani G, *et al.* Calcineurin inhibitor-free immunosuppression in dual kidney transplantation from elderly donors. Clin Transplant 2007; 21: 57-62.

[34] Schiffrin EL, Lipman ML, Mann JFE. Chronic kidney disease: effects on the cardiovascular system. Circulation 2007; 116: 85-97.

CHAPTER 7

Kidney Transplantation from Donors with Hepatitis

Massimiliano Veroux*, Daniela Corona and Pierfrancesco Veroux

Vascular Surgery and Organ Transplant Unit, Department of Surgery, Transplantation and Advanced Technologies, University Hospital of Catania, Catania, Italy

Abstract: The increasing demand of organ donors to supply the increasing number of patients on kidney waiting list, has led most of the transplant centers to develop protocols that allow safe utilization from donors with special clinical situation, which heretofore were regarded as contraindication. Deceased donors with previous hepatitis may represent a safe resource to expand the donor pool. When allocated to serology-matched recipients, kidney transplantation from donors with hepatitis may result in excellent short term outcome. However, many concerns may arise in the long term outcome, and studies must be addressed to the evaluation of the progression of liver disease and to the rate of reactivation of liver disease in the recipients. An accurate selection of both donor and recipient is mandatory to achieve a satisfactory long term outcome.

Keywords: Kidney Transplantation, Deceased Donor, Hepatitis C Virus, Hepatitis B Virus, Hepatitis B Surface Antigen, Hepatitis B Core Antigen, Chronic Hepatitis, Interferon, Lamividine, Entecavir, Ribavirin.

INTRODUCTION

The increasing demand for available organ donors for kidney transplantation has led many transplant centers to expand their acceptance criteria, by including deceased donors with special clinical situations, such as potentially transmittable infections.

Kidney transplantation is nowadays considered the best replacement therapy for patients with End-stage renal disease (ESRD), so that there is a clear need to expand the current donor pool. One strategy focuses on the use of donor kidneys with viral hepatitis, and several organ procurement associations have adopted the policy to accept deceased donor kidneys with viral C or B hepatitis.

The aim of this paper is to review the current status of kidney transplantation from donors with Hepatitis B and C or with a previous Hepatitis B infection (Anti-HBc positive organ donor).

HCV-POSITIVE DONORS

Defining the natural history of Hepatitis C infection (HCV) in ESRD patients remains difficult for several reasons: the disease extends for several years, and the onset of the disease is frequently unknown [1]; moreover, the infection is likely to be asymptomatic with an apparently indolent course.

HCV infection has been estimated to occur in 7.8-9.2% of the ESRD population, and fortunately its incidence is slowly declining all over the world [2-5]. ESRD patients have an increased risk of death when compared to non-HCV positive dialysed population [5-7], and a recent metanalysis quantified as 1.57 the relative risk of death in ESRD patients with HCV infection [8].

Natural history of HCV infection in renal transplant recipients is not well known [9]: most transplant centers do not perform liver biopsy before transplant and in addition, compared to those with normal renal function, ESRD patients with HCV have lower serum alanine aminotransferase (ALT), aspartate

***Address correspondence to Massimiliano Veroux:** Vascular Surgery and Organ Transplant Unit, Department of Surgery, Transplantation and advanced Technologies, University Hospital of Catania, *Via* Santa Sofia, 86, 95123 Catania, Italy; Fax: +39 095 3782358; Phone: +39 095 3782206; E-mail: veroux@unict.it

Massimiliano Veroux and Pierfrancesco Veroux (Eds)

aminotransferase (AST) and albumin levels, lower viral loads (usually <1 million copies/mL), and less hepatic steatosis [10-34]; moreover, HCV-positive renal transplant recipients may have higher morbidity and mortality, making long-term consequences difficult to assess [1].

The presence of anti-HCV antibody is an independent and significant risk factor for death and graft failure in renal transplant recipients [10], and many transplant centers have recently reported a lower graft and patient survival in HCV-positive recipients [2-5, 11-25]. Multicentre surveys [26-28] confirmed that HCV-seropositivity confers an additional risk for death in renal transplant recipients.

There are several factors that may influence the patients survival in HCV-seropositive patients: the progression of liver disease [34-36], although all studies did not incorporate liver biopsy in the pre-transplant work-up, immunosuppression, the development of new-onset diabetes mellitus after transplantation and the higher risk of cardiovascular disease [1].

However, the benefit in term of survival advantage of renal transplantation in patients with HCV infection *versus* long-term dialysis has been demonstrated in many retrospective studies [32-34], and no studies have demonstrated a diminished survival after kidney transplantation, so that kidney transplantation should be now considered the treatment of choice for ESRD patients with HCV infection.

While survival is improved in this group of patients compared to HCV infected patients with ESRD who do not undergo renal transplantation, debate in the literature continues as to the short and long-term outcome of patients with chronic HCV infection undergoing renal transplantation compared with ESRD patients without HCV infection who are transplanted. It is known that viral loads increase following renal transplantation (1.8- to 30.3-fold), the prevalence of diabetes mellitus is higher in HCV infected patients post-transplant and chronic HCV infection is associated with decreased patient and graft survival when compared with patients that are not infected with HCV [35, 36]. Additionally, liver failure has been implicated as the cause of death in 8–28% of renal transplant recipients long term [37] and death from hepatocellular carcinoma and cirrhosis was notably higher among hemodialysed patients who were HCV antibody positive [8].

While short term results are similar to those who are not infected with HCV, data about long term outcome of HCV infected kidney transplant showed a lower graft and patient survival among HCV recipients, with liver failure being the first cause of death in these patients (10-22%) [38, 39].

The widely accepted opinion that the HCV infection may be transmitted with 100% of frequency from donor with HCV-infection [40], has yielded opinion that HCV-positive kidney should not be transplanted. However, this policy could determine a discard of about 5% of organ donors, aggravating the organ shortage. A recent survey [7] demonstrated that of 93, 825 deceased donors performed in the USA between 1995 and 2009, HCV-positive kidneys were 2.60-times more likely to be discarded. Interestingly, only 29% of HCV-positive recipients received HCV-positive kidneys, and more than 50% of HCV-positive kidneys were discarded [7].

Nowadays, many transplant centers have adopted the policy of accepting kidneys from HCV-positive organ donors for HCV-positive recipients, even if the safety of the use of kidneys from HCV-infected donors is not fully elucidated [41-43]. Evidence suggests that outcomes of HCV-positive recipients who receive kidneys from HCV-positive donors are slightly worse than outcomes of HCV-positive recipients who receive kidney from similar HCV-negative donors [7]. However, HCV-positive recipients who received HCV-positive kidneys have a significant lower waiting time than their counterparts HCV-negative recipients [7], with no adverse effects on the short-term patient and graft survival [44-47]. Although some authors advocated to avoid the use of HCV-positive kidney in recipients older than 65 years, due to the higher risk of infectious complications [3], there are not clear evidences that older age may have an impact on graft survival in patients receiving kidney transplantations from HCV positive donors [47]. However, up to 20% of patients may have reactivation of the disease after transplantation [47] and the time of reactivation may be shorter in renal transplant recipients of HCV-positive kidneys. The clinical importance of HCV-reactivation following kidney transplantation from HCV-positive donors is controversial and, although some studies demonstrated a higher rate of liver disease in recipients of HCV-positive kidneys compared to recipients of HCV-negative recipients, graft survival was not different between the two groups [48, 49].

While kidney transplantation confers a significant advantage in term of patient survival in ESRD patients with HCV infection when compared to maintenance hemodialysis, donor HCV serologic status is independently associated with increased risk of mortality [50]. Abbot *et al.* [51], evaluated 38, 270 USRDS Medicare beneficiaries awaiting kidney transplantation, and demonstrated that transplantation from HCV positive donors is associated with improved survival when compared with patients on the waiting list, although this advantage was not as substantial as transplantation with all deceased donors. However, a recent survey by Kucirka *et al.* [7] showed that kidney transplantation from HCV-positive donors was associated with 1.29 times the hazard of death, this reflected only in a difference of 1% in 1-year survival and 2% of difference in 3-year survival.

A historical cohort study of 36, 956 U.S. adult deceased donors renal transplant recipients over a 5-year period from 1996 to 2001 demonstrated that HCV(+) donor kidney was independently associated with increased mortality, primarily as a result of non-HCV infection, presumably due to the theory that acute HCV infection places transplant patients at risk for over-immunosuppression as a direct inhibitory effect of HCV on T-cell function [52].

Recent evidences suggested that kidney transplantations from HCV-positive donors may have a worse graft outcome when compared with HCV-negative recipients [4, 55-57], and eradication of HCV infection before transplantation seems to reduce the risk for HCV-associated renal dysfunction after transplantation and may reduce the risk for HCV disease progression, thereby providing the rationale for treatment of HCV before transplantation.

The issue of transplanting kidneys from HCV positive organ donors into HCV positive/HCV RNA negative recipients has not been fully addressed: in a retrospective study, Morales *et al.* [53] demonstrated a higher rate of viral reactivation among anti-HCV positive/HCV RNA negative recipients who received a kidney from an anti-HCV positive donor. Basing on these findings, many transplant centers adopted the policy of transplanting kidneys from anti-HCV positive donors into HCV RNA positive recipients, restricting the use of HCV-positive donors to recipients with active viremia [1, 47]. The use of organs from viremic HCV positive donors into HCV-RNA negative recipients would have the effect of reintroducing HCV infection, whereas using HCV positive kidneys in HCV RNA positive recipients can determine a superinfection with a different genotype [1], with many important clinical consequences.

Ideally, donor and recipients should be matched for HCV genotype to minimize the risk of superinfection, even if this procedure is performed rarely during a deceased donor evaluation.

HCV-RNA positive organ donors should be offered only to viremic recipients or even discarded, due to the high rate or viral reactivation after the transplantation [47].

However, a large multicentre trial demonstrated that the type of genotype may not have a significant role on survival among patients with ESRD, since the survival in patient with mixed infection was similar to that of patients with a single HCV infection [54].

Pretransplant Evaluation and Treatment

All kidney transplant candidates undergo a fully evaluation of serologic markers, including anti-HCV serology.

In dialysis patients with chronic HCV infection, serum aminotransferase levels are not reliable in determining disease activity and fibrosis severity , and uremic patients are more likely than nonuremic patients to have persistently normal serum aminotransferase levels Therefore, the presence of persistently normal serum aminotransferase levels does not exclude the presence of significant liver disease [58], and all ESRD patients anti-HCV positive should undergo an HCV-RNA dosage, and all HCV-RNA positive patients should undergo a liver biopsy (Fig. **1**).

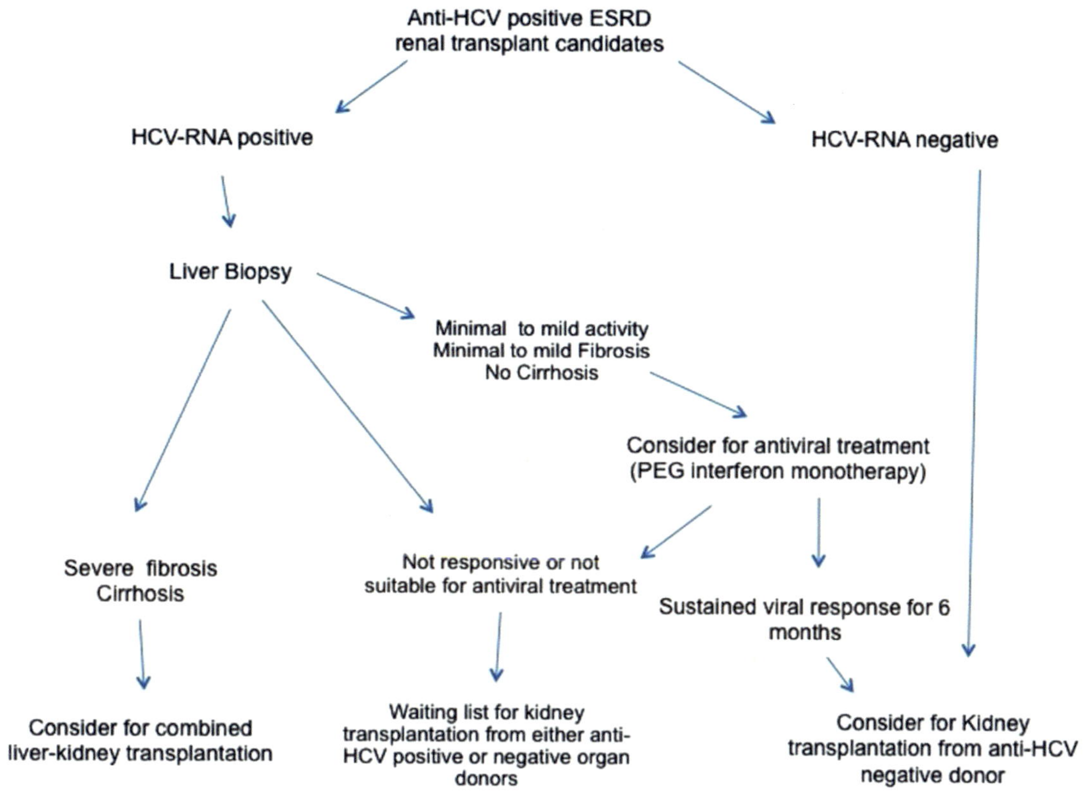

Figure 1: Proposed algorithm for the evaluation and allocation of renal transplant candidates with HCV infection; ESRD: end-stage renal disease.

The information obtained from liver biopsy are mandatory in the decision making to accept an anti-HCV positive ESRD patient for waiting list for a kidney transplantation. In fact, biochemical test are not useful to reflect the histological severity of liver damage, and liver disease may progress rapidly after transplantation.

While the finding of pretransplant cirrhosis has been clearly associated with a strong reduction of survival in renal transplant recipients [58], and now it is considered a contraindication to kidney transplantation alone, information about the progression of liver disease after transplantation are lacking. In fact, most of the studies demonstrated the progression of liver disease in kidney transplant recipients, but data on pre-transplant biopsy are not reported.

Cross-sectional studies suggest that about 25% of HCV+ patients with ESRD have significant fibrosis pretransplant [1]. Zylberberg *et al.* [59] retrospectively compared liver histopathology of 28 HCV (+) kidney recipients to 28 controls. Over a period of 7 yr, hepatic fibrosis worsened in 50% of patients, and 21% developed cirrhosis. In a prospective cohort study by Alric *et al.* serial liver biopsies in 30 renal transplant recipients, performed at 4 and 7 yr following renal transplant, demonstrated a progression of liver fibrosis in the 30% of the renal transplant patients [60]. However a recent study demonstrated no progression of liver fibrosis in the 50% of patients [61]. The rate of progression among kidney transplant recipients was lower than HCV –infected patients without ESRD, probably due to immunosuppressant effects that result in less inflammation and subsequent fibrosis in response to HCV infection [59-61].

Basing on liver histology, kidney transplant candidates with severe fibrosis or compensated cirrhosis should not be considered for kidney transplantation due to the high risk of evolution of liver damage after transplantation: these patients should be evaluated for a combined liver-kidney transplantation.

Since most studies [62-66] demonstrated a rate of 20-100% of acute rejection in HCV positive kidney transplant recipients treated with interferon alfa, post-transplant treatment is now contraindicated, and the only therapeutic management of HCV infection in ESRD patients listed for kidney transplantation remains the pre-transplant treatment, whenever possible. Optimal management of HCV infection should occur prior to the development of ESRD, when both interferon and ribavirin can be used to maximize viral response. However, for those patients who are not diagnosed until after they have reached ESRD or contract HCV after ESRD develops, treatment options are more limited given the relative contraindication to ribavirin in the setting of renal failure and the need for close monitoring for hemolysis and anemia in the event of ribavirin use [67]. In addition, ESRD patients have a lower tolerability of interferon, and two meta-analyses that showed a 17–30% dropout rate in this patient population *versus* a standard non-ESRD dropout rate of about 3–10% [68].

Many small studies demonstrated the efficacy of interferon monotherapy in the treatment of HCV infection in ESRD patients. Two recent meta-analyses assessing the efficacy of interferon monotherapy have shown sustained viral response (SVR, defined by an undetectable HCV RNA <50 IU/ml in serum at least 6 months after stopping treatment) rates of 33–37% [68, 69] and this SVR appears to be durable post-transplant, minimizing the effect of post-transplant HCV glomerulonephritis.

The combination of ribavirin and interferon is problematic in ESRD patients, due to the low clearance of ribavirin by dialysis, exacerbating the risk of hemolysis in patients already at higher risk of anemia. Small studies demonstrated a sustained viral response of 66% in ESRD [65], but and the risk/benefit ratio related to adding ribavirin has not been established. Given the difficulty with hemolysis when using ribavirin in ESRD, extreme caution with close monitoring of ribavirin levels is recommended [3].

At this time, there are data, albeit limited, supporting the safety of pegylated interferon as monotherapy for the treatment of hepatitis C in patients with ESRD. Gupta *et al.* [70] showed that less than 50% of pegylated interferon alfa-2b is renally cleared and hemodialysis did not appear to affect its clearance. Unfortunately, there are little data on tolerability, with a wide range of withdrawal rates in the three studies performed above from 0% to 73% [3]. However, recently, Werner *et al.* [71] reported a 45% of SVR among 22 ESRD HCV-positive patients treated with PEG-IFN monotherapy.

In patients with normal renal function, the similar enhancement in SVR rates are seen when pegylated interferon is combined with ribavirin. Due to this finding, the most promising recent development in the treatment of chronic HCV-infected patients with ESRD is the use of pegylated interferon combined with low-dose ribavirin, despite the known risks with ribavirin use in patients with chronic renal failure.

Rendina *et al.* completed a randomized, controlled trial involving 35 patients treated with 135μg/week of pegylated interferon alpha-2 a and low-dose ribavirin of 200 mg daily to every other day for 48 wk [72]. The study showed a 97% SVR rate despite an early withdrawal rate of 15% with only 6% withdrawal due to lack of tolerability and no adverse events reported.

In summary, recent evidences suggest that the standard of care for treatment of HCV ESRD patients is Interferon monotherapy. Whether pegylated IFN offers advantages over nonpegylated IFN is unknown [72, 73]. The treatment duration with IFN monotherapy is typically 48 wk [72, 73], but non responder may be identified even after 3-6 months of treatment. Genotypes 1, 4, 5 and 6 are more resistant to IFN therapy and need longer course of treatment [74]. Patients who fail to achieve HCV RNA of <50 IU/ml after 6 months of treatment should be considered as nonresponsive and generally should have treatment discontinued.

Post-Transplant Treatment and HCV Glomerulonephritis

Treatment of HCV in kidney transplant recipients is not routinely recommended [75, 76] because of concerns about IFN precipitating acute rejection. However, there are clinical circumstances in which a risk– benefit assessment may favor treatment. HCV-associated glomerulonephritis can recur after kidney transplantation and cause progressive renal dysfunction, and antiviral therapy may be needed to prevent graft loss; moreover, patients with advanced fibrosis or severe cholestatic hepatitis warrant consideration of treatment to prevent death as a result of liver-related complications. Some data suggest that these transplant recipients will benefit from treatment with IFN monotherapy or IFN plus ribavirin combination therapy [74-78].

Kidney injury in HCV-positive patients may be mediated through immunological and non immunological mechanisms. HCV-RNA and related proteins have been found in mesangial cells, tubular epithelial cells and endothelial cells of glomerular and tubular capillaries, and this was associated with higher proteinuria, possibly reflecting direct mesangial injury by HCV infection [79].

Kidney injury may be mediated by systemic immune response to HCV infection, that is mediated by cryoglobulins, HCV-antibody immune complexes or amyloid deposition [80]. Persistence of HCV leads to chronic overstimulation of the B-lymphocytes and production of mixed cryoglobulins, that are deposited in the mesangium and glomerula capillaries [80]. This is usually associated with histologic signs of vasculitis and downstream fibrinoid necrosis of the glomeruli.

Nonimmunologically mediated kidney injury may be related to high levels of fasting serum insulin and insulin resistance, that promote proliferation of renal cells [81].

This histological kidney injury represents the HCV-related glomerulonephritis, which may develop many years after initial infection with HCV [73]. The most common HCV-related nephropathy is membranoproliferative glomerulonephritis (MPGN), usually in context of cryoglobulinemia. Most patients has no clear symptoms, but the triad of purpura, asthenia and arthralgia is evident in 30% of cases [82]. Renal involvement is reported in one third of patients with cryoglobulinemia [83]. Glomerular disease may manifest acutely in 5% of cases and the majority of patients develop hypertension: renal biopsy shows a pattern of MPGN [83], and the diagnosis of HCV-related MPGN is made by positive test for serum HCV antibodies and HCV RNA.

The long-term outcome of HCV-related nephropaties is still not clear defined: however, HCV-positive patients had a 40% higher likelihood for developing renal insufficiency compared with seronegative patients [84].

Hypertension, proteinuria and progressive renal failure are the main clinical manifestation of HCV-associated chronic kidney disease. Thus, renoprotection with either angiotensin-converting enzyme inhibitors or angiotensin II receptor blockers must be applied [74]. Antiviral therapy should be attempted in hemodialysed patients [74]. In kidney transplant recipients with *de novo* glomerulonephritis (GN) with low proteinuria and stable renal function, initiation of antiviral therapy should be based on degree of liver damage. Patients with severe *de novo* GN and high risk of chronic graft failure, antiviral therapy (IFN alone or in combination with ribavirin) should be initiated as soon as possible [74].

Immunosuppressive treatment should be adapted to prevent rejection while minimizing viral replication. Experimental studies [85] have shown that cyclosporine may inhibit the intracellular replication of HCV, independently of its immunosuppressive activity. However, in the clinical setting, this antiviral effect of cyclosporine remains controversial [85, 86].

Findings of the USRDS registry reported a better graft survival in recipients treated with mycophenolate mofetil than those on other immunosuppressive therapy [87]. However, a recent prospective study reported an increase in viral replication in patients on MMF therapy [88], suggesting that the immunosuppressive therapy should be adapted to patients clinical conditions.

HBV-POSITIVE DONORS

HBcAb Positive Donors

The prevalence of hepatitis B virus core antibody (HBcAb) in the population of deceased organ donors is 24% in geographic area endemic for hepatitis B virus (HBV) infection [89, 90]. In about 10% of these individuals, HBV DNA is detected by polymerase chain reaction [91, 92].

The detection of HBcAb in the blood of a potential organ donor may increase the risk for donor infectivity and the risk of transmission of HBV to the recipient [93-95]. The risk of transmission of HBV is more accurately determined by measuring HBV-DNA than anti-HBc, but HBV-DNA measurement is not routinely recommended in standard deceased donors. In an interesting study by Cirocco *et al.* [96], HBV-

DNA measured by PCR was negative in all HBsAg negative, anti-HBc positive donors. Moreover, in the 9 transplanted kidneys that were tested, the kidney tissue was also negative for HBV-DNA, suggesting that HBc-positive HBV-DNA donors are unlikely to transmit infection to recipients.

Liver transplant recipients of HBcAb+ donors may have up to 70% of risk to develop a *de novo* HBV infection after transplantation [95, 97, 98]. Despite the impact of HBcAb+ donors in renal transplantation appears low to negligible [90, 99, 100], some authors emphasized the risk of seroconversion or *de novo* HBV after kidney transplantation from HBcAb+ deceased donors, particularly in HBcAb+ recipients [101, 102].

Kidney transplantation from HBcAb+ donors seems to confer a minimal risk of transmission of HBV to the recipient [90, 98-100]. In experimental models, hepadnaviruses have a strong preference for infecting liver cells and infection at this site is not linked to extra -hepatic disease [103]: this hypothesis was confirmed by Wachs *et al.* [95], who reported a HBcAb+ multiorgan donor who transmitted HBV to liver allograft recipient without apparent transmission to the two kidney recipients.

In a recent report by De Feo *et al.* [90], analyzing the risk of disease transmission of HBcAb+ donors in a population of 356 kidney transplant recipients, none of the recipients acquired a positive hepatitis B surface antigen: however, 4/10 vaccinated patients seroconverted from HBcAb- to HBcAb+, without any clinical or biochemical signs of hepatitis. In our recent experience, among 42 kidney transplant recipients who received a graft from a HBcAb-positive donor, none of naïve or vaccinated recipients developed HBsAg seroconversion: however, 4 of 28 (14.2%) vaccinated patients seroconverted from HBcAb- to HBcAb+, but HBV-DNA levels were undetectable in the follow up, suggesting that prophylaxis in these recipients is probably not warranted.

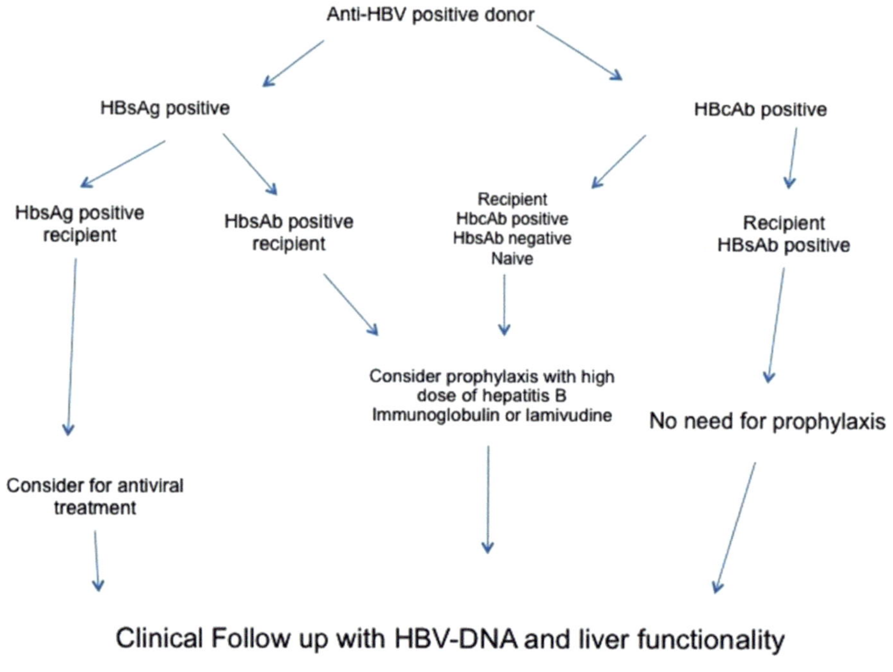

Figure 2: Proposed algorithm for the management of deceased kidney donor with HBV infection.

There are no current guidelines on the need for a prophylaxis in kidney transplant recipients of grafts from HBcAb+ donors (Fig. **2**).

Kidneys from HBcAb+ donors are preferably allocated to successfully immunized patients [90, 99, 100]. The HBsAb positive serologic status, from previous exposure or after vaccination, had a variable effect on serologic conversion, and after transplantation with a HBc-positive kidney, recipients HBsAb-positive were not completely protected [90, 99, 101, 104].

All end-stage renal disease candidates to kidney transplantation should receive hepatitis B vaccine. In recipients of HBc-positive kidneys with protective anti-HBs concentration, the seroconversion to HBc-positive was only 4% compared with 10% in recipients with no protective levels of HBsAb (< 10 mIU/mL) [90].

In a review article, Chung *et al.* [94] recommended a 7-day high dose (10000 units intravenously daily for the first 7 days then monthly) HBIg or 12-month lamivudine (100 mg every day) prophylaxis in all recipients without evidence of HBV immunity. In the series of Akalin *et al.* [105], 50 renal transplant recipients of HBcAb+ kidneys received a 1 yr lamivudine prophylaxis after transplantation without requiring HBIg, suggesting that this approach may protect against the risk of HBV transmission.

Although the very low level of transmitted virus in this settings, the theoretical risk for selection of lamivudine-resistant HBV exists; on contrast, long-term prophylaxis with HBIg may be very expensive [95].

Basing on the experience on liver transplantation, where HBIg prophylaxis has been shown to be effective in reducing the rate of HBV recurrence after liver transplantation [97, 98], we recently applied a prophylaxis with a single dose of 2000 IU of HBIg in all recipients who were not immunized against HBV, and this resulted in a very low incidence of seroconversion when compared with patients who did not receive prophylaxis. All our HBcAb+ patients who have undergone prophylaxis did not have HBV reactivation, while we observed a subclinical reactivation in two patients who did not undergo prophylaxis.

Ouphen *et al.* [92], recently proposed a different approach: recipients of HBc-positive kidneys start prophylaxis with lamivudine or HBIg. If the recipients have been vaccinated and the titer is protective, HBV-DNA is monitored every three months, and prophylaxis suspended when HBV-DNA is undetectable.

If the recipients are not vaccinated and the HBV-DNA is negative, the HBV-DNA is followed monthly, and the recipient revaccinated with 3 doses.

Graft and patient survival in kidney transplantation from HBcAb+ donors are similar to those from HBcAb- donors. This findings are consistent with previous reports [90, 100, 101], but are in contrast with the results of Fong *et al.* [99], which demonstrated that graft and patient survival at 1 and 3 years were significantly lower in kidney recipients of HBcAb+ donors compared to those from HBcAb- donors. However, the reduction in survival was attributable to donor and recipient factors independent to anti-HBc status.

In the study by Fong *et al.* [99], the incidence of anti-HBc conversion in recipients of anti HBc positive and anti HBc- negative kidneys was 0.011 and 0.005 per year, respectively. In other retrospective studies, the incidence of seroconversion varied between 0% and 27 % [90, 93, 95, 99-101, 104], but these data must be interpreted cautiously because patients who are immunosuppressed may not develop detectable antibody levels post-transplant [92].

Most of the clinical studies reported an increase in transaminase levels in 0-26% of patients [90, 93, 95, 99-101], and Alkalin *et al.* suggested that the recipients at higher risk for elevated transaminase levels were those who were co-infected with hepatitis C [105].

In summary, existing data support the use of HBc-positive organ donors for kidney transplantation. Anti-HBc positive kidney should be used in vaccinated patients. Current evidences do not suggest to use extensively prophylaxis for recipients of HBcAb-positive kidneys: however, a strict surveillance serologies is mandatory and a prophylaxis with a single shot of hepatitis B immunoglobulin may be effective in reducing the risk of HBV seroconversion or reactivation in all naïve or HBcAb+ transplant recipients.

HBsAg –Positive Donors

In geographic areas endemic for hepatitis B virus (HBV) infection, hepatitis B surface antigen (HBsAg) carrier rates are so high (10%–20%) [106] that exclusion of HBsAg donors from the donor pool would significantly reduce the supply of kidney allografts.

It is generally accepted that transplanting a HBsAg positive allograft into a HBsAg negative recipient carries a significant risk of the novo infection, so that most of the study investigating the use of HBsAg positive kidney donors have shown that the policy of transplanting such kidneys to HBsAg-positive recipients with natural immunity is reasonable and seems to be safe [107-113].

A study from Taiwan has compared patient survival among 24 HBsAg-positive recipients of kidneys from HBsAg-positive donors with that among 42 HBsAg-positive recipients of kidneys from HBsAg-negative donors [114]. The results of this study showed that there were no statistically significative differences between the 2 groups with respect to the number of episodes of hepatitis. However, among recipients from deceased donors, recipients of kidneys from HBsAg-negative donors had significantly higher 1- and 5-year survival rates than recipients of kidneys from HBsAg positive donors. We have previously showed that short-term results among recipients of HBsAg-positive kidneys are acceptable, and these kidney should be used for highly selected recipients.

Recent observations suggests the opportunity to transplant HBsAg positive kidneys into HBsAb-positive recipients, and recipients were given hepatitis B immunoglobulin at the time of and after transplantation. Lamivudine was also recommended for these recipients [110, 113, 115].

Treatment of HBsAg+ renal transplant recipients with nucleoside/nucleotide analogues confers long-term survival benefit, and that rescue therapy with adefovir or entecavir is effective and well tolerated in patients who had developed resistance to lamivudine [116].

In a recent study, Jiang *et al.* [117] compared the clinical outcomes in 373 HBsAb-positive kidney transplant recipients receiving a kidney from either HBsAg-postive donors (n=65) or HBsAg-negative donors: patients receiving HBsAg-positive graft underwent a prophylaxis with 400 IU of anti-hepatitis B immunoglobulin on the day of surgery and again 1-month after procedure. Recipients who received HBV DNA-positive grafts were administered lamivudine 100 mg daily for 6 months.

There was no differences in graft and patient survival among the two groups, and none of the seven recipients receiving a graft from a HBV DNA-positive donor displayed evidence of HBV infection for 20 months after transplantation. Thus, kidney grafts from HBsAg-positive donors can be use safely in anti-HBs positive recipients, with post-transplant prophylaxis with HBIg and/or lamivudine.

In summary, kidney transplantation from HBsAg positive donor kidneys may be safely allocated in HBsAg positive recipients. All transplant recipients should undergo a prophylaxis with lamivudine or, in case of failure, with adefovir or entecavir which can confer long-term survival benefit.

Kidney transplantation in HBsAb-positive recipients, although some promising results, needs further data to be extensively adopted.

REFERENCES

[1] Fabrizi F, Messa P, Martin P. Current status of renal transplantation from HCV-positive donors. Int J Artif Organs 2009; 32: 251-261.

[2] Finelli L, Miller JT, Tokars JI, *et al.* National surveillance of dialysis-associated diseases in the United States, 2002. Semin Dial 2005;18:52–61.

[3] Okoh EJ, Bucci JR, James F. Simon JF, Harrison SA. HCV in Patients With End-Stage Renal Disease. Am J Gastroenterol 2008;103:2123–2134.

[4] Domínguez-Gil B, Morales JM. Transplantation in the patients with hepatitis C. Transplant Int 2009: 22; 1117-1131.

[5] Kalantar-Zadeh K, Kilpatrick RD, McAllister CJ, *et al.* Hepatitis C virus and death risk in hemodialysis patients. J Am Soc Nephrol 2007; 18: 1584-1593.

[6] Berenguer M. Treatment of chronic hepatitis C in hemodyalised patients. Hepatology 2008; 48:1690-1699.

[7] Kucirka LM, Singer AL, Ros RL, *et al.* Underutilization of hepatitis C-positive kidneys for hepatitis C-positive recipients. Am J Transplant 2010; 10: 1238-1246.

[8] Fabrizi F, Martin P, Dixit V, *et al.* Meta-analysis: Effect of hepatitis C virus infection on mortality in dialysis. Aliment Pharmacol Ther 2004;20:1271–1277.

[9] Kidney Disease: Improving Global Outcomes. KDIGO clinical practice guidelines for the prevention, diagnosis, evaluation, and treatment of Hepatitis C in chronic kidney disease. Kidney Int 2008; 73 (Suppl. 109): S1-S99.

[10] Fabrizi F, Martin P, Dixit V, *et al.* Hepatitis C virus antibody status and survival after renal transplantation: meta-analysis of observational studies. Am J Transplant 2005; 5: 1452-1461.

[11] Giblin L, Clarkson MR, Conlon PJ, *et al.* Impaired renal allograft, but not patient survival, in patients with antibodies to hepatitis C virus. Irish J Med Sci 2004; 173: 82-84.

[12] Manga Sahin G, Sahin S, Kantarci G, Ergin H. Impact of hepatitis C virus infection on patient and graft survival in kidney transplantation. Transplant Proc 2006; 38: 499-501.

[13] Pedroso S, Martins L, Fonseca I, *et al.* A. Impact of hepatitis C virus on renal transplantation: association with poor survival. Transplant Proc 2006; 38: 1890-1894.

[14] Mitwalli AH, Alam A, Al-Wakeel J, *et al.* Effect of chronic viral hepatitis on graft survival in saudi renal transplant patients. Nephron Clin Pract 2006; 102: c72-c80.

[15] Ozdemir BH, Ozdemir FN, Sezer S, *et al.* *De novo* glomerulonephritis in renal allografts with hepatitis C virus infection. Transplant Proc 2006; 38: 492-495.

[16] Unal E, Trukmen F, Sevinc C, Kiziler AR. Outcome of renal allograft in Turkish patients with pretransplantation hepatitis C virus infection. Transplant Proc 2006; 38: 3448-3450.

[17] Ingsathit A, Thakkinstian A, Kantachuvesiri S, Sumenthkul V. Different impacts of hepatitis B virus and hepatitis C virus on the outcome of kidney transplantation. Transplant Proc 2007; 39: 1424-1428.

[18] Gheith OA, Saad MA, Hassan AA, *et al.* Hepatic dysfunction in kidney transplant recipients: prevalence and impact on graft and patient survival. Clin Exp Nephrol 2007; 11: 309-315.

[19] Einollahi B, Pourfarziani V, Ahmadzad-Asl M, *et al.* Iranian model of renal allograft transplantation in 3028 recipients: survival and risk factors. Transplant Proc 2007; 39: 907-910.

[20] Ridruejo E, Cusumano A, Diaz C, *et al.* Hepatitis C virus infection and outcome of renal transplantation. Transplant Proc 2007; 39: 3127-3130.

[21] Ghafari A, Sanadgol H. Impact of hepatitis B and hepatitis C virus infections on patients and allograft outcomes in renal transplant recipients. Transplant Proc 2008; 40: 196-198.

[22] Arango J, Arbelaez M, Henao J, *et al.* Kidney graft survival in patients with hepatitis C: a single-center experience. Clin Transplant 2008; 22: 16-19.

[23] Kliem V, Burg M, Haller H, *et al.* Relationship of hepatitis B or C virus prevalences, risk factors, and outcomes in renal transplant recipients: Analysis of German data. Transplant Proc 2008; 40: 909-914.

[24] Romero E, Galindo P, Bravo JA, *et al.* Hepatitis C virus infection after renal transplantation. Transplant Proc 2008; 40: 2933-2935.

[25] Minz M, Sharma A, Das A, Chawla Y. Impact of anti-hepatitis C virus antibody on outcomes in renal transplant recipients infected with HCV. Transplant Proc 2008; 40: 2386-2388.

[26] Meier-Kriesche HU, Ojo AO, Hanson JA, Kaplan B. Hepatitis C antibody status and outcomes in renal transplant recipients. Transplantation 2001; 72: 241-244.

[27] Batty DS, Swanson SJ, Kirk AD, *et al.* Hepatitis C virus seropositivity at the time of renal transplantation in the United States: associated factors and patient survival. Am J Transplant 2001; 1: 179-184.

[28] Luan FL, Schaubel DE, Zhang H, *et al.* Impact of immunosuppressive regimen on survival of kidney transplant recipients with hepatitis C. Transplantation 2008; 85: 1601-1606.

[29] Hu KQ, Lee SM, Hu SX, *et al.* Clinical presentation of chronic hepatitis C in patients with end-stage renal disease and on hemodialysis *versus* those with normal renal function. Am J Gastroenterol 2005;100:2010–2018.

[30] Sterling RK, Sanyal AJ, Luketic VA, *et al.* Chronic hepatitis C infection in patients with end-stage renal disease: Characterization of liver histology and viral load in patients awaiting renal transplantation. Am J Gastroenterol 1999;94:3576–3582.

[31] Luzar B, Ferlan-Marolt V, Brinovec V, *et al.* Does end-stage kidney failure influence hepatitis C progression in hemodialysis patients? Hepatogastroenterology 2003;50:157–160.

[32] Maluf DG, Fisher RA, King AL, *et al.* Hepatitis C virus infection and kidney transplantation: predictors of patient and graft survival. Transplantation 2007; 83: 853-857.

[33] Sezer S, Ozdemir FN, Akcay A, *et al.* Renal transplantation offers a better survival in HCV-infected ESRD patients. Clin Transplant 2004; 18: 619-623.

[34] Bloom RD, Sayer G, Fa K, *et al.* Outcome of hepatitis C virus-infected kidney transplant candidates who remain on the waiting list. Am J Transplant 2005; 5: 139-144.

[35] Montori VM, Basu A, Erwin PJ, *et al.* Posttransplantation diabetes: A systematic review of the literature. Diabetes Carc 2002;25:583–592.

[36] Fabrizi F, Martin P, Dixit V, *et al.* Post-transplant diabetes mellitus and HCV seropositive status after renal transplantation: Meta-analysis of clinical studies. Am J Transplant 2005;5:2433–2440.

[37] Einollahi B, Hajarizadeh B, Bakhtiari S, *et al.* Pretransplant hepatitis C virus infection and its effect on the posttransplant course of living renal allograft recipients. J Gastroenterol Hepatol 2003;18:836–840.

[38] Aroldi A, Lampertico P, Montagnino G, *et al.* Natural history of hepatitis B and C in renal allograft recipients. Transplantation 2005;79:1132–1136.

[39] Pedroso S, Martins L, Fonseca I, *et al.* Renal transplantation in patients over 60 years of age: A single-center experience Transplant Proc 2006;38:1885–1889.

[40] Pereira BJ, Wright TL, Schmid CH, *et al.* Screening and confirmatory testing of cadaver organ donors for hepatitis C virus infection: A U.S. National Collaborative Study. Kidney Int 1994;46:886–892.

[41] Botero RC. Should patients with chronic hepatitis C infection be transplanted? Transplant Proc 2004; 36: 1449-1454.

[42] Avery R, Preiksaitis J, Green M. Use of anti-HCV positive donor organs. Am J Transplant 2005; 5: 1579 .

[43] Kiberd BA. Should hepatitis C-infected kidneys be transplanted in the United States? Transplantation 1994; 57: 1068-1072.

[44] Mandal AK, Kraus ES, Samaniego M, *et al.* Shorter waiting times for hepatitis C virus seropositive recipients of cadaveric renal allografts from hepatitis C virus seropositive donors. Clin Transplant 2000; 14: 391-396.

[45] Morales JM, Campistol JM, Castellano G, *et al.* Transplantation of kidneys from donors with hepatitis C antibody into recipients with pretransplantation anti-HCV. Kidney Int 1995; 47: 236-240.

[46] Woodside KJ, Ishihara K, Theisen JE, *et al.* Use of kidneys from hepatitis C seropositive donors shortens waitlist time but does not alter one-year outcome. Clin Transplant 2003; 17: 433-437.

[47] Veroux P, Veroux M, Sparacino V, *et al.* Kidney transplantation from donors with viral B and C hepatitis. Transplant Proc 2006; 38: 996-998.

[48] Pereira BJ, Wright TL, Schmid CH, *et al.* A controlled study of hepatitis C transmission by organ transplantation The New England Organ Bank Hepatitis C Study Group. Lancet 1995;345:484–487.

[49] Bouthot BA, Murthy BV, Schmid CH, *et al.* Long-term follow-up of hepatitis C virus infection among organ transplant recipients: Implications for policies on organ procurement. Transplantation 1997;63:849–853.

[50] Abbott KC, Bucci JR, Matsumoto CS, *et al.* Hepatitis C and renal transplantation in the era of modern immunosuppression. J Am Soc Nephrol 2003; 14: 2908-2918.

[51] Abbott KC, Lentine KL, Bucci JR, *et al.* The impact of transplantation with deceased donor hepatitis C-positive kidney on survival in wait-listed long-term dialysis patients. Am J Transplant 2004; 4: 1032-2037.

[52] Chan TM, Wu PC, Lok AS, *et al.* Clinicopathological features of hepatitis C virus antibody negative fatal chronic hepatitis C after renal transplantation. Nephron 1995; 71: 213-217.

[53] Morales JM, Campistol JM, Castellano G, *et al.* Transplantation of kidneys from donors with hepatitis C antibody into recipients with pretransplantation anti-HCV. Kidney Int 1995; 47: 236-240.

[54] Natov SN, Lau JY, Ruthazer R, *et al.* Hepatitis C virus genotype does not affect patient survival among renal transplant candidates. The New England Organ Bank Hepatitis C Study Group. Kidney Int 1999; 56: 700-706.

[55] Scott DR, Wong JK, Spicer TS, *et al.* Adverse Impact of Hepatitis C Virus Infection on Renal Replacement Therapy and Renal Transplant Patients in Australia and New Zealand. Transplantation. 2010; 90:1165-1171.

[56] Ridruejo E, Díaz C, Michel MD, *et al.* Short and long term outcome of kidney transplanted patients with chronic viral hepatitis B and C. Ann Hepatol. 2010;9:271-277.

[57] Morales JM, Marcén R, Andres A, *et al.* Renal transplantation in patients with hepatitis C virus antibody. A long national experience. NDT Plus. 2010;3(Suppl_2):ii41-ii46.

[58] Mathurin P, Mouquet C, Poynard T, *et al.* Impact of hepatitis B and C virus on kidney transplantation outcome. Hepatology 1999; 29: 257-263.

[59] Zylberberg H, Nalpas B, Carnot F, *et al.* Severe evolution of chronic hepatitis C in renal transplantation: a case control study. Nephrol Dial Transplant 2002; 17: 129-133.

[60] Alric L, Kamar N, Bonnet D, Danjoux M, *et al.* Comparison of liver stiffness, fibrotest and liver biopsy for assessment of liver fibrosis in kidney-transplant patients with chronic viral hepatitis. Transplant Int. 2009 May;22:568-573.

[61] Kamar N, Rostaing L, Selves J, *et al.* Natural history of hepatitis C virus-related liver fibrosis after renal transplantation. Am J Transplant 2005;5:1704–1712.

[62] Therret E, Pol S, Legendre C, *et al.* Low-dose recombinant leukocyte interferon-alpha treatment of hepatitis C viral infection in renal transplant recipients. A pilot study. Transplantation 1994;58:625–628.

[63] Harihara Y, Kurooka Y, Yanagisawa T, *et al.* Interferon therapy in renal allograft recipients with chronic hepatitis C. Transplant Proc 1994;26:2075.

[64] Magnone M, Holley JL, Shapiro R, *et al.* Interferon-alpha induced acute renal allograft rejection. Transplantation 1995;59:1068–1070.

[65] Ozgur O, Boyacioglu S, Telatar H, *et al.* Recombinant alpha-interferon in renal allograft recipients with chronic hepatitis C. Nephrol Dial Transplant 1995;10:2104–2106.

[66] Rostaing L, Modesto A, Baron E, *et al.* Acute renal failure in kidney transplant patients treated with interferon alpha 2b for chronic hepatitis C. Nephron 1996;74:512–516.

[67] Bruchfeld A, Lindahl K, Stahle L, *et al.* Interferon and ribavirin treatment in patients with hepatitis C-associated renal disease and renal insufficiency. Nephrol Dial Transplant 2003;18:1573–1580.

[68] Fabrizı F, Dulai G, Dixit V, *et al.* Meta-analysis: Interferon for the treatment of chronic hepatitis C in dialysis patients. Aliment Pharmacol Ther 2003;18:1071–81.

[69] Russo MW, Goldsweig CD, Jacobson IM, *et al.* Interferon monotherapy for dialysis patients with chronic hepatitis C: An analysis of the literature on efficacy and safety. Am J Gastroenterol 2003;98:1610–1615.

[70] Gupta SK, Pittenger AL, Swan SK, *et al.* Single-dose pharmacokinetics and safety of pegylated interferon-alpha2b in patients with chronic renal dysfunction. J Clin Pharmacol 2002;42:1109–15.

[71] Werner T, Aqel B, Balan V, *et al.* Treatment of hepatitis C in renal transplantation candidates: a single-center experience. Transplantation. 2010;90:407-411.

[72] Rendina M, Schena A, Castellaneta NM, *et al.* The treatment of chronic hepatitis C with peginterferon alfa-2 a (40 kDa) plus ribavirin in haemodialysed patients awaiting renal transplant. J Hepatol 2007;46: 768–774.

[73] Terrault NA, Adey DB. The Kidney Transplant Recipient with Hepatitis C Infection: Pre- and Posttransplantation Treatment. Clin J Am Soc Nephrol 2007; 2: 563-575.

[74] Durlik M, Gaciong Z, Rowinska D, *et al.* Long-term results of treatment of chronic hepatitis B, C and D with interferon-alpha in renal allograft recipients. Transpl Int 1998; 11[Suppl 1]: S135–S139.

[75] Perico N, Cattaneo D, Bikbov B, Remuzzi G. Hepatitis C Infection and Chronic Renal Diseases. Clin J Am Soc Nephrol 2009; 4: 207–220.

[76] Shu KH, Lan JL, Wu MJ, *et al.* Ultralow-dose alpha-interferon plus ribavirin for the treatment of active hepatitis C in renal transplant recipients. Transplantation 2004; 77: 1894–1896.

[77] Tang S, Cheng IK, Leung VK, *et al.* Successful treatment of hepatitis C after kidney transplantation with combined interferon alpha- 2b and ribavirin. J Hepatol 2003; 39: 875–878.

[78] Poynard T, Yuen MF, Ratziu V, Lai CL. Viral hepatitis C. Lancet 2003; 362: 2095–2100.

[79] Sansonno D, Gesualdo L, Manno C, *et al.* Hepatitis C virus-related proteins in kidney tissue from hepatitis C-virus infected patients with cryoglobulinemic membranoproliferative glomerulonephritis. Hepatology 1997; 25: 1237–1244.

[80] Barsoum RS. Hepatitis C virus: From entry to renal injury— Facts and potentials. Nephrol Dial Transplant 2007; 22: 1840–1848.

[81] Sarafidis PA, Ruilope LM. Insulin resistance, hyperinsulinemia, and renal injury: Mechanisms and implications. Am J Nephrol 2006; 26: 232–244.

[82] Monti G, Galli M, Invernizzi F, *et al.* Cryoglobulinaemias: A multi-centre study of the early clinical and laboratory manifestations of primary and secondary disease. Italian Group for the Study of Cryoglobulinaemias. QJM 1995; 88: 115–126.

[83] Meyers CM, Seeff LB, Stehman-Breen CO, Hoofnagle JH. Hepatitis C and renal disease: An update. Am J Kidney Dis 2003; 42: 631–657.

[84] Dalrymple LS, Koepsell T, Sampson J, *et al.* Hepatitis C virus infection and the prevalence of renal insufficiency. Clin J Am Soc Nephrol 2007; 2: 715–721.

[85] Fabrizi F, Bromberg J, Elli A, *et al.* Review article: Hepatitis C virus and calcineurin inhibition after renal transplantation. Aliment Pharmacol Ther 2005; 22: 657–666.

[86] Fagiuoli S, Bruni F, Bravi M, *et al.* Cyclosporin in steroid-resistant autoimmune hepatitis and HCV-related liver diseases. Dig Liver Dis 2007;39[Suppl 3]: S379–S385.

[87] Abbott KC, Bucci JR, Matsumoto CS, *et al.* Hepatitis C and renal transplantation in the era of modern immunosuppression. J Am Soc Nephrol 2003; 14: 2908–2918.

[88] Rostaing L, Izopet J, Sandres K, *et al.* Changes in hepatitis C virus RNA viremia concentrations in long-term renal transplant patients after introduction of mycophenolate mofetil. Transplantation 2000; 69: 991–994.

[89] Lee KH, Wai CT, Lim SG, *et al.* Risk of *de novo* hepatitis B from antibody to hepatitis B core antigen-positive donors in liver transplantation in Singapore. Liver Transplant 2001; 7: 469-470.

[90] De Feo TM, Grossi P, Poli F, *et al* . Kidney transplantation from anti-HBC^+ donors: results from a retrospective Italian study. Transplantation 2006; 81: 76-80.

[91] Grob P, Jilg W, Bornhak H, *et al.* Serological pattern "Anti-HBc alone": report on a qorkshop. J Med Virol 2000; 62: 450-455.

[92] Ouseph R, Eng M, Ravindra K, *et al.* Review of the use of hepatitis B core antibody-positive kidney donors. Transplant Rev 2010: 24: 167-171.

[93] Fytili P, Ciesek S, Manns MP, *et al.* Anti-HBc seroconversion after transplantation of Anti-HBc positive nonliver organs to anti-HBc negative recipients. Transplantation 2006; 81: 808-809.

[94] Chung RT, Feng S, Delmonica FL. Approach to the management of allograft recipients following the detection of hepatitis B virus in the prospective organ donor. Am J Transplant 2001; 1:185-191.

[95] Wachs ME, Amend WJ, Ascher NL, *et al.* The risk of transmission of hepatitis B from HBsAg(-), HBcAb (+), HbIgM (-) organ donors. Transplantation 1995; 59: 230-234.

[96] Cirocco R, Zucker K, Contreras N, *et al.* The presence of hepatitis B core antibody does not preclude kidney donation: lack of viral DNA in the serum and biopsies of core antibody-positive donors and clinical follow-up. Transplantation 1997;63:1702-1703.

[97] Donataccio D, Roggen F, De Reyck C, *et al.* Use of AntiHBc positive allografts in adult liver transplantation: toward a safer way to expand the donor pool. Transplant Int 2006;19: 38-43.

[98] Takemura N, Suguwara Y, Tamura S, *et al.* Liver transplantation using hepatitis B core antibody – positive grafts: review and university of Tokyo experience. Dig Dis 2007; 52 : 2472-2477.

[99] Fong TL, Bunnapradist S, Jordan SC, *et al.* Impact of hepatitis B core antibody status on outcomes of cadaveric renal transplantation: analysis of United Network of Organ Sharing Database between 1994 and 1999. Transplantation 2002; 73:85-89.

[100] Veroux M, Puliatti C, Gagliano M, *et al.* Use of hepatitis B core antibody-positive donor kidneys in hepatitis B surface antibody-positive and -negative recipients. Transplant Proc 2005; 37:2574-2575.

[101] Madayag RM, Johnson LB, Bartlett ST, *et al.* Use of renal allografts from donors positive for hepatitis B core antibody confers minimal risk for subsequent development of clinical hepatitis B virus disease. Transplantation 1997; 64:1781-1786.

[102] Knoll A, Pietrzyk M, Loss M, *et al.* Solid –organ transplantation in HbsAg-negative patients with antibodies to HBV core antigen: low risk of HBV reactivation. Transplantation 2005; 79: 1631-1633.

[103] Ganem D, Prince AM. Hepatitis B virus infection – natural history and clinical consequences. N Engl J Med 2004; 350: 1118-1129.

[104] Satterthwaite R, Ozgu I, Shidban H, *et al.* Risks of transplanting kidney from hepatitis B surface antigen-negative, hepatitis B surface antibody-negative, hepatitis B core antibody-positive donors. Transplantation 1997; 64: 432-435.

[105] Akalin E, Ames S, Sehgal V, *et al.* Safety of using hepatitis B virus core antibody or surface antigen-positive donors in kidney or pancreas transplantation. Clin Transplant 2005; 19: 364-366.

[106] Lai MK, Chang SC, Chueh CC, *et al.* Kidney transplantation from hepatitis B surface antigen (HBsAg)-positive donors: change of relative genome copy number after transplantation. Transplant proc 1996; 28:1518-1520.

[107] Berber I, Aydin C, Yigit B *et al.* The effect of HBsAg-positivity of kidney donors on long-term patient and graft outcome. Transplant Proc 2005; 37: 4173–4175.

[108] Kim JA, Huh W, Lee KW, *et al.* Cadaveric renal transplantation in hepatitis B antigen-positive recipients using hepatitis B antigenpositive donor organs with lamivudine treatment. Transplant Proc 2004; 36: 1434–1437

[109] Veroux M, Puliatti C,Macarone M, *et al.* Kidney transplantation from hepatitis B surface antigen-positive donors into hepatitis B surface antigen-positive recipients: Preliminary findings. Transplant Proc 2005; 37: 2467–2468.

[110] Chan PC, Lok AS, Cheng IK, *et al.* The impact of donor and recipient hepatitis B surface antigen status on liver disease and survival in renal transplant recipients. Transplantation 1992; 53: 128–131.

[111] Chan MK, Chang WK. Renal transplantation from HbsAg positive donors to HbsAg negative recipients. Br Med J 1988; 297: 522– 523.

[112] Bedrossian J, Akposso K, Metivier F, *et al.* Kidney transplantation with HbsAg positive donors. Transplant Proc 1993; 25: 1481–1482.

[113] Okamoto M, Yoshimura N, Nakai I, *et al.* Kidney transplantation from a hepatitis B surface antigen-positive donor to a HBSAG-negative recipient. Transplant Proc 1999; 31: 2869.

[114] Lai MK, Chang SC, Chueh CC, *et al.* Kidney transplantation from hepatitis B surface antigen (HbsAg)- positive donors: changes of relative HBV genomic copy number after transplantation. Transplant Proc 1996; 28:1518.

[115] Chung RT, Feng S, Delmonico FL. Approach to the management of allograft recipients following the detection of hepatitis B virus in the prospective organ donor. Am J Transplant 2001; 1: 185–191.

[116] Yap DY, Tang CS, Yung S, *et al.* Long-term outcome of renal transplant recipients with chronic hepatitis B infection-impact of antiviral treatments. Transplantation 2010;90:325-330.

[117] Jiang H, Wu J, Zhang X, *et al.* kidney transplantation from hepatitis B surface antigen positive donors into hepatitis B surface antibody positive recipients: a prospective nonrandomized controlled study from a single centre. Am J Transplant 2009; 9:1583-1858.

CHAPTER 8

Perioperative Anaesthesiologic Management During Kidney Transplantation

Massimiliano Sorbello[1,*], Laura Parrinello[1], Jessica Giuseppina Maugeri[1], Alessandro Laudani[1], Mirko Tindaro Sidoti[1] and Gianluigi Morello[2]

[1]Anaesthesia and Intensive Care Unit, University Hospital of Catania, Italy and [2]Vittorio Emanuele Hospital, Gela, Italy

Abstract: Acute kidney injury in the critically ill patient represents a serious danger for the patients' survival, and is probably one of the most challenging fields for ICU physicians, as renal physiology is very well known and different drugs and molecules are available to try to perform an effective nephroprotection.

The main goals to achieve before any pharmacological attempt for nephroprotection are represented by fluid balance optimization and by hemodynamic sustain, which, together with the internal renal hemodynamic and oxygen imbalance of nephrons and tubules, represent the target of any available or potential nephroprotective strategy: most of the studies support many different nephroprotective drugs, including dopamine, dopexamine, N-Acetyl-Cisteine (NAC), prostaglandins and fenoldopam.

This chapter is devoted to the analysis of all potential nephroprotective strategies, focusing on the different phases in the field of kidney transplantation.

Keywords: Kidney Transplantation, Anaesthesiology, Fenoldopam, N-Acetyl-Cisteine, Nephroprotection, Ischemia-Reperfusion Injury, Deceased Donor, Brain Death, Living Donor, Delayed Graft Function.

INTRODUCTION

The patient undergoing kidney transplantation can be considered as a two-phase patient: in the early phase he is a chronic end stage kidney patient, often receiving dialysis and affected by complications of chronic kidney disease accordingly to length of his disease.

On the anaesthesiological and preoperative point of view, these considerations become of paramount importance, deserving specific and well scheduled approach and preparation.

In the post-transplantation phase he can be compared with an Intensive Care Unit (ICU) patient at risk or immediately after an acute kidney injury, so any treatment or prophylaxis strategy could someway be referred to postoperative or ICU strategies for nephroprotection.

Acute kidney injury in the critically ill patient represents a serious danger for the patients' survival, and is probably one of the most challenging fields for ICU physicians, as renal physiology is very well known and different drugs and molecules are available to try to perform an effective nephroprotection.

The main goals to achieve before any pharmacological attempt for nephroprotection are represented by fluid balance optimization and by hemodynamic sustain, which, together with the internal renal hemodynamic and oxygen imbalance of nephrons and tubules, represent the target of any available or potential nephroprotective strategy: most of the studies support many different nephroprotective drugs, including dopamine, dopexamine, N-Acetyl-Cisteine (NAC), prostaglandins and fenoldopam.

***Address corresponding to Massimiliano Sorbello:** Anaesthesia and Intensive Care Unit, University Hospitalof Catania, *Via* Santa Sofia, 86, 95123, Catania, Italy; Tel: + 39 095 3782307; E-mail: massimilianosorbello@libero.it

Massimiliano Veroux and Pierfrancesco Veroux (Eds)

The last step is represented by renal replacement therapies such as hemodialysis and peritoneal dialysis. Data coming from kidney transplantation and from contrast dye induced acute kidney injury highlight new research fields for nephroprotection, represented by ischemia-reperfusion injury, oxidative imbalance, heme-oxygenase chain modulation, protein expression and programmed cell death (apoptosis): this is probably the next future of nephroprotection.

Finally, to underline how scientific reality dramatically changes in the round of few years, different studies show that both dopamine [1] or conventional diuretics [1] such as furosemide either lack in terms of nephroprotective effect during conditions of potential kidney damage (such as ischemia, hypoperfusion, nephrotoxic agents or contrast dye) or might even show detrimental effects on renal function recovery or maintenance. Moreover, many controversies have been recently introduced regarding dopamine pharmacokinetics in different patients.

Many studies are actually focusing the role of anti-oxidant agents such as N-acetyl-cisteine [1], but to date the pivotal role in renal protection seems to be played by agents able to promote renal blood flow, glomerular filtration rate and diuresis, to recover the oxygen delivery/oxygen consumption (DO_2/VO_2) imbalance and to reduce renal medullary VO_2 especially in conditions of low DO_2.

We'll try to analyze all potential nephroprotective strategies, focusing on the different phases in the field of kidney transplantation, starting from the optimal preparation of patient scheduled for kidney transplantation going through the perioperative period with some considerations for the potential deceased organ donor in ICU.

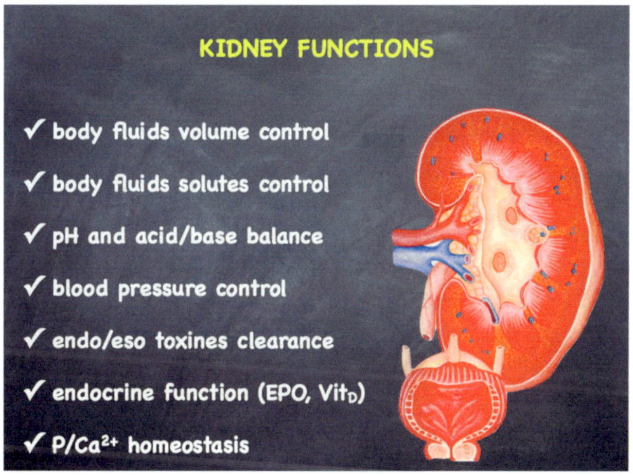

Figure 1: Kidney functions.

PREOPERATIVE EVALUATION AND PREPARATION FOR KIDNEY TRANSPLANTATION

The kidney performs many functions, such as filtering blood, removing nitrogenous waste, maintaining the balance of sodium and water, regulating acid–base balance, electrolyte homeostasis, bone metabolism, regulating red blood cells production and controlling blood pressure *via* water readsorption and renin-angiotensin-aldosterone system (Fig. **1**). Renal impairment, whether acute or chronic, affects many organs and reduces the body's ability to regulate these functions, resulting in many important implications for the patient undergoing general anesthesia [1].

Careful evaluation of any renal replacement therapy, such as haemodialysis or peritoneal dialysis, or history of a previous renal transplant is of paramount importance, especially for determination of correct perioperative fluid balance and for patient preparation, including immediate preoperative dialysis [1].

Systemic conditions, such as diabetes mellitus [2], hypertension, systemic lupus erythematosus, rheumatoid arthritis, thyroid disease [3] and spina bifida or other rare diseases (Fabry disease, Kimura Disease,

Sarcoidosis, *etc.*) [4] can be associated with renal failure. Each of these conditions will present difficulties specific to anaesthesia, including association with difficult airway management, which has been revealed in our experience (unpublished data), as shown in Fig. **2**, and which results someway linear depending on dialysis severity and duration [5].

A detailed patient history is thus very important for diagnostic and management considerations, with particular reference to patients' fluid tolerance in terms of maximal admitted weight before dialysis: these important data would allow optimal and safe patient filling during transplantation for an optimal status favouring graft perfusion [6]. Preoperative electrolytes evaluation and correction, if needed, is mandatory, and similarly glucose control should be tight and accurate, especially in resistant diabetes or combined kidney pancreas transplantation.

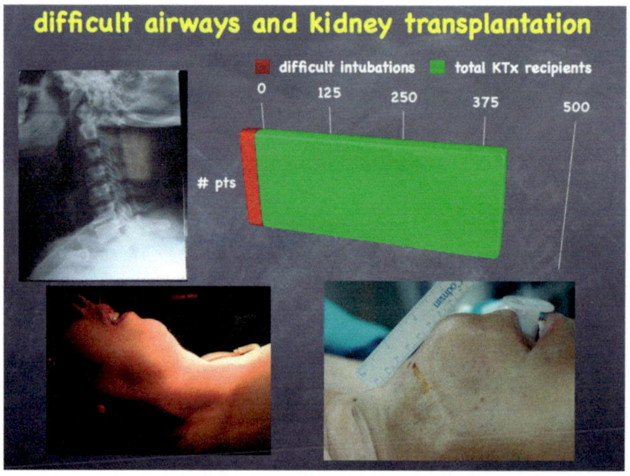

Figure 2: Difficult oro-tracheal intubation and end-stage renal disease patients candidates to kidney transplantation.

An accurate drug history remains important, too, and reduces the risk of harmful drug interactions. and pharmacokinetic or pharmacodynamic problems, including considerations about a decrease in drug excretion because of reduced or absent kidney function. Drugs evaluation is important also to determine which drugs should be continued (*i.e.* beta-blockers), switched (*i.e.* oral anticoagulants for heparine) or discontinued (*i.e.* ACE-inhibitors) before surgery.

Cardiac comorbidity is very frequent in renal patient, and a careful and detailed evaluation (including coronarography, stress tests or echocardiography) should be considered according to disease severity [7], and opportune precautions should be undertaken at anaesthesia induction and for postoperative care, with particular reference to hypertensive crisis or ischemic cardiac complications [8, 9].

The arterio-venous (AV) fistula for hemodialysis, if present, should be considered and protected during surgery; any decision regarding pressure cuff position, arterial line and central venous lines should be balanced against the position of the AV) fistula and risks of postoperative dysfunction. Similarly postoperative dialysis should be planned in advance, if needed postoperatively.

Anaesthesia can be safely induced with propofol, fentanil, remifentanil and non-depolarizing neuromuscular blocking agents, adjusting doses on renal function and taking account of possible residual activity within the end of surgery [10]. Neuromuscular reversal should be avoided, and adequate analgesia should be granted with advance respect the end of surgery. Fig. **3(a)** and **(b)** show our anaesthetic protocol for kidney transplantation recipients.

Analgesia could be provided *via* IV/IM morphine at fixed hours [11] with implementation with paracetamol [12], avoiding non-steroidal anti inflammatory drugs (NSAIDs) which are well known to be nephrotoxic and interphering with delicate local autoregional mechanisms [13].

In our experience with living kidney donors, which can be extended also to kidney transplanted patient, direct wound infusion of local anaesthetic, such as levobupivcaine or ropivacaine, can be a safe and clinically effective strategy to minimize systemic drug administration [14].

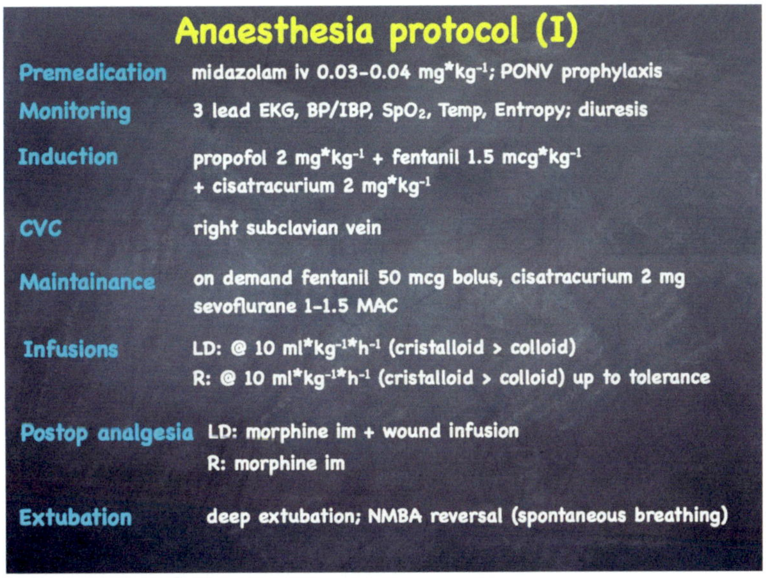

Figure 3(a): Anaesthesiologic protocol at University Hospital of Catania for kidney transplant candidates.

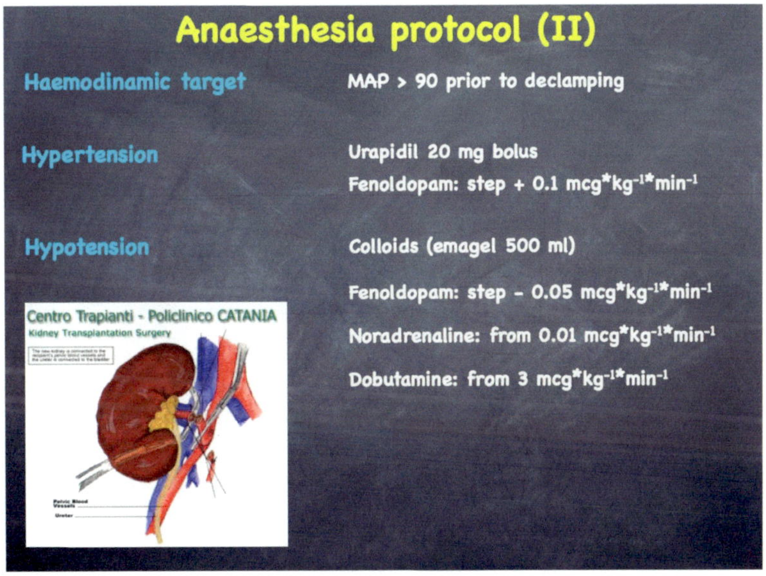

Figure 3(b): Hemodynamic support in kidney transplant candidates.

Nephroprotective Agents

The ideal characteristics of a nephroprotective agent should be on one hand capability of maintaining or increasing renal blood flow and glomerular filtration rate, granting renal perfusion, and on the other the ability of reducing oxygen consumption, especially in case of renal hypoxemia or hypoperfusion.

Normally a certain amount (around 20%) of cardiac output reaches kidney *via* renal arteries; such a flow is used maximally for urine production (around 90%), while the remaining part is addressed to medullary structures in order to provide oxygen and metabolites to all active systems aimed to concentrate urine ("counter-current multiplication") and to promote water and electrolytes re-absorption (Fig. **4**).

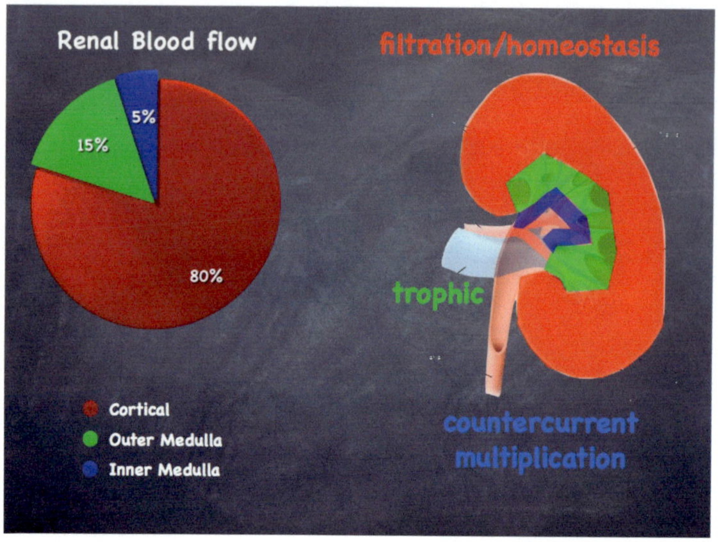

Figure 4: Renal blood flow and kidney filtration.

In such a system, a sudden decrease of renal blood flow, such as in case of hypotension, means a dramatic reduction of oxygen partial pressure and availability, especially in the less perfused and highly-consuming areas of the kidney, particularly medullary structures, with risk of acute tubular necrosis (Fig. **5**).

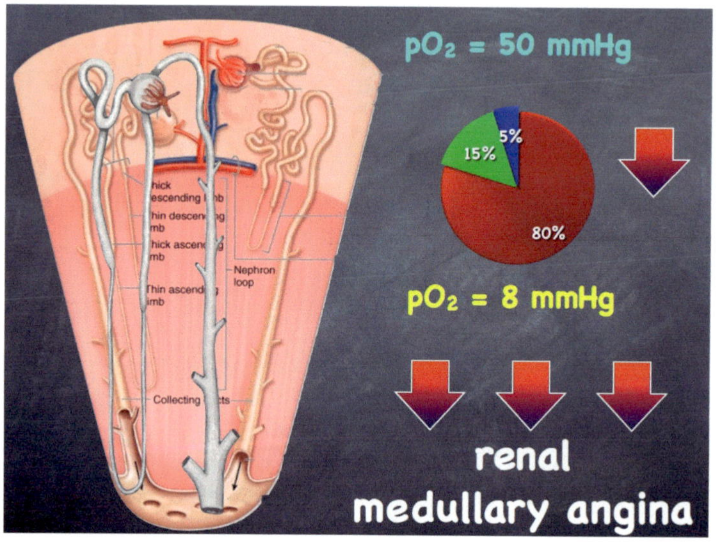

Figure 5: Role renal perfusion and risk of kidney injury.

In the healthy patient, the kidney receives about 20% of the total cardiac output (about 1 litre*min^{-1}), with an oxygen delivery in excess of 80 ml min^{-1}*100 g^{-1} tissue. The distribution of blood flow within the kidney is not uniform, with the cortex receiving more than 90% of total blood flow. On the other hand, oxygen consumption usually does not exceed about 10% of total body utilization, such that there is a low arteriovenous oxygen content difference (1.5 ml oxygen per 100 ml blood). The low fraction of oxygen extraction by the kidney should suggest that there is an adequate and ample oxygen reserve. However, the kidney is highly sensitive to hypoperfusion, with acute renal failure being a frequent complication of hypotension. This apparent paradox (of high blood supply and low extraction of oxygen, yet high incidence of renal damage to hypoperfusion) is related to the physiological gradient of intra-renal oxygenation with the renal medulla able to function at ambient oxygen tensions of 2–3 kPa. This low oxygen tension results from the high oxygen requirement for tubular reabsorptive activity of sodium and chloride. Although a high percentage of blood goes to the cortex (about 5 ml*min^{-1}*g^{-1}), the cortex extracts only about 18% of total oxygen delivered to it. On the other hand, the medullary region has a far smaller blood flow (0.03 ml*min^{-1}*g^{-1}), but has a far greater extraction (of about 79% of the delivered oxygen). Medullary oxygenation is normally strictly balanced by a series of control mechanisms, which match regional oxygen supply and consumption. Failure of these controls renders the outer medullary region susceptible to acute or repeated episodes of hypoxic injury, which may lead to acute tubular necrosis especially of the thick ascending limbs and the straight proximal segments, or to chronic tubulo-interstitial changes respectively.

As a result of the heterogeneity of flow and oxygen requirement, the oxygen tension in the cortex is about 50 mmHg higher than that of the inner medulla. This explains why the thick ascending limbs region is extremely vulnerable to hypoxic injury and why acute tubular necrosis can be induced by as little as a 40–50% decrease in renal blood flow.

Medullary hypoxic injury is characterized by necrosis of those renal tubules that are farthest away from the blood vessels. The main determinant of medullary oxygen requirement is the rate of active reabsorption of salt and water in the thick ascending limbs region. When this process is inhibited by loop diuretics, there is an increase in the medullary tissue oxygen partial pressure from 2 to about 4 kPa.

Providing that in any case blood pressure and circulating volume should be adequately restored, and considering the paramount importance of local autoregulation mechanisms (Fig. **6**), the goal of any effective nephroprotective agent should be helping in maintaining or increasing renal blood flow (meaning maintenance or increase of oxygen delivery), helping in maintenance or increase of glomerular filtration rate (meaning restoring, maintenance or increase of urinary output) and finally optimizing oxygen consumption in the "high-risk" zones. With reference to this last point, decreasing oxygen consumption *via* inhibition of oxygen-consuming structures seems more important than providing pharmacological attempts to increase regional blood flow.

On this point of view, the main and "historical" goal of diuretics was represented by their capability of inhibiting Na-K ATPases and consequentially reduce oxygen consumption, thus resulting in increased urine output because of natriuresis, but without any effect on renal blood flow and glomerular filtration rate.

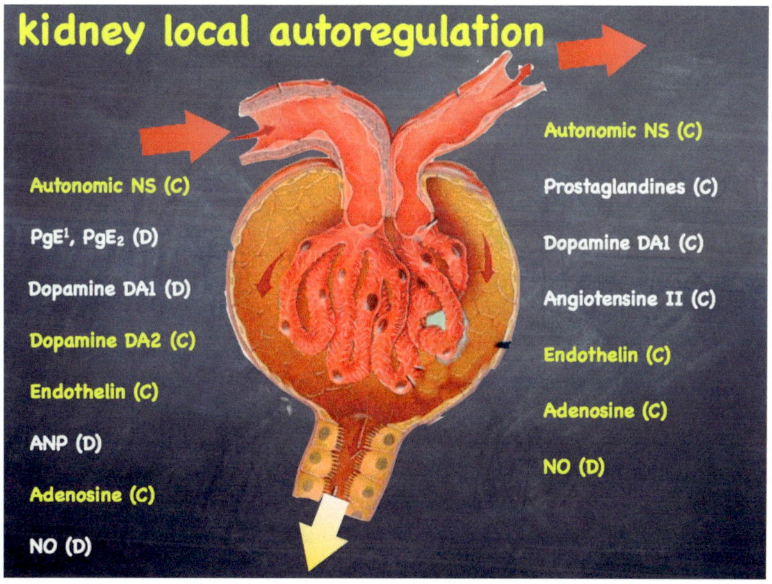

Figure 6: Local autoregulation of kidney in response to hormones.

Most current practices used to provide 'renal protection' are based on tradition, anecdotal information, or extrapolation from animal models. There are few double-blinded, randomized studies in man of sufficient power to allow a definitive assessment of efficacy [15, 16].

Adequate hydration: The most extensive evidence for the role of fluid balance in the development of renal dysfunction is based on studies of radiocontrast nephropathy. These dyes can cause severe intra-renal haemodynamic disturbances, which may result in an ischaemic injury comparable with that seen after major cardiac and aortic surgery. One of the important conclusions of these studies is that pre-contrast hydration reduces the incidence of renal injury.

Diuretics: Molecules such as acetazolamide, furosemide or bumetanide exert a theoretical nephroprotective effect *via* inhibition of medullary structures (resulting in lowering of oxygen consumption) and promoting natriuresis.

Mannitol: Mannitol acts by a number of separate mechanisms: first, as an osmotic diuretic, it causes renal vasodilation through increased prostaglandin production and thereby promotes renal tubular urine flow. This protects against injury by reducing tubular obstruction. It also acts as a free radical scavenger, reducing the effects of hydroxyl and other free radicals in causing ischaemia–reperfusion injury. However, in a recent randomized prospective clinical trial in 28 patients undergoing infra-renal aortic surgery the combination of mannitol (0.3 $g*kg^{-1}$) and saline resulted in no differences in postoperative serum creatinine or urea, or creatinine clearance, with a greater first day diuresis and less glomerular and tubular damage for the mannitol group. To be effective, the mannitol must be given before the ischaemic episode, whereas mannitol can be injurious in large doses causing intra-renal vasoconstriction.

Dopexamine: This synthetic sympathomimetic agonist has a number of different properties but is mainly a b2 agonist synthetic agent, developed as alternative to dopamine to overcome dopamine limits, with particular reference to dopamine induced tachycardia or to detrimental postoperative effects on renal function. In volunteers, dopexamine acts as a positive inotrope to increase the heart rate and decrease the systemic vascular resistance. In animals, dopexamine increases renal blood flow by DA1 agonist to cause intra-renal vasodilatation; an increased cortical but not medullary blood flow; and an increase in urine flow as a result of increased renal blood flow and thence glomerular filtration rate (GFR). However, in human the effects on diuresis and natriuresis are small, and may solely reflect the increase in renal blood flow from the increased cardiac output. Up to date no large studies support or recommend use of dopexamine for nephroprotection.

Dopamine: Dopamine has been historically identified as nephroprotective agent due to its effects on dopaminergic receptors; dopamine has been identified has multi-receptorial agonist on dopaminergic, beta and alpha receptors accordingly to different administration doses.

Recent studies have shown dopamine limits on three different points of view: first of all, not all patient show a linear dose-response curve after dopamine administration; some patient do show tachycardia with low doses while some others do not show any natriuretic effect even on high doses. The second element is that different studies have shown poor or no effect for dopamine in terms of urine output and tubular structures inhibition, so that its effect on oxygen delivery/consumption imbalance has been deeply reviewed. Finally recent papers comparing dopamine with furosemide and placebo have shown some potential detrimental effects on postoperative renal outcome, due to possible down-regulation of dopamine DA1 receptors (with loss of vasodilatative effect on afferent arteriole) and probable dopamine DA2 up-regulation (with possible vasoconstrictive effect on afferent arteriole and lowering of renal blood flow and glomerular filtration rate).

Fenoldopam: Fenoldopam is a selective DA1 agonist born as anti-hypertensive agent (Fig. **7**) with potential nephroprotective capabilities; several studies show that fenoldopam grants normal or increased renal blood flow and glomerular filtration rate despite anti-hypertensive effect if compared with other drugs; other studies indicate that fenoldopam exerts diuretic effect *via* DA_1-mediated tubular Na-K ATPases blockade. These two elements satisfy the concept of DO_2/VO_2 imbalance recovery, suggesting a potential role for fenoldopam use as nephroprotective pharmacologic strategy.

Further, there is robust evidence of renal protection during experimental hypotension [17] or evidence of contrast dye induced nephropathy protection [18] when using fenoldopam; finally it seems that all dopamine-like negative effects, probably due to non selective DA receptors subtypes activation, are not present with fenoldopam because of its DA1 selectivity without any intrinsic activity [19].

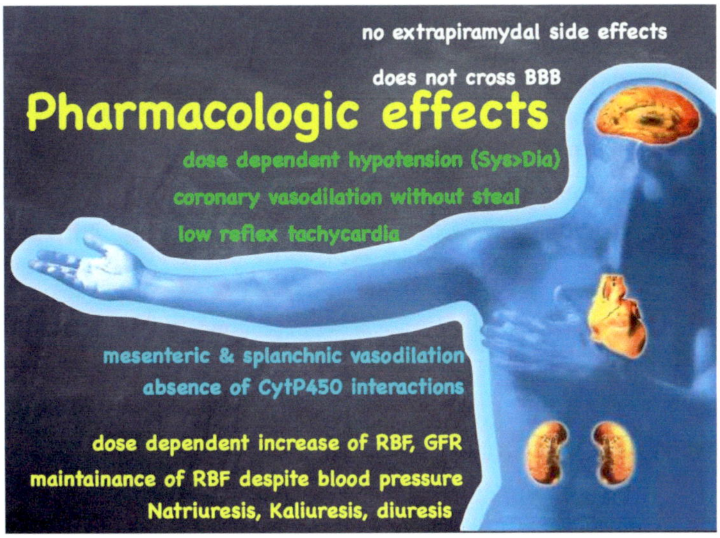

Figure 7: Pharmacological effects of fenoldopam.

The fenoldopam "nephroprotective dose" was fixed in 0.1 mcg*kg^{-1}*min^{-1} continuous infusion, according to Mathur experience [20], providing this dose as the one able to grant renal blood flow and glomerular filtration rate increase, NA-K ATPases blockade without any significant effect on systemic blood pressure and heart rate.

Calcium Antagonists: Molecules such as nifedipine or verapamil were supposed to be potential nephroprotective agents because of their capability of increasing regional blood flow, thus decreasing oxygen imbalance thanks to increased availability. On such basis, some papers showed verapamil to significantly reduce the incidence of acute tubular necrosis following kidney transplantation by presumably increasing renal blood flow and glomerular filtration rate. There are, however, few data examining the possible effects of calcium channel blocking drug on postoperative renal dysfunction, and no major studies have supported such hypothesis, resulting in no evidence to support calcium antagonists use for nephroprotection.

ACE Inhibitors: Some papers showed that increases in renal vascular resistance associated with cross-clamping can be prevented by pre-treatment with ACE-Inhibitors; however, further double-blind controlled studies are needed to support these data and show whether these drugs alter the incidence of perioperative renal dysfunction.

Atrial Natriuretic Peptide: Atrial natriuretic peptide increases glomerular filtration rate by vasodilation of the afferent arterioles and constriction of the efferent arterioles. Atrial natriuretic peptide also increases glomerular permeability and promotes tubular sodium and water loss. To date there are very few studies evaluating the effects of infusions of ANP. The synthetic agent urodilatin has ANP-like activity, but is more haemodynamically stable. There have been a number of studies examining its utility in post-cardiac bypass surgery, but no studies to date of its efficacy in patients undergoing other high-risk surgeries [21-23].

N-Acetyl-Cisteine and Other Agents: NAC and other anti-oxidant agents have been used to prevent contrast-induced nephropathy thanks to its powerful anti-oxidant effect, basing on the concept that kidney injury might be prevented improving renal perfusion and modulating intrarenal pathophysiological mechanisms, first of all formation of free oxygen radicals, inflammation, tubular cast formation and renal (tubular) regeneration. Up to now prospective randomised controlled trials on selective renal vasodilatation have turned out rather unsuccessful, with the exception of the adenosine antagonist theophylline, in certain indications like drug-induced renal failure or contrast nephropathy. Studies in humans on pharmacological interventions interfering with intrarenal pathophysiological mechanisms of acute kidney injury are also sparse. Investigated compounds comprise N-acetyl-cysteine, sodium bicarbonate, prostaglandin E1 and E2 agonists, mannitol and antioxidants like selenium or vitamin C. The results are heterogeneous and a significant beneficial effect of either substance could not yet be convincingly demonstrated. A recent paper from our group [21] further shows that NAC, when added to fenoldopam continuous infusion during kidney transplantation, someway modulates ischemia-reperfusion injury better pH values and better hemodynamics after declamping.

Fenoldopam and Kidney Transplantation

Assuming that an effective nephroprotective strategy, provided an adequate volume support, should promote urine output (indirect result of renal blood flow and glomerular filtration rate maintenance) while inducing urinary electrolytes modifications (as the result of tubular ATPases blockade), what is crucial is the DO_2/VO_2 imbalance. Whenever renal blood flow and/or glomerular filtration rate decrease, a complex neuro-endocrine and humoral response triggers local and systemic hydroelectrolytic and haemodynamic changes aimed to preserve hydroelectrolytic function, even if paying the due of potential kidney damage.

In effect, in a moment in which renal blood flow decreases (thus renal DO_2 decreases), the kidney itself increases its workload (thus renal VO_2 increases), as ATP and oxygen are necessary to let tubular pumps work. This might become a kind of "renal medullary angina" with potential damage and acute tubular necrosis.

Analyzing literature data, different positive results for perioperative renal protection with fenoldopam were identified, including extended indications for fenoldopam use during postoperative phase are available [22].

In our experience, fenoldopam has been used in more than 300 living and deceased donor kidney transplants, and different aspects of fenoldopam continuous infusion have been explored to assess its role in terms of nephroprotection (partially unpublished data).

Fenoldopam has shown a potentially nephroprotective drug turning off medullary oxygen consumption while increasing renal blood flow, glomerular filtration rate and urine output, as demonstrated measuring urine output and modifications in urinary electrolytes excretion during living kidney transplantation [23, 24].

We have previously shown that fenoldopam, added to NAC, was able to modulate ischemia-reperfusion injury during kidney transplantation with positive effects on pH values and hemodynamic performance during intraoperative phase [25].

Further, fenoldopam was compared with dopamine on the same endpoints, resulting in a better and more constant nephroprotective effect in terms of urine output, electrolytes urinary concentrations and avoidance of haemodynamic effects.

Preliminary data in ICU show interesting effects for fenoldopam infusion in potential organ donors; if comparing urine output in the first hours after transplantation, incidence of early graft function and recurrence to dialysis, patients receiving fenoldopam showed better parameters in terms of potential nephroprotective effect.

Finally, our data from long term follow up in patients receiving either living or deceased donor kidney transplantation suggest an interesting and long-lasting effect for patients treated with fenoldopam in the perioperative period of kidney transplantation.

Interestingly, all patients receiving fenoldopam, compared with a historical group of patients, treated with either dopamine or simple fluid expansion, showed a lower recurrence to dialysis, a lower incidence of delayed graft function and better mean scores whenever kidney biopsy was performed during follow up.

A possible hypothesis, requiring experimental animal studies, is that fenoldopam infusion someway might modify expression of surface proteins responsible for partial rejections and, out of all, for delayed graft function or graft failure [24]. When stratifying patients by HLA match, our results show that patients with the same degree of HLA mismatch result in different outcomes if considering those receiving fenoldopam and those who did not receive it.

In some terms, fenoldopam infusion might either improve graft perfusion, minimizing ischaemia-reperfusion damage and consequent expression of Heat Shock Proteins (which have been demonstrated to act as potential rejection source molecules), or act directly *via* dopaminergic receptors stimulation thus modifying expression of surface or intracellular proteins, including HLA complexes and Heat shock Proteins. Interestingly, very recent studies suggest a potential role of fenoldopam in modulation of Heme-Oxygenase expression with potential positive effects on tubular cells apoptosis and ischemic cell death [25] (Fig. **8**).

Definitively further studies are necessary to confirm our data, including important potential implications on early graft function and graft outcome as consequences of improved or poorly compromised O_2 balance and extracellular proteins expression.

Finally, independently on results on fenoldopam effectiveness, which has yet to be studied, our data could be considered as a further indication to abandon daily use of "renal dose" dopamine and to introduce fenoldopam as a pivotal drug for nephroprotection, at least in the field of living and deceased donor kidney transplantation.

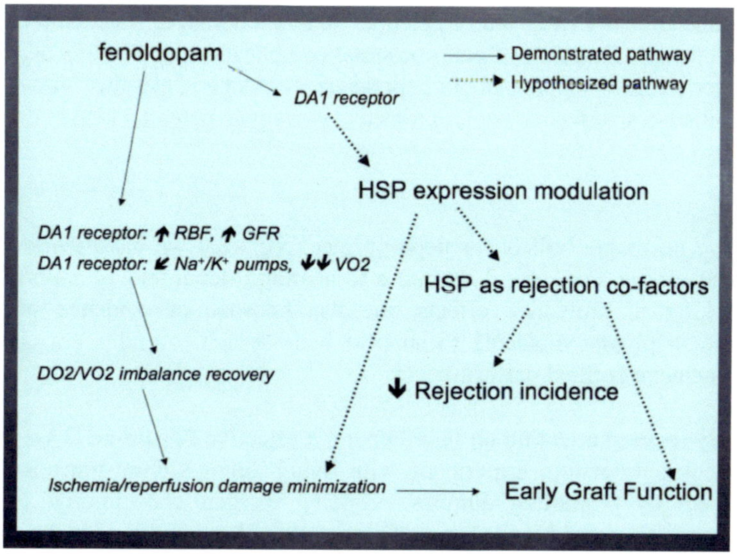

Figure 8: Relationship between fenoldopam, heat shock proteins and acute rejection in kidney transplantation.

Organ Donor

One possible extended use for fenoldopam is nephroprotection in the potential organ donor. Fenoldopam use in ICU *per se* might represent an interesting opportunity, especially taking account of epidemiological data; a recent systematic review [26] found that the overall mortality rate from acute renal failure was relatively unchanged between 1956 and 2003 and remained at approximately 50%.

An interesting and well designed study, investigating the role of fenoldopam in critically patients [27], performed on one hundred adult patients with early renal dysfunction (intensive care unit stay <1 wk, hemodynamic stability, and urine output <0.5 mL/kg over a 6-hr period and/or serum creatinine concentration >1.5 mg/dL and < 3.5 mg/dL) randomized to receive 2 mcg/kg/ min dopamine or 0.1 mcg/kg/min fenoldopam continuous infusion over a 4-day period, demonstrated that fenoldopam at 0.1 mcg/kg/min did not cause any clinically significant hemodynamic impairment and improved renal function compared with renal dose dopamine in the setting of acute early renal dysfunction, resulting effective in the attempt to early reverse of renal hypoperfusion.

Remembering these data, we should underline that organ donor management starts with surveillance to identify ICU patients with severe neurological injury likely to progress to brain death, in order to sustain organ functions and act towards donation consent and organ retrieval as soon as possible.

Aggressive medical management should be maintained throughout the period between brain death and organ retrieval, in order to ensure organ preservation, particularly from ischemic injury.

Within ICU stay particular care should be applied accordingly to donors potentialities, thus choosing for a restricted fluid support in case of lung donation, for a less sustained amine support in case of hearth donation or for a generous volume support and hypotension control in case of kidney donation.

In a preliminary pilot study (unpublished), our group tested the hypothesis of using fenoldopam in a group of ICU brain dead patients received high standard supportive care [28, 29] including amines (dobutamine, noradrenaline), hormones (tiroxine, cortisole, desmopressine), protective ventilation (according to ARDSnetwork standards) comparing fenoldopam 0,1 mcg*Kg*min^{-1} continuous infusion and renal-dose dopamine 3 mcg*Kg*min^{-1} as a nephroprotective strategy. All donors eligible for kidney donation were followed during transplantation, observing no cases of delayed graft function except for one case in dopamine group D.

Our results, with all limitations which might be drawn on a small number of patients, led us to consider as paramount the importance of early detection of potential donors in terms of successful organ maintenance and retrieval, resulting in a lower occurrence of periprocedural complications and in less organ function worsening if compared with longer artificial support. In our experience fenoldopam, together with an aggressive and high standard ICU care resulted in an effective nephroprotective strategy in potential kidney donors.

CONCLUSIONS

To conclude, there are no magic bullets for nephroprotection; what we have learnt is probably what we should not do: there is strong evidence in literature to abandon dopamine as nephroprotective agent, not only because of lacking of protective effects but also because of evidence of detrimental effects; noradrenaline becomes a pivotal molecule to support hemodynamics and a correct fluids management remain mandatory to achieve optimal performance.

Our group has recently focused attention on fenoldopam, a selective dopamine DA-1 receptor agonist with potential effect on nephroprotection. Experience with living donor kidney transplantation indicated that Fenoldopam should act by promoting diuresis, reducing oxygen consumption in the medullary and maintaining, if not increasing, renal blood flow and glomerular filtration rate (Fig. **9**).

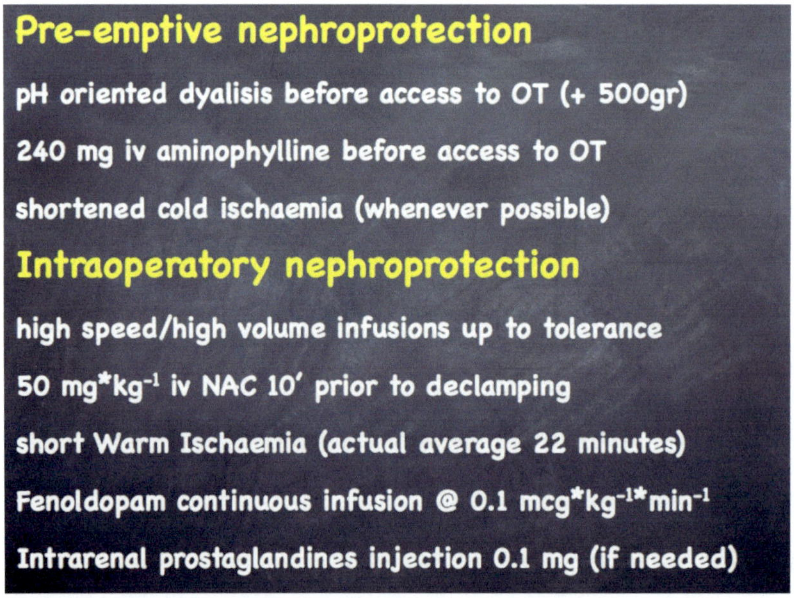

Figure 9: Nephroprotection in living donor kidney transplantation.

Interesting potential effects, which deserve further and methodologically correct studies, seem to affect also heat shock protein expression in the transplanted organ, with great implications on early graft function, need for post-transplant dialysis and long term outcome.

In any case no organ protective strategy is possible if fundamentals of a correct and high standard ICU and perioperative treatment are respected; only if we respect the basics of physiology and pharmacology we would be allowed to think of advanced nephroprotective strategies. Up to then, the main organ to be preserved is always the anaesthesiologists brain.

REFERENCES

[1] Sarinkaapor H, Kaur R, Kaur H. Anaesthesia for renal transplant surgery. Acta Anaesthesiol Scand 2007; 51: 1354–1367

[2] Joyce AT, Iacoviello JM, Nag S, *et al.* End-stage renal disease-associated managed care costs among patients with and without diabetes. Diabetes Care 2004; 27: 2829–2835.

[3] Veroux M, Giuffrida G, Gagliano M, *et al.* Evaluation of thyroid disease in kidney transplantation candidates: management and follow up. Transplant Proc 2009; 41: 1142-1144.

[4] Sorbello M, Veroux M, Cutuli M, *et al.* Anaesthesiologic protocol for kidney transplantation in two patients with Fabry Disease: a case series. Cases Journal 2008, 18; 1: 321.

[5] Goldfarb-Rumyantzev A, Hurdle JF, Scandling J, *et al.* Duration of end-stage renal disease and kidney transplant outcome. Nephrol Dial Transplant 2005; 20: 167–175.

[6] Schnuelle P, Johannes van der Woude F. Perioperative fluid management in renal transplantation: a narrative review of the literature. Transpl Int 2006; 19: 947–959.

[7] Pilmore H. Cardiac Assessment for Renal Transplantation. Am J Transplant 2006; 6: 659–665.

[8] Foley RN, Parfrey PS, Sarnak MJ. The clinical epidemiology of cardiovascular disease in chronic renal disease. Am J Kidney Dis 1998; 32: 112–119.

[9] Locatelli F, Bommer J, London GM, *et al.* Cardiovascular disease determinants in chronic renal failure. Clinical approach and treatment. Nephrol Dial Transplant 2001; 16: 459–468.

[10] Ma H, Zhuang X. Selection of neuromuscular blocking agents in patients undergoing renal transplantation under general anaesthesia. Chin Med J 2002; 11: 1692–1696.

[11] Osborne R, Joel S, Grebenik K, *et al.* Thepharmacokinetics of morphine and morphine glucuronides in kidney failure. Clin Pharm Ther 1993; 54: 158–167.

[12] Martin U, Temple RM, Venkat-Raman G, Prescott LF. Paracetamol disposition in renal allograft recipients. Eur J Clin Pharmacol 2002; 57: 853–856.

[13] Gooch K, Culleton BF, Manns BJ, *et al.* NSAID use and progression of chronic kidney disease. Am J Med 2007; 120: e1–7.

[14] Sorbello M, Paratore A, Morello G, *et al.* Wound levobupivacaine continuous infusion for postoperative analgesia in living to living kidney donors: case-control study. Transplant Proc 2009; 41: 1128-1131.

[15] Sear JW. Kidney dysfunction in the postoperative period. British Journal of Anaesthesia 2005; 95: 20–32.

[16] Thomsen HS. Current evidence on prevention and management of contrast-induced nephropathy. Eur Radiol. 2007;17, Suppl 6: F33-37.

[17] Halpenny M, Markos F, Snow HM, *et al.* Effects of prophylactic fenoldopam infusion on renal blood flow and renal tubular function during acute hypovolemia in anesthetized dogs. Crit Care Med 2001; 29:855–860.

[18] Tumlin JA, Wang A, Murray PT, *et al.* Fenoldopam mesylate blocks reductions in renal plasma flow after radiocontrast dye infusion: A pilot trial in the prevention of contrast nephropathy. Am Heart J 2002; 143: 894–903.

[19] Brienza N, Malcangi V, Dalfino L, *et al.* A comparison between fenoldopam and low-dose dopamine in early renal dysfunction of critically ill patients. Crit Care Med 2006; 34:707–714.

[20] Mathur VS, Swan SK, Lambrecht LJ, *et al.* The effects of Fenoldopam, a selective dopamine receptor agonist, on systemic and renal hemodynamics in normotensive subjects. Crit Care Med 1999; 27: 1832–1837.

[21] Sorbello M, Morello G, Parrinello L, *et al.* Effect of N-acetyl-cysteine (NAC) added to fenoldopam or dopamine on end-tidal carbon dioxide and mean arterial pressure at time of renal artery declamping during cadaveric kidney transplantation. Transplant Proc 2010; 42:1056-1060.

[22] Jones DR, Thomas Lee H. Perioperative renal protection. Best Pract Res Anaest 2008;22: 193–208.

[23] Sorbello M, Morello G, Paratore A, *et al.* Fenoldopam *vs.* Dopamine as a Nephroprotective Strategy During Living Donor Kidney Transplantation: Preliminary Data. Transplant Proc 2007; 39: 1794 –1796.

[24] Trieb K, Dirnhofer S, Krumbock N, *et al.* Heat Shock Protein expression in the transplanted human kidney. Transpl Int 2001; 14: 281-286.

[25] Salahudeen AK, Yang M, Huang H, *et al.* Fenoldopam preconditioning: role of heme oxygenase-1 in protecting human tubular cells and rodent kidneys against cold-hypoxic injury. Transplantation 2011;91:176-182.

[26] Ympa YP, Sakr Y, Reinhart K, Vincent JL. Has mortality from acute renal failure decreased? A systematic review of the literature. Am J Med 2005; 118: 827–832.

[27] Brienza N, Malcangi V, Dalfino L, *et al.* A comparison between fenoldopam and low-dose dopamine in early renal dysfunction of critically ill patients. Crit Care Med 2006; 34:707–714.

[28] DuBose J, Salim A. Aggressive organ donor management protocol. J Intens Care Med 2008; 23:367-375.

[29] Karcioğlu O, Ayrik C, Erbil B. The brain-dead patient or a flower in the vase? The emergency department approach to the preservation of the organ donor. Eur J Emerg Med 2003;10:52-57.

CHAPTER 9

Surgical Techniques of Living Donor Nephrectomy

Ugo Boggi*, Fabio Vistoli, Carlo Moretto, Marco Del Chiaro, Chiara Croce, Stefano Signori, Nelide De Lio, Vittorio Perrone and Gabriella Amorese

Operative Unit Chirurgia Generale e Trapianti nell'Uremico e nel Diabetico Università di Pisa, Azienda Ospedaliero Universitaria Pisana; Ospedale di Cisanello, Pisa, Italy

Abstract: A variety of surgical techniques are currently available for live donor nephrectomy (LDN). The surge of laparoscopic LDN (LLDN) has promoted the reduction of the invasiveness of open donor nephrectomy (ODN). Overall, LDN is a safe operation, the risk of donor death being 0.03%. Long-term complications are rare, and actually live renal donors have a lower risk of end-stage renal failure and live longer as compared with aged-matched individuals who do not donate.

Advantages of LLDN are mostly faster recovery, shorter sick leave, reduced incidence of wound-related complications, and improved cosmetic result. On the other hand, safety is the main advantage of ODN. No donor death has been reported since 1991 following ODN. LLDN increases operative costs, especially when combined with hand assistance, but decreases overall hospital costs and indirect costs.

Bleeding, mostly caused by failure of methods used to seal renal vessel, remains the main surgical complication of LDN. Transfixion ligature is currently recommended for renal arteries, while the use of any type of clips, including locking clips, is banished by the manufacturers themselves. Effective post-operative analgesia also plays an important role since it reduces the arising of hypertensive peaks. Awareness of the risk of massive hemorrhage after LDN is fundamental to reduce the risk of this dramatic complication.

Overall, based on current information no technique of LDN is definitely superior. Transplant surgeons should therefore be familiar with multiple methods of LDN in order to be able to select the one that best fits the needs of each individual donor.

Keywords: Live Donor Nephrectomy, Open Live Donor Nephrectomy, Laparoscopic Live Donor Nephrectomy, Laparo-Endoscopic Single Site Surgery Live Donor Nephrectomy, Robot-Assisted Live Donor Nephrectomy, Complications of Live Donor Nephrectomy.

INTRODUCTION

Compared with dialysis, kidney transplantation improves quality of life [1], facilitates social rehabilitation [2], reduces death rate [3, 4], and diminishes the costs put on health reimbursement systems [5]. Live donor kidney transplantation (LDKT), in particular, is the ideal solution to end-stage renal disease since, compared with deceased donor kidney transplantation (DDKT), it offers substantially superior graft function and survival [6]. These considerations, along with the ever increasing gap between demand and number of kidneys available for transplantation, have led to a considerable increase in LDKT activity in most western countries. In 2001 in the United States, for the first time, the number of living donors exceeded the number of deceased donors for kidney transplantation (http:/www.unos.org). Although this result has not been duplicated yet in Europe (Fig. **1**), in many European countries the rate of LDKT currently exceeds 10 LDKT pmp per year (Denmark 11 LDKT pmp; Iceland 26 LDKT pmp; Netherlands 17 LDKT pmp; Norway 17 LDKT pmp; Sweden 14 LDKT pmp; Switzerland 16 LDKT pmp; UK 11 LDKT pmp) [7]. Growth of LDKT has paralleled that of DDKT and countries with the highest rate of kidney transplantation are very active and successful in both live and deceased donor programs [7].

***Address correspondence to Ugo Boggi:** University of Pisa, Genaral Surgery and Transplantation Unit, Azienda Ospedaliero Universitaria Pisana, Ospedale di Cisanello *Via* Paradisa 2, 56124 PISA, Italy; Phone:+39 050 996926; Fax: +39 050 996800; E-mail: u.boggi@med.unipi.it

Massimiliano Veroux and Pierfrancesco Veroux (Eds)

It has been estimated that 27,000 live donor nephrectomies (LDN) are performed annually worldwide, accounting for some 40% of all kidney transplants. These estimates do not include an additional 10% of LDKT performed under illegal conditions, including commercialism. The greatest number of LDKT are performed in the US (with some 6500 cases per year), followed by Brazil (n ~1800), Iran (n ~1600), Mexico (n ~1500), and Japan (n ~900). The highest rate of LDKT per million population, however, is achieved in Saudi Arabia (32 pmp) followed by Jordan (29 pmp), Iceland (26 pmp), Iran (23 pmp) and the US (21 pmp) [7].

In this chapter we present the surgical techniques of LDN. Possible complications and safety issues are emphasized since the health and well being of live donors remains the main outcome of LDKT and accepts no compromise.

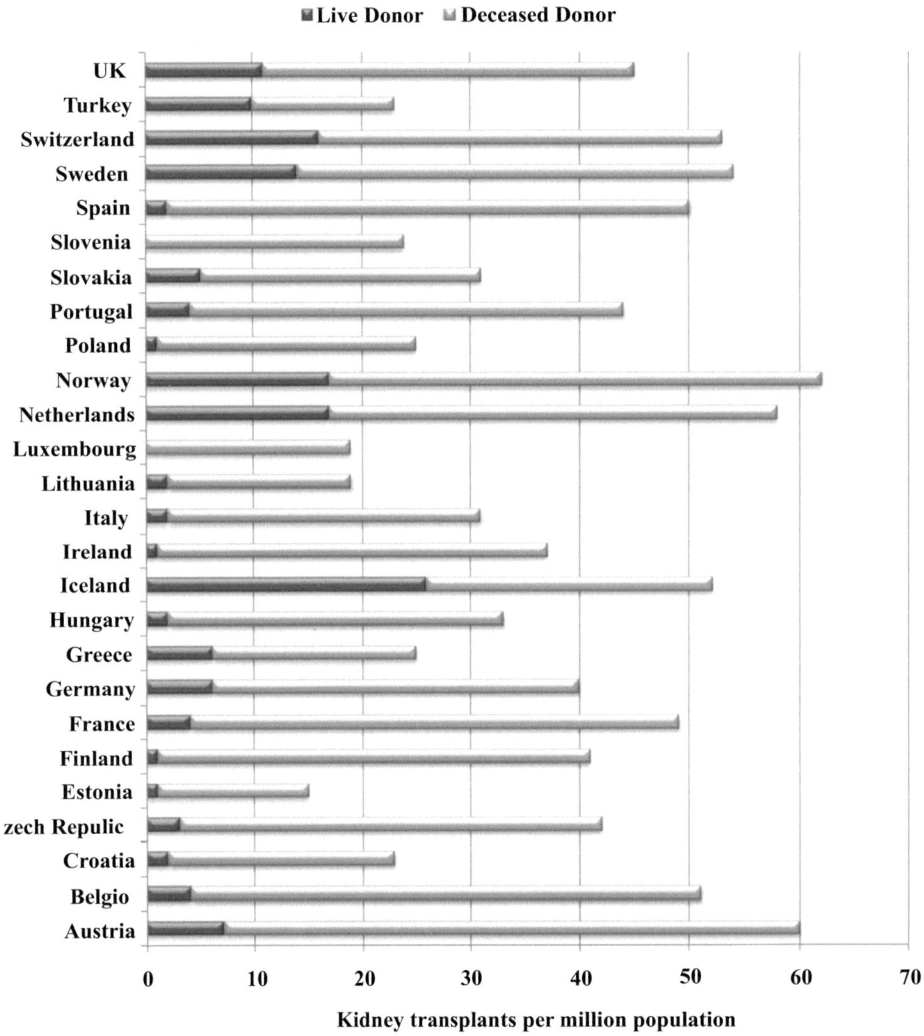

Figure 1: Rate of kidney transplants in Europe, per million population, in the year 2006.

DONOR SAFETY

Overall, the expected rate of donor death following renal procurement is 0.03% [8]. This rate has substantially not changed with time. It should however be noted that, no deaths have been reported as a consequence of open donor nephrectomy (ODN) since 1991, while a total of 11 donor deaths have been reported following the introduction of laparoscopic live donor nephrectomy (LLDN) in 1995. Pulmonary embolism is the leading cause of donor death but arterial hemorrhage also plays an important role [8]. In a recent survey, Matas *et al.* reported two donor deaths and one persistent vegetative state, all from hemorrhagic shock, in 10,828 LDN [9]. According to these figures the risk of donor death is 1 out of 5,414 LDN (0.018%), but a more realistic appraisal including the patient in persistent vegetative state brings the risk back to the "historical" risk of 0.03% (0.027%). In a UK survey no donor deaths were reported after 2509 LDN. A more detailed analysis, however, showed that one donor had died 3 months after LDN from myocardial infarction. This donor, discharged after an uneventful course on the 6th post-donation day, had already suffered a first myocardial infarction on the 10th post-operative day. Presuming that this death was related to the recent surgery, the rate of donor death in the UK survey is 0.04% [10].

Non fatal perioperative complications occur in 0.3% to 3% of donors after ODN, and in 1% to 17% of donors following LLDN. Blood transfusions are required in up to 5% of ODN intraoperatively and in a further 5% postoperatively. Equivalent rates for LLDN are 10% and 7%, respectively [8]. Frequent surgical complications include: bleeding (1-6%), wound infection (0.6% - 21%), pneumonia (2.5% - 10%), urinary tract infection (~ 7%), and pneumothorax (0.6% - 9%) [11].

In general, LDN is a safe procedure, although it entails a very low risk of donor death and a more realistic risk of postoperative complications.

DONOR WORK-UP

Donor safety begins with meticulous pre-donation work-up. In part because of this initial screening living kidney donors live longer than the age-matched general population. Fehrman-Ekhom *et al.* showed that 85% of donors were alive 20 years after nephrectomy, while expected survival was 65% [12].

Approximately 50% of potential donors will not be declared suitable. The majority of unsuitable donors are healthy subjects that could donate safely, but that are not compatible with their intended recipient due to AB0 incompatibility or positive (T cell) crossmatch reaction. Positive B cell crossmatch is a relative contraindication, since it decreases 5 year graft survival by 4-6% only [13]. Tissue compatibility is not an issue, unless the recipient is immunized, and can be used to select one donor when multiple subjects are willing and otherwise suitable [14]. Survival of grafts from fully HLA unmatched live donors equals survival of grafts from fully HLA matched deceased donors [15, 16]. In other instances the donor is discarded because of presence of transmittable diseases (infection o cancer) or other medical problems (diabetes, sever hypertension, insufficient renal reserve, *etc.*). Absolute surgical contraindications are rarely encountered, in seemingly healthy persons, and are often relative and operator dependant. Absolute surgical contraindications include bilateral fibromuscular dysplasia (prevalence in kidney donors 4.4%) [17], and renal stones at high risk of recurrence (such as those caused by inherited disorders, inflammatory bowel disease, or systemic disease) [14]. Obesity makes LDN more troublesome and may significantly increase operative times, but it has not been clearly associated with increased morbidity or mortality. Donors with a body mass index exceeding 35 kg/m^2 should be encouraged to lose weight since obesity has been associated with proteinuria and hypertension, and includes the risk for diabetes [14, 15].

The field of donor evaluation is really vast and beyond the specific purposes of this chapter. A summary of stepwise evaluation of candidates to live kidney donation is shown in Table **1**. More insights are provided by the Amsterdam forum [14], although not all possible issues are covered and "uncommon" situations are often encountered in clinical practice and challenge the experience of transplant teams.

Autopsy studies have shown that multiple renal arteries are found in 18% to 30% of subjects, being bilateral in 15% [18]. Venous variations are also very frequent. Multiple renal veins are encountered in some 10% of renal donors [19], but their prevalence on the right side ranges between 15% and 28% [20]. Circumaortic left renal veins have a prevalence of 8%-17% and retroaortic renal veins are seen in 3% of donors [20]. Since renal veins collateralize, small accessory veins can be ligated and are of no concern for transplantation. Unrecognized accessory renal veins, however, may be incidentally injured or torn during procurement potentially causing severe bleeding, requiring either transfusion or conversion to open surgery. Radiologists should be therefore aware of the relevance of accessory renal veins, especially in the current era of minimally invasive surgery, and use appropriate technology and methodology to maximize their identification.

Table 1: Main investigations for potential living donors

STEP 1	
Anamnesis	
Physical examination	
STEP 2	
Laboratory tests	Blood type, T and B cell cross-match reaction, tissue typing (HLA-DR, A, B)
	Urinalysis, urine culture
	Serum creatinine, urea nitrogen
	Cell counts (erythrocytes, leukocytes total, leukocytes differential, platelets)
	Hemoglobin, hemoglobin A_{1C}, hematocrit
	Coagulation tests (partial thromboplastin time, prothrombin time, fibrinogen)
	Electrolytes(Na, K, Cl, Ca, Mg, P)
	Liver tests (bilirubin, ALT, ALP, AST, γ-glutamyltransferase, LDH)
	Serum proteins, glucose, Creatine kinase, pancreatic enzymes (amylase, lipase)
	Lipids (total cholesterol, HDL cholesterol, LDL cholesterol, tryglicerides)
	Serology (HIV, HBAg, HCV, CMV, EBV, VDRL)
	Tumor markers (CEA, Ca 19.9, PSA [males > 40 years], Ca 125 [females > 40 years
	Serum pregnancy test (pre-menopausal females)
Non-invasive instrumental investigations	Electrocardiogram
	Chest X-ray
	Abdominal ultrasound
	Pap test (cervical smear) (> 30 years)
STEP 3	
Creatinine clerance	
Special consultations	Cardiologist
	Gynecologist (> 40 years)
	Physcologist
	Others (as required)
Non-invasive instrumental investigations	Mammography
	Ecochardiogram
	Sequential renal scintigraphy
	Others (as required)
STEP 4	
Invasive/sophisticated instrumental investigations	Gastroscopy
	Colonoscopy
	Multislice CT (with multiplanar vascular reconstruction and pyelographic images)
	(or) Magnetic resonance angiography
	(Angiography)
	Others (as required)

Assessment of Vascular Anatomy and its Practical Implications

Although the number of renal arteries is not an absolute contraindication to LKDT, number, size and location of renal arteries should be known before LDN. Further, in case of single artery the level of first branching is also important. The course of vessels (*e.g.,* retroaortic renal vein, precaval right renal artery) should also be known [21]. These information will be evaluated also in the light of recipient status (*e.g.,* presence of calcified or diseased vessels precluding some reconstruction options, small size pediatric recipients) to select the kidney to be procured. Some surgeons may prefer to discard a donor because of multiple vessels and/or early branching. Actually, the presence of accessory arteries to the lower renal pole may be associated with an increased rate of ureteral complications [19].

Angiography has dominated the evaluation of vascular anatomy of live donor kidneys for a long period. Current availability of alternative, non-invasive, methods has reduced the use of angiography to well selected cases. In general angiography beautifully depicts arterial anatomy while is less reliable for the veins [22]. Its ability to detect and define fibromuscular dysplasia is unchallenged by other imaging modalities [20].

Computed tomography (CT) angiography is highly efficient in defining vascular anatomy of kidney grafts. In a study from Lewis *et al.* 48 renal arteries and 41 renal veins were detected at surgery. Using spiral technology, CT angiography had predicted 47 arteries (98%) and 40 veins (98%). The missed accessory artery, was a third artery of less than 2 millimeters in diameter [23]. Further, CT gives a comprehensive assessment of kidneys and other abdominal organs. Although, as compared with angiography, the arterial anatomy is not quite as defined, CT offers a superior view of veins, requires only a peripheral intravenous injection (rather than an arterial puncture) and does not require bed rest and puncture site compression, so that the donor can leave the hospital immediately [22].

Kok *et al.* compared vascular anatomy at operation with preoperative imaging by magnetic resonance (MR) angiography and digital subtraction angiography in 288 LDKT. MR imaging failed to predict arterial anatomy in 23 of 220 donors (10%) compared with 3 of 101 (3%) after angiography. In this study the sensitivity of MR angiography and digital subtraction angiography in depicting renal arteries was 0.61 and 0.81, respectively (specificity 0.98 and 1.00, respectively) [19].

The main drawback of MR are motion artifacts. Hence, donors should fully understand instructions before being imaged by MR angiography or should undergo CT angiography [19].

Renal Artery Aneurysm

Renal artery aneurysms (RAA) occur in approximately 0.09% of the general population [24]. In an institutional survey, Henke *et al.* reported on 252 RAA in 168 patients (mean age 51 years). The majority of patients were asymptomatic (55%), although often hypertensive (73%), and females were more frequent than males (107:61). RAA were multiple in 53 patients (31,5%) and bilateral in 32 (19%). The right kidney was affected more often (60%) than the left one (40%). RAA were saccular in 79% of patients, the remaining being fusiform, 63% were noncalcified, and were located more often at the bifurcation of the main renal artery (60%). First order renal branches were also involved frequently [24].

Kidneys from donors with RAA have been successfully transplanted [24-29]. Subjects with RAA can be accepted as living kidney donors if there are no other signs of vascular disease, if the etiology of the aneurysm is different from fibromuscular dysplasia, and if the RAA can be resected and safely reconstructed [26-29]. Specific informed consent should be obtained from both donor and recipient. The recipient, in particular, should be aware of the fact that graft suitability can only be defined after reconstruction of the renal artery at the back table. The authors of this chapter have a rather vast experience with *ex vivo* excision of RAA, reconstruction of renal artery and renal autotransplantation. We have also successfully procured (laparoscopically), repaired *ex vivo*, and transplanted a kidney graft with single RAA from a father into his son.

Fibromuscular Dysplasia

In a recent survey of 716 donor angiographies, Neymark *et al.* found abnormal findings in 78 subjects (10,9%), which were unilateral in 51 persons (65%) and bilateral in 27 (35%). In unilateral lesions the right kidney was involved more often than the left one (75% *vs.* 25%). Overall in 47 patients (47/716; 6,6%) abnormal arteriographic findings were attributed to fibromuscular dysplasia [30]. Thus, it is expected that approximately 1 out of 22 renal donors have fibromuscular dysplasia. The lower diagnostic power of CT and MR, as compared to angiography, makes it likely to miss diagnosis in donors with unilateral mild findings, especially if located in the mid-to-distal portion of the renal artery [30, 31]. Despite these donors could be deemed suitable anyway, missing the diagnosis does not allow the transplant team to properly select the side of LDN. Notably, fibromuscular dysplasia occurs more frequently in young and middle-aged women, who currently constitute a relevant proportion of potential live donors [31].

Highly selected subjects with mild anatomic abnormalities have been accepted for kidney donation with good LDKT results [32]. However, bilateral disease and severe anatomic abnormalities (irregularity with greater than 50% stenosis or aneurysm) represent a formal contraindication to donation [16]. Undetected or untreated fibromuscular dysplasia may induce hypertension and ischemic renal failure both in the recipient, if transplanted with the lesion, and in the donor, if the remaining single kidney is affected [31].

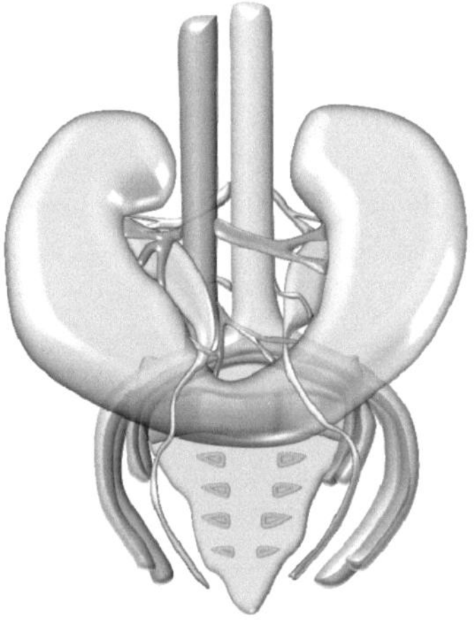

Figure 2: Horsheshoe kidney.

Horseshoe Kidney

Horsheshoe kidney (HK) is the most common variation of renal anatomy with an incidence of one in 600-800 population, are more frequent in males than in females (2:1), and may occur familial [33-36]. In the majority of cases HKs are joined to the lower poles [37], although in 5% of subjects are united to the upper poles [36]. Two patterns of fusion of the renal units are recognized: midline fusion and lateral fusion. In the latter instance, the calyceal system may drain a portion of the contralateral renal unit [36]. The vascular anatomy of HKs is highly variable, in number, origin and size of both arteries and veins. Some 30% of HKs, however, are supplied by single renal arteries. Since the ascent of HKs is limited by the inferior mesenteric vein, HKs are located lower than expected, the isthmus being usually located at the level of sacral promontory. Because of fusion of lower poles and the consequent lack of medial rotation during embryogenesis, the renal pelvis are located in a rather ventral position and ureters hence course in front, rather than behind, the lower poles (Fig. **2**) [36].

Split HKs have been successfully transplanted from both deceased [33, 35, 36, 38] and living renal donors [36-38]. Actually, the first HK that was transplanted was a split graft from a living donor [36]. A questionnaire survey sent to members of the European Society for Organ Transplantation shows that most European surgeons (71.4%) consider post-transplant results of HKs to be equal to those of "normal" kidneys [34]. However, while HKs from deceased donors can be transplanted either en-bloc or as split grafts, organs procured form live donors must be split. Division of HKs from live donors requires that graft procurement does not compromise the function of the kidney remaining with donor. The decision to accept HKs for LDKT, although clearly demanding, is not forced by time constraint or limitation in diagnostic studies. Exclusion criteria for live donation of split HKs are a donor history of urinary tract disease (*i.e.* recurrent urinary tract infections, renal stones, and hydronephrosis) a communicating calyceal system, and complex vascular anatomy [34, 37]. Venous anatomy should also be considered [34] and presence of a fibrous (15% of cases) [36] or thin isthmus is preferable [34].

The authors of this chapter have transplanted one split HK from a live donor. The decision to accept the donor was based on the aforementioned criteria. Although at the authors' institution all kidney grafts from live donors are currently procured by laparoscopy, in this donor we have preferred a conventional transperitoneal approach through a midline incision. We acknowledge that HK can be split and procured by laparoscopy [39, 40]. Our decision was based on the fact that through an open approach we were fully capable of splitting the HK maximizing the safety of the donor while preserving the anatomic integrity of either HK halves.

PREOPERATIVE MANAGEMENT

Donors are usually admitted the day before surgery and are quickly, but comprehensively, reassessed (chest radiograph, electrocardiogram, and standard biochemistry and hematology tests). At most centers donors receive overnight hydration with intravenous infusion of dextrose (5%) and saline solution at the rate of approximately 2 ml/kg/hr [41]. The rest of preoperative management is identical to standard practice in patients requiring nephrectomy because of renal disease.

ANESTHESIA AND INTRAOPERATIVE MANAGEMENT

The operating table is equipped with a heating blanket. A CO_2 heater is also useful in case of LLDN.

Anesthesia is induced using fentanyl (0.2 mg), sodium thiopental (3 mg/kg^{-1}) and atracurium besilate, and it is maintained using sevofluorane in a 50% air oxygen low flow (2 L/min) respiratory mixture delivered by a volumetric ventilator. Atracurium besilate is used in a continuous infusion (0.01 mg/kg^{-1}/min^{-1}) to achieve the necessary neuromuscular blockade [42]. Intraoperative hemodynamic monitoring includes ECG, mean arterial pressure, and central venous pressure. Respiratory monitoring includes end tidal CO_2 and pulse O_2. At the end of operation donors are closely observed for the first 12 hours with special attention to hemodynamic stability and pain control. Effective post-operative analgesia avoids high peaks of hypertension and significantly reduces the risk of post-operative hemorrhage.

After administration of anesthesia, a Foley catheter is introduced aseptically into the bladder. The legs are wrapped with compressive banding or with sequentially squeezing stockings to reduce venous pooling in the lower extremities. The donor is then placed in the planned operative position. Pillows and foam are used liberally to prevent undue pressure lesions. The patient is then secured to the table using wide banding or strips of adhesive tape. Although anticipated blood loss during donor nephrectomy is minimal and the need for intraoperative blood transfusion does not exceed 5-7% [8], packed red blood cells should be available in the operating room before starting with donor surgery. Preoperative blood banking is not standard and complicates the organization of the procedure. It can be considered in selected patients, although it does not seem to be really useful since renal donors must not be anemic at baseline, intraoperative blood loss is usually limited and when it rarely occurs it is sudden and massive almost certainly exceeding the amount of banked autologous blood. Likewise, it is not standard to use intraoperative blood salvage since the amount of bleeding is expected to be minimal and routine use of intraoperative blood salvage would be cost-ineffective.

As soon as vital signs are stabilized, efforts of anesthesia team are focused on maintaining proper hydration and brisk diuresis. Hydration, key for all donors, is especially important to counterbalance the effects of pneumoperitoneum on kidney perfusion [43]. Although diuretics are not recommended routinely, mannitol is frequently used mostly as a cytoprotectant before kidney manipulation. Small doses of intravenous furosemide (20 mg) may occasionally be needed.

Once the kidney has been completely dissected, and the surgeon is ready for vascular cross-clamping, the anesthesiologist is asked to deliver a systemic bolus of sodium heparin (70 U/kg) which will be reversed, by slow infusion of an equivalent dose of protamine sulfate, immediately after closure of renal vessels [41].

BASIC SURGICAL CONCEPTS

Regardless of the methods used for LDN there are several principles that must be respected to properly procure kidney grafts, maximize their chance of immediate function, and reduce the risk of long-term urologic and vascular complications. Some of these caveats should also be used in renal procurement from deceased donors, but others are unique to LDN since dissection is carried out while the kidney is perfused and because the surgeon must respect at the same time graft integrity and donor safety.

Handling of Urether

Some urologic complications are prompted by inappropriate handling of donor ureter resulting in acute or chronic ischemia.

Native ureters derive their blood supply from several sources with which they are closely associated anatomically as they descend from the hilus of the kidney. Branches may be obtained from the suprarenal, renal, gonadal, common iliac and internal iliac arteries. In general, the proximal and the distal ends of the ureter receive a greater number of branches.

In the isolated kidney graft the ureter receives its entire blood supply from descending vessels that emanate in the hilar and upper periareaolar tissue. These sites are vulnerable to injury during donor nephrectomy.

To reduce the possibility of devascularization, the ureter should be mobilized en-bloc with surrounding adipose tissue. The gonadal vein should also be kept adherent to the ureter. Attention should also be paid to avoid thermal injury. Using the harmonic scalpel, for instance, the increase of tissue temperature 1.0 centimeter away from the tips of the instrument exceeds 140 degrees Celsius, if the device is activated for 15 seconds at a power level of 5 [44]. Thus, especially when dissection is closer to the ureteral adventia, such as at the level of the iliac vessels, cold dissection techniques are preferable. If the kidney is procured laparoscopically, use of a dissecting hook connected to a low-energy electrocautery may be an alternative to pure cold dissection.

Finally, blood supply may also be compromised if the ureter in the recipient is left either too long or too short.

Multiple Renal Arteries

Considering the high sensitivity of the current state of the art imaging, most of vascular variations are known when planning donor surgery. However, renal transplant surgeons should be mentally and technically prepared to face unexpected hilar vascular anomalies. Presence of multiple renal arteries complicates donor and recipient surgery. It is clear that handling multiple vessels prolongs operative times, and increases warm ischemia time [45], possibly resulting in higher rates of delayed graft function and triggering late rejection episodes. Further, especially if the diameter of the accessory artery (or arteries) is small the risk of vascular complications is expected to increase, and may possibly result in higher risk of urological complications [46-48].

Because of these considerations, we prefer to revascularize all accessory arteries irrespective of their diameter. Other authors, however, have reported that revascularization of arteries supplying less than 5% to 10% of the renal parenchyma or less than 2 millimeters in diameter is not mandatory [49]. As specifically regards the incidence of urologic complications, however, it is important to note that the risk of anastomotic fistula o stricture increases when grafts with lower pole arteries are considered [50].

Techniques for Vascular Control

The technique used for vascular control is of overwhelming importance.

In October 2003 Friedman *et al.* sent a 33-question survey to all 893 surgeon-members of the American Society of Transplant Surgeons. Questions posed included details about member training in ODN or LLDN, as well as the techniques used to control the renal artery and vein during donor nephrectomy. Two hundred and thirteen surveys (24%) were returned. In ODN artery control was more commonly achieved with a simple tie plus suture ligature (85 surgeons; 40%) and oversewing (52 surgeons; 24%) while in laparoscopy most surgeons used the gastro intestinal anastomosis (GIA) stapler (64 surgeons, 30%) or multiple locking clips (39 surgeons, 18%). Sixty-six episodes of arterial hemorrhage and 39 of venous hemorrhage were disclosed. Two patients (3%) died as a consequence of arterial bleeding, 2 (3%) developed end-stage renal failure, 19 (29%) required blood transfusions, and 29 (44%) required repeat surgery or conversion to open nephrectomy. Arterial hemorrhage occurred more frequently when artery occlusion employed nontransfixion techniques (45; 68%). In the two fatal cases and in the two patients developing end-stage renal failure the renal artery had been managed by multiple locking clips (hem-o-lok) [51].

Teleflex MEDICAL

2345 Waukegan Road, Suite 120
Bannockburn, IL 60015 USA

Phone (USA): (800) 334-9751
International: (919) 433-4952

www.teleflexmedical.com

Important Product Safety Information

April 11, 2006

Re: Contraindication For Use of Hem-o-lok Ligating Clips in Laparoscopic Donor Nephrectomy

Catalog Number (REF)	Description
544250	Hem-o-lok XL
544240	Hem-o-lok L
544230	Hem-o-lok ML
543965	Hem-o-lok ML automatic endoscopic applier

Dear Valued Customer and Healthcare Provider:

The purpose of this communication is to provide you with important information regarding the use of our Hem-o-lok® Non-absorbable Polymer Ligating Clips in laparoscopic donor nephrectomy. Teleflex Medical has been made aware of rare incidents in which the ligating clips (sizes L and XL) were reported to have become dislodged following ligation of the renal artery after laparoscopic donor nephrectomy.

Our preliminary assessment is that none of the incidents appears to have involved any defect in or malfunction of the Hem-o-lok® ligating clips. We are aware, however, that laparoscopic donor nephrectomies pose special surgical challenges, including the surgeon's desire to maximize the length of the renal artery removed from the donor in order to facilitate the arterial anastomosis of the transplanted kidney. In rare instances, misapplication of the Hem-o-lok® clips during such laparoscopic procedures may not immediately be apparent, but can have serious, even life-threatening consequences post-operatively. Because of the nature of this risk and the surgical challenges posed by ligation of the renal artery during laparoscopic donor nephrectomies, we are adding a contraindication to the Instructions for Use accompanying Hem-o-lok® Polymer Ligating Clips specifically directed to this procedure—ligation of the renal artery during laparoscopic nephrectomies in living donor patients.

Our decision to contraindicate is limited solely to the use of Hem-o-lok Polymer® Ligating Clips for ligating the renal artery in laparoscopic donor nephrectomies. We recognize that the clips are used in many other types of surgical procedures, and we continue to believe that the clips offer unique advantages when used as directed in other procedures.

A sample of a revised Instructions for Use is attached for your convenience, and the two modified sections now read as follows:

> **"CONTRAINDICATIONS":**
> **Hem-o-lok® ligating clips are contraindicated for use in ligating the renal artery during laparascopic nephrectomies in living donor patients.**
>
> **"CAUTION":**
> **The clip must be latched to ensure proper ligation of the vessel or tissue. Inspect the ligation site after application to ensure proper closure of the clip. Security of the closure should be confirmed after ligation. The Hem-o-lok Polymer Ligating Clip is not designed for use as a tissue marker. Weck recommends that more than one clip be used to ligate the renal artery in procedures other than laparoscopic donor nephrectomy (see CONTRAINDICATION, above). Application of more than one clip to all other vessels should be left to the surgeon's judgment.**

Figure 3: Product safety information from Teleflex Medical, prohibits the use of hem-o-lok on renal arteries in laparoscopic donor nephrectomy.

Between January 1992 and March 2006 the Manufacturer and User Facility Device Experience (MAUDE) database, that catalogs complications involving medical devices reported to the Food and Drug Administration (FDA) recorded 2172 kidney-related complications. A total of 352 (16%) of these complications involved failures of hemostatic devices during laparoscopic surgery. The endovascular staplers had the greatest number of total failures (223; 63%), followed by titanium clips (111; 33%). Locking clips had the fewest reported complications with 18 (5%) failures. All device types had specific mechanisms of failure, including the human error [52]. Consequences of device failure, however, were very much different. Indeed, probably because of the often delayed arising of hemorrhage [53, 54], 3 patients treated with locking clips (3/18 17%) died [52]. Although the percentages obtained from the MAUDE database should be interpreted with caution, because of the voluntary nature of report and the consequent lack of reliable denominator, as a matter of fact, use of both titanium clips and polimer locking clips on renal artery is banished by manufacturer themselves (Fig. **3**) [52].

Although considering the Teleflex safety information there seems to be little room to use hem-o-lok clips on renal arteries, Ponsky *et al.* reported 1695 laparoscopic nephrectomies without hem-o-lok failures [55]. These authors emphasized the importance of proper selection of clip size (L-purple for the artery, and XL-gold for the vein) and accurate preparation of the vessel before placing the clip [55].

The occurrence of failures can also be reduced by avoiding the use of energy sources (such as harmonic scalpel and monopolar cautery) close to hem-o-lok clips, since the thermal injury may weaken the polymer, possibly resulting in delayed failure of the clip [53]. Finally, when using any kind of clips judicious placement is required also because they may preclude later application of vascular stapler or cause device malfunction [53].

Left or Right Kidney

The kidney that remains with the donor must be completely normal and fully functional. Thus, when there is a significant disparity in the function donor's kidneys, it is mandatory to leave the best functioning organ with the donor [56-58]. In the other cases the selection of which kidney to procure is mostly a surgeon's decision.

Many surgeons prefer the left kidney because the vein is longer and has thicker walls when compared with the right one. Some 30% of European centers accept only left kidneys [58], mostly because of the reported higher risk of venous thrombosis when using right kidney grafts [59] and the greater technical challenge posed by vein control close to the inferior vena cava in the donor and possible need for vein elongation in the recipient [60]. Some authors, on the contrary, preferentially procure the right kidney because on this side the renal vein usually has fewer and smaller posterior branches [57]. Most experiences actually show equivalent success of LDKT using either left or right kidney grafts [57, 60, 61], making the decision of which kidney to procure mostly a matter of surgeons' preference.

When both kidneys have single renal vessels, the left kidney is usually preferred because of the more favorable vein [56]. Some surgeons, however, prefer to have the left kidney even when this graft has anatomic variations and the right one has one artery and one vein [56]. In case of ureteral duplication the kidney with a single ureter is preferentially selected for LDKT because of the lower risk of urologic complications in the recipient. Other, minor, practical considerations are the risk of splenic tears on the left side, occasionally requiring splenectomy [57], and the risk of hepatic injury [60] on the right side, secondary to liver retraction. In female donors of childbearing age the right kidney may be preferred, because the left kidney is often spared by hydronephrosis during pregnancy [62].

In case of LLDN, strategies have been developed to maximize the length of the right renal vein. Some authors, after complete dissection of the kidney, perform short incisions in the right upper abdominal quadrant or flank region, and introduce a Satinski clamp onto the vena cava (Fig. **4a**). The same incision is used to extract the kidney. The limited length of the incision, however, makes suture of the caval defect challenging, especially in heavy donors. Under these circumstances, slippage of Satinsky clamp results in significant hemorrhage which may be difficult to control without quick extension of surgical incision. Use of an endo-GIA stapler (Fig. **4b**), armed with a vascular cartridge (white), is less troublesome.

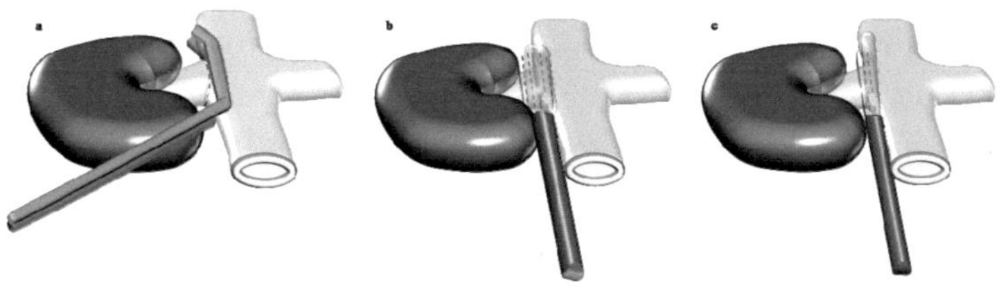

Figure 4: (A) The right renal vein, along with a cuff of inferior vena cava, is closed using a Satinski clamp; (B) The right renal vein is closed and sectioned using an endo-GIA staler; (C) The right renal vein is closed using an endo-TA staler.

To maximize the length of the renal vein, however, the device should be oriented parallel to the inferior vena cava (Fig. **5**). Further, since a row of staples is fired also on the side of the graft, a few of millimeters of vein are necessarily sacrificed when using a GIA stapler. Using an endo-TA stapler (Fig. **4c**) spares these millimeters, but requires that after firing the stapler the vein is cut using scissors.

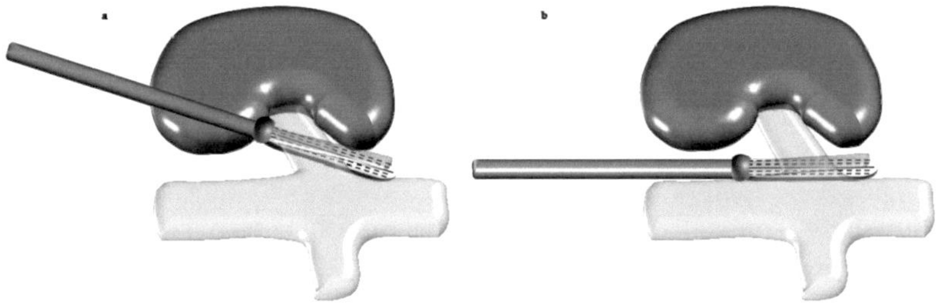

Figure 5: (A) If the GIA stapler is not oriented parallel to the inferior vena cava, a variable length of the right renal vein will remain on the caval side and will not be available for transplantation; (B) When the GIA stapler is oriented parallel to the course of the inferior vena cava, the length of the right renal vein is maximized.

If on one hand, the need for separate cutting of the vein prolongs of few seconds the period of warm ischemia of the graft, on the other, it enhances the safety of the procedure. Indeed, malfunction of GIA stapler results in massive bleeding after releasing the jaws. Malfunction of TA staplers is not associated with any consequences, because the device is designed only to suture.

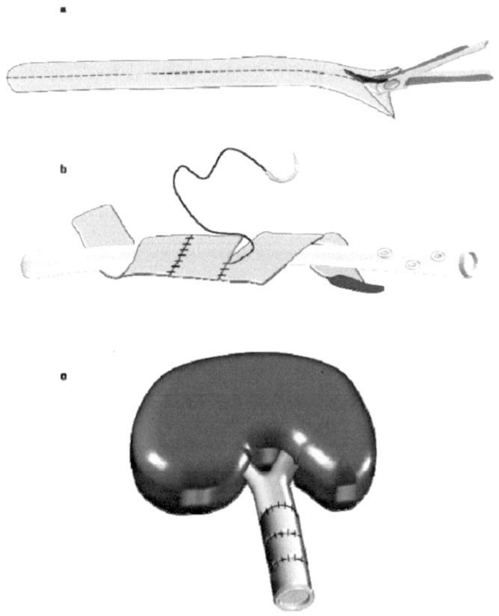

Figure 6: Elongation of the right renal vein using a spiralized saphenous graft: (A) The saphenous vein is filleted; (B)The saphenous vein is fashioned as a spiral-tube graft over a chest tube or large bore catheter; (C) Spiral vein graft in place.

Dols *et al.* suggest that the right kidney should be preferred since it can be procured more easily than the left one. The opinion of these authors is based on several considerations. In the first place, the right kidney is located more caudal in the abdomen, being covered by the right flexure of the colon that is easier to mobilize than the left colonic flexure. Second, the venous anatomy is simpler due to lack of significant posterior branches. Third, liver retraction is unlikely to cause significant bleeds even in case of hepatic tears, as opposed to the spleen. Fourth, hand-assistance is particularly suitable for the right kidney and greatly reduces operative times. Fifth, dissection of the right artery and vein is far from periaortic lymphatics, possibly reducing the chance of lymphatic leak and/or chylous ascites [57].

The main disadvantage of using right kidneys is the length of the renal vein, which is approximately one centimeter shorter than the contralateral (27 mm *vs.* 38 mm; $p < 0.05$) [60]. Elongation of the renal vein, however, is rarely required [60]. As described by Veroux *et al.* [63], and recently reported also by Nghiem [64], the renal vein of live donor kidney can be elongated using spiral saphenous vein grafts (Fig. **6**).

WHICH APPROACH IS THE BEST: OPEN SURGERY OR LAPAROSCOPY?

The kidney donor is a healthy volunteer undergoing major surgery for altruistic reasons. Safety is therefore the main goal of LDN. Reduced pain, earlier recovery, quicker return to everyday activities, better cosmetic results, and reduction of long-term morbidity caused by the surgical incision are other important endpoints, but cannot be exchanged for safety. As long as safety is the main, inalienable, goal of LDN, ODN, usually through a flank approach, remains the standard technique. However, since laparoscopy has proven to be consistently safe, LLDN has become an attractive alternative to ODN. The success of laparoscopic methods, and their appeal on donors [6], have promoted refinement of ODN with the aim of reducing surgical trauma and its long-term consequences. In general, incisions have been placed more anteriorly and more medially, as compared with the classic flank incision; the length of the incision itself has been reduced, and muscles are preferentially split, rather than transected [50].

As already noted in the paragraph on "donor safety", LDN is remarkably safe with an expected rate of donor death of approximately 0.03% [8]. No death after ODN has been reported since 1991, while 11 deaths have been reported after the introduction of LLDN in 1995 [8]. In a review from Davis and Delmonico [15], including 10828 LDN, no donor deaths were noted in 5660 ODN, one donor died out of 2239 hand-assisted LLDN (0.04%), and two donors died after 2929 LLDN (0.07%). Likewise, donors undergoing ODN required fewer reoperations (0.4% *vs.* 1.0% and 0.9%, respectively) and hospital readmissions (0.6% *vs.* 1.6% and 1.6%, respectively), and experienced fewer nonoperative complications (0.3% *vs.* 1.0% and 0.8%, respectively) and bleeding episodes (0.1% *vs.* 0.45% and 0.2%, respectively). Additionally, the incidence of deep venous thrombosis and/or pulmonary embolism was lower after ODN (0.02% *vs.* 0.09% and 0.1%, respectively), as it was the rate of rhabdomyolysis (0 *vs.* 0.09% and 0.13%, respectively) [15].

A recent questionnaire survey of 12 European Countries showed that LLDN was performed in 41 centers out of the 92 responding and practicing LDKT (45%). In particular, hand-assisted LLDN was performed in 20 centers, LLDN was performed in 19 centers, and one center used both laparoscopic techniques and the retroperitoneoscopic LDN [58]. Overall, 51 centers (55%) reported to perform ODN exclusively, and 73 centers (79%) in addition to LLDN. Main incentives for ODN were increased safety, lack of striking evidence favoring LLDN, lack of experience with LLDN, reduced costs [65] and greater confidence in dealing with difficult anatomy/vascular variations and/or with omental obesity [58].

The fact that LDN employs different techniques (*i.e.* pure laparoscopy *vs.* hand-assisted laparoscopy, and transperitoneal laparoscopy *vs.* retroperitoneal laparoscopy) further complicates the field and, probably, makes it impossible to reach conclusions that would be universally accepted. Hadjianastassioua *et al.* estimated that a prospective randomized study comparing ODN and LLDN, having post-operative morbidity as the primary endpoint, should enroll 650 donors in each arm to achieve a power of 80% (alpha = 0.05) [10]. Consequently, the few prospective randomized comparisons that are available [65-70] are mostly inconclusive.

In summary, there is no sound evidence (*i.e.* evidence based on large prospective randomized studies) demonstrating which method of LDN is preferable. ODN is very safe, but also LLDN is safe and there is no proof that the few donor deaths recorded since 1995 would not have occurred anyway if all procurement had been done by open methods. Laparoscopy, on the other hand, reduces operative trauma and is more easily accepted by donors and by their intended recipients. Renal transplant surgeons should therefore be accustomed to all methods of LDN, have no preconceived opinions, and maintain a flexible attitude when choosing the approach for LDN.

OPEN SURGERY

The first LDN was performed through a flank approach in 1954 [71]. For many years little has changed in the technique of ODN but recently refinements have been implemented mostly as a consequence of the advent of laparoscopy.

In a recent questionnaire survey on practice of LDN in Europe, ODN was practiced in 73 centers (79%). Techniques used for ODN included: classic lumbotomy (defined as a 15-20 cm flank incision) (n= 28; 38%), minimal incision flank approach (n= 24; 33%), anterior vertical pararectal incision (n= 9; 12%), anterior horizontal incision (n= 8; 11%), and median laparotomy (n=1; 1%). Three centers (4%) used other open techniques [58].

Flank Approach (Loin Incision)

The patient is placed in the lateral decubitus position. The table is flexed to exaggerate the distance between the twelfth rib and the iliac crest to afford ample exposure. A sandbag may be used to increase the flexion. The lower knee is flexed along with thight and leg, while the upper thight and leg are kept straight with a pillow supporting them. The upper arm may be supported on pillows or fixed to a support. The dependent arm and axilla are protected by placing an axillary roll to avoid injury to the brachial plexus. In any case, upper limbs must be positioned to afford easy accessibility by the anesthetist for fluid replacement and blood pressure monitoring. Once the desired position has been reached the patient must be securely fixed to the table by using wide banding or strips of adhesive tape.

A subcostal, intercostal or transcostal approach may be used. The length of the incision depends on the body structure of the donor. Usually, a 10 to 12 centimeters incision is sufficient and the length of the incision should not be reduced at the expenses of donor safety.

For the subcostal incision, muscles are divided starting with the external oblique anteriorly and the latissimus dorsi posteriorly. The internal oblique muscle and the transversus abdomini are then divided. Care is taken to separate the peritoneum from the trasversalis fascia. The retroperitoneal space is entered and the kidney identified within Gerota's fascia. The surface of the kidney should be explored at this stage, to identify small subcapsular lesions that may have been missed at preoperative studies. If a malignant tumor is discovered, or other findings precluding donation are identified, the procedure can be aborted at this stage with minimal risk to the donor.

For the intercostal approach the appropriate space is identified and intercostal muscles are divided taking care to avoid injury to intercostal nerves.

For the transcostal approach, the appropriate rib is identified and the incision made directly on it. The latissimus dorsi and the serratus posterior inferior muscles are divided. The fascial attachments to the rib are removed using a periosteal elevator and the rib is resected. The incision is then deepened and extended anteriorly until the retroperitoneum is entered.

After the retroperitoneum is entered, a self-retaining retractor is placed. On the left side care is taken to avoid injury to the spleen. The parietal peritoneum is reflected anteriorly until the left renal vein is visible. The kidney is then dissected from the posterior abdominal wall and the renal artery is identified, dissected and encircled with a vessel loop. The same is done anteriorly for the renal vein. On the left side the adrenal vein is cut between ties. On the right side the gonadal vein is also tied (suture-ligated) and divided close to the inferior vena cava. The ureter and the gonadal vessels are identified, mobilized en-bloc off the psoas muscle, and divided at the level where they cross the iliac vessels. Following injection of an intravenous bolus of sodium heparin (70 U/Kg), the renal artery and the renal vein are sequentially cross-clamped and divided. While the anesthesiology team reverse sodium heparin with an equivalent dose of sulphate protamine, the kidney graft is retrieved and immediately immersed in a basin containing ice slushed saline solution. The graft is hence perfused with a cold solution through the artery until clear perfusate is noted on the venous side (Fig. **7**).

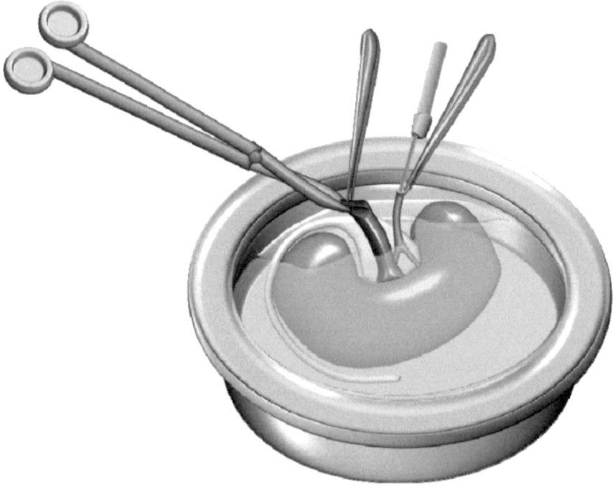

Figure 7: The kidney graft is placed in a basin containing ice slushed saline solution. The surgeon, holding the staple line with his/her left hand, makes and incision on the renal artery through which a cannula is inserted. Kidney perfusion is hence started. The staple line is not removed at this time, but it is used as an handle to hold the renal artery during kidney perfusion. In the meanwhile, the assistant surgeon makes an incision on the venous side, close to the staple line, to allow the perfusate to pour freely.

According to a recent European survey, transcostal lumbotomy is used by few centers, while approximately 50% of centers split muscles without transecting them [58]. Transcostal lumbotomy, provides excellent exposure but up to 30% of donors develop pneumothorax and require a chest tube [72]. Currently, 77.5% of LDN *via* a flank incision is performed without rib resection and 22,5% with rib resection [10].

Long-term morbidity of flank incision was evaluated by Duque *et al.* in a questionnaire sent to 100 consecutive renal donors [72]. Replies were received from 52 donors. After a median follow-up of 27.5 months, 13 patients (25%) were complaining of a painful discomfort at the incision that, although not interfering with daily activities, was persistent in 6 of them. No patient was taking pain medications chronically. Post-operative pain had disappeared by the end of the 4th week in 25% of donors, but it was completely gone only by the end of the 3rd month in 81% of donors. Fifty-four percent of donors, however, had discontinued pain medications by the end of the 2nd week, and only 3 patients had needed pain medications for more than 6 weeks. Sixty-two percent of donors had returned to daily activities within 4 weeks after surgery and 50% had returned to work by the end of the 6th week. The incision was felt as bothering by 35% of donors, very bothering by 6% of donors, and not disturbing at all by the remaining donors (60%). Eighty-three percent of donors, however, declared that the incision had no impact on their self-esteem or quality of life. Fifteen percent of donors disclosed little impact on the same targets, while self-esteem and quality of life of one donor were significantly affected by the incision [72].

Anterior Approaches

Anterior approaches for LDN have been developed to avoid complications specifically caused by lumbotomy, such as chronic neuralgia and abdominal wall relaxation. It may be a necessity in patients with skeletal deformities who cannot be placed in the flexed lateral decubitus position. Since the kidney is located posteriorly, anterior approaches may entail additional difficulties because of the greater space between the site of incision and the kidney. Vascular control, however, may be actually easier [50].

The patient is positioned in a supine position, padded and fixed in a standard fashion. A sandbag may be placed behind the spine, at the level of the 11-12th thoracic vertebra to elevate the kidneys.

The incision is either longitudinal, pararectal, or subcostal. Longitudinal incisions start below the costal arch and extend for 8-12 centimeters. Subcostal incisions, often curvilinear, are made few centimeters below the costal arch, to ensure adequate fascia for closure. The fascia and muscle are divided either by muscle transection or splitting. Irrespective of the type of incision used the retroperitoneal space is hence developed by separating the parietal peritoneum from the anterior and lateral abdominal walls over the area from diaphragm to pelvic brim (Fig. **8**) [73]. Once this working space has been developed the kidney is dissected free from all its attachments, the renal vessels are dissected and encircled with a vessel loop, and the ureter and the gonadal vessels are mobilized en-bloc. Kidney retrieval, vessel management, and back-table procedures are not different from flank incision procedures.

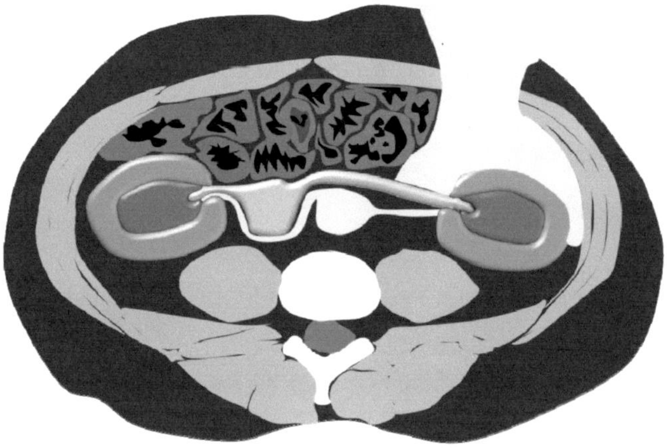

Figure 8: Cross sectional cartoon, demonstrating the anterior route for LDN.

LAPAROSCOPY

The first LLDN was performed in 1995 by Ratner *et al.* [74] at the University of Maryland. At this Institution, where a formal family education program was in force since October 1994, the introduction of LLDN in March 1996 increased the rate of recipients having at least one potential donor from 39% to 50%, thus increasing LDKT rate from 16.5% to 24.7% (p< 0.001). More detailed analysis, demonstrated that LLDN increased the rate of LDKT among Caucasians (p=0.008), but not among African-Americans (p= 0.14), and among recipients aged 55 years or less (p= 0.0001), but not among older recipients (0.10). Overall, regression analysis showed that availability of LLDN was independently associated with a 1,9 relative risk of receiving a LDKT [6]. The fact that starting from 2001 in the USA the number of live donors exceeds that of deceased donors for kidney transplantation (http:/www.unos.org), despite the high annual rate of cadaveric renal donation (ranging from 49 donors pmp in 2001 to 57 donors pmp in 2006) [7], is probably the most convincing proof that LLDN has at least increases the number of LDKT.

Transperitoneal or Retroperitoneal

LLDN can be performed either by a retroperitoneal or by a transperitoneal approach. Proponents of retroperitoneal LLDN underscore that since the kidney is a retroperitoneal organ, the retroperitoneal approach provides direct access to the graft and avoids unnecessary manipulation of intraperitoneal organs thus reducing the risk of intestinal injury. On the other hand, opponents of retroperitoneal laparoscopy argue that working space is limited and prone to collapse when suction is needed, and that repeat fogging of the lens makes dissection more tedious.

Retroperitoneoscopy has been described with and without hand-assistance. The retroperitoneal space may be developed manually or by inflating a balloon (Fig. **9**) [75], and it is insufflated with CO_2. The peritoneal sac and the intestine are displaced medially and several trocars are placed. The kidney can be extracted *via* either a muscle splitting loin incision or a Pfannenstiel, bikini-type, incision. The main advantage of the retroperitoneoscopic technique is that the peritoneum is left intact [50].

In the European questionnaire survey the retroperitoneoscopic access was used only in one center out of 41 practicing LLDN [58]. Therefore, this technique has yet to be fully developed and evaluated and does not currently play a major role in LLDN.

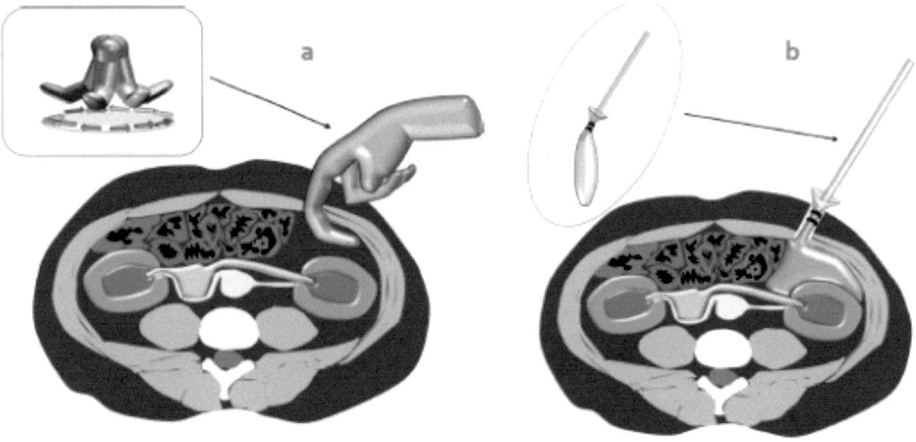

Figure 9: Development of retroperitoneal space for LLDN. (A) Surgeon's forefinger is introduced through a small incision, to be used for port placement, and is moved circumferentially to develop the retroperitoneal working space. (B) A hand-made balloon, consisting of a gloove's finger secured to the tip of a catheter, is introduced through a small incision, to be used for port placement, and is inflated to develop the retroperitoneal working space.

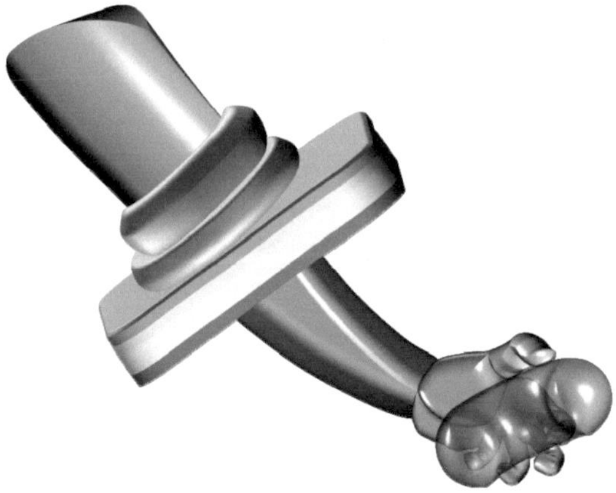

Figure 10: Surgeon's hand, introduced through a hand-port device, is used to grasp the kidney thus improving exposure and facilitating dissection.

Hand Assisted or Pure Laparoscopy?

Hand assisted LLDN was first described in 1998 [76], three years after the first LLDN [74].

Hand-assisted LLDN may enhance the safety of donor nephrectomy since the surgeon retains his/her tactile sensory feedback. By having a hand in the operative field, the surgeon can indeed palpate, control bleeding by digital pressure, dissect bluntly, and improve exposure by direct tissue retraction (Fig. **10**). These advantages, in comparison with pure laparosocopy, result into significant reduction of operative times (by some 45-60 minutes) [77] and warm ischemia time of the graft, because the kidney is readily extracted after division of renal vessels. In obese patients, especially if they are males with omental obesity, hand assistance clearly speeds up LLDN, mainly by improving the otherwise difficult exposure and facilitating dissection of the upper renal pole [77].

Arguments against routine use of hand assistance in LLDN mainly include increased operative costs, higher incidence of incisional hernia, and worse cosmetic result (when the hand assisted device cannot be placed through a Pfannienstel incision). Operative costs, as compared with pure laparoscopy, are increased by the cost of the hand port device, which averages about 400-500 US dollars [77]. Hand assisted LLDN, however, spares the costs of both Verres needle and endobag for kidney extraction. Considering these indirect savings, Lindström *et al.* estimated that hand assistance is more cost-effective than pure laparoscopy in LDN [78].

From a surgical point of view, most of the debate revolves around the optimal site for placement of the hand port device. For left LLDN placing the hand port device in the supraumbelical region, either in the midline or in the upper left quadrant, is ergonomically convenient and allows the surgeon to use his/her left hand with ease. However, especially in young female donors, who may desire optimal cosmestic result, the hand may still be inserted through a Pfannienstel incision. The use of the right hand for kidney retraction will be still ergonomically convenient during dissection of upper renal pole, although the surgeon needs to have a good degree of dexterity using his/her left hand for dissection. Alternatively, an assistant may introduce his/her hand while the surgeon proceeds with bimanual dissection, as in pure laparoscopy. For right-sided nephrectomy placement of the hand port device in the Pfannienstel incision is feasible and less traumatic than placing it in the lower right abdominal quadrant. Even in obese patients the upper pole can be reached with the hand. Slipping of surgeon's forearm through the hand port device is facilitated by wrapping it within a film dressing and its greasing with liquid paraffin.

Technique of Left Transperitoneal Donor Nephrectomy

The patient is positioned in the lateral decubitus position and the table is slightly flexed to open the angle between the 12th rib and the pelvis. Legs and upper arms are positioned, padded and fixed as described for ODN through flank incision. Since laparoscopy requires elevation and titling of operation table, the patient must be securely fixed so that no accidental injury can occur. To do so, besides standard maneuvers, two wide bands are passed across pelvic and shoulder girdles and secured to the table.

Pneumopertitoneum can be created using a Verres needle or by the open technique [19, 79]. Insufflators should be set to maintain the pressure at 12 mmHg. There is no actual need for using higher pressures, which may have negative effects on kidney perfusion. Both surgeon and camera person stand to the patient's side opposite to the kidney to be procured. We currently use pure LLDN for the left kidney and hand-assisted LLDN for the right kidney, although hand-assistance is sometimes used also for left nephrectomies.

According with our method of left LDN [80], three trocars are needed to complete the procedure (Fig. **11**). Pneumoperitoneum is created in the left iliac fossa, where a 12 mm trocar is placed. This trocar will be used for stapling renal vessels. A 30°-video-endoscope is advanced through this port for the initial exploration. The other two trocars are then placed under view: a 10 mm port is placed in the periumbelical region, to be used for the optics, and a 5 mm port is positioned in the left upper quadrant, in the subxyphoid area.

Dissection begins with wide mobilization of splenic flexure, descending colon, and sigmoid colon. The spleno-phrenic ligament should also be incised at this stage to facilitate dissection of the upper renal pole and to avoid splenic tears, especially when the kidney is loaded in the endo-bag and pulled apart to expose renal vessels for stapling (Fig. **12**). Once the left colon has been reflected medially the gonadal vessels, the ureter and the left renal vein are readily identified. Starting at the level of iliac vessels ureter and gonadal vessels are mobilized en-bloc. Attention should be paid to avoid stripping of the ureter which might result in ischemic damage. Likewise, dissection near to the ureter should not be carried out using surgical energy devices, which are known to have lateral energy spread resulting in tissue heating within several centimeters from the cutting blade [44, 81].

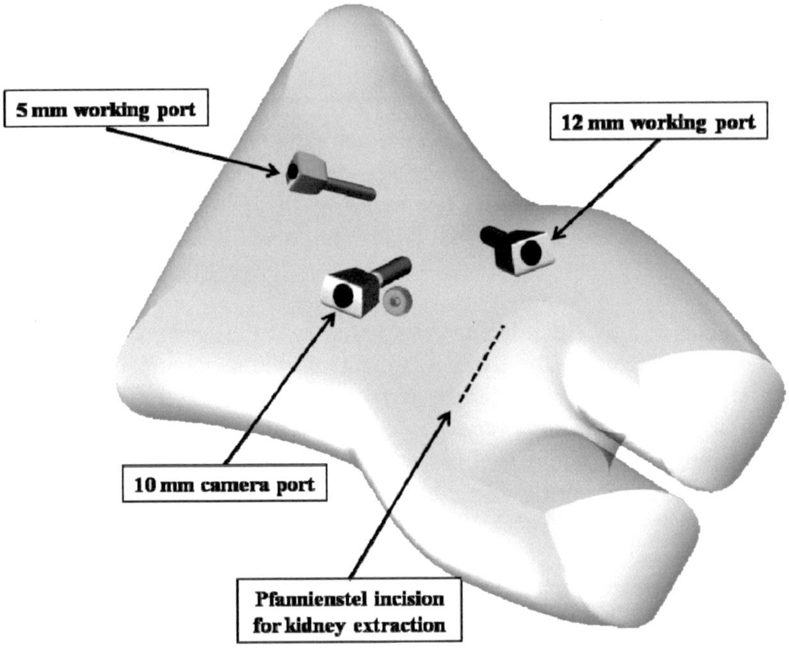

Figure 11: Sites for port placement and incision for kidney extraction in left LLDN.

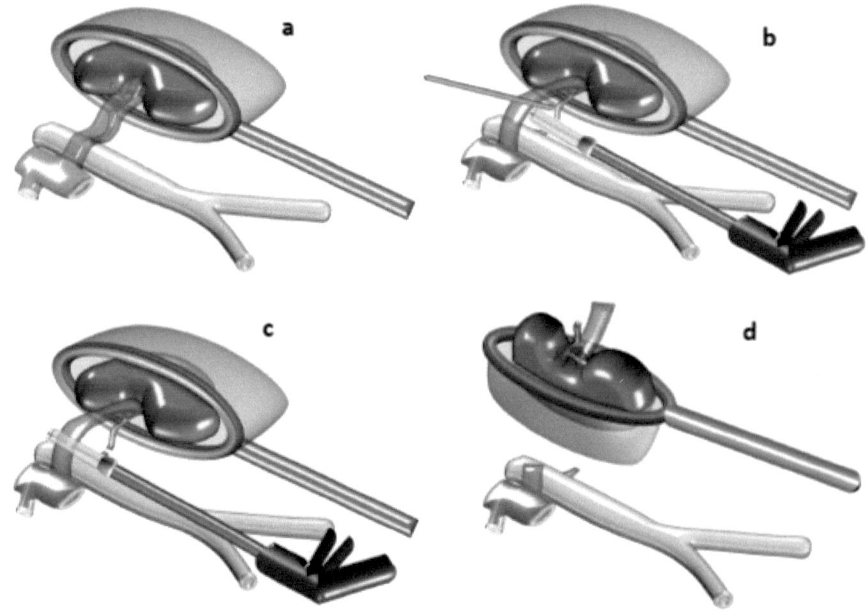

Figure 12: (A) The kidney is preloaded into an endo-bag introduced through the suprapubic incision. Pulling the endo-bag laterally and cephalad exposes the renal vessels. (B) An endo-GIA stapler, introduced through the 12 mm port, is fired on the renal artery. (C) An endo-GIA stapler, introduced through the 12 mm port, is fired on the renal artery. (D) The kidney graft, entrapped into the endo-bag, is ready for retrieval.

As dissection proceeds cephalad, in the setting of "normal anatomy" (*i.e.* anteaortic left renal vein, and single renal artery), the left renal vein is encountered at the end of the gonadal vein and dissected medially up to the level where it crosses the aorta. During periaortic dissection attention should be paid to lymphatics, especially above the renal vein in the region where the superior mesenteric artery and the left renal vein originate from the aorta. However, until the renal vessels have been stapled, no clip should be placed on lymphatics since clips could entrap within staple jaws causing device failure. For the same reason, posterior branches of left renal vein and adrenal vein are best managed by intracorporal ligature. Clips may actually be applied on the side of the vessel that does not remain with the renal vein, since these clips are not expected to interfere with vascular stapler function. Once the renal vein has been completely dissected off, attention is turned to the renal artery. This vessel, in the usual anatomic configuration, appears behind and cranially to the left renal vein. When the artery is difficult to identify from this perspective the kidney can be fully mobilized, leaving the Gerota's fascia with the donor, and rotated medially. Dissection of the upper renal pole may be rather tedious. Sometimes, placement of a further, 5 mm, trocar may be required. This additional port is placed in the left flank region and is used to introduce the harmonic scalpel and other dissecting instruments. It can be also used to introduce an instrument to pull the colon medially thus maintaining good exposure of the operative field.

Once the kidney is completely freed from all attachments, except renal vessels, gonadal vessels, and ureter, a Pfannienstel type incision, measuring approximately 7 centimetres, is made in the suprapubic region. The transverse incision is deepened by longitudinal division of the linea alba and lateral muscle splitting. A purse-string suture is made on the intact peritoneum around the passage of the shaft of the endo-bag, to prevent loss of pneumoperitoneum. After division of the ureter and the gonadal vessels the retrieval bag is advanced and open inside the abdomen. The kidney is caught by the bag (Fig. **12a**) and, following systemic heparinization, the renal artery and the vein are divided sequentially using a endo-GIA stapler loaded with vascular (white) cartridges (Fig. **12b** and **12c**). The bag is closed and delivered through the Pannienstel incision (Fig. **12d**), after digital dilatation of the small peritoneal defect. After extraction the kidney is transferred to a back table, put in a basin containing ice slushed saline solution and flushed using cold lactated Ringer solution (Fig. **7**).

Immediately after kidney extraction, heparin is reversed by an equivalent dose of sulphate protamine and a wet laparotomic pad is pressed onto the suprapubic incision to restore the pneumoperitoneum. The field is quickly checked for major bleeding sites. If nothing are discovered, the Pfannienstel incision is closed in layers. Now the field is systematically searched for all bleeding points as well as for lymphatic leaks. Large lymphatic channels can now be secured by clips or hem-o-lok. If the endo-GIA stapler has functioned properly, no further intervention on renal vessels is necessary. Occasionally the surgeon can elect to place a large (purple) or extra-large (gold) hem-o-lok on renal vessels. When the field is dry, a 10-12 Fr closed suction drain is placed in the renal bed.

Some authors prefer to divided the ureter early during dissection to facilitate elevation of the lower renal pole and exposure of renal vessels [75]. In our experience this maneuver has not been necessary. Furthermore, since brisk diuresis should be maintained during LLDN, early division of ureter results in urine spillage during kidney dissection. Although the ureter may be clipped to avoid urine spillage, we see no obligation for cutting the ureter before the kidney is ready for extraction.

Technique of Hand-Assisted Laparoscopic Donor Nephrectomy

For right LLDN there is no good reason to withhold hand assistance, the real practical matter being the site for hand port placement (*i.e.* through a McBurney-type right lower quadrant incision, or a Pfannienstel-type transverse suprapubic incision). For left LLDN the hand port device is almost necessarily placed in the supra-umbilical region (through either a longitudinal or transverse incision) or infraumbilical region [82]

In right LLDN we prefer to place the hand port device through a Pfannienstel incision. The upper renal pole can be reached anyway if the left forearm of the surgeon is wrapped within a dressing film and greased with liquid paraffin. Pneumoperitoneum is created through the hand port device that is placed at the beginning of the operation. A 30° endoscope may also be advanced through the hand port device for initial abdominal inspection and placement of three ports under view. The camera port is placed in the peri-umbelical region, usually immediately above the umbilicus and a couple of centimeters to its right. A 5 mm operative port is placed in the right subcostal region. An additional 5 mm port is placed in the subxyphoid area to be used for liver retraction (Fig. **13**).

The ascending colon and the second duodenal portion are mobilized until the inferior vena cava is exposed. The ureter and the gonadal vessels are hence elevated en-bloc off the psoas muscle, starting at the level of the iliac vessels.

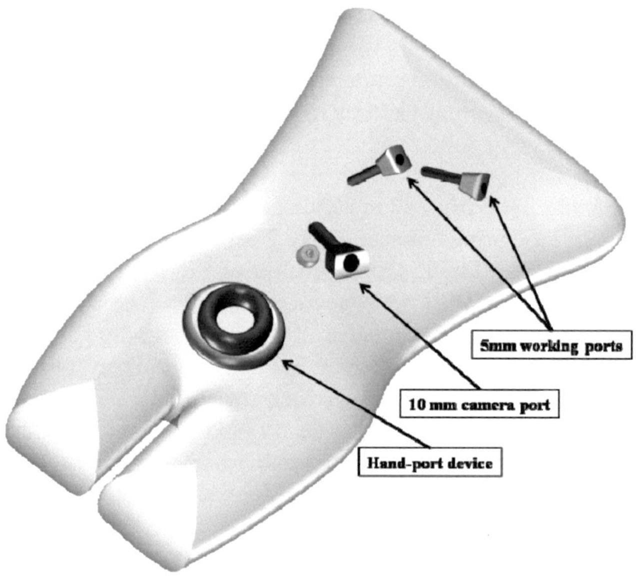

Figure 13:.Sites for port placement and incision for hand-port device placement in right LLDN.

As dissection proceeds cephalad the right gonadal vein is ligated, using hem-o-lok clips, and divided near to its junction to the inferior vena cava. The renal vein is identified next and encircled. The right renal vein, usually, has no large posterior branches but attention should be paid to tear small posterior veins that may bleed extensively and be difficult to control. The renal artery is hence identified behind the renal vein and it is also encircled. Dissection of the upper renal pole is greatly facilitated by hand assistance.

To maximize the length of the renal vein, the vascular stapler should reach the vessel in a plane parallel to the inferior vena cava (Fig. **5**). The use of articulating staplers may help in this respect. Our preference goes to the use a straight endo-TA stapler which is advanced through the hand port device while the left surgeon hand holds the kidney in a lateral position, thus providing for optimal exposure of renal vessels. This maneuver is facilitated by the use of a gel-port device. Indeed, while the surgeon's hand is placed in the central defect an additional small defect can be created peripherally and be used to introduce the stapler. Since the hand port is placed in the lower abdomen, the stapler is easily oriented parallel to the inferior vena cava and thus in the ideal position to maximize the length of the renal vein (Fig. **14**). Using this method an assistant should place and fire the TA stapler, but the surgeon will cut the renal vessels using scissors inserted through the right subcostal port. The kidney will be quickly extracted through the hand port device.

In the right side lymphatic leak is a minor concern, since dissection does not reach the large periaortic channels. However, after kidney removal, it is prudent to check the field accurately and seal all large lymphatic channels.

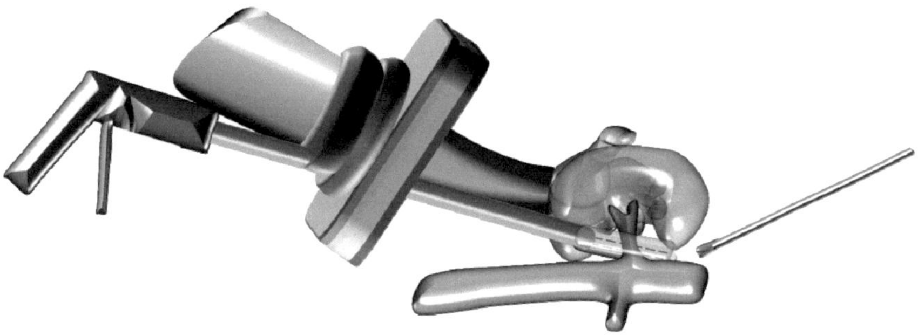

Figure 14: While the surgeons holds the kidney in optimal position to expose the renal vessels, an assistant surgeon advances an endo-TA vascular stapler through the gel-port device. During stapler firing the surgeon uses his/her right hand for suction, keeping the field clear. After closure of both renal vessels, scissors are introduced through the 5 mm working port to divide the vessels. The kidney is hence quickly retrieved through the gel-port device.

Robot-Assisted Laparoscopy

Although surgical robotics is in its infancy, the rapid development of robotic technology attests the fact that this new tool is here to stay.

Surgical robotics systems, that have been used for operations in humans, are the Zeus (Computer Motion Inc.) and the daVinci surgical system (dVss) (Intuitive Surgical, Sunnyvale, CA, USA). These systems were initially developed as a military project by the Pentagon's Defense Advanced Research Projects Agency with the purpose of allowing a remote surgeon to treat wounded soldiers on the battlefield. Since robotic surgery is basically an expansion of laparoscopic surgery, it was not practically feasible to use a robot for military purposes on the battlefield. On the contrary, the potential for widespread clinical application of surgical robotics was soon recognized, and in 1997 the dVss was first used to perform a cholecystectomy in Belgium [83].

Zeus and dVss mainly differ in the configuration of the surgeon's workstation, but are both designed for telerobotic surgery. Computer Motion Inc. was acquired by Intuitive Surgical in 2003 and the Zeus system is no longer commercially available. Thus the only robotic surgical system that is currently available is the dVss [83].

The greatest practical advantage of the dVss is that it allows surgeons to perform laparoscopic operations without giving up the dexterity, precision, and instinctive movements of open surgery [84]. The dVss consists of a console, used by the operating surgeon as a workstation, an operating tower, driving both robotic instruments and endoscope, and a control tower, housing technology equipment (Fig. **15**) [83, 84]. Since the surgeon operates from a remote site, a surgical assistant is required at the patient-side to operate suction/irrigation, to change surgical instruments, to place clips, and to retrieve the kidney graft [85].

In the console the surgeon rests his/her head between sensors on either sides of a viewport consisting of two viewers, one for each eye, which provide true three-dimensional view of the operating field and fully restore hand–eye coordination. The surgeon controls instrument movements *via* two hand-controlled masters, allowing for arm, wrist and pincer movements, and that are directly linked *via* electronics to motordriven arms of the operating tower, holding and moving surgical instruments. The surgeon's hands, which rest in line with the visual axis, control the seven degrees of freedom of the wristed instruments. The video system provides 10X to 15X magnification and true 3D vision.

The robotically controlled instrument drive system is a tower with four multiply jointed arms, three of which control a variety of 8 mm while the fourth drives a binocular video endoscope. The wristed instruments track the surgeon's movements 1,300 times per second and provide for tremor filtration and scaled motion, translating larger movements of the surgeon's hands into finer movements of the wristed instrumentation.

The dVss has been used for LLDN only by few centers [56, 84-87]. The group of the University of Illinois (Chicago, USA) has added hand assistance to the use of the robot [56, 84, 86]. The group of the University Hospital of Nancy (France) has employed the robot in a purely laparoscopic approach, the renal graft being retrieved through a Pfannienstel incision [85, 87].

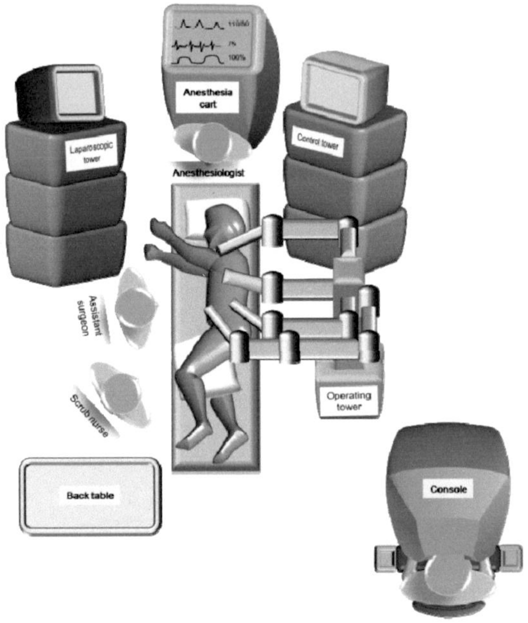

Figure 15: Operating room set up for donor nephrectomy using the dVss.

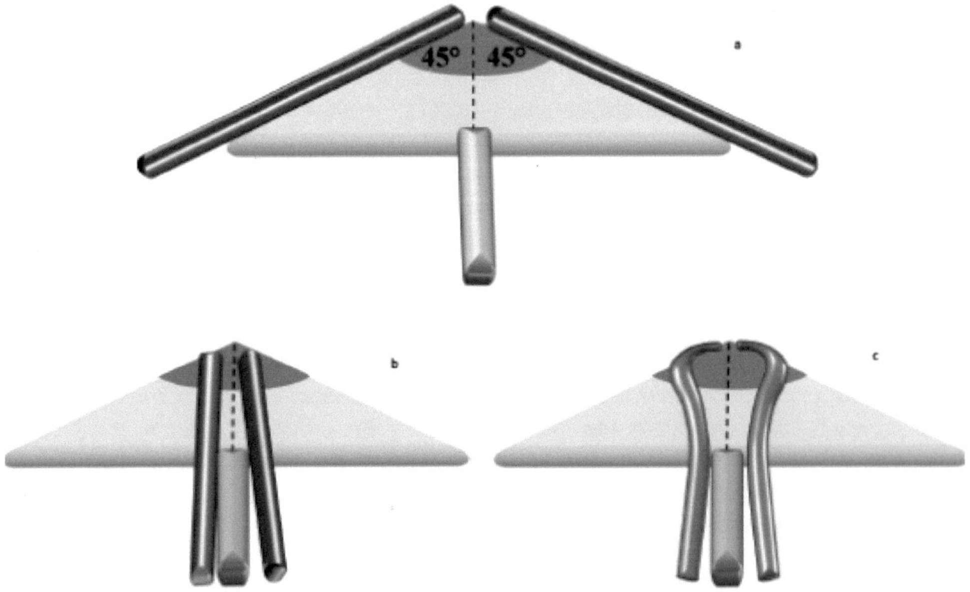

Figure 16: Instrument triangulation. (A) In conventional laparoscopy, camera is placed halfway between the two working instruments. (B) In LESS surgery, camera and working instruments course parallel and reach the working site without forming a triangulation. (C) Use of curved instruments restores a variable degree of triangulation in LESS surgery.

Laparo-Endoscopic Single Site Donor Nephrectomy

Traditional laparoscopy requires placement of, at least, three ports to achieve optimal instrument triangulation (Fig. **16a**).

Laparo-endoscopic single site (LESS) surgery is a newly developed technique that allows surgeons with advanced laparoscopic skills to perform major operations through a single, small, incision and nearly scar-free results. The single incision is indeed frequently placed within the umbilicus that conceals much, if not all, of the scar. Complex abdominal operations have been carried out successfully by LESS surgery, including nephrectomy [88-92] and LDN [89, 90, 94, 95].

This new approach is appealing for LDN, since it can further reduce the invasiveness of the operation, but has several intrinsic difficulties. Indeed, since endoscope and working instruments are all inserted through the same site, triangulation cannot be achieved (Fig. **16b**), instrument maneuverability is greatly limited, and the laparoscope often clashes with instruments [88]. Use of curved, and/or articultating, instruments is thought to restore an acceptable degree of triangulation and improve instrument maneuverability (Fig. **16c**). However, these new instruments may be difficult to master. Current experience with LESS surgery in LDN is limited.

Canes *et al.* reported on 18 consecutive LESS LDN. The single incision was made at the level of the umbilicus (Fig. **17a** and **17b**) and a needlescopic grasper was inserted, through a 2 millimeters port, in the hypochondrium to aid in tissue retraction and dissection. The donor was placed in the lateral decubitus position and the pneumoperitoneum was created by either Verres needle puncture or open Hasson technique. A 2–2.5-cm vertical intraumbilical skin incision was used to insert the single port device (Fig. **17c**). Dissection then proceeded as in standard LDN but the lateral attachment of the kidney were not released until completion of hilar dissection. After division of gonadal vessels and ureter the kidney was preloaded in an endo-bag device. The artery was divided after placing two hem-o-lok clips proximally and one titanium clip distally. The renal vein was handled using an endo-GIA stapler. The port was hence removed, the skin incision extended to approximately 4 centimeters and the linea alba divided beneath the skin cranially and caudally. The kidney was hence extracted (Fig. **17d**). Using this method, Canes *et al.* demonstrated that LDN is feasible using LESS techniques and, although the mean duration of warm ischemia is doubled (6.1 min *vs.* 3 min; $p < 0.0001$) as compared with standard LLDN, renal function at 3 months is not worsened [93].

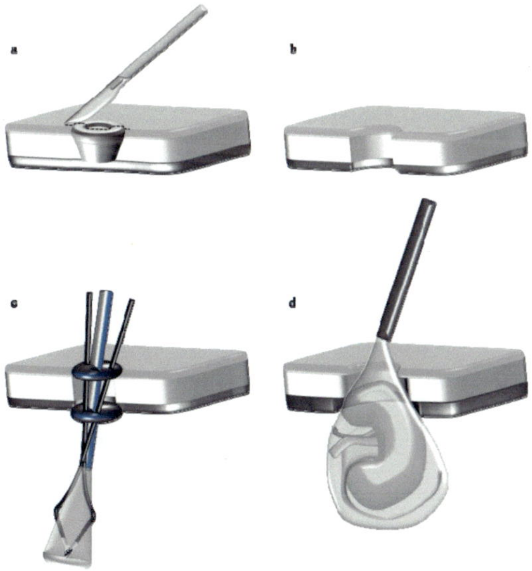

Figure 17: Laparo-endoscopic single site live donor nephrectomy. (A) A small vertical incision is made in the umbilicus. (B) Incision of linea alba and peritoneum creates room for placement of LESS port device. (C) A laparoscope and a pair of instruments are advanced through the LESS port. (D) The kidney graft is preloaded in an endo-bag device. After division of all attachments and vessels, the graft is extracted through the umbilical incision.

Andonian *et al.* have described six LESS LDN (5 left and 1 right). Working through a Pfannienstel incision, these authors have placed 3 trocars through the intact fascia and rectal muscles (Fig. **18**). Namely, two ports were placed along the midline, and one through the rectal muscle to the side of the kidney planned for LDN. Overall, the three ports were placed in a triangular configuration. The inferior midline port was used for the laparoscope (a 5 mm, flexible tip, laparoscope) and the other two ports for surgical instruments (both articulating and standard laparoscopic instruments). After dissection of the kidney and section of renal vessels using an endo-GIA stapler, the kidney was entrapped within an endo-bag device and retrieved through the Pfannienstel incision after incising the anterior rectal fascia and the peritoneum between the two midline ports. All procedures were successful. Median operative time was 142 minutes with a median warm ischemia time of 5 minutes [94].

White *et al.* have recently reported 19 LESS LDN. The single port was placed through the umbilicus. Two procedures were converted to standard LLDN. Mean operative time was 199 minutes, and mean warm ischemia time was 5.29 minutes [90].

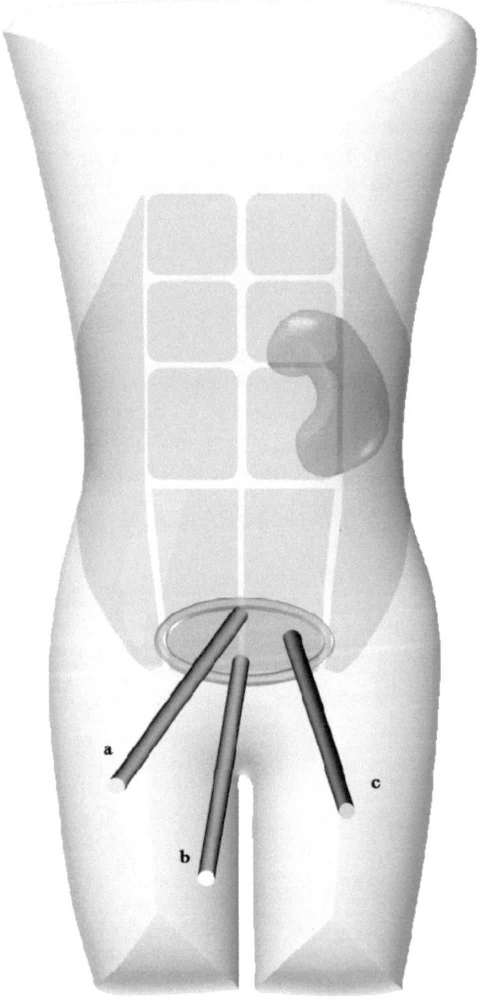

Figure 18: LESS LDN through a Pfannienstel incision.

FLUSHING/PRESERVATION FLUID

Immediately after procurement the kidney graft is placed in a basin filled with ice slushed saline solution and perfused by a gravity system (Fig. 7). Differently from deceased donor kidney grafts, that are expected to be preserved for several hours, live donor kidneys are usually reperfused after a short period of cold ischemia, that does not usually exceeds one hour. Thus, there seems to be no actual need for true preservation of live donor kidneys, graft flushing with cold (4 degrees Celsius) lactated Ringer's solution (containing 5000 U of sodium heparin per liter) plus surface cooling being sufficient. The authors, using this policy, have had no cases of preservation injury in more than 200 consecutive LDKT.

Most authors, however, prefer to use formal preservation solutions such as Euro-Collins solution [93], University of Wisconsin solution [84-86], or Custodiol solution [43, 73, 96, 97].

POSTOPERATIVE MANAGEMENT AND PAIN CONTROL

The management of uncomplicated course of LDN entails no specific challenge. Pain control, however, should be particularly stringent, since pain-induced hypertension facilitates post-operative bleeding and, occasionally, have been credited of the blowing out of renal artery closure.

Patients must also be encouraged to ambulate as early as possible. Ideally they should be out of their bed within the first 6 hours after the end of the operation.

COMPLICATIONS

The risks to live kidney donors are small, but real. Persons selected for kidney donation are truly healthy individuals and they have been shown to live longer than non-donating age cohorts [12]. The risk of death is approximately 0.03% and the risk of major life-threatening complications appears to be small. There have been reports of an increased risk of hypertension and a non-progressive mild proteinuria [98], but the long term risk of end stage renal failure is not increased after unilateral nepherectomy [99].

In a recent survey of the UK experience with 2509 LDN, as reported to the Living Donor Registry between November 2000 And June 2006, the overall risk of a donor experiencing major morbidity was 4.9% and the risk of having any morbidity at all was 14.3% [10]. Overall morbidity was higher after ODN (15,7%) as compared with LLDN (10,3%) ($p< 0.001$), but the rate of major complications was equivalent with the two techniques (5.1% *vs.* 4.5%, respectively). In the 14 donors requiring tube thoracostomy to drain a pneumothorax (0.8%), LDN was done through a flank incision, that in 13 of them included rib resection. Other complications were: need for blood transfusions (ODN 2.3% *vs.* laparoscopic 1.5%), wound infection (ODN 2.9% *vs.* LLDN 1.3%), need for reoperation (ODN 1.1% *vs.* LLDN 1.5%), pneumonia (ODN 1.5% *vs.* LLDN 1.3%), pulmonary embolism (ODN 0.2% *vs.* LLDN 0.2%), deep venous thrombosis (ODN 0.4% *vs.* LLDN 0.2%), need for splenectomy (ODN 0.1% *vs.* LLDN 0.2%).

Medical Complications

The greater medical concern with LDN is the risk that unilateral nephrectomy increases the risk of end stage renal failure in the donor. From a physiologic point of view, hyperfiltration damage is a real threat only in subjects with a single kidney after removal of more than 75% of the renal parenchyma [100]. After unilateral nephrectomy the average decrease in glomerular filtration rate is 17,1 ml/min, but tends to improve in the long-term period [101]. A study on 28 veterans of second World War, who had lost a kidney due to military injury, shows that creatinine clearance is still 75 ml/min, 45 years after nephrectomy [102]. Many other studies have confirmed no evidence of progressive deterioration of kidney function up to, and beyond, 20 years after renal donation [11].

According to a recent survey of the OPTN database, that identified 56 kidney donors out of 6371 who were subsequently listed for a renal transplant, the rate of end stage renal disease in donors is estimated to be 0.04%. This rate is comparable to the rate observed in the general US population (0.03%). It is also important to note that 16 of these 56 donors developed end-stage renal failure as a consequence of nephropathies that would have led them to the same stage anyway. Indeed 9 donors were diagnosed with focal sclerosis and 7 with chronic glomerulonephritis [99]. Thus the risk of long-term end stage renal failure does not seem to be a real concern in live kidney donors.

Rhabdomyolysis is a rare but serious complication of laparoscopic nephrectomy. Reisiger *et al.* in a series of more than 700 nephrectomies, reported 7 cases of rhabdomyolysis all occurring after prolonged surgery (average operation time: 7.5 hours; range 5.8 to 9.4 hours) [103]. The risk that rhabdomyolysis results in acute renal failure, that would be particularly worrisome in live renal donors, depends on early recognition and immediate implementation of specific treatment. Excessive gluteal muscular pain, arising early after LDN, is an important diagnostic clue that requires immediate evaluation of serum creatinine kinase. Aggressive hydration and maintenance of a brisk diuresis are recommended to minimize renal injury [8, 104].

Ischemic optic neuropathy is also an exceedingly rare, but severe, complication that has been reported after LLDN [8, 105].

Deep venous thrombosis and pulmonary embolism are infrequent, but dreadful, complications of LDN. Several cases of donor death were caused by massive pulmonary embolism. Prevention, besides adequate pharmacologic prophylaxis and intraoperative use of compressive stockings, largely depends on early patient ambulation.

Surgical Complications

The most dreadful surgical complication of LDN is delayed bleeding. These hemorrhages are often of arterial origin, and hence massive. Without immediate reintervention, immediate control of the bleeding vessel, and vigorous resuscitation maneuvers, the donor cannot survive or will eventually remain in persistent vegetative conditions. As discussed in a previous section of this chapter, all forms of vascular control are liable to failure and may result in bleeding, morbidity, and death. It is responsibility of the surgical team to be fully aware of the limitation of current technology, to be continuously updated with newer methods, and coordinate the overall management of the live donor as to reduce the incidence of surgical complications.

Intestinal complications, including bowel perforation and bowel obstruction, have been reported more frequently after LLDN and often require reoperation.

Chylous ascites is a rare complication of LLDN, occurring in about 0.6% of donors [104]. Because of the anatomic disposition of large periaortic lymphatic channels, this complication typically follows left LDN. Although often responsive to conservative treatment, chylous ascites may be difficult to treat and, when persistent, can have serious nutritional and immunologic consequences caused by loss of protein and lymphocytes, respectively. Conservative treatment is typically based on dietary intervention (high-medium chain triglyceride diet with low-fat and high-protein content) plus diuretics. The site of lymphatic leak can be identified by means of bipedal lymphangiogram. Surgical repair can be implemented in patients refractory to conservative treatment [106].

It is interesting to note that extraction of kidney grafts from a suprapubic incision entails a risk of bladder injury [8].

CONCLUSIONS

Various techniques are currently available for LDN. Although each transplant surgeon may be more familiar with a given method or have a preference for one approach, all validated methods should be known and available in order to select the one that best fits the needs of each donor. In taking this difficult decision, donor safety must be considered first. Next, the selected technique should permit procurement of a viable graft in which renal vessels and ureter are suitable for successful LDKT. Lastly, considerations such as faster recovery, hospital costs, and improved cosmetic results should also be considered, although by no means they can be exchanged for either donor safety or success of LDKT.

REFERENCES

[1] Keown P. Improving quality of life. The new target of transplantation. Transplantation 2001; 72 (suppl 12): S67-74.

[2] Matas AJ, Lawson W, McHugh L, *et al.* Employment patterns after successful kidney transplantation. Transplantation 1996; 61: 729-733.

[3] Ojo AO, Hanson JA, Meier-Kriesche H, *et al.* Survival in recipients of marginal cadaveric donor kidneys compared with other recipients and wait-listed transplant candidates. J Am Soc Nephrol 2001; 12: 589-597.

[4] Wolfe RA, Ashby VB, Milford EL, *et al.* Comparison of mortality in all patients on dialysis, patients on dialysis awaiting transplantation and recipients of a first cadaveric transplant. N Engl J Med 1999; 341: 1725-1730.

[5] Whiting JF, Woodward RS, Zavala EY, *et al.* Economic cost of expanded criteria donors in cadaveric renal transplantation: analysis of Medicare payments. Transplantation 2000; 70: 755-760.

[6] Schweitzer EJ, Wilson J, Jacobs S, *et al.* Increased Rates of Donation With Laparoscopic Donor Nephrectomy. Ann Surg 2000; 232: 392-400.

[7] Horvat LD, Shariffl SZ, Garg AX, for the Donor Nephrectomy Outcomes Research (DONOR) Network. Global trends in the rates of living kidney donation. Kidney International 2009; 75: 1088–1098.

[8] Shokeir AA. Open versus laparoscopic live donor nephrectomy: a focus on the safety of donors and the need for a donor registry. J Urol 2007; 178: 1860-1866.

[9] Matas AJ, Bartlett ST, Leichtman AB, *et al.* Morbidity and mortality after living kidney donation, 1999–2001: survey of United States transplant centers. Am J Transplant. 2003; 3:830–834.

[10] Hadjianastassioua VG, Johnsonb RJ, Rudgeb CJ, Mamodea N. 2509 Living Donor Nephrectomies, Morbidity and Mortality, Including the UK Introduction of Laparoscopic Donor Surgery. Am J Transplant 2007; 7: 2532–2537.

[11] Gaia M, Giunti S, Lanfranco G, Segoloni GP. Potential risks of living kidney donation—a review. Nephrol Dial Transplant 2007; 22: 3122–3127.

[12] Fehrman-Ekhom I, Elinder CG, Stenbeck M, *et al.* Kidney donors live longer. Transplantation 1997; 64: 976-978.

[13] Cho YW, Cecka JM. Cross-match tests. An analysis of UNOS data from 1991-2000. In Cecka JM, Terasaki PI, eds. Clinical Transplants 2001. Los Angeles: UCLA Tissue Typing Labaratory, 2002: 237-246.

[14] Delmonico F, Council of the Transplantation Society. A report of the Amsterdam forum on the care of live kidney donor: data and medical guidelines. Transplantation 2005; 79 (suppl 6): S53-66.

[15] Davis CL, Delmonico FL. Living-Donor Kidney Transplantation: A Review of the Current Practices for the Live Donor. J Am Soc Nephrol 2005; 16: 2098–2110.

[16] Selection and preparation of the donor. In Ponticelli C, ed. Medical Complications of kidney transplantation. Informa healthcare, UK, 2007: 1-30.

[17] Andreoni KA, Weeks SM, Gerber DA, *et al.* Incidence of donor renal fibromuscular dysplasia: does it justify routine angiography? Transplantation 2002; 73: 1112–1116.

[18] Roza AM, Perloff LJ, Naji A, *et al.* Living-related donors with bilateral multiple renal arteries: a twenty-year experience. Transplantation. 1989; 47: 397-399.

[19] Kok NFM, Dols LFC, Hunink MGM, *et al.* Complex Vascular Anatomy in Live Kidney Donation: Imaging and Consequences for Clinical Outcome. Transplantation 2008; 85: 1760–1765.

[20] Holden A, Smith A, Dukes P, *et al.* Assessment of 100 Live Potential Renal Donors for Laparoscopic Nephrectomy with Multi–Detector Row Helical CT. Radiology 2005; 237: 973–980.

[21] Modi PR, Rizvi SJ, Gupta R, *et al.* Retroperitoneoscopic right-sided donor nephrectomy with pre- and postcaval renal arteries. Urology 2008; 72: 672–674.

[22] Jacobs SC, Flowers JL, Dunkin B, *et al.* Living donor nephrectomy. Curr Opin Urol 1999; 9: 115-120.

[23] Lewis G, Mulcahy K, Brook NR, Veitch PS, Nicholson ML. A prospective study of the predictive power of spiral computed tomographic angiography for defining renal vascular anatomy before live-donor nephrectomy. BJU Int 2004; 94: 1077-1081.

[24] Henke PK, Cardneau JD, Welling III TH, *et al.* Renal artery aneurysms A 35-year clinical experience with 252 aneurysms in 168 patients. Ann Surg 2001; 234: 454–463.

[25] Gravante G, Pisani F, D'Angelo M, *et al.* Renal artery aneurysms in kidney grafts. Am J Surg 2008; 196: 46-47.

[26] Kadotani Y, Okamoto M, Akioka K, *et al.* Renovascular reconstruction of grafts with renal artery variations in living kidney transplantation. Transplant Proc. 2005; 37: 1049-1051.

[27] Nahas WC, Lucon AM, Mazzucchi E, *et al.*Kidney transplantation: the use of living donors with renal artery lesions. J Urol. 1998; 160:1244-1247.

[28] Maciel RF, Branco AJ, Branco AW, *et al.* Renal artery aneurysm in hand-assisted laparoscopic donor nephrectomy: case report. Transplant Proc. 2003; 35: 2858-2859.

[29] Desgrandchamps F, Jabbour ME, Gossot D, *et al.* Hand-assisted laparoscopic live donor nephrectomy in a patient with renal artery aneurysm. Surg Endosc. 2001; 15: 101.

[30] Neymark E, LaBerge JM, Hirose R, *et al.* Arteriographic detection of renovascular disease in potential renal donors: incidence and effect on donor surgery. Radiology 2000; 214: 755-760.

[31] Parasuraman R, Attallah N, Venkat KK, *et al.* Rapid progression of native renal artery fibromuscular dysplasia following kidney donation. Am J Transpl 2004; 4: 1910–1914.

[32] Kolettis PN, Bugg CE, Lockhart ME, *et al.* Outcomes for live renal donor transplantation using kidneys with medial fibroplasias. Urology 2004; 63: 656-659.

[33] Königsrainer I, Knubben K, Thiel C, *et al.* Successful transplantation to two recipients after splitting a large horseshoe kidney with complicated anatomy. Transpl Int 2006; 19: 521–522.

[34] Stroosma OB, Wilhelmus G, Schurink H, Kootstra G. Current opinions in horseshoe kidney transplantation Transpl Int 2002; 15: 196-199.

[35] Salehipour M, Bahador A, Salahi H, *et al.* Transplantation of a horseshoe kidney. Arch Iranian Med 2007; 10: 239–241.

[36] Stroosma OB, Scheltinga MRM, Stubenitsky BM, Kootstra G.Horseshoe kidney transplantation: an overview. Clin Transplant 2000: 14: 515–519.

[37] Hüser N, Gerauer KE, Novotny AR, *et al.* Successful living donor transplantation of a kidney with horseshoe malformation: extending the donor pool. Transpl Int 2005;18: 761–762.

[38] Dinckan A, Tekin A, Turkyilmaz S, *et al.* Horseshoe kidney for transplant: report of 3 cases. Exp Clin Transplant. 2007; 5: 716-719.

[39] Hayakawa K, Baba S, Aoyagi T, *et al.* Laparoscopic heminephrectomy of a horseshoe kidney using microwave coagulator. J Urol 1999; 161: 1559.

[40] Donovan JF, Cooper CS, Lund GO, Winfield HN. Laparoscopic nephrectomy of a horseshoe kidney. J Endourol 1997; 11: 181-184.

[41] Selection and operative approaches for cadaveric and living donors. In Kahan BD, Ponticelli C, eds. Principles and practice of renal transplantation. Martin Dunitz ltd, London UK, 2000: 145-190.

[42] Biancofiore G, Amorese G, Lugli D, *et al.* Perioperative management for laparoscopic kidney donation. Min Anestesiol 2003; 69: 681-689.

[43] Paul A, Treckmann J, Gallinatc A, *et al.* Current concepts in transplant surgery: laparoscopic living donor of the kidney. Langenbecks Arch Surg 2007; 392:501–509.

[44] Eman TA, Cuschieri A. How safe is high-power ultrasonic dissection? Ann Surg 2003; 237:186-191.

[45] Kuo PC, Cho ES, Flowers JL, *et al.* Laparoscopic living donor nephrectomy and multiple renal arteries. Am J Surg. 1998;176: 559-563.

[46] Carter JT, Freise CE, McTaggart RA, *et al.* Laparoscopic procurement of kidneys with multiple renal arteries is associated with increased ureteral complications in the recipient. Am J Transplant. 2005; 5: 1312-1318.

[47] Fuller TF, Deger S, Büchler A, *et al.* Ureteral complications in the renal transplant recipient after laparoscopic living donor nephrectomy. Eur Urol. 2006; 50: 535-540.

[48] El-Mekresh M, Osman Y, Ali-El-Dein B, *et al.* Urological complications after living-donor renal transplantation. BJU Int. 2001; 87: 295- 306.

[49] Saidi R, Kawai T, Kennealey P, Tsouflas G, Elias N, Hertl M, Cosimi AB, Ko DSC. Living Donor Kidney Transplantation With Multiple Arteries. Recent Increase in Modern Era of Laparoscopic Donor Nephrectomy. Arch Surg. 2009; 144: 472-475.

[50] Dols LF, Kok NF, IJzermans JN. Surgical aspects of live kidney donation. Front Biosc 2009; 14: 4746-4757.

[51] Friedman AL, Peters TG, Jones KW, Boulware LE, Ratner LE. Fatal and Nonfatal Hemorrhagic Complications of Living Kidney Donation. Ann Surg 2006; 243: 126–130.

[52] His RS, Saint-Elie DT, Zimmerman GJ, Baldwin DD. Mechanisms of Hemostatic Failure During Laparoscopic Nephrectomy: Review of Food and Drug Administration Database. Urology 2007; 70: 888-892.

[53] Meng MV. Reported Failures of the Polymer Self-Locking (Hem-O-Lok) Clip: Review of Data from the Food and Drug Administration. J Endourol 2006; 20: 1054-1057.

[54] Dekel Y, Mor E. Hem-o-lok clip dislodgment causing death of the donor after laparoscopic living donor nephrectomy. Transplantation 2008; 86: 887.

[55] Ponsky L, Cherullo E, Moinzadeh A, Desai M, Kaouk J, Haber G-P, Chen D, Ng C, Fuchs G, Singh D, Finelli A, Frank I, Matin S. The Hem-o-Lok Clip is safe for laparoscopic nephrectomy: a multi-institutional review. Urology 2008; 71: 593-596.

[56] Gorodner V, Horgan S, Galvani C, Manzelli A, Oberholzer J, Sankary H, Testa G, Benedetti E. Routine left robotic-assisted laparoscopic donor nephrectomy is safe and effective regardless of the presence of vascular anomalies. Transpl International 2006; 19: 636-640.

[57] Dols LFC, Kok NFM, Alwayn IPJ, Tran TCK, Weimar W, Ijzermans JNM. Laparoscopic Donor Nephrectomy: A Plea for the Right-Sided Approach. Transplantation 2009; 87: 745–750.

[58] Kok NFM, Weimar W, Alwayn IPJ, IJzermans JNM The current practice of live donor nephrectomy in Europe. Transplantation 2006; 82: 892–897.

[59] Mandal AK, Cohen C, Montgomery RA, *et al.* Should the indications for laparascopic live donor nephrectomy of the right kidney be the same as for the open procedure? Anomalous left renal vasculature is not a contraindiction to laparoscopic left donor nephrectomy. Transplantation 2001; 71: 660-664.

[60] Kay MD, Brook N, Kaushik M, Harper SJF, Bagul A, Nicholson ML. Comparison of right and left laparoscopic live donor nephrectomy.BJU Int 2006; 98: 843 –844.

[61] Boorjian S, Munver R, Sosa RE, Del Pizzo JJ. Right laparoscopic live donor nephrectomy: a single institution experience. Transplantation 2004; 77: 437-440.

[62] Riehle RA, Steckler R, Naslund EB, Riggio R, Cheigh J, Stubenbord W. Selection criteria for the evaluation of living related renal donors. J Urol 1990; 144: 845-848.

[63] Veroux P, Veroux M, Puliatti C. Complete renal vein disruption during living kidney transplantation: successful repair with spiral vein graft. Surgery. 2003;134: 511-512.

[64] Nghiem DD. Use of spiral vein graft in living donor renal transplantation. Clin Transplant 2008: 22: 719–721

[65] Hamidı V, Andersen MH, Øyen O, Mathisen L, Fosse E, Kristiansen IS. Cost Effectiveness of Open Versus Laparoscopic Living-Donor Nephrectomy. Transplantation 2009; 87: 831–838.

[66] Wolf JS Jr, Merion RM, Leichtman AB *et al.* Randomized controlled trial of hand-assisted laparoscopic versus open surgical live donor nephrectomy. Transplantation 2001; 72: 284–290.

[67] Andersen MH, Mathisen L, Oyen O, *et al.* Postoperative pain and convalescence in living kidney donors-laparoscopic versus open donor nephrectomy: A randomized study. Am J Transplant 2006; 6: 1438–1443.

[68] Simforoosh N, Basiri A, Tabibi A, *et al.* Comparison of laparoscopic and open donor nephrectomy: A randomized controlled trial. BJU Int 2005; 95: 851–855.

[69] Brook NR, Harper SJ, Bagul A, *et al.* Laparoscopic donor nephrectomy yields kidneys with structure and function equivalent to those retrieved by open surgery. Transplant Proc 2005; 37: 625–626.

[70] Kok NF, Lind MY, Hansson BM, *et al.* Comparison of laparoscopic and mini incision open donor nephrectomy: Single blind, randomised controlled clinical trial. BMJ 2006; 333: 221.

[71] Molmenti EP, Pinto PA, Montgomery RA, *et al.* Concomitant surgery with laparoscopic live donor nephrectomy. Am J Transplant 2003; 3: 219-223.

[72] Duque JLF, Loughlin KR, Kumar S. Morbidity of flank incision for renal donors. Urology 1999; 54: 796–801.

[73] Schnitzbauer AA, Loss M, Hornung M, *et al.* Mini-incision for strictly retroperitoneal nephrectomy in living kidney donation *vs.* flank incision. Nephrol Dial Transplant 2006; 21: 2948–2952.

[74] Ratner LE, Ciseck LJ, Moore RG, *et al.* Laparoscopic live donor nephrectomy. Transplantation 1995; 60: 1047–1049.

[75] Srivastava A, Gupta N, Kumar A. Evolution of the Technique of Laparoscopic Live Donor Nephrectomy at a Single Center: Experience with More than 350 Cases. Urol Int 2008; 81: 431–436.

[76] Wolf JS Jr, Tchetgen MB, Merion RM. Hand-assisted laparoscopic live donor nephrectomy. Urology 1998; 52: 885–887.

[77] Giessing M, Turk I, Roigas J, *et al.* Laparoscopy for living donor nephrectomy–particularities of the currently applied techniques. Transplant International 2005;18: 1019–1027

[78] Lindström P, Häggman M, Wadström J. Hand-assisted laparoscopic surgery (HALS) for live donor nephrectomy is more time- and cost-effective than standard laparoscopic nephrectomy. Surg Endosc 2002; 16: 422-425.

[79] Kok NFM, van der Wal JBC, Alwayn IPJ, *et al.* Laparoscopic kidney donation: The impact of adhesions. Surg Endosc 2008; 22: 1321–1325.

[80] Boggi U, Pietrabissa A, Vistoli F, *et al.* Laparoscopic live donor nephrectomy. Organs and tissues 2003; 3: 155-160.

[81] Hruby GW, Marruffo FC, Durak E, *et al.* Evaluation of Surgical Energy Devices for Vessel Sealing and Peripheral Energy Spread in a Porcine Model. J Urol 2007; 178: 2689-2693.

[82] Kokkinos C, Nanidis T, Antcliffe D, *et al.* Comparison of Laparoscopic Versus Hand-Assisted Live Donor Nephrectomy. Transplantation 2007; 83: 41–47.

[83] Hockstein NG, Gourin CG, Faust RA, Terris DJ. A history of robots: from science fiction to surgical robotics. J Robotic Surg 2007; 1: 113-118.

[84] Horgan S, Vanuno D, Silieri P, *et al.* Robotic-assisted laparoscopic donor nephrectomy for kidney transplantation. Transplantation 2002; 73: 1474–1479.

[85] Hubert J, Renoult E, Mourey E, *et al.* Complete robotic-assistance during laparoscopic living donor nephrectomies: An evaluation of 38 procedures at a single site. Int J Urol 2007; 14: 986–989.

[86] Horgan S, Benedetti E, Moser F. Robotically assisted donor nephrectomy for kidney transplantation. Am J Surg 2004; 188: 45S–51S.

[87] Louis G, Hubert J, Ladriere M, *et al.* Robotic-assisted laparoscopic donor nephrectomy for kidney transplantation. An evaluation of 35 procedures. Néphrologie & Thérapeutique 2009; 5: 623—630.

[88] Stein RJ, White WM, Goel RK, *et al.* Robotic laparoendoscopic single-site surgery using gel-port as the access platform. Eur Urol 2010; 57: 132–137.

[89] Ponsky LE, Steinway ML, Lengu IJ, *et al.* A Pfannenstiel single-site nephrectomy and nephroureterectomy: a practical application of laparoendoscopic single-site surgery. Urology 2009; 74: 482–485.

[90] White WM, Haber G-P, Goel RK, *et al.* Single-port urological surgery: single-center experience with the first 100 cases. Urology 2009; 74: 801–804.

[91] Rais-Bahrami S, Montag S, Atalla MA, *et al.* Laparoendoscopic single-site surgery of the kidney with no accessory trocars: an initial experience. J Endourol 2009; 23: 1319–1324.

[92] Stolzenburg J-U, Kallidonis P, Hellawell G, *et al.*Technique of laparoscopic-endoscopic single-site surgery radical nephrectomy. Eur Urol 2009; 56: 644-650.

[93] Canes D, Berger A, Aron M, *et al.* Laparo-endoscopic single site (LESS) versus standard laparoscopic left donor nephrectomy: matched-pair comparison. Eur Urol 2010; 57: 95 –101.

[94] Andonian S, Herati AS, Atalla MA, *et al.* Laparoendoscopic single-site Pfannenstiel donor nephrectomy. Urology 2010; 75: 9-12.

[95] Gill IS, Canes D, Aron M, *et al.* Single port transumbilical (E-NOTES) donor nephrectomy. J Urol 2008; 180: 637-641.

[96] Saad S, Paul A, Treckmann J, *et al.* Laparoscopic live donor nephrectomy: Are ten cases per year enough to reach the quality standards? A report from a single small-volume transplant center. Surg Endosc 2009.

[97] Sener A, Uberoi V, Bartlett ST, *et al.* Living-donor renal transplantation of grafts with incidental renal masses after *ex vivo* partial nephrectomy. BJU Int 2009; 104: 1655–1660.

[98] Ratner LE, Hiller J, Sroka M, *et al.* Laparoscopic live donor nephrectomy removes disincentives to live donation. Transplant Proc 1997; 29:3402-3403.

[99] Ellison MD, McBride MA, Taranto SE, *et al.* Living kidney donors in need of kidney transplants: A report from the organ procurement and transplantation network. Transplantation 2002; 74: 1349–1351.

[100] Novick AC, Gephardt G, Guz B, *et al.* Long-term follow-up after partial removal of a solitary kidney. N Engl J Med 1991; 325: 1058–1062.

[101] Kasiske BL, Ma JZ, Louis TA, Swan SK. Long term effects of reduced renal mass in humans. Kidney Int 1995; 48: 814–819.

[102] Narkun-Burgess DM, Nolan CR, Norman JE, *et al.* Forty-five year follow-up after uninephrectomy. Kidney Int 1993; 43: 1110–1115.

[103] Reisiger KE, Landman J, Kibel A, Clayman RV. Laparoscopic renal surgery and the risk of rhabdomyolysis: diagnosis and treatment. Urology 2005; 66 (5 suppl): 29–35.

[104] Breda A, Veale J, Liao J, Schulam PG. Complications of Laparoscopic Living Donor Nephrectomy and Their Management: The UCLA Experience. Urology 2007; 69: 49-52.

[105] Metwalli AR, Davis RG, Donovan JF. Visual impairment after laparoscopic donor nephrectomy. J Endourol 2004; 18: 888-890.

[106] Caumartin Y, Pouliot F, Sabbagh R, Dujardin T. Chylous ascites as a complication of laparoscopic donor nephrectomy. Transplant International 2005; 18: 1378–1381.

CHAPTER 10

A Market in Organs

Miran Epstein*

Barts and The London School of Medicine and Dentistry, Queen Mary University of London, United Kingdom

Abstract: This chapter presents a critical overview of the relationship which transplant medicine has had with the market as a source of organs for transplantation. It has three parts. The first two parts discuss the increasing appeal of the market option in practice and theory against the backdrop of the worsening organ crisis and the intensification of pro-transplant interests. The emerging trend suggests that the recent achievements in the struggle against international organ trafficking do not herald the abolition of the organ market but rather presage its reconfiguration in deglobalized, more or less regulated, forms. The third part rephrases the market question. It concludes that the struggle against a market in organs could make sense, let alone stand a chance, only as part of a general struggle against the conditions that have made it so appealing in the first place.

Keywords: Ethics, Commodification, Market in Organs, Transplant Tourism.

INTRODUCTION

The relationship of transplant medicine with the market as a source of organs for transplantation has taken place in two different social tiers: the *commercial tier* where people actually trade in organs, and the *discursive tier* where people justify and criticize actual and theoretical models of the organ market, including the very principle of buying and selling body parts.

This chapter presents a critical overview of this two-tier relationship. It has three parts. The first two parts discuss the increasing appeal of the market option in both tiers against the backdrop of the worsening organ crisis and the intensification of pro-transplant interests. The emerging trend suggests that the recent achievements in the struggle against international organ trafficking do not herald the abolition of the organ market but rather presage its reconfiguration in deglobalized, more or less regulated, forms. The first part describes and explains the evolution of the organ market in practice. It shows that the market has so far been quick to adapt to the restrictions that had been imposed on it. The second part addresses the discursive manifestations of this process and their reciprocal effects thereon. It shows that the anti-market case and the pro-market case have both been distorted by counter-interests in ways that conceal and thereby reaffirm the hegemony of pro-market interests. The third part rephrases the market question in light of these conclusions. It constructs a value-neutral, ideology-free, representation of the question and sets forth the social implications of the choices to which it gives rise. This representation entails, among other things, that the struggle against a market in organs could make sense, and perhaps stand a chance, only as part of a general struggle against the conditions that have made it so appealing in the first place.

Two comments before we start. First, since the kidney happens to be by far the most common commercial solid organ, the chapter will focus largely on its specific market. Having said that, it will also discuss the organ market question in general, that is to say, regardless of any specific organ or tissue. Second, the terminology that prevails in the discourse about the organ market is often vague, inaccurate, prone to equivocation and, above all, biased and possibly misleading. The following glossary seeks to maximize accuracy, maintain neutrality, and minimize the risk of confusion and misunderstanding. Above all, it aims to clarify the terms as they are to be used in this chapter.

***Address correspondence to Miran Epstein:** Barts and The London School of Medicine and Dentistry Queen Mary, University of London, United Kingdom; Tel: +44 (0) 20 7882 7086; Fax: +44 (0) 20 7882 2552; E-mail: m.epstein@qmul.ac.uk

Massimiliano Veroux and Pierfrancesco Veroux (Eds)

Glossary (in Alphabetical Order)

Alienation. The state of being estranged from one's own life, body, soul, actions, products, family, or community. The opposite of attachment. Alienation presupposes and implies some sort of *coercion*.

Autonomy. Self-determination. Decision-making and acting under *freedom*. The opposite of *heteronomy*.

Altruistic donation. Non-alienated organ donation, *i.e.* one in which the donor continues to care about the organ, now in the recipient's body, as if he/she never lost it.

Coercion. The condition of *heteronomy*. Any condition that restricts or distorts choice, information, rationality and action. The opposite of *freedom*. It can be non-social (not man-made) or social (man-made).

Commerce. Exchange of *commodities*.

Commercialism. Any practice, policy, or discourse that support any particular kind of *commerce*; *e.g.*, organ commercialism.

Commodification. A value-laden term denoting any kind of *commoditization* of which the speaker is critical. Usually refers to commoditization that involves *alienation*; *e.g.*, commoditization of body and soul.

Commoditization. A value-neutral term denoting the act of turning an object, which has not previously been a commodity, into a *commodity*. For example, the kidney has already been commoditized, as opposed to the heart which has not been commoditized as of yet.

Commodity. The object of *commerce*. Any object that has an exchange value; *i.e.* that can be exchanged for another object, thereby switching ownerships. Money, for example, is currently the most common commodity.

Exploitation. As a value-neutral term, exploitation denotes extraction of benefit from the use of an object. For example, a machine or an opportunity can be exploited. As a value-laden term, exploitation denotes a consent-mediated act of capitalizing on the other's weakness for one's own interest in a way that reaffirms one's domination over the other. Unfair exchange, where the commodities that switch hands are not equivalent in value, is an example of this form of exploitation. Slavery and robbery are not exploitative in this sense, assuming that they are not mediated by the consent of the victim.

Freedom. The condition of *autonomy*. Absence of restrictions on and distortions of rationality, information, choice, and action. The opposite of *coercion*.

Heteronomy. Decision-making and acting under *coercion*. The opposite of *autonomy*.

Market. The social sphere where commercial dealings are taking place.

Pseudononcommercialism. Any practice, policy or discourse that purports to be noncommercialist, but in fact tends to pass commercial transactions for altruistic donations.

Regulated market in organs. A market in organs, in which one or more of the following are regulated by the state: eligibility to trade, price of the organ, quality of the organ, care of recipients and vendors, allocation of organs.

Trafficking. Originally a value-neutral term (yet currently used in a derogatory sense) denoting any practice that facilitates a particular kind of commerce but is external to the transaction itself, *e.g.*, brokering, couriering, advertising, *etc.*

Transplant tourism. Travel of recipient, donor, organ, or some/all of them, across national boundaries, for transplantation. One should distinguish between transplant tourism that involves *commerce* in organs from such that does not. The latter may either be a particular form of medical tourism or take place in the context of inter-national agreements of cooperation.

Unfettered market in organs. An unregulated market in organs. An organ market whose transactions are governed solely by the power relations between the parties. An unfettered market can be either legal (a 'free' market) or illegal (a 'black' market).

THE KIDNEY MARKET IN PRACTICE

A systematic analysis of the actual kidney market requires consideration of four points. First, this market is a *social fact*, not merely a theoretical possibility. It actually accounts for a certain volume of all kidney transplants. Second, it has taken several *different forms* that need to be acknowledged and identified. These forms pertain to its legal status, economic confines, identifiability, and the sources of the organs it utilizes. Third, it is not a stable endemic phenomenon, but rather *a practice in flux*. It changes in form, volume, and social status. Fourth, it *has a history*. That is not merely to say that it has a past or that it has changed over time (which is trivially true), but rather that it has been shaped and continues to be shaped by certain social circumstances that are in flux too. Moreover, it has a reciprocal effect on these circumstances. Understanding this dialectical process is a necessary precondition of any rational intervention therein.

The Kidney Market is a Social Fact

At the Second Global Consultation on Human Transplantation of the World Health Organization's (WHO) in March 2007 it was estimated that commerce in organs accounts for 5-10% of kidney transplants performed throughout the world [1, 2]. These figures may not seem very high. However, the tendency of the market to concentrate in certain places, that is to say, to involve buyers and vendors from certain countries, communities and even genders, suggests that even low rates may have significant local, national, and international, implications.

Having said that, there are two good reasons to suspect that the actual figures are significantly higher. Firstly, the estimate is based on known data only. An unknown number of transactions remains clandestine owing to illegality and stigmatization. Secondly, the estimate pertains solely to global variants of the organ market, where individual transactions involve at least two countries at a time. It ignores local markets altogether. The volume of such markets and the global-to-local ratio are yet to be gauged. However, the socioeconomic distribution of potential buyers and vendors, inter-national differences in the implementation and enforcement of anti-commerce norms, and differences in the nature and intensity of transplant pressures, suggest that, at least until recently, the global variant had predominated, notwithstanding the fact that it contravenes international conventions and notwithstanding the political stigma it carries [3-11].

The global market involves transplant tourism with the most common form being that of a rich (or insurance-funded) recipient travelling to a poor country for transplantation of a kidney purchased from a local subject. The Sindh Institute of Urology and Transplantation (SIUT) in Pakistan reveals that at least 2000 commercial kidney transplants had been performed in this country until 2007 with virtually all buyers being tourists, including 80 coming from the small country of Trinidad alone. In the Philippines, the number of kidney sales to foreign patients until 2007 was said to be over 3000 [12]. In 2007, Israel imported at least 20 commercial kidneys from the Philippines every month *via* transplant tourism [13]. The Egyptian Society of Nephrology estimates that at least 500 commercial kidney transplants are performed in the country annually, mostly for foreign patients [14]. At least 100 nationals from countries such as Saudi Arabia (700 in 2005), Taiwan (450 in 2005), Malaysia (131 in 2004) and South Korea (124 in the first eight months of 2004) went abroad annually for a commercial kidney transplant. At least 20 nationals from Australia, Japan, Oman, Morocco, India, Canada and the United States travelled as transplant tourists to buy organs.

In this context, the story of China warrants a special discussion. In 2006, 11, 000 transplants were performed there: 8000 kidney transplants, 3000 liver transplants, and approximately 200 heart transplants. The majority of the organs were obtained from executed prisoners. According to Amnesty International, China has executed thousands of offenders annually with figures shifting between 1700 and 10, 000 [15]. The use of executed prisoners as a source of organs raises many issues that cannot be addressed in a chapter that deals with organ commercialism only. Jefferies estimates that approximately 4, 500 executed prisoners per year generate between 2, 000 and 3, 000 commercial organs [16].

Culminating in the 2008 Declaration of Istanbul, the recent international campaign against organ commercialism has had some significant achievements [17, 18]. Often mediated by new legislation and tightened enforcement, the campaign appears to have caused some decline in the volume of the global variant of the organ market [19]. Whether it has affected the total volume of the market as well is unclear, but it has certainly made thing more difficult for the stakeholders. As we shall see, however, there are signs that the market is quickly adapting to the new restrictions: it changes its form.

The Kidney Market takes Different Forms

The kidney market takes several different forms largely depending on the prevailing local and international political, legal, declarative and regulatory constraints. These forms pertain to its *legal status*, *economic confines*, *identifiability* and the *source of the organs*.

(a) Legal status. Iran is the only country so far to have legalized and partly regulated the kidney market. The trade is controlled by two nongovernmental organizations—the Charity Association for the Support of Kidney Patients (CASKP) and the Charity Foundation for Special Diseases (CFSD)—both endorsed by the government. The CASKP connects potential recipients and donors, and organizes tests to ensure compatibility. The regulations assert that both vendor and buyer must be Iranians. The vendor must be 20-35 of age, healthy, and provide a written consent also from a spouse or parent. The donor will receive an equivalent of €900 (2007) from the government in addition to one year free health insurance, a fixed payment from the recipient (a similar sum), and any extra payment from the recipient achieved through direct or mediated negotiation. The last point indicates that the Iranian model is a hybrid of a regulated market and a free market [20-22]. In other countries, organs are being traded in the black market only.

In most countries the organ market still has no legal status at all. In other words, they have not criminalized commerce and trafficking in organs. Having said that, the majority have some laws and/or mechanisms in place that are supposed to ensure that transplantation involves altruistic donations only. Whether or not these mechanisms do what they are supposed to do is a different matter.

Several countries have so far criminalized organ trafficking, but actual commerce remains largely decriminalized. This means that buyers and sellers are not regarded as having committed a criminal offence, whereas brokers are. Countries such as U.S.A. (1985), [23] India (1994), Pakistan (2007), and Israel (2008), have banned organ trafficking (interestingly, the Chinese law too regards organ trafficking as a severe offence carrying capital punishment). Enforcement varies greatly from one place to another. However, conviction rates are generally very low. There is currently no international law forbidding organ trafficking.

(b) Economic confines. We have already seen that a large part of the organ market is globalized, involving various forms of transplant tourism: (1) recipient from country A travelling to country B for an organ purchased in country B; (2) vendor from country B travelling to country A where the transplant takes place in a recipient from country A; (3) both vendor and buyer travelling to another country for the transplant. Local markets exist as well, and not just in Iran where the market is legal. Countries with extreme economic gaps plus deep-rooted cultural reluctance to use cadaveric organs, like India, have quite an extensive local market in organs from living vendors. This is in addition to their involvement in the global market as well.

(c) Identifiability. Although the organ market in Iran is legal, the individuals involved often conceal what has happened of fear of stigmatization. This is to show that legalization does not necessarily imply normalization and moralization. In this context, it is noteworthy that the right to confidentiality plays a complex role. On the one hand, it protects the parties from stigmatization. Yet on the other hand, in doing so, it reaffirms and perpetuates the market and the stigma associated with it.

In contrast to the legal market, the black market shows a prominent tendency to conceal itself behind legalistic and linguistic non-commercial façades. Referred to as *pseudononcommercialism*, this phenomenon is likely to evolve, or should at least be suspected, under the following circumstances: (1) commerce in organs is the object of some strong social interests, and (2) oversight mechanisms are in place to ensure that organ donations are exclusively altruistic, and (3) these mechanisms are lax [24].

Pseudononcommercialism has different expressions. Most generally speaking, it takes the form of *legal fiction*, namely, a presumption that is taken to be true, irrespective of whether it is true or false, and even though it might be false (see 'fiction' in The Concise Dictionary of Law and Merriam-Webster's Dictionary of Law) [25, 26]. In this respect, there are two fictions which often supplement each other. The most common one capitalizes on the presumptions that 'professed altruism necessarily reflects altruism', or, alternatively, that 'professed altruism necessarily rules out organ vending'. These presumptions almost beg organ vendors to lie to the oversight committees [27]. The other fiction builds on various material benefits, which are openly offered to donors, plus a narrow and exclusive definition of organ commercialism that regards these benefits as essentially altruistic. In this case then, the market capitalizes on the presumption that 'the benefits can never be regarded by the donor as a kind of payment', or, in other words, that 'they can never motivate the donation'. The typical way this fiction works in practice is through a set of euphemisms describing material benefits as anything but commercialism. These euphemisms include 'stimuli', 'ethical incentives', 'rewards', 'gratuity packages', 'removal of disincentives', 'compensation', 'reimbursement of expenses with fixed components', 'reimbursement of lost earnings for the unemployed', 'repatriation of corpse', 'funeral expenses', 'memorialisation benefits', 'health tax relief', 'health care coverage', 'life insurance', 'furloughs for prisoners-donors', *etc.* For example, the new Israeli transplant law now allows the Ministry of Health and certain nongovernmental organisations to offer donors stimuli of potentially commercial nature, including 'reimbursement of lost earnings' for unemployed donors. Until recently, up to $13, 400 could be paid directly to families for memorialisation. However, from now on the money could only be paid to the providers of the memorialization project, and not directly to the family (as if it really matters). Let it be noted that the very same law regards organ trafficking as a punishable criminal offence [28].

(d) The source of the organ. The organ market takes its particular forms also depending on the source of its commodities. Two general points need to be acknowledged in this respect. The first point is that there is no source or form of organ donation that precludes the possibility of commerce. Even living non-directed donations, where organs are donated to a pool rather than to designated individuals, are not immune from commercialization. In such cases, the doctors involved may act either as middlemen/brokers or even as dealers. Relatedness does not preclude commercialization either. It only makes it easier to conceal. The second point is that, notwithstanding what has been said, the vast majority of commercial organs comes from living vendors, typically unrelated to the recipient. This fact can be attributed to several factors including cultural reluctance to accept commercial or non-commercial cadaveric organs, higher quality of organs from the living, emotional detachment from the vendor, and the relative ease of concealing such transactions behind the cloak of altruism. Having said that, organs from cadaveric sources can be commoditized as well. Indeed, some of the aforementioned pseudononcommercialist measures clearly pertain to such sources.

The Organ Market is in Flux

A detailed chronicle outlining the evolution of the organ market is beyond the scope of this chapter. However, some major milestones need to be mentioned if only to emphasize the fact that the organ market is not a stable endemic phenomenon but rather a process in flux.

The organ market (mainly for *ritual purposes*) has a very long past, dating many centuries back [29]. Needless to say, however, a market in organs for *transplantation* could not have emerged before the advent of modern transplant technology. The story of the eighteenth century Scottish surgeon, John Hunter (1728-1793), furnishes probably the earliest evidence of commerce in body parts for this particular purpose. In the 1770s, Hunter had advocated the transplantation of teeth, a practice that was rapidly adopted by high-class dentists, first using teeth supplied by grave-robbery, then from living children-vendors [30, 31].

Owing to high rejection rates, a significant market in organs for transplantation emerged only after the advent of cyclosporine in 1971. In fact, the ethical debate on the market arose only in the early 1980s. Until the mid 1990s, the organ market had existed in some countries with transplant services as a largely silent, relatively unorganized, sporadic phenomenon. It typically took the form of a black market involving living vendors, buyers, brokers and transplant teams, all from the same country. Its yet largely undefined legal status combined with virtually no enforcement at all meant that most transactions concealed themselves behind some of the aforementioned pseudononcommercialist loopholes. Although the state turned a blind eye to the phenomenon, it did not support it actively.

For reasons that will be discussed later on, this has changed. Since the mid 1990s, the organ market has become largely globalized. Albeit tacitly, some governments and health insurers in rich countries were urging their kidney patients to obtain a transplant abroad, preferably even before the latter were to be put on dialysis. In fact, they often supported this outbound tourism financially [32]. In parallel, governments and medical institutions in some poor countries encouraged this inbound tourism [33-41]. At first, China was the major organ-exporting centre (similar practices have also taken place in other countries, including Pakistan, Turkey, India, Egypt, Iraq, Moldova, Latvia, South Africa, and several countries in Latin America). However, it toned down this activity largely of fear that international outcry would interfere with the 2008 Olympic Games in Beijing. The Philippines was quick to fill in the void, but it was forced to revoke its pro-tourism policy shortly thereafter following an international campaign against transplant tourism conducted by The Transplantation Society (TTS) and the World Health Organization (WHO) [42-44]. Recently, however, the new Health Secretary of the country announced his intention to lift the ban on selling organs to foreigners and offer 'donors' a 'gratuity package'. Culminating in the Declaration of Istanbul (2008), the effect of this campaign was immediate and impressive, with several countries that had been heavily involved in transplant tourism—Israel and Pakistan, for example—enacting fairly radical anti-commercialist transplant laws and closing (albeit not hermetically) their gates to outbound and inbound transplant tourism. Moreover, the Declaration of Istanbul Custodian Group (DICG), an oversight forum aiming to enforce the implementation of the Declaration, has established a global network of 'emissaries', whose task is to report violations of the principles of the Declaration.

But notwithstanding these developments, transplant tourism that involves organ trafficking and commerce is still taking place in one way or another. The death of this phenomenon is thus still too early to pronounce. For example, in March 2009, Singapore was about to brand itself as a pseudononcommercialist international transplant centre inviting 'donors' and 'recipients' from other countries. With a similar rationale in mind, China is currently demanding the right to allocate up to 5% of its national organ pool to foreigners. (The '5% rule' is a completely arbitrary American standard that was allocated years ago for medical tourism and international aid, not for organ commercialism. Ironically, it now turns out to have a pseudononcommercialist potential, which threatens to undermine the achievements entire anti-tourism campaign.) Recently, the DICG complained to the Israeli Ministry of Health that, in breach of the new Israeli transplant law, Israeli couples of donor and recipient had been travelling to the Philippines for the transplant, receiving a certificate from the Israeli Embassy in Manila attesting to their 'relatedness' and declaring 'relatedness' to meet the requirements of the local law [45]. In April 2009, Israeli health care providers and insurers reinterpreted the Declaration of Istanbul as if it only banned transplant tourism that involves trafficking in organs from the *living*, not the *deceased*. In accordance with this interpretation, they started sending transplant tourists to a hospital in Quito, Ecuador, for commercial deceased donor organ transplant.

In parallel, the relative success of the anti-tourism campaign is now giving rise to intensive attempts to deglobalize the organ market and confine it to national bounds. For example, in 2008, U.S. Senator Arlen Specter (D-Pa.) proposed an amendment in the existing National Organ Transplantation Act (NOTA) that would allow financial incentives for deceased and living donors [46]. In 2009, the American Society of Transplant Surgeons made it clear that while it supported the particular position of the Declaration of Istanbul on international organ trafficking, it did not accept its sweeping rejection of all other forms of organ commercialism, notably local ones [47]. Moreover, the Council and Ethics Committee of the Society conducted a survey of its members' views on strategies to increase organ donation, which showed that the majority supported material incentives for both deceased and living donation. Moreover, there was strong support for a government-regulated trial to evaluate the potential benefits and harms of financial incentives for both deceased and living donation [48]. In May 2010, the British Nuffield Council on Bioethics published a consultation paper on organ sales [49]. Considering the prevailing trend, the final report (which is to become policy) is very likely to support some forms of local commercialism. In November 2010, the International Forum on the Legal and Ethical Issues of Gifted/Rewarded/Incentivized Organ Donation from Living and Deceased Donors, a forum of proponents of localized markets, will hold a meeting in Manila, the Philippines. It will probably attempt to revise the Declaration of Istanbul. Like the latter, it will reject global organ commercialism; however, unlike it, it will embrace some forms of local organ commercialism.

The Kidney Market has a History

In the previous section, we saw that the organ market has a past (it has existed for some time now) and that it has been in flux (it has changed in form and extent). However, we said nothing about the circumstances that had given rise to it and have sustained it ever since as an *abstract* phenomenon. Nor did we say much about the circumstances that have shaped its *concrete* expressions as it evolved.

The History of the Organ Market in the Abstract

Most generally speaking, one may plausibly assume that the organ market exists because it meets the interests of certain social stakeholders. This truism is not very informative, however. We need to identify (1) these stakeholders, (2) their particular interests, and (3) the social circumstances that have given rise to their interests.

a) The **patient** who suffers from end-stage renal disease (ESRD) regards the market as a potential *source of healthy kidneys*. This interest builds on two accurate premises: first, transplantation is better than dialysis, and second, the market can meet the demand for the organs. Underlying this interest are rising morbidity rates increasingly caused by certain profit-driven forms of production and consumption [50] and failure to obtain kidneys from other sources.

b) The **doctor** whose business is to treat patients regards the market as a potential *source of transplants*. This interest also builds on the premises that transplantation is better than dialysis and that the market can meet the demand for the organs. At any rate, it reflects the failure to control morbidity and obtain kidneys from other sources.

c) Other players regard the organ market as a potential source of *profit or funding*, depending on whether the system in question is private or public, respectively. This group includes the

hosting medical institution, the **transplant system**, its **supporting technological and pharmaceutical industries**, and, under certain circumstances, even **organ brokers** and the **travel and tourism business**. Some of these stakeholders may have some direct interest in the organ market. Put differently, the benefit they expect to extract from this market may not be related to any failure to obtain organs from other sources. In fact, they would favour the market even if there were no shortage of organs from other sources.

d) Payers and purchasers of health care—**states**, **insurers**, **providers**, and **taxpayers**—are interested in the *cost-saving potential* of the organ market. Kidney transplant, for example, has the biggest cost-saving capacity of all organs, considering the relatively large number of patients with renal failure and the high cost of dialysis per patient. Although its cost per patient (around £46, 000) is more than the annual cost of dialysis (around £25, 000), once the transplantation has been done, annual treatment expenses drop to £7, 000 each year, a saving of £18, 000 per patient per annum. The overall saving is more than double, however. Thus every 2, 400 kidney transplantations done in a certain year would save the payer a total of one billion pounds over the next decade [51, 52]. Underlying the cost-saving interest is an increasingly intensifying global economic competition and an overwhelming neo-liberal policy advocating abolition of the welfare state.

e) For **those who can sell nothing but their body parts**, the organ market promises *financial deliverance*. Poverty and financial distress are largely the outcomes of unequal distribution and redistribution of socially produced wealth.

We have mentioned the failure to obtain organs from other sources as one of the factors that have given birth to various interests in the market. This point warrants a brief discussion concerning its dimensions and causes.

In general, the organ crisis reflects a gap between demand and supply. This crisis seems to be getting worse. The U.S., for example, saw a 46% increase in the absolute number of donors between 1995 and 2008, but the patient to donor ratio has increased at a much faster rate (142%) and continues to grow. In 2009, the number of patients with end-stage renal disease (ESRD) listed for transplantation stood at just over 77, 000 with only 16, 000 receiving transplantation in that year. Another 25, 000 patients were waiting for other organs, mainly heart, lung, liver and pancreas [53]. The British experience is essentially similar. In March 2008, 7, 500 patients were on the active transplant lists, and a further 2, 000 were on the temporarily suspended transplant lists. This represents an increase of 6% and 10%, respectively, compared to the corresponding figures from the previous year [54]. The trend in Europe is somewhat different with a slight drop in the patient to donor ratio, but the number of patients on the waiting list saw a thirtyfold increase from 1969 to 2006.

The causes of this trend are complex. On the one hand, the increasing demand for organs is related both to rising rates of morbidity as well as to intensifying financial interests. On the other hand, declining and at any rate insufficient supply has several reasons too. Socioeconomic-cultural circumstances affecting social solidarity and mutual aid, including willingness to donate organs, are often implicated in this respect.

For example, some communities of Jewish Orthodox conviction forbid both deceased and living organ donation, but not reception [55]. In other societies, reluctance to sign a donor card or donate organs of deceased relatives may be secondary to cultural reluctance to receive cadaveric organs. Misunderstanding of the way death is established, distrust in the motivations of the medical authorities, and perhaps even awareness of the inferiority of cadaveric organs relative to organs from the living are negative factors as well. In addition, reluctance to sign a donor card is commonly attributed to laziness, indifference, and unawareness. These phenomena are known to thrive in the absence of effective donor recruitment programmes. Indeed, the efficiency of such programmes has a direct bearing on the supply of organs.

The commercial option may perhaps compensate for the any decreased willingness to donate organs. However, in doing so, it creates a viscous cycle. At first it decreases such willingness even further ('why should I donate a kidney to my brother, if I can help him buy a kidney from a stranger'). In turn, the decreasing willingness to donate makes the market even more attractive an option.

The History of the Concrete Expressions of the Organ Market

The emergence of a black market in organs reflects a social compromise between interests in a market in organs in the abstract on the one hand and interests in protecting the traditional non-commercialist ethos of transplant medicine on the other hand. The emergence of *global organ commercialism*, the hitherto dominant form of the black organ market, is not surprising. In offering virtually unlimited supply of kidneys, global organ commercialism brings together the diverse interests of many stakeholders: patients on the waiting lists in rich countries and the parsimonious payers of their expensive dialysis (states, insurers, and providers), the middlemen involved (brokers, officials, and doctors), the hosting medical centres, the organ-exporting countries, the travel and tourism industries, and, finally, the impoverished men and women who can sell nothing but their body parts. On a more general note, global organ commercialism tallies with the economic zeitgeist known as 'neoliberal globalization', the conception that purports to enhance competitiveness, among other things, by shopping around the globe for the cheapest commodities available, while promising that wealth will eventually 'trickle down' to benefit the poor too [56].

But if this is the case, then how are we to explain the emergence of an *organized campaign against this trend*, let alone a somewhat successful one? The answer is simple: global organ commercialism has failed to deliver on its promises. As it grew, it transpired to be a double-edged sword: it has spared none of the stakeholders but the various intermediaries [57].

Rich countries that have been spellbound by its promises may have had no qualms about its morality, but they did find its practical drawbacks disturbing at times. Many of them are now experiencing a deepening shortage in organs. True, it is largely the result of increasing morbidity and could thus be depicted as the outcome of too little 'outsourcing' rather than too much. But this is apparently just a partial picture. Global organ commercialism is said to have had a direct negative effect on local donation rates. It has thus sidelined the patients who could not 'outsource' and thereby increased the financial burden on their healthcare payer.

Global organ commercialism has also sparked global competition for patients, organs, and investments between transplant services of rich and poor countries. In this competition, the former are increasingly disadvantaged (it may be of interest to note that the representation of this victim in the campaign against global organ commercialism is particularly prominent) [58].

Moreover, global organ commercialism has failed to deliver on its promises to the 'tourists' (transplant recipients) themselves, with outcome studies indicating increased morbidity mainly due to poor vendor screening, selection, and matching in the organ-exporting country complicated even further by poor record keeping. In fact, the possibility that transplant tourists import not just kidneys but perhaps some transmissible infections as well has become a public health hazard [59-62]. Such upshots and perils do not affect individual and public health only. They also call the very financial logic of outgoing transplant tourism into question. Global transplant commercialism has affected poor countries too. Diverting organs and scarce public resources to the incoming transplant tourism industry, it has elbowed aside both the local patients on the waiting lists as well as the public services that should have treated them. And last but not least, whatever its benefits, few, if any, have trickled down to the impoverished vendors. On the contrary, the latter often fall victim to manipulation, fraud, and physical violence. At any rate, their post-transaction health and financial status tend to worsen [63-68].

All these failings were reflected in a remarkable phenomenon: the campaign against global organ commercialism has become an ad hoc alliance between proponents of local organ commercialism and opponents of any organ commercialism. The two things that unite these strange bedfellows are their hostility towards global organ commercialism and their desire to meet the local demand for organs. Otherwise, there is a war going on between them, a war about the appropriate solution to the organ crisis. Interestingly, this partnership-rivalry knows no bounds; it exists in rich and poor countries alike [69-71].

As we have seen, the results of the campaign have so far been mixed: on the one hand, a certain decline in the volume of the global market, but on the other hand, a rise in pseudononcommercialist practices and increased attempts to deglobalize, legitimize and localize the market in some more or less regulated form.

The Ethical Discourse

So far, our discussion about the organ market has been sociological-historical, not judgmental. We have seen that the emergence of a market in kidneys and its evolution reflect a dynamic compromise among agonistic and antagonistic interests. We have also seen that these interests have evolved under certain historical, man-made, circumstances and that the market, now absorbed into these circumstances, reaffirms these interests even further. Above all, we have seen that the very existence of the market and its progressive legitimization reflect the domination of those interests that derive some benefit from it. Interestingly but not surprisingly, the same domination is also reflected in the discourse about the market. As we shall see, both the anti-market side of this discourse as well as the pro-market one have been shaped not just by the interests which each would be expected to promote, but also by the interests of the other. In other words, each one of them is making some compromise with the other. As it happens, however, the concessions, which the pro-market case has made to the other side, are minor. In fact, they are exclusively terminological. In contrast, the concessions, which the anti-market case has made, are significant. They reflect embarrassment and, more important, misunderstanding of the faults of the market. In other words, the entire pros and cons discourse reflects the increasing hegemony of pro-market forces.

The Pro-Market Discourse

The pro-market discourse maintains that, however efficient, a transplant donor programme that only appeals to social solidarity and the goodwill of individuals will inevitably fail to meet the increasing demand for organs. It asserts that letting patients suffer and die on the waiting lists, when so many organs are out there just begging to be harvested, is morally unacceptable, and so is wasting public resources. Non-commercial systems are thus both ineffective as well as immoral [72, 73].

The pro-market discourse also holds that the market, and only the market, can provide unlimited access to these organs and be moral at the same time. Not any market, though. The global organ market, for example, is not just counterproductive but also immoral. This is because it creates, as its practical drawbacks clearly reflect, severe inequities in the distribution of power, benefit, and risk. Such faults, the pro-market discourse contends, result from the essentially unfettered nature of this particular market. A global organ market cannot be tamed and is thus bound to remain both counterproductive as well as immoral.

That said, the pro-market discourse argues that an organ market that is free from any practical drawbacks and inequities is feasible within the bounds of a national market or an economic union. Such a market must adhere to certain regulatory principles, which were outlined already in the mid 1990s [74]. As far as the protection of recipients is concerned, the principles include a single buyer, mechanisms assuring safety and quality, and systems that guarantee equitable, non-means-based, allocation of the organs. The principles are no less attentive to the welfare of the vendors. In addition to the single buyer, they include mechanisms validating consent requirements, safeguards against buying organs from vulnerable people, strict prohibition of brokering, and systems assuring competitive remuneration, life insurance, continuous healthcare, and priority in transplant waiting lists [75-82].

Otherwise, the pro-market discourse sees no essential moral problem with trading in organs. Firstly, body parts are private property. In the name of liberty, their owners should be free to do with them as they like [83-89]. Secondly, both parties can make a free choice, at least in principle. The unpleasant nature of the dilemma each one of them is facing does not by itself render their choices heteronomous. On the contrary, it is rather the existing prohibition of commerce in organs that limits their freedom, often with dire consequences for both of them. Thirdly, the generally accurate classification of buyers and vendors as rich and poor, respectively, may perhaps seem to reflect inequities and suggest relations of power and exploitation. However, this does not have to be the case. In the regulated market, the pro-market discourse holds, the parties would maintain perfectly symmetrical relations vis-à-vis each other. Their complementary deficiencies and surpluses would guarantee 'mutual exploitation' and hence equal distribution of benefits and risks. Fourthly, proponents of the market remind us that many instances involving commerce in the body are already legitimate. Making the kidney an exception would be ethically inconsistent. Fifthly, the real choice we are facing, and the only one, is between a regulated market and a black market, so they are saying. Considering the interests of buyers and vendors, the former is not only by far the better option. It is also the remedy against the black market. To sum up, the pro-market discourse argues that a regulated market is feasible, that it entails nothing but benefit to all stakeholders, and that it is ethical.

The concessions, which the pro-market case is making to its rival are merely terminological. In attempt to convince the public to accept its position, it employs pseudononcommercialist tokens, such as 'incentives', 'gifted rewards' and 'compensation'. Interestingly, it is not willing to wait until the local market becomes fully regulated. Its use of pseudononcommercialist tricks suggests that its proponents are really interested in one thing only—increasing the organ pool. All the other things, which the ideally regulated market purports to guarantee, are apparently just lip service.

The Anti-Market Discourse

While the pro-market discourse is robust in its own terms, its rival is not. Firstly, it directs its moral critique at the grotesque features of what might be described rather as the unfettered market ('exploitation' of 'vulnerable' vendors). Ironically, this is exactly what the proponents of the regulated market do, which explains why they too accepted the recent international declarations and how seriously anti-commercialist (not just anti *global* organ commercialism) the latter really are.

Secondly, it fails to tackle the essence of organ commercialism, that is, the very principle of trade in body parts. In other words, it fails to challenge the ideally regulated market on its own terms. Occasionally, it attacks the financial element of the transaction for being either coercive when it involves a lot of money ('undue inducement') or exploitative when it involves little money, and at any rate humiliating. In truth, the financial element may be exploitative for both parties (for example, if the kidney is sold for a price that is above or below its real value, whatever that is), but not coercive. In itself, money simply allows the potential vendor to make the choice whether to sell the organ or not. Without pointing at whatever *essential* faults commerce in organs might have, the use of expressions such as 'commodification of the body' and 'violation of human dignity' becomes mere sentimentalism. The same goes for the psychological argument of 'repugnance' [90].

Thirdly, the pragmatic objection of the anti-market case to the regulated market, which maintains that regulation would be counterproductive, if not altogether impossible, may or may not make sense. However, it is no less problematic. With so much money at stake, it posits, the regulatory mechanisms that purport to assure liberty, quality, and safety are bound to fail. Doctor-patient relationship would be harmed, and people would start selling what they currently donate, which would rather increase public spending [91-99]. On top of that, there is a serious risk that once rich countries introduce a regulated market, poor countries will immediately follow suit. In such countries, the prospects of ideal regulation are very low (as the Iranian model clearly shows). Whether such fears are sound or not is beside the point. The problem with this essentially empirical criticism is that it actually invites the proponents of the market to try to prove their case. They will not turn this invitation down. Who knows, they might also succeed. And even if they don't, there will be no easy way back.

Fourthly, the anti-market discourse tends to identify and denounce pseudononcommercialist practices only when these are overly blatant. It is usually silent about the more subtle fictions, notably 'altruistic-directed living unrelated donation' [100]. This situation may suggest that the anti-market campaign is willing to make a compromise with the market, as long as the compromise allows it to pretend that it has made no compromise. Another problem with the anti-market discourse concerns its recent appeal to all countries to assume enduring responsibility for healthcare and financial welfare of local organ donors. This plea, which purports to protect organ vendors in poor countries and 'remove disincentives' to donation in rich countries, is certainly compassionate and rational, respectively. At the same time, however, it makes organ vending even more attractive.

Fifthly, the anti-market discourse tends to squirm whenever its rival invokes the 'precedent argument'. This argument rightly maintains that your case against the commoditization of the kidney would fall flat, if you accepted other instances of commoditization of the body. On the medical side, such instances include paid participation in clinical trials, commerce in reproductive tissue, reproductive surrogacy, commerce in blood, and sexual surrogacy. Non-medical instances pertain to commerce in sex and labour power, the latter being not only the most widespread form of commoditization of the body, but arguably also the ethical paradigm for all future commoditizations of the body. The fact that most anti-market campaigners condone at least some of these practices is yet another evidence that commercialist ideas have pervaded their discourse.

Rephrasing the Market Question

We have seen that the proponents and the opponents of the organ market are united on one basic premise: if an organ market involves any coercion/exploitation, then the latter should be sought *in the act of exchange*. This premise explains why both parties reject the unfettered market. After all, transactions that take place in that market typically involve coercion/exploitation. The premise is also the source of the controversy on the very principle of buying and selling body parts, a principle that is best reflected in the concept of an ideally regulated organ market. Proponents of the market argue that ideally regulated exchange involves no coercion/exploitation, whereas opponents of the market regard such transactions as intrinsically coercive/exploitative. The views of both parties on this matter seem to be mutually exclusive. If one is correct, then the other is wrong, and vice versa.

And yet both are right and both are wrong at the same time, albeit in different respects. Proponents of the organ market are right in asserting that organ-money transactions do not have to involve coercion/exploitation. However, they are wrong in assuming that the absence of exchange-related coercion/exploitation precludes extra-transactional coercion/exploitation. Similarly, opponents of the market are right in assuming that any organ-money exchange presupposes some sort of coercion/exploitation. However, they are wrong in confining their search of the fault to the sphere of exchange.

Indeed, one prominent fact suggests that organ-money transactions presuppose coercion/exploitation, even if they are intrinsically flawless: they always involve *alienation* (see definition in the glossary section of the introduction). Indeed, it is a well-documented fact that kidney vendors typically wish that their kidney be rejected (The only exception to this rule is an altruistic, *i.e.* non-alienated, donation, which coincidentally involves payment to the donor). The point is that the coercion is to be found not in the sphere of exchange, but rather in the social circumstances that have made the exchange possible and attractive to begin with. To be more specific, it is to be found in the vectors that have shaped the particular options of each party: *buying or dying* for the patient, and *selling or dying* for the potential vendor (the term 'dying' is used here as a metaphor standing for dreadful options in general). These vectors have been discussed above in the section dealing with the history of the organ market.

To sum up: both parties, buyer and vendor, may perhaps make a completely free choice whether or not to enter the respective transaction. Indeed, in the ideally regulated market they do. That having been said, none of them has chosen freely to face the respective dilemma in the first place. Both were forced to face it. Both are victims of social, man-made, coercive circumstances.

Three important conclusions can be drawn at this point. The first conclusion pertains to the nature of the ethical debate in general: it transpires to be ideological to the bone. Preoccupied exclusively with the nature of the organ-money transaction (whether it is coercive or not), it ignores the fundamental source of the coercion and thereby reaffirms it even further [101, 102]. The second conclusion pertains to the ideally regulated market: it transpires to be an ethical façade of coercive social circumstances. Those who are either happy with these circumstances or just regard them as unchangeable should certainly support this market. The third conclusion pertains to the anti-market case: it could certainly make sense, but only as part of a greater struggle against these coercive circumstances. This road may not guarantee success, but failure to follow it will most likely result in defeat.

CONCLUSION

This chapter has shown that both the organ market as well as its satellite ethical discourse have evolved under coercive social circumstances. One might perhaps wish to ignore them. In such case, the organ market should receive full support. On the other hand, rejecting this market would only make sense as part of a greater struggle against these circumstances. If it succeeds, it will save more lives than the market could ever dream of saving.

REFERENCES

[1] Shimazono Y. The state of the international organ trade: a provisional picture based on integration of available information. Bull World Health Organ 2007; 85:955-962.

[2] Budiani-Saberi DA, Delmonico FL. Organ trafficking and transplant tourism: a commentary on the global realities. Am J Transplant 2008; 8:925-929.

[3] Leung G. Fun, sun, get a surgery done! The growing trend of transplant tourism. Issues Berkeley Med J 2006; 13:7-8.

[4] Milstein A, Smith M. America's new refugees: seeking affordable surgery offshore. N Engl J Med 2006; 355:1637-1640.

[5] Watkins C. 3 ways to cash in on the growth of offshore surgery alternatives. Managed Care Rep 2006; 21:146-149.

[6] Bramstedt KA, Xu J. Checklist: passport, plane ticket, organ transplant. Am J Transplant 2007; 7:1698-1701.

[7] Freeman RB. 'Transplant tourism' in the United States? Transplantation 2007; 84:1559-1560.

[8] Delmonico FL. The Pakistani revelation. Transplant Int 2007; 20:924-925.

[9] UNOS board further addresses transplant tourism; 2007. http://www.unos.org/newsDetail.asp?id=891.

[10] Merion RM, Barnes AD, Lin M, *et al.* Transplants in foreign countries among patients removed from the US transplant waiting list. Am J Transplant 2008; 4:988-996.

[11] Surman OS, Saidi R, Purtilo R, *et al.* The market of human organs: a window into a poorly understood global business. Transplant Proc 2008; 40:491-493.

[12] RP admits 'rampant' traffic in human organs. http://www.manilatimes.net/national/2007/feb/07/yehey/topstories/20070207top1.html.

[13] Israel citizens organ transplant in Columbia - Medellin. http://www.happylife.co.il/main eng.html.

[14] El-Agroudy AE, Sabry AAl, *et al.* Long-term follow-up of living kidney donors: A longitudinal study. BJU International 2007; 100:1351-1355.

[15] Amnesty International. The death penalty in Asia in 2009. http://www.amnesty.org/en/death-penalty/death-sentences-and-executions-in-2009/asia

[16] Jefferies DE. The body as commodity: The use of markets to cure the organ deficit. International Journal of Global Legal Studies 1998; (5)2:621-658.

[17] Steering Committee of the Istanbul Summit. Organ trafficking and transplant tourism and commercialism: the Declaration of Istanbul. Lancet 2008; 372:5-6.

[18] WHO. WHO guiding principles on human cell, tissue and organ transplantation. EB123/5 2008:1-8.

[19] Delmonico FL. The implications of Istanbul Declaration on organ trafficking and transplant tourism. Curr Opin Organ Transplant 2009;14:116-119.

[20] Ghods AJ, Savaj S. Live kidney organ donation: is it time for a different approach? Iranian model of paid and regulated living-unrelated kidney donation. Clin J Am Soc Nephrol 2006; 1:616-625.

[21] Iran's market in human organs. The Economist. Nov16th, 2006.

[22] Griffin A. Iranian organ donation: Kidneys on demand. BMJ 2007; 334:502-505.

[23] National Organ Transplantation Act 1985. 42 U.S.C.A. § 274(e).

[24] Epstein M. Pseudononcommercialism: The Trojan horse of the organ market. In Organ transplantation: Ethical, legal and psychological aspects. Expanding the European platform. Pabst Science Publishers.

[25] The concise dictionary of law. Oxford: Oxford University Press 1983.

[26] Merriam-Webster's dictionary of law. MA: Springfield, 1996.

[27] Epstein M, Danovitch GM. Is altruistic directed living unrelated organ donation a legal fiction? Nephr Dial Transplant 2009; 24: 357-360.

[28] Organ Transplantation Law 5768-2008. Israeli book of laws. http://www.justice.gov.il/NR/rdonlyres/F8E6E7B8-D67A-475A-B64A-F9B86797F282/9952/2144.pdf (in Hebrew).

[29] Scott R. The body as property. New York:Viking Press, 1981.

[30] Richardson R. Transplanting teeth: reflections on a cartoon by Thomas Rowlandson. Lancet 1999; 354:1740.

[31] Richardson R. A necessary inhumanity? Med Humanities 2000; 26:104-106.

[32] Resnik R. Half of the Israeli kidney recipients—commerce in organs. Ha'aretz, 2003; 1 (in Hebrew).

[33] Leung G. Fun, sun, get a surgery done! The growing trend of transplant tourism. Issues Berkeley Med J 2006; 13:7-8.

[34] Milstein A, Smith M. America's new refugees: seeking affordable surgery offshore. N Engl J Med 2006; 355:1637-1640.

[35] Watkins C. 3 ways to cash in on the growth of offshore surgery alternatives. Managed Care Rep 2006; 21:146-149.

[36] Bramstedt KA, Xu J. Checklist: passport, plane ticket, organ transplant. Am J Transplant 2007; 7:1698-1701.

[37] Freeman RB. 'Transplant tourism' in the United States? Transplantation 2007; 84:1559-1560.

[38] Delmonico FL. The Pakistani revelation. Transplant Int 2007; 20:924-925.

[39] UNOS board further addresses transplant tourism; 2007. http://www.unos. org/newsDetail.asp?id=891. [Accessed 30 October 2008].

[40] Merion RM, Barnes AD, Lin M, *et al.* Transplants in foreign countries among patients removed from the US transplant waiting list. Am J Transplant 2008; 4:988-996.

[41] Surman OS, Saidi R, Purtilo R, *et al.* The market of human organs: a window into a poorly understood global business. Transplant Proc 2008; 40:491-493.

[42] Republic of the Philippines, Department of Health, Office of the Secretary. Revised national policy on kidney transplantation from living nonrelated organ donor and its implementing structures. Administrative Order No. 2008-0004; 2008.

[43] Philippine Society of Nephrology. Statement on Department of Health Administrative Order 2008-0004; 2008.

[44] The Transplantation Society and the International Society of Nephrology. The Transplantation Society and the International Society of Nephrology support the Philippine Society of Nephrology. Letter sent to the Philippine Government and the office of the President; 2008.

[45] Hibner Har'el M. Legal Advisor to the Israeli Ministry of Health. Letter of complaint to Ehud Keinan, Legal Advisor to the Ministry of Foreign Affairs, 22 March 2010 (in Hebrew).

[46] Organ Donation Clarification Act of 2008: Proposed Specter Bill. 8 September 2008. http://www.asts.org/Advocacy/Legislative.aspx.

[47] Reed AI, Merion RM, Roberts JP, Klintmalm GB, Abecassis MM, Olthoff KM, Langnas AN. The Declaration of Istanbul: Review and commentary by the American Society of Transplant Surgeons Ethics Committee and Executive Committee. Am J Transplant 2009; 9:2466-2469.

[48] Rodrigue, JR, Crist K, Roberts JP, *et al.* Stimulus for organ donation: A survey of the American Society of Transplant Surgeons membership. Am J Transplant 2009; 9:2172-2176.

[49] Nuffield Council on Bioethics. Give and take? Human bodies in medicine and research. May 2010. https://consultation.nuffieldbioethics.org/fileLibrary/pdf/Human_bodies_in_medicine_and_research_consultation_paper.pdf.

[50] Wenying Y, Juming L, Jianping W, *et al.* Prevalence of diabetes among men and women in China. N Engl J Med 2010; 362:1090-1101.

[51] About Operations. Organ donation: facts and figures. http://www.aboutoperations.co.uk/organ-donation-facts-figures.html.

[52] NHS Blood and Transplant (2009). The cost-effectiveness of transplantation.http://www.uktransplant.org.uk/ukt/newsroom/fact_sheets/cost_effectiveness_of_transplantation.jsp.

[53] Organ Procurement and Transplantation Network. 2009. http://www.optn.org/latestData/rptData.asp.

[54] NHS Blood and Transplant. 2008. Transplant activity in the UK 2007-2008.http://www.uktransplant.org.uk/ukt/statistics/transplant_activity_report/transplant_activity_report.jsp.

[55] Gal I. Heart recipient's father: We'll never donate organs. Yedioth Ahronot 29.1.09. http://www.ynet.co.il/english/articles/0,7340,L-3663653,00.html.

[56] Epstein M. Sociological and ethical issues in transplant commercialism. Curr Opin Organ Tran 2009; 14(2):134-139.

[57] Turner L. Let's wave goodbye to 'transplant tourism'. BMJ 2008; 336:1377.

[58] Budiani-Saberi DA, Delmonico FL. Response to: Will transplant tourism erode the surgical skills of transplant surgeons in Israel? Am J Transplant 2008; 8:1964.

[59] Prasad GV, Shukla A, Huang M, *et al.* Outcomes of commercial renal transplantation: a Canadian experience. Transplantation 2006; 82:1130-1135.

[60] Canales MT, Kasiske BL, Rosenberg ME. Transplant tourism: outcomes of United States residents who undergo kidney transplantation overseas. Transplantation 2006; 82:1658-1661.

[61] Levine GN, Port FK, Burdick J. Transplants in foreign countries among patients removed from the US transplant waiting list. Am J Transplant 2008; 8:988-996.

[62] Gill J, Madhira BR, Gjertson D, *et al.* Transplant tourism in the United States: a single-center experience. Clin J Am Soc Nephrol 2008; 3:1820-1828.

[63] Noorani MA. Commercial transplantation in Pakistan. BMJ 2008; 336:1378.

[64] Budiani D. Consequences of living kidney donors in Egypt. Presentation at the Middle East Society on Organ Transplants (Mesot) meetings; November 2006; Kuwait.

[65] Naqvi SAA, Ali B, Mazhar F, *et al.* A socioeconomic survey of kidney vendors in Pakistan. Transpl Int 2007; 20:934-939.

[66] Naqvi SAA, Rizvi SAH, Zafar MN, *et al.* Health status and renal function evaluation of kidney vendors: a report from Pakistan. Am J Transplant 2008; 8:1444-1450.

[67] Sajjad I, Baines LS, Patel P, *et al.* Commercialization of kidney transplants: a systematic review of outcomes in recipients and donors. Am J Nephrol 2008; 28:744-754.

[68] Stephan A, Barbari A, Younan F. Ethical aspects of organ donation activities. Exp Clin Transplant 2007; 5:633-637.

[69] Laurance J. Surgeon: organ trade should be legalized. The Independent June 2008. http://www.independent.co.uk/life-style/health-and-wellbeing/health-news/surgeon-organ-trade-should-be-legalised-846234.html.

[70] Danovitch GM, Leichtman AB. Kidney vending: the 'Trojan horse' of organ transplantation. Clin J Am Soc Nephrol 2006; 1:1133-1135.

[71] Satel S, Hakim N. 'What's wrong with selling kidneys?' International Herald Tribune 20 June 2008. http://www.iht.com/articles/2008/06/20/opinion/edsatel.php.

[72] Brennan T. Markets in healthcare: the case of renal transplantation. J Law Med Ethics 2007; 35:249-255.

[73] Novelli G, Rossi M, Poli L, *et al.* Is legalizing the organ market possible? Transplant Proc 2007; 39:1743-1745.

[74] Erin CA, Harris J. A monopsonistic market: or how to buy and sell human organs, tissues and cells ethically. In: Robinson I, editor. Life and death under high technology medicine. Manchester: Manchester University Press in association with the Fulbright Commission, London; 1994. pp. 134-153.

[75] Friedman AL. Payment for living organ donation should be legalized. BMJ 2006; 333:746-748.

[76] Friedman E, Friedman AL. Payment for donor kidneys: pros and cons. Kidney Int 2006; 69:960-962.

[77] Daar AS. The case for a regulated system of living kidney sales. Nat Clin Pract Nephrol 2006; 2:600-601.

[78] Hippen B. The case for kidney markets. The New Atlantis Fall 2006:47-61.

[79] Satel S. Paying for kidneys. The Washington Post 30 April 2007. http://www.washingtonpost.com/wp-dyn/content/article/2007/04/29/AR2007042901321.html.

[80] Abouna GM. Organ shortage crisis: problems and possible solutions. Transplant Proc 2008; 40:34-38.

[81] Matas AJ. Should we pay donors to increase the supply of organs for transplantation? Yes. BMJ 2008; 336:1342.

[82] Godlee F. Is it time to pilot paying for organs? BMJ 2008; 336.

[83] Humber JM. Coercion, paternalism, and the buying and selling of human organs. In: Humber JM, Almeder RF, eds. Biomedical ethics reviews. New Jersey: Humana Press, 1985:13-25.

[84] Andrews LB. My body, my property. Hastings Cent Rep 1986; 16:28-38.

[85] Campbell C. Body, self, and the property paradigm. Hastings Cent Rep 1992; 22:34-42.

[86] Childress JF. The body as property: some philosophical reflections. Transplant Proc1992; 24:2143-8.

[87] Radcliffe Richards J. Nepharious goings on: kidney sales and moral arguments. J Med Philos1996; 21:375-416.

[88] Radcliffe-Richards J, Daar AS, Guttmann RD, Hoffenberg R, Kennedy I, Lock M, Sells RA, N Tilney. The case for allowing kidney sales. Lancet 1998; 351 (9120):1950 - 1952.

[89] Taylor JS. Autonomy and organ sales, revisited. Journal of Medicine and Philosophy 2009; 34(6):632-648.

[90] Roth AE. Repugnance as a constraint on markets. Journal of Economic Perspectives 2007; 21(3):37-58.

[91] Chapman J. Should we pay donors to increase the supply of organs for transplantation? No. BMJ 2008; 336:1343.

[92] Danovitch GM. The doctor/patient relationship in living donor kidney transplantation. Curr Opin Nephrol Hypertens 2007; 16:503-505.

[93] Paramesh AS, Killackey MT, Zhang R, *et al.* Living donor kidney transplantation: medical, legal, and ethical considerations. South Med J 2007; 100:1208-1213.

[94] Danovitch GM. Cultural barriers to kidney transplantation: a new frontier. Transplantation 2007; 84:462-463.

[95] Zargooshi J. Iran's commercial renal transplantation program: results and complications. In: Weimar W, Boss MA, Busschbach JJ, editors. Organ transplantation: ethical, legal and psychosocial aspects. Lengerich: Pabst Science Publishers 2008; 80-94.

[96] Danovitch GM. Who cares? A lesson from Pakistan on the health of living donors. Am J Transplant 2008; 8:1-2.

[97] Danovitch GM, Delmonico FL. The prohibition of kidney sales and organ markets should remain. Curr Opin Organ Transplant 2008; 13:386-394.

[98] Delmonico FL, Danovitch GM. Regulated market for organs is unattainable. Minn Med 2008; 91:6.

[99] Tilney NL, Chapman JR, Delmonico FL. Debate on financial incentives is off the mark of national and international realities. Transplantation 2010; 89:906-907.

[100] Epstein M. The Declaration of Istanbul on Organ Trafficking and Transplant Tourism: an important international achievement with one disturbing loophole. BMJ 2008. http://www.bmj.com/cgi/eletters?lookup=by_date&days=1#198338.

[101] Epstein M. The ethics of poverty and the poverty of ethics: the case of Palestinian prisoners in Israel seeking to sell their kidneys in order to feed their children. J Med Ethics 2007; 33:473-474.

[102] Epstein M. Pros and cons of a regulated market in organs. Lancet 2009; 374:2049-2050.

CHAPTER 11

Pediatric Renal Transplantation

Kar-Hui Ng, Wee-Song Yeo and Hui-Kim Yap*

Department of Pediatrics, Yong Loo Lin School of Medicine, National University of Singapore and University Children's Medical Institute, National University Health System, Singapore

Abstract: Renal transplantation is the treatment of choice for children with end-stage renal disease as it results in better survival rates and quality of life compared to dialysis. The pediatric transplant population represents a unique population whereby patients undergo rapid phases of growth and development, not only physically but also mentally and psychologically. This chapter provides an overview of the current trends and issues pertaining to pediatric renal transplantation. These issues include the discrepancy in size between the young recipient and the large adult-sized kidney, variations in the development of the immune response, specific pediatric considerations in immunosuppressive regimens, non-adherence in adolescence, and the greater propensity for infections and viral-driven lymphoproliferative disorders, growth failure and long-term cardiovascular disease. Recurrence of the primary renal disease, especially focal segmental glomerulosclerosis, is a significant concern in pediatric renal transplantation, as this often results in graft loss. Patients with abnormal urinary tracts will need evaluation and often surgical correction prior to transplant. Advances in immunosuppression regimens and surgical techniques in the last two decades have dramatically improved short and medium-term patient and graft survival outcomes in pediatric renal transplantation. Long-term graft survival, however, remains suboptimal, due to calcineurin inhibitor toxicity, cardiovascular disease, infections and non-adherence. Therefore the current challenge in pediatric renal transplantation will be to improve long-term graft survival by minimizing the side effects of immunosuppression while preventing rejections. There are trends towards steroid and/or calcineurin inhibitor-sparing immunosuppressive regimens, with the use of non-depleting or depleting monoclonal and polyclonal antibodies as induction therapy.

Keywords: Immunosuppressive Regimens, Induction Therapy, Monoclonal Antibodies, Polyclonal Antibodies, Growth Failure, Non-Adherence, Tacrolimus, Cyclosporine, Acute Rejection, Living Donor.

INTRODUCTION

End-stage renal disease (ESRD) is an important cause of morbidity and mortality in both developing and developed countries, resulting in significant economic burden. Renal transplantation is the treatment of choice for children with ESRD, as it results not only in better survival rates but also better quality of life compared to dialysis [1]. Moreover, it alleviates the medical complications associated with ESRD, and facilitates significant improvement in cognition and psychosocial functioning [2]. Renal transplantation is more cost-effective compared to dialysis in the long term [3]. Nevertheless, access to renal transplantation is variable across the different countries in the world, and is influenced by several factors such as patient demographics [4], patient race/ethnicity [5-7], etiology of ESRD [4], geographical location [8-10], and the local incidence of ESRD [8]. In addition, socioeconomic, religious and cultural attitudes, availability of funding, local experience and national policies on deceased donor transplantation and organ allocation also affect access to a renal transplant [11].

The current success in pediatric renal transplantation is a culmination of improvements in pre-transplant evaluation, operative techniques, post-transplant care, and immunosuppression regimens as well as early diagnosis and treatment of, and prophylaxis against, potential opportunistic infections [12]. Though the success rates in pediatric renal transplantation have been encouraging, the process remains a challenge. The pediatric transplant population represents a unique population whereby patients undergo rapid phases of

***Address correspondence to Hui-Kim Yap:** Division of Pediatric Nephrology, University Children's Medical Institute, Yong Loo Lin School of Medicine, National University of Singapore, Singapore; Tel: +65 67724411; Fax: +65-67797486; E-mail: hui_kim_yap@nuhs.edu.sg

Massimiliano Veroux and Pierfrancesco Veroux (Eds)

growth and development, not only physically but also mentally and psychologically [13]. This chapter provides an overview of the current trends and issues pertaining to pediatric renal transplantation. These issues include the discrepancy in size between the young recipient and the large adult-sized kidney, variations in the development of the immune response, specific pediatric considerations in immunosuppressive regimens, non-adherence in adolescence, and the greater propensity for infections and viral-driven lymphoproliferative disorders, growth failure and long-term cardiovascular diseases. These issues must be properly addressed for maximal patient and graft outcomes.

EPIDEMIOLOGY

In North America, the incidence and prevalence of ESRD in the pediatric population, defined as age 0 to 19 years, has been steadily increasing since 1980 [14]. The pediatric ESRD incidence rate has increased by 3.5% from 14.1 per million age-related population in 2000 to 14.6 per million age-related population in 2007 [14]. In addition, the pediatric ESRD prevalence rate has nearly tripled since 1980, albeit with some slowing in recent years as the increase was modest at only 11.4% since 2000. In 2007, 7,209 pediatric patients were receiving ESRD treatment, with an adjusted rate of 84.6 per million age-related population. Since the establishment of the North American Pediatric Renal Transplant Cooperative Society (NAPRTCS) in 1987, there were 9854 pediatric patients who have received a renal transplant compared to 6491 patients who have received dialysis [15]. Approximately 800 kidney transplants are performed annually in children below 18 years of age in North America [15]. The number of pediatric renal transplant patients has also increased by almost 19% since 2000.

Most developed nations have the resources to provide for sufficient funds and organized deceased donor networks for renal transplantation to be offered uniformly to all patients who need it. Hence, a relatively higher proportion of children with ESRD in these countries have received a transplant. In the United Kingdom, there are between 700 and 800 children on renal replacement therapy, about two thirds of whom have renal transplants [16]. Collective data from 28 European countries showed an overall point prevalence of 20.1 per million age-related population for pediatric transplant recipients with functioning grafts in 2007. This was more than half of all pediatric patients with ESRD (33.6 per million age-related population) [17].

In contrast, in many developing countries such as Pakistan [18], Sri Lanka [19], Vietnam [20], and South Africa [21], renal replacement for children is nonexistent or poorly developed due to limited resources, funding and expertise. Even if available, challenges such as delayed referral and poor patient compliance make transplantation difficult [22]. Hence, it is not surprising that less than 1% of children with ESRD in the developing world receive transplants [18], and that the transplantation rates for children in developing nations are low at less than 5 per million age-related population [19]. Interestingly, the donor types within these developing nations differ due to cultural and social attitudes, as well as availability of dialysis facilities and deceased donor programs. In countries where there are no deceased donor programs such as India [23], Pakistan [18], Sri Lanka [19] and Egypt [24], transplants are exclusively from living related donors, mainly parents. In countries with established deceased donor programs such as South Africa [21], Chile [25] and Thailand [26], deceased donor rates are much higher at 61 to 79%, comparable to 50% in North America [15]. Iran with its regulated living paid donor program, reports 80% of transplants from living unrelated paid donors, of which more than 40% are preemptive [27]. Indeed, rates of preemptive transplants vary greatly in developing nations from 2.6% in Turkey [28] to almost 50% in Sri Lanka [19], where dialysis facilities are absent. Comparatively, 26% of pediatric renal transplants in North America are preemptive [15].

UNDERLYING CAUSES OF ESRD IN PEDIATRIC RENAL TRANSPLANT RECIPIENTS

The causes of ESRD in the pediatric population are different from adults. In the adult population, the majority of ESRD are due to diabetes and hypertension [14]. On the other hand, congenital structural abnormalities of the urinary tract and glomerulonephritis predominate in the pediatric population [15]. Data from the USRDS as well as other developed countries [15, 29] showed that congenital structural abnormalities of the kidney and urinary tract, including renal hypoplasia-dysplasia, obstructive uropathies as well as reflux nephropathy occur in more than 35% of children with ESRD. Of the glomerulopathies, focal segmental glomerulosclerosis (FSGS) is the most common cause of ESRD, occurring in at least 10%. Other causes including hemolytic uremic syndrome, polycystic kidney disease, juvenile nephronophthisis, Alport's syndrome, congenital nephrotic syndrome and cystinosis form 2 to 3% of the causes. Less common causes include other glomerulopathies such as membranoproliferative glomerulonephritis types I and II, crescentic glomerulonephritis, lupus nephritis, Henoch-Schönlein purpura nephritis, immunoglobulin A (IgA) nephropathy and systemic polyarteritis including Wegener's granulomatosis, forming 1 to 2% of the causes of ESRD. Other rare causes pertinent to pediatric patients include primary hyperoxaluria type 1, Wilms' tumor and Denys-Drash syndrome, comprising less than 1% of cases. In addition, sickle cell nephropathy and diabetic nephropathy must be considered in susceptible populations.

On the other hand, in some parts of the world, glomerulopathies are the more important causes of ESRD in children. In Finland, congenital nephrosis (Finnish type) remains the most common cause of ESRD in children younger than 15 years of age [30]. Japan reports a very high proportion (34%) of cases secondary to glomerulopathies, namely FSGS and IgA nephropathy in their pediatric ESRD population [31], while the Australia and New Zealand Dialysis Registry reported that glomerulonephritis accounts for the majority (42%) of causes of ESRD in children and adolescents [32].

Because CKD is diagnosed in its earlier stages in developed countries, congenital causes predominate in most countries. In contrast, in developing countries where patients are referred in the later stages of CKD, infectious or acquired causes such as chronic glomerulonephritis predominate [33] due to a higher prevalence of bacterial, viral and parasitic infections such as hepatitis C, malaria, schistosomiasis, tuberculosis and human immunodeficiency virus [34]. This high prevalence of glomerulonephritis may also be related to a better diagnosis rate due to obvious clinical features and more rapid progression. In addition, children with 'unknown' cause of ESRD constitute up to half of all the transplanted children in the developing world; a rather rare entity in developed world [22]. This is mainly due to the very late diagnosis in most of the patients as well as the lack of available investigation facilities, such as renal biopsy and imagery [33]. In addition, certain causes of ESRD may be more common in some countries than others. For example, hereditary disorders such as polycystic kidney disease, primary hyperoxaluria, Alport syndrome and congenital nephrotic syndrome are more prevalent in countries like Jordan and Iran where consanguinity is common. Lastly, the data depicting causes of ESRD in developing countries are mainly reports from single centers and are of only those children who were transplanted. These numbers can by no means be confidently considered as representative of the general population [22].

Renal replacement therapy should be considered in all children with ESRD, defined as a glomerular filtration rate of less than 15 ml/min/1.73m^2 [35]. However, not all ESRD patients are suitable candidates for renal transplantation, and the outcome of renal transplantation depends to some extent on the underlying cause. One possible contraindication to renal transplantation is the presence of an active malignancy and especially so if it has metastasized. In patients with Wilms' tumor, current recommendation with regards to the timing of renal transplantation is to wait for one to two years after completion of treatment in view of the increased risk of mortality from sepsis secondary to immunosuppression following chemotherapy and radiation therapy, as well as the published findings of an increased incidence of recurrence of tumor or metastases in children transplanted within one year of treatment of the disease [36]. A recent review of the NAPRTCS database comparing the outcomes of renal transplantation between children with a primary diagnosis of Wilms' tumor and children with other diagnoses, demonstrated comparable outcomes [37]. In children with XO/XY gonadal dysgenesis and renal failure (Denys-Drash syndrome), there is a high frequency of Wilms' tumor if the native kidney is left *in situ*. Current recommendations therefore include native nephrectomy prior to transplantation.

Patients with bladder dysfunction such as neurogenic bladder, Prune-Belly syndrome and posterior urethral valves have to undergo thorough evaluation, including urodynamic studies, prior to transplantation. They may require augmentation cystoplasty with appendicovesicostomy (Mitrofanoff) so that clean intermittent catheterization can be performed adequately to prevent damage due to high bladder pressures [35-37]. Patients with dilating vesicoureteric reflux may require ureteric reimplantation to prevent recurrent urinary tract infections post-transplant, whereas those with massive reflux may require nephroureterectomy.

Recurrence of the primary renal disease is a significant concern in pediatric renal transplantation. The overall risk of graft loss due to disease recurrence is 7 to 8%, the majority of which are due to primary glomerulonephritis [38]. Glomerulopathies that have a high risk of graft loss include FSGS (14 to 50% risk of recurrence and 40 to 60% risk of graft loss) [38-40], membranoproliferative glomerulonephritis type 2 (30 to 100% risk of recurrence and 17 to 61% risk of graft loss) [38, 41-43] and membranous nephropathy (30% risk of recurrence and 50% risk of graft loss) [38]. Other glomerulonephritis that may recur include IgA nephropathy, lupus nephritis, and anti-neutrophilic cytoplasmic antibody (ANCA)-associated glomerulonephritis (Table 1) [38]. Patients with ESRD due to Alport syndrome and congenital nephrotic syndrome, strictly-speaking, are not at risk of recurrence of the original disease, but are, however, at risk of development of anti-GBM disease and *de novo* nephrotic syndrome respectively. Other diseases that have a high risk of graft loss include atypical hemolytic uremic syndrome (20 to 80% risk of recurrence and 10 to 83% risk of graft loss) [44, 45] and primary hyperoxaluria type 1 (80 to 100% risks of recurrence and graft loss in the absence of a liver transplant). Additional strategies should be considered for patients with underlying disease that may recur after transplantation, such as donor selection, concomitant liver transplantation, plasmapheresis or specific immunosuppression protocols. Patients are rarely excluded from renal transplantation unless the risk of disease recurrence is very high and there have been repeated graft losses [38].

Table 1: Risks of disease recurrence and graft loss for various primary renal diseases (Adapted from Reference [38])

Primary Renal Disease	Risk of Disease Recurrence	Risk of Graft Loss
Focal segmental glomerulosclerosis	14-50%	40-60%
Membranoproliferative glomerulonephritis	30-100%	17-61%
Membranous nephropathy	30%	50%
Lipoprotein glomerulopathy	~100%	~100%
Atypical hemolytic uremic syndrome	20-80%	10-83%
Primary hyperoxaluria type 1	80-100%	80-100%
IgA nephropathy	36-60%	7-10%
Lupus nephritis	0-30%	0-5%
Wegener granulomatosis	-	0-6%
Overall	-	7-8%

Inborn errors of metabolism such as cystinosis may also lead to progressive renal injury. Cystinosis is a rare autosomal recessive disorder affecting primarily tubular function. Its major manifestations are early-onset Fanconi syndrome [46], and progressive renal glomerular deterioration culminating in ESRD at seven to twelve years of age [47]. Early treatment with cysteamine, a cystine-depleting agent, can delay glomerular deterioration and accumulation of cystine in other organs. Renal transplantation in these children has significantly prolonged their survival, however, cystine continues to accumulate unabated in most organs post-transplantation, leading to late systemic complications [38]. Hence, cysteamine should be continued after renal transplantation. There is no risk of recurrence of the primary disease in the graft, even though protocol biopsies have shown cystine crystals deposited within the interstitial tissue without any clinical or biological manifestations [38].

The two most common indications for combined liver and kidney transplantation in children are primary hyperoxaluria type 1 and autosomal recessive polycystic kidney disease [48, 49]. When patients with primary hyperoxaluria type 1 develop ESRD, systemic oxalosis rapidly develops due to insufficient oxalate excretion with conventional dialysis. Isolated renal transplantation does not correct the underlying metabolic defect and generally has a poor outcome due to deposition of oxalate crystals in the graft [50]. Combined liver and kidney transplantation is now generally accepted as the treatment of choice, especially in children, and outcomes have been good [51, 52]. In patients with ESRD due to autosomal recessive polycystic kidney disease with concurrent congenital hepatic fibrosis or Caroli's disease, combined liver and kidney transplantation has been performed with good results [53, 54].

DONOR-RECIPIENT SIZE MISMATCH

The optimal moment to transplant a child with ESRD is preemptively just before dialysis becomes necessary, provided there is an available donor. This avoids complications associated with dialysis such as peritonitis or venous access problems, as well as loss of precious years of growth potential [55]. However, early transplantation may be challenging for the very young due to, among other factors, the disparity in size between the adult donor and young pediatric recipient. Many centers prefer an age above two years and a weight above 15 kg before proceeding with renal transplantation [56], though some centers will perform transplant surgery on children at least 6 months of age, and a minimum weight of approximately 10 kg [55, 57]. Previously, infants and younger children were rarely transplanted in view of the greater incidence of early graft loss and mortality in this age group [58, 59]. However, this has since changed with the improvement in surgical techniques and immunosuppressive strategies.

In small children, some consideration must be given to the site where the transplant kidney is to be placed. The traditional extraperitoneal approach in the iliac fossa is often not suitable in small children due to lack of physical space for the large adult kidney. This can potentially cause significant pressure on the transplant kidney upon wound closure, resulting in vascular compression and compromise. In addition, anastomosis to the external iliac artery and vein can be challenging due to the small size of the recipient vessels compared to the donor renal vessels. Therefore, kidney transplantation in children below the age of five years is generally done through a midline incision, where the graft is placed into the peritoneal cavity, with vascular anastomosis to the recipient's caval vein and either the distal aorta or one of the common iliac arteries, depending on the size of the arteries and position of the renal graft [56]. Some young children with ESRD may have had previous intra-abdominal procedures, peritonitis or vascular access difficulties. In such patients, thrombosis of the major intra-abdominal vessels should be excluded, and if present, the donor kidney selected may have to be smaller to accommodate the small collateral vessels in the abdomen [60].

Another potential problem in small children is the relatively lower blood volume and cardiac output. Adult kidneys in small children can take up a large proportion of the cardiac output, resulting in a drop in blood pressure at reperfusion of the graft. This can cause insufficient perfusion of the graft, which has been used to the higher blood pressure of the donor. Such inadequate perfusion pressure in the early post-transplant period can result in poor graft function [61]. To circumvent this, it is important when dialyzing the patient on the day prior to transplant, to keep the patient slightly above his dry weight so as to facilitate post-transplant diuresis. Intraoperatively, it is crucial to over-hydrate the small recipient prior to reperfusion of the graft, keeping the central venous pressure between 12 to 15 cm water, as well as maintaining the systolic blood pressure above 100 mmHg. Fluid management in the early postoperative period is also critical and is determined by the urine output. There must be adequate volume loading especially during the diuretic phase of acute tubular necrosis, so as to ensure continued perfusion of the renal graft. Generally, total or almost total replacement of the urine output is necessary for at least the first few days post-transplant.

Ensuring adequate hydration to optimize perfusion of the disproportionately large donor kidney, and avoidance of compression of the new graft anastomosis are important measures that also help to minimize the risk of vascular thrombosis, a complication which is highest in the youngest age group. Despite the technical difficulties in transplanting an adult-size kidney into a small child, it is still crucial to use adult donors as opposed to pediatric donors as the former provides the young recipient with a large renal mass and is relatively less surgically complex [62]. Indeed adult-sized kidneys without acute tubular necrosis provide the best outcomes for infants and young children [63]. This explains why living donors, even if unrelated, are always preferred in a young child as delayed graft function is less likely to occur [62].

IMMUNOSUPPRESSIVE PROTOCOLS IN THE PEDIATRIC RENAL TRANSPLANT RECIPIENT

Advances in immunosuppressive regimes have significantly decreased the incidence of acute rejection episodes in both adult and pediatric renal transplantation, and as a result, short- and medium-term graft survival has significantly improved. However, long term graft survival has not improved dramatically in the last two decades [12], mainly due to the side effects of immunosuppression such as calcineurin inhibitor

(CNI) toxicity, infections, malignancy, diabetes and hypertension. The latter two also contributes to graft loss due to recipient mortality from cardiovascular events [15]. The current challenge in pediatric renal transplantation will be to improve long-term graft survival by minimizing the side effects of immunosuppression while preventing rejection, and nowhere is this more important than in children who have the lifetime risk of potential consequences of immunosuppression related to malignancy, infections, cardiovascular disease, growth and fertility. Additionally, the transplant physician is faced with management challenges arising from childhood obesity and diabetes mellitus. Another consideration specific to pediatric recipients is the problem of ontogeny, which may affect drug disposition and response.

Children under five years of age who received an adult-sized kidney are probably the best group to attempt immunosuppression minimization strategies, as these patients have the lowest risk of acute rejection, and the best graft survival rates [64]. However, the group of patients likely to benefit the most from immunosuppression minimization strategies is the adolescent group who is also more prone to non-adherence to medications. Immunosuppression minimization will minimize cosmetic effects from drugs and reduce the number of daily medications, thereby increasing the likelihood of adherence and extending graft survival.

Induction Agents

Current induction strategies aim to minimize acute rejection episodes and prolong long term graft survival by induction of immune tolerance or 'prope tolerance' (near tolerance) towards allografts. Induction therapy may involve non-depleting or depleting monoclonal and polyclonal antibodies, plasmapheresis, immunoadsorption and/or intravenous immunoglobulins. Not uncommonly, a biologic agent is used during induction, especially in individuals who are at high risk for rejection, such as in deceased donor graft recipients and sensitized patients. These are commonly used in conjunction with corticosteroids, anti-proliferative agents and CNIs, agents also used for maintenance therapy, albeit at lower dosages. According to the NAPRTCS 2008 Annual Report, induction therapy with a biologic agent is employed in approximately 53.6% of transplant recipients [15].

Peripheral T-cell/B-cell depleting agents are primarily monoclonal or polyclonal antibodies which are targeted against T- or B-cells and hence work primarily *via* inhibiting signal 1 of the immune response. Antithymocyte globulins (ATG) are polyclonal antibodies derived from either rabbit (Thymoglobulin®) or horse (Atgam®) sera, with broad T-cell specificity and is said to be the most potent polyclonal antibody to date [65]. Use of antilymphocyte antibody induction in young children allows for the delayed introduction of CNIs until graft function is well-established. Early introduction of these potentially nephrotoxic agents may increase the incidence, or prolong the duration of delayed graft function [62]. In the NAPRTCS 2008 Annual Report, ATG was used in 14% of living donor transplants, decreasing from 28% in 1996; and in 20% of deceased donor transplants, decreasing from 36% in 1996 [15]. This decrease in the use of ATG was associated with increasing utilization of monoclonal antibodies (both lymphocyte-depleting and non-lymphocyte depleting), from 21% in 1996 to 51% in 2006/2007 for living donor transplants and from 30% in 1996 to 50% in 2006/2007 for deceased donor transplants [15].

In a study by Olaitan *et al.* [66] which examined the long-term outcomes of intensive initial immunosuppression protocol using rabbit ATG in 75 pediatric recipients receiving deceased donor renal transplants, it was noted that only one (1.2%) recipient developed post-transplant lymphoproliferative disease (PTLD). The actuarial one and ten-year patient survival rates were 99% and 94% respectively, while the actuarial one and ten-year immunological graft survival rates were 91% and 63% respectively. The results of this study suggest that rabbit ATG as an induction agent is safe and effective in pediatric recipients of deceased donor kidneys with excellent immunological graft survival, without an increase in the incidence of PTLD.

Alemtuzumab (CAMPATH-1H) is a humanized CD52-specific complement fixing (cytotoxic-lymphodepleting) IgG1 monoclonal antibody first introduced in hemato-oncology by Waldmann and Hale [67] and then in renal transplantation by Calne [68]. This antibody is directed against the membrane glycoprotein CD52, which is found on T-cells, B-cells, monocytes/macrophages, natural killer cells,

CD34+ stem cells and granulocytes [66]. Originally approved for use in patients with chronic lymphocytic leukemia, alemtuzumab is increasingly being used as an induction agent in renal transplant, especially in adult recipients. In the initial studies by Calne *et al.* [68] where adult transplant recipients given two doses of Alemtuzumab as induction therapy followed by cyclosporine monotherapy, there was a lower incidence of acute rejection initially, compared to the control group. However, with the 5-year follow-up [69], the incidence of acute rejection equaled that of the control group and was approximately 30%. This was due to an increase in late (1 to 3 years post-transplant) rejections.

Experience in the use of alemtuzumab in pediatric renal transplantation remains limited. In a study by Tan *et al.* [70], who analyzed the first 42 pediatric consecutive living donor kidney transplants given alemtuzumab induction followed by tacrolimus monotherapy and subsequent spaced weaning, the actuarial one and four-year patient and graft survivals were 97.6% and 97.6%, and 93.5% and 85.4%, respectively. The incidence of cumulative acute cellular rejection at one, two and four years was 0%, 2.4% and 4.8%, respectively. The mean serum creatinine (mg/dL) and glomerular filtration rate (ml/min/1.73m^2) at 3 years were 0.9 ± 0.4 and 95.0 ± 21.7, respectively. Weaning to spaced dose (alternate day or less) tacrolimus monotherapy was attempted in 16 (38%) and was successful in 12 (26%) patients. There was no tissue invasive cytomegalovirus (CMV) disease or infection, BK/polyoma viral nephropathy, or PTLD, thus supporting the efficacy and safety of alemtuzumab in pediatric renal transplant recipients. Some of the adverse effects reported with alemtuzumab included mild cytokine-release syndrome, neutropenia, anemia, autoimmune thrombocytopenia, and thyroid disease.

Rituximab is a chimeric monoclonal antibody that contains murine heavy and light chain variable regions directed against CD20 plus a human IgG1 constant region. The CD20 antigen is found on both immature and mature B-cells. CD20 mediates both B-cell proliferation and differentiation. Following treatment with rituximab, B cells are prevented from proliferating and undergo apoptosis and lysis through complement-dependent and complement-independent mechanisms. B-cell depletion generally lasts 6 to 9 months in over 80% of patients, although the degree of depletion is highly variable [71]. Initially approved for the treatment of B-cell lymphoproliferative diseases in non-transplant patients and PTLD after organ transplantation, it is now being increasingly used for treatment of antibody-mediated rejection and for the suppression of preformed alloantibodies in sensitized patients (re-transplant, ABO-incompatible) before transplant, together with other immunosuppressive drugs, plasmapheresis and/or intravenous immunoglobulin [72].

Non-depleting antibodies currently in use in renal transplantation are the interleukin-2 receptor (IL-2R) monoclonal antibodies. Complete T-cell activation leads to the secretion of IL-2, a key autocrine growth factor that induces T-cell proliferation (signal 3). Hence, a possible mode of therapy would be abrogation of IL-2 activity *via* the administration of anti-IL-2R antibody. Daclizumab and basiliximab are humanized and chimeric IgG monoclonal antibodies, respectively, with a high specificity and affinity for the α-subunit of the IL-2 receptor (CD25). By binding to IL-2R, they prevent IL-2 from binding to these receptors, hence preventing the clonal expansion of activated T-cells. However, as IL-2R has overlapping functions with other interleukin receptors, the binding of IL-2R by these antibodies produces a relatively mild immunosuppression and is effective only in combination with other immunosuppressive agents.

Since daclizumab and basiliximab were introduced, they have been used increasingly as induction agents. In the NAPRTCS Annual Report 2008, the usage of these two antibodies increased from 5.6% in 1997 to 33.7% in 2007. In a recent meta-analysis by Webster *et al.* [73] which included 71 studies in adults and children (306 reports, 10,537 participants), IL-2R antagonists (IL-2RAs) were compared with placebo (32 studies; 5,784 participants). It was noted that graft loss including death with a functioning graft was reduced by 25% at one year (24 studies: RR 0.75, 95% CI 0.62 to 0.90), but not beyond this. Similarly, biopsy-proven acute rejection was reduced by 28% and CMV disease by 19% at one year. When IL-2RAs were compared to ATG (16 studies, 2211 participants), there was no difference in graft loss at any time point or incidence of acute rejection diagnosed clinically. However, there was benefit of ATG therapy over IL-2RA for biopsy-proven acute rejection at one year, but at the cost of a 75% increase in malignancy and a 32% increase in CMV disease. Moreover, ATG patients experienced significantly more fever, cytokine release syndrome and other adverse reactions to drug administration and more leukopenia but not thrombocytopenia. IL-2RAs appear to be as effective as other antibody therapies and with significantly fewer side effects.

The advent of these newer induction agents namely daclizumab, basiliximab and alemtuzumab, together with the increasing use of tacrolimus, mycophenolate and sirolimus, offers options of new combinations of drugs for steroid or CNI minimization regimens. Immunosuppression minimization strategies place the greatest emphasis on minimization or avoidance of CNIs and/or steroids, as elimination of their side effects will probably have the greatest benefit on improvement of patient and graft survival, and in the case of steroids, on growth. It may be that effective induction is the key; however opinion is currently divided about the optimal induction agent for such regimens, be it ATG, IL-2R blockade or alemtuzumab. Moreover, many of these strategies have been based on an increased dose or duration of the drugs used for induction. Such an approach has not been shown to impact significantly on infection or PTLD rates [64].

Maintenance Immunosuppression

Typically, maintenance immunosuppression utilizes a combination of immunosuppressive agents with different mechanisms of action, so as to fully harness their synergistic effects on immunosuppression and to minimize the adverse effects associated with each agent. Many transplant centers utilize a triple immunosuppressive regimen comprising corticosteroids (prednisolone or methylprednisolone), an antimetabolite (mycophenolate or azathioprine) and a CNI (tacrolimus or cyclosporine). Sirolimus is also being increasingly used in recent years, often substituting the CNI or antimetabolite. Data from NAPRTCS showed that almost 75% of pediatric transplant recipients received triple immunosuppressive therapy at one-year post-transplant [15], with an increasing number of centers favoring the use of mycophenolate and tacrolimus.

Corticosteroids

Glucocorticoids remain an integral part of the immunosuppressive regimens in most transplant centers. Binding to the glucocorticoid receptor results in migration of the active glucocorticoid-glucocorticoid receptor complex across into the nucleus, and binding to the promoter region of target genes, leading to induction or suppression of gene transcription. The immunosuppressive effects of glucocorticoids are complex, reflecting the summation of its effects on lymphocyte proliferation, apoptosis, expression of cell adhesion molecules and cytokine production.

Adverse effects of corticosteroids are well-known. In children, growth retardation, osteopenia, infections and lifelong cardiovascular risk associated with hypertension, diabetes mellitus and lipid abnormalities are particularly worrying. Nevertheless, steroids remain as part of the standard maintenance therapy for transplant patients due to their ability to prevent acute rejection. There have been trends towards minimization of steroids in both adult and pediatric transplant recipients due to the long-term morbidity associated with their side effects, and also availability of other more potent immunosuppressive agents.

Steroid-sparing strategies include alternate day dosing regimens, rapid or late steroid withdrawal post-transplantation and complete steroid avoidance. The safety of these strategies, especially in relation to acute rejection episodes, has not been unambiguously proven. However, recent studies have shown promising results in children. The Stanford study demonstrated that a complete steroid-free regimen comprising tacrolimus, mycophenolate mofetil and extended daclizumab induction for six months was very effective in causing sustained post-transplant growth in children up to 12 years of age at the time of transplantation, while achieving an acute rejection rate that was significantly lower in the steroid-free patients [74]. This regimen has been extended to a larger population of children and adolescents in a large multicentre trial in North America. Its preliminary results have not confirmed the effects of steroid avoidance on growth at one year post-transplant, although the incidence of acute rejection was comparable between the arms [75]. Another promising trial is the European TWIST (Tacrolimus and Withdrawal of STeroids) study, a multicentre randomized study that evaluated a tacrolimus-based regimen combined with mycophenolate mofetil and early steroid withdrawal at day five post-transplant, together with two doses of daclizumab, compared to standard triple therapy. The preliminary results demonstrated significant growth improvement as early as six months post-transplant, while the acute rejection rates and renal function were comparable between the two groups [76].

Anti-Metabolites (Azathioprine and Mycophenolate)

Azathioprine and mycophenolate are anti-proliferative agents that block *de novo* purine synthesis. Azathioprine is a purine analog derived from 6-mercaptopurine (6-MP) and has been used in renal transplantation for more than four decades. Azathioprine is metabolized in the liver to 6-MP and then subsequently converted to the active metabolite thioinosinic acid (TIMP). Its immunosuppressive action results from inhibition of proliferation of activated T and B lymphocytes [77]. Major adverse effects of azathioprine include that of bone marrow suppression with resultant leukopenia, anemia and thrombocytopenia, and hepatotoxicity. The toxic effects of azathioprine are augmented with the concurrent use of drugs like allopurinol, which increases the levels of TIMP.

Mycophenolate mofetil is a noncompetitive inhibitor of inosine monophosphate (IMP) dehydrogenase, a key enzyme in "*de novo*" synthesis of guanosine nucleotides, with resultant inhibition of proliferation of activated T- and B-lymphocytes. Because lymphocytes cannot efficiently utilize the salvage pathway of guanosine synthesis catalysed by hypoxanthine-guanine phosphoribosyltransferases, the anti-proliferative action of mycophenolate is lymphocyte-specific. Compared to azathioprine, it has less bone marrow toxicity, the major side effects being mainly gastrointestinal such as gastric discomfort and diarrhea.

In view of the success of mycophenolate in adult transplant recipients, this drug was subsequently investigated for its efficacy and safety profile in pediatric renal transplant recipients. Data from seven studies provided the evidence for the safety and efficacy of mycophenolate mofetil for use in pediatric transplant recipients [78-80]. The incidence of acute rejection at six to twelve months post-transplant in patients receiving mycophenolate mofetil in these studies ranged from 21 to 44% and was significantly better than previous conventional protocols. In a recent systematic review performed by Knight *et al.* [81], it was noted that mycophenolate mofetil significantly reduced the risk of acute rejection when used in combination with any CNI (relative risk 0.62, 95% CI 0.55 to 0.87). The hazard for graft loss, including death with a functioning graft, was also significantly reduced in patients treated with mycophenolate mofetil (hazard ratio 0.76, 95% CI 0.59 to 0.98). There was, however, no significant difference in patient survival or graft function between groups. Risk of adverse events, including CMV infection, anemia, leukopenia or rates of malignancy, did not differ significantly. A greater risk of diarrhea was seen in mycophenolate-treated patients. Unfortunately, children appeared to have a higher risk of side effects, requiring discontinuation of the drug [82]. Population pharmacokinetic-pharmacogenetic studies in pediatric renal transplant recipients have shown that inter-individual variability of mycophenolate disposition was contributed by body weight, UGT2B7 genotype and concomitant immunosuppressive medications [83]. Tacrolimus co-administration, unlike cyclosporine, results in delayed clearance of mycophenolate, requiring a reduction in the mycophenolate dose by at least half.

In another meta-analysis looking at the role of mycophenolate as the sole adjunctive immunosuppression in CNI minimization or elimination regimens, 19 randomized controlled trials in adults were assessed. There was some, albeit weak, evidence of improved graft survival with mycophenolate in CNI sparing regimens (odds ratio 0.72, 95% CI 0.52-1.01) [84]. Some studies in pediatric transplant recipients have also suggested that substituting azathioprine for mycophenolate mofetil may have a role to play in the prevention and treatment of chronic rejection [85].

Calcineurin Inhibitors

The introduction of cyclosporine as an immunosuppressive agent in transplant patients in the early 1980s has greatly improved outcomes in solid organ transplantation, mainly by reducing acute rejection episodes [86]. Immunosuppressive protocols using a CNI together with other immunosuppressants have been the mainstay of pediatric renal transplantation for more than two decades.

Both cyclosporine and tacrolimus are immunosuppressants which work *via* inhibition of the calcium-dependent serine phosphatase calcineurin, which is the rate-limiting step in T-cell activation. Both cyclosporine and tacrolimus cross the cell membrane freely and bind respectively to the immunophilins, cyclophilin and FK-binding protein 12 (FKBP12), which are intracellular proteins with isomerase activity. The complex then binds to calcineurin and blocks its interaction with nuclear factor of activated T cells (NFAT), preventing the transcription of many genes associated with T-cell activation.

Both CNIs have similar and different adverse effect profiles. Both agents can cause nephrotoxicity, hyperkalemia, hyperuricemia, hypomagnesemia, arterial hypertension, and tremor, albeit to different extents. For example, the incidence of hypomagnesemia is higher in the tacrolimus-treated group as compared to the cyclosporine-treated group [87]. The side effects of hypertrichosis and gum hyperplasia were only reported in the cyclosporine-treated group.

Tacrolimus is now the preferred CNI for maintenance immunosuppression in pediatric renal transplantation because of better graft survival and lower acute rejection rates, in addition to its lack of cosmetic side effects. A Cochrane review involving 4102 patients from 30 studies showed that at six months post-transplant, graft loss was significantly reduced in tacrolimus-treated (RR 0.56, 95% CI 0.36 to 0.86) compared to cyclosporine-treated recipients, and this effect was persistent up to three years. At one year, tacrolimus patients suffered less acute rejection (RR 0.69, 95% CI 0.60 to 0.79), and less steroid-resistant rejection (RR 0.49, 95% CI 0.37 to 0.64), but more insulin-requiring diabetes mellitus (RR 1.86, 1.11 to 3.09) [88]. There were no differences in infection or malignancy.

With better graft survival, the major focus in transplantation is the management of CNI-related adverse effects [89]. In pediatric renal transplantation, the major risk factor for reduced long-term graft survival is CNI-induced renal impairment [90], which is secondary to their effect on reduction of vascular perfusion [91] and upregulation of fibrogenic genes [92]. Elimination of CNI may also minimize hypertension, diabetes and hyperlipidemia. CNI-sparing immunosuppressive regimens aim to decrease the non-immune CNI-related injury while not increasing the acute rejection incidence which will result in immune-related chronic graft injury. At the same time, any increase in other immunosuppressive agents should not counterbalance the anticipated decrease in CNI-related side effects.

Studies on CNI-sparing strategies in pediatric patients suggested that reducing CNI doses had no beneficial effect on long term renal function and that total CNI withdrawal may be more beneficial [93]. However, the latter must be accompanied by addition of the new agents in renal transplantation. This can be in the form of induction with antibodies depleting T and/or B cells or targeting lymphocyte receptors and inhibiting function, or replacement of the CNI with other drugs that have distinct mechanisms of action, such as mycophenolate or sirolimus [93]. Unfortunately, there are very few studies reporting the use of ATG, alemtuzumab, or IL-2RA (basiliximab or daclizumab) for CNI-sparing regimens in pediatric renal transplant recipients. Three small studies showed that following induction with ATG or alemtuzumab, tacrolimus dosage could be significantly reduced with subsequent benefit to renal function, while the incidence of acute rejection remained low at 9 to 12% [70, 94-96]. However, when daclizumab induction was used with sirolimus, mycophenolate mofetil and prednisone maintenance immunosuppression in a CNI-sparing regimen in 34 pediatric renal transplant patients, the acute rejection rate at one year was high at 32% [97].

Mammalian Target of Rapamycin (mTOR) Inhibitors

Sirolimus is a macrocytic triene antibiotic produced by the actinomycete *Streptomyces hygroscopicus*. Sirolimus exerts its activity *via* binding to FKBP12 which in turn binds to and inhibits the activation of the mammalian target of rapamycin (mTOR). This suppresses the progression from the G1 phase to the S phase of the cell cycle and hence suppresses cytokine-mediated cellular proliferation. In view of its unique properties, sirolimus can be used in conjunction with CNIs to produce a synergistic effect [98].

Since its introduction in 1998, the use of sirolimus increased from 0.2% in 1998 to a peak of 25.8% in 2002 and subsequently declined to 3.4% in 2007 [15], as its initial promise compared to the CNIs did not hold out in larger studies. Clinically significant adverse effects of sirolimus included hypercholesterolemia, hypertriglyceridemia, infectious and non-infectious pneumonia, anemia, impaired wound healing and lymphocele formation. Moreover, caution needs to be exercised in the use of sirolimus in patients with delayed graft function or immunologic rejection in view of its anti-proliferative effects on the recovering renal tubular epithelial cells.

In pediatric patients, sirolimus is primarily used as a rescue therapy especially in CNI toxicity. In a case-control study on 10 pediatric renal transplant recipients with biopsy-proven CNI-induced nephrotoxicity, Höcker *et al.* [99] analyzed the efficacy and safety of a sirolimus-based immunosuppressive regimen plus mycophenolate mofetil and corticosteroids *versus* CNI minimization (mean dose reduction by 39%) plus mycophenolate mofetil and corticosteroids, and observed that the sirolimus group had a similar improvement in glomerular filtration rate at one year post-entry into the study compared to the CNI minimization group. No patient in either group experienced an acute rejection episode. The main adverse event under sirolimus therapy was transient hyperlipidemia in 70% of patients.

OUTCOMES AND COMPLICATIONS

Patient and Graft Survival

The life expectancy of pediatric ESRD patients is shorter compared to the corresponding age-related population [100, 101]. Amongst the pediatric ESRD population, patient survival in the transplant group is superior to that of the dialysis group over all pediatric age groups [102, 103]. Five-year patient survival rates amongst pediatric renal transplant recipients vary between 70 to 100% [21, 27, 59, 100, 104-107]. The NAPRTCS data reported patient survival rates of 97.8%, 94.5% and 92.4%, at one, five and seven years respectively [15]. The patient survival rates in living donor transplants and that of deceased donor transplants were comparable, however, the survival rate in the infant cohort was lower compared to the other age groups. The predominant causes of death in pediatric transplant recipients were infections, malignancy and cardiopulmonary disease.

Graft survival rates, in both living donor and deceased donor recipients, have been improving over the years, with one-year graft survival rates of 75.2% (deceased donor) and 89.4% (living donor) in the 1987 to 1990 NAPRTCS cohort, as compared to 94.4% (deceased donor) and 96.1% (living donor) in the 2003 to 2007 cohort [15]. There was also an improvement in the three-year graft survival rates with rates of 63.5% (deceased donor) and 81.2% (living donor) in the 1987 to 1990 cohort as compared to 81.1% (deceased donor) and 90.6% (living donor) in the 2003 to 2007 cohort. The improvement in survival rates was attributable to changes in the immunosuppressive regimens, decreased blood transfusions in recipients and decreased use of young deceased donors. On the other hand, the most important and common cause of late graft failure is chronic rejection which accounts for an estimated 35% of graft loss [15]. Long-term graft survival further depends on the underlying original renal disease. Recurrence of the original disease accounts for an estimated 6.8% of graft failures [15].

In many developing countries, access to renal replacement therapy for children is poor, and many of these patients tend to present late with serious co-morbidities, increasing the morbidity of renal transplantation [19]. In a review by Rizvi *et al.* which looked at ten reports from developing countries, comprising 300 transplants followed up for a period ranging from one to 28 years, more than 94% were living-related, and recipients tended to be older than six years [22]. The mainstay of immunosuppression therapy in these centers was cyclosporine, azathioprine and steroids. Unfortunately, the high costs of drugs and non-adherence resulted in a high acute rejection rate of more than 40%, and discontinuation of therapy in many cases. One-year and five-year graft survival rates ranged from 89 to 98% and 67 to 84% respectively, while patient survival rates ranged from 88 to 98% and 65 to 90% respectively. The major causes of graft and patient loss were acute and chronic rejection, and infections.

Donor Source

Donor source is an important determining factor in graft survival with living donor recipients having better graft survival as compared to deceased donor recipients. Both short and long-term graft survival and patient survival rates are better in living donor recipients compared to deceased donor recipients [15, 57, 100, 106-108]. Registry data showed that patient survival rates in living donor recipients are 1 to 3% better than deceased donor recipients. Graft survival rates in living donor recipients are also better than deceased donor recipients, with a 2 to 20% advantage [80, 100, 109]. Moreover, experience from the Eurotransplant group also demonstrated an improvement in graft survival in preemptive renal transplant recipients [109]. Possible contributing factors for better graft and patient survival rates in living donor recipients include shorter cold ischemia time, lower acute rejection rates as well as more time for pre-operative preparation.

Donor Age

Kidneys from deceased donors aged 11 to 17 years of age provide the best graft survival with a five-year survival rate of 73% [57]. Grafts from donors less than five years of age fare poorly, associated with the increased risk of graft thrombosis [78, 110]. More recently, however, the five-year graft survival rate from donors less than one year of age has risen to 60% and more impressively, to 70% for donors aged one year to five years [57], which is approaching the long-term graft survival seen with adolescent donors. Hence, kidneys from very young donors can be performed in selected recipients [111, 112].

Recipient Age

Recipient age has an important influence on transplant outcome. Previous reports have demonstrated a lower graft survival especially in children under two years of age, with a one and five-year graft survival of 71% and 60%, respectively [113, 114]. The increased risk of graft loss was possibly attributable to technical difficulties encountered in the every young recipient, as well as increased risk of graft thrombosis. Despite the higher incidence of graft thrombosis in the very young recipients, children aged five years or less have an excellent long-term graft outcome as demonstrated by the United Network for Organ Sharing (UNOS) data, with an estimated graft half-life of greater than 26 years in living graft recipients [63]. This is in contrast to the half-life of less than ten years for a living donor graft in adolescents, which is less than the graft survival in adults and children six to twelve years of age. Possible contributing factors could be non-adherence to medications [113] and the vigorous immune response in adolescents as compared to other age groups [115, 116], as well as the higher incidence of FSGS with decreased graft survival [117].

Race

Analysis of the North American registries demonstrated poorer outcomes for African American recipients compared to white recipients [118]. Five-year graft survival rates in African Americans for living donor transplants and deceased donor transplants were 71.2% and 57.5%, respectively. This was in contrast to the 83.7% and 72.3% observed in whites and 83.4% and 67% observed in Hispanics respectively [15]. In fact, African American race was the single most influential prognostic variable in multivariate proportional hazards models, with relative hazards ratio of 1.54 to 1.99, compared to the whites.

Antibody Induction Therapy

Data from the NAPRTCS 2008 Annual Report demonstrated a favorable effect on graft survival in those who received antibody induction therapy compared to those who did not receive induction therapy (living donor: relative hazard 0.83, p=0.003; deceased donor: relative hazard 0.90, p=0.0807) [15]. Unfortunately, interpretation of the use of induction antibody therapy is hampered by selection factors that motivate its usage.

HLA-Match

Donor-specific HLA mismatch appears to be a risk factor for poor outcome [119, 120]. Graft survival was better in recipients with one to two HLA-B mismatches compared to no mismatch (relative hazard 1.4, p=0.006) [15]. Sensitized individuals with high panel reactive antibody levels of greater than 40% also had a poorer outcome [113], while recipients with donor antigen-specific hyporeactivity had better long term graft function [121].

Rejection

Data from earlier years suggested that younger children had a higher risk of acute rejection episodes which are more likely to be irreversible, suggesting a heightened immune response [122-124]. However, experimental evidence to convincingly confirm or refute this suggestion is scarce [124]. Over the last two decades, advances in immunosuppressive agents have decreased the rates of acute rejection, such that this risk is now the lowest in the youngest age group [15, 64]. This could be explained in part by the high medication adherence in this age group compared to older children, and in part by the postulate that infants have a less well-developed immune system [62]. It is also possible that mild acute rejection episodes in infants are not easily detected clinically without a protocol biopsy, as serum creatinine may not be significantly elevated early on, related to the proportionately larger renal mass of an adult-sized kidney. However, given the fact that the incidences of both acute and chronic rejection are lower in infants, failure to detect acute rejection is an unlikely explanation, since the most significant risk factor for chronic rejection is previous acute rejection episodes [125].

Vascular Thrombosis

Vascular thrombosis is an important cause of early graft loss, accounting for 3 to 12.5% of cases [126-130]. Some of the associated risk factors for vascular thrombosis include young age of recipients (less than two years of age), recipients of kidneys from deceased donors less than five years of age, history of prior transplantation, organ cold ischemia time greater than 24 hours [126] and previous peritoneal dialysis [131].

Non-Adherence

The highest acute rejection rates occur in adolescents [15]. Indeed, adolescence is the only age group where graft survival has not improved in concert with the last two decades of advancement in immunosuppression strategies, due to non-adherence [132]. Adolescence is a time of major transformation involving educational and vocational decisions, establishing a new and more equal relationship with their parents, discovering their sexual identity and taking increasing responsibility for their health [133]. Adolescents are much more likely to be non-adherent to medication regimens compared to the younger pediatric patients [134]. A recent meta-analysis showed the weighted mean of prevalence for medication non-adherence in adolescents to be 43.2%, which was significantly higher than the weighted mean of 22.4% in younger recipients only or a mixed pediatric/adolescent population [134]. Non-adherence is also more common during the transition from pediatric to adult-centered care [135] with anecdotal evidence that graft function deteriorates after transition [136, 137].

Non-adherence to the immunosuppressive regimen is an important predictor of poor long-term post-transplant outcome [138, 139]. In a systematic review, medication non-adherence was associated with 14.4% of grafts lost in pediatric kidney transplant recipients and 23.2% of late acute rejection episodes [134]. In those studies focusing exclusively on adolescents, the percentage of graft loss because of non-adherence was higher at 31.8% [140, 141]. Non-adherence is also associated with increased serum creatinine level [142], and a poorer perceived health status in children [143]. Two meta-analyses in chronically ill pediatric patients found that multi-component interventions including education, parental involvement, self-monitoring, reinforcement, and problem-solving have been most successful, with small to moderate effect sizes, in promoting adherence to chronic regimens, subsequently leading to improved health outcomes [144, 145]. Interventions should be tailored individually and should be a collaborative effort between the adolescent, family and healthcare providers [146].

Growth Issues

The need to maximize growth and developmental potential in children is one of the most important issues distinguishing pediatric from adult renal transplantation. Normal adult height attainment is one of the determining issues for the overall success of a pediatric kidney transplant program [147]. The problem of growth retardation, which often accompanies chronic kidney disease in children, can persist even after a renal transplant, largely due to the use of corticosteroids [148]. Attainment of optimal final adult height is predicated on minimal height deficits at the time of transplantation, persistent good allograft function, and minimization or avoidance of corticosteroid treatment [147-150]. Recent data involving both *in vitro* work and clinical trials have indicated that recombinant human growth hormone, in supra-physiological doses, may partially overcome the growth-inhibiting effects of glucocorticoid treatment, and improve growth velocity in the persistently growth-retarded allograft recipient [147, 150]. It is especially useful in maximizing the pubertal growth spurt [148]. However, growth hormone may affect the immune system and hence, patients with previous frequent acute rejections may have increased risk of acute rejection during growth hormone treatment.

Infectious Complications

While new immunosuppressive drugs have considerably reduced the incidence of rejection, they have also increased the susceptibility of patients to opportunistic infections [151]. The success of transplantation therefore depends in part on effective prevention, diagnosis, and treatment of infectious diseases after transplantation. The main causes of death in children with a functioning graft after renal transplantation are infections and malignancies [152]. Bacterial and viral infections account for 1.8% of all graft failures, and are one of the leading causes of hospitalizations in the transplant recipient [15]. Indeed, children are at higher risk of infections after transplantation compared to adult recipients. This is because young children often lack immunity to many pathogens before transplantation, if they have not completed their primary immunization series, or if they have not had exposure to common community pathogens, in particular Epstein-Barr virus (EBV) and CMV. Accordingly, young children are at higher risk of acquiring primary infections after they are immunosuppressed, and these tend to be of greater severity compared to reactivation disease [153]. The principles of management of these infections involve prevention (*via* prophylactic antibiotics and update of vaccinations prior to transplant) and early identification and aggressive treatment of these infections. In fact, there is now increasing emphasis on the role of prevention [151].

Bacterial Infections

Urinary tract infections and pneumonias are two of the commonest bacterial infections in recipients post-transplant. Pediatric renal transplant recipients with underlying neuropathic bladders or residual gross dilatation of the urinary tract secondary to previous reflux nephropathy or obstructive uropathies are at higher risk of acute pyelonephritis. In the immediate post-transplant period, urinary tract infections are mostly related to the presence of double-J stents [138]. Patients at high risk of recurrent pyelonephritis may benefit from prophylactic antibiotics. The exception to this are transplant recipients who have had augmentation cystoplasty and appendicovesicostomies done for neuropathic bladders, as the routine use of prophylactic antibiotics may result in colonization by multi-resistant bacteria or fungal infections. These patients should empty the bladder frequently, by performing clean intermittent catheterizations five times or more daily, to prevent ascending infections.

Of the opportunistic pneumonias, *Pneumocystis jiroveci* is a serious cause of morbidity and mortality in immunosuppressed patients. In some of the earlier studies, *Pneumocystis jiroveci* pneumonia (PCP) occurred in 3 to 6.5% of transplant recipients with mortality rates of up to 60% [154-156]. The incidence of PCP was increased in transplant recipients who received maintenance immunosuppression regimens containing the combination of tacrolimus and sirolimus, cyclosporine and mycophenolate, and sirolimus and mycophenolate. Prophylaxis against PCP with cotrimoxazole is therefore recommended, at least up to three months post-transplant. However, studies have shown that the median time to development of PCP after transplant was 0.80 ± 0.95 years [157], suggesting the need for longer period of prophylaxis against PCP. Treatment options for PCP include cotrimoxazole or pentamidine, especially in patients with glucose-6-phosphate dehydrogenase deficiency.

Viral Infections

Herpesviruses, namely CMV, EBV, herpes simplex virus and varicella zoster virus (VZV) are some of the more important viral infections that occur after pediatric renal transplantation. There is evidence that subclinical CMV and EBV viremia are associated with adverse outcomes in the pediatric transplant recipient [158, 159]. As such, routine surveillance for subclinical infections with CMV and EBV has become the standard of care in many pediatric renal transplant programs. Recent steroid avoidance immunosuppressive protocols have been shown to markedly reduce the incidence of sub-clinical viral replication for CMV and EBV [158].

CMV infection and disease are important causes of mortality and morbidity among pediatric organ transplant recipients [160]. CMV disease was reported in 22% of adult kidney transplant recipients before the widespread use of ganciclovir prophylaxis, however data in pediatric renal transplant recipients are limited by non-uniform laboratory diagnosis and definition [151]. Pediatric patients are more likely to be seronegative for CMV, placing them at greatest risk of CMV disease when they receive allografts from the largely seropositive adult donors. These tend to be primary CMV infections and have the highest morbidity and mortality [161]. The use of ATG and anti-CD3 monoclonal antibody also increases the risk of CMV disease [162].

CMV disease typically presents 30 to 90 days after transplantation, but can be delayed if the recipient has been given CMV prophylaxis [163]. It may manifest as CMV syndrome where fever, malaise, leukopenia, and/or thrombocytopenia occur in the absence of end organ involvement, while CMV tissue invasive disease involves end organ involvement such as pneumonitis, hepatitis, gastrointestinal disease, myocarditis, and less frequently encephalitis or retinitis [153]. There is a predilection for CMV to invade the allograft. CMV also has indirect immunomodulatory effects leading to enhanced susceptibility to other opportunistic infections including aspergillus, EBV-related PTLD, and an increased risk of graft rejection [164]. The method of choice for diagnosis and monitoring in CMV disease are quantification of CMV DNA by polymerase chain reaction, or the pp65 antigenemia assay that detects the late structural protein pp65 produced in leukocytes. Histopathologic examination of involved organs is essential to confirm the diagnosis of invasive CMV disease.

Intravenous ganciclovir, together with judicious reduction of immunosuppression, is the therapy of choice for CMV disease in pediatric transplant recipients. This is accompanied by CMV hyperimmune globulin therapy in some centers [151], though its benefit remains uncertain [165]. There is data emerging on the use of valganciclovir both in the prevention and treatment of CMV infection/disease among adult transplant recipients [166]. Unfortunately there is less data available in children [167]. Foscarnet and cidofovir may be considered in ganciclovir resistance, but both agents have significant nephrotoxicity.

Another worrying infection in pediatric renal transplantation is EBV infection. Because approximately half of the children are EBV naïve at the time of transplantation, they are more likely to develop primary EBV infections when receiving an allograft from a seropositive donor. Concurrent immunosuppressive therapy in these children impairs the ability of the cytotoxic T lymphocyte response to inhibit the proliferation of immortalized B cells. As such, children are at considerably higher risk of developing PTLD than adults. Indeed, primary EBV infection is the most clearly defined risk factor for the development of early PTLD (less than 12 months after transplant) [168] and PTLD is the most common post-transplant malignancy in pediatric solid organ transplant patients [169]. PTLD can range from a benign self-limited form of polyclonal proliferation to true malignancies containing clonal chromosomal abnormalities [170]. Reduction of immunosuppression is the initial strategy and additional therapy, such as antiviral agents, intravenous immunoglobulin, monoclonal antibodies such as rituximab, and chemotherapy, remain controversial.

In the last decade, the advent and utilization of more potent immunosuppression drugs have decreased the rates of acute rejection in kidney transplantation [171] but on the other hand have also led to the emergence of polyomavirus associated nephropathy [172-174] associated with increased graft loss. Infection with *Polyomavirus hominis* type 1, better known as BK virus (BKV) is also an important consideration in pediatric renal transplantation. Pediatric patients are more likely to be naïve to BKV, and pre-transplant BKV seronegative status has been associated with increased risk of primary infection with subsequent BKV nephropathy [175]. BKV infections in pediatric transplant recipients are generally primary infections, as opposed to reactivation disease in adults [151]. The major clinical manifestations in the renal transplant recipient are tubulointerstitial nephritis and ureteral stenosis. In addition, persistent BKV infection has been associated with an increased risk of urological malignancies [176]. Renal biopsy is required for definitive diagnosis. There is no firm consensus on the management of BKV nephropathy, but early detection is generally most desirable to allow for modulation of immunosuppression. As such, quantitative PCR monitoring for BKV DNA is performed in some centers. Pharmaceutical agents which have been tried in the treatment of BK nephropathy include the use of leflunomide, cidofovir, fluoroquinolones, and intravenous immunoglobulins [177], but there have been no consensus on their therapeutic efficacy.

Immunization

Because of the increased risk of infections among pediatric renal transplant recipients, the transplant physician should ensure that transplant candidates and their household members are given the full complement of recommended vaccinations prior to transplantation. While inactivated vaccines are generally safe after transplantation, they may not be sufficiently immunogenic. In addition, since the response to many vaccines is diminished in ESRD, potential transplant candidates should be immunized early in the course of their disease [178].

Live vaccines such as measles, mumps, rubella (MMR) and varicella should be given prior to transplantation as these are contraindicated in the immunosuppressed patient. While MMR is most effective after a year of age when maternal antibody has waned, it can be administered as early as six months of age for pediatric patients who may require a kidney transplant. A minimum of four weeks between live-virus vaccine administration and transplantation is suggested. In addition, pediatric renal transplant candidates, especially if splenectomy is being considered, should be immunized against encapsulated bacterial pathogens, namely pneumococcal, meningococcal, and *Haemophilus influenzae* (Hib) vaccinations.

Pediatric transplant candidates and recipients should also receive the seasonal influenza vaccine, as well as the H1N1 vaccine as they are known to be at increased risk of severe outcomes from pandemic H1N1. They are candidates for treatment with oseltamivir or zanamivir (where appropriate) if they have acute respiratory illness that is suspected or confirmed to be caused by H1N1 [179]. They are also at an increased risk of prolonged viral shedding and the harboring of drug-resistant strains of influenza A, including pandemic H1N1 [151].

Renal transplant recipients, due to their immunosuppressed state, have an increased risk of cancer, which is a major cause of premature death in transplant recipients with a functioning graft [180, 181]. The preliminary findings of a prospective study evaluating the incidence of human papillomavirus (HPV) infection and cervical carcinoma in 35 kidney transplant recipients showed that although no cytologic anomalies were detected in Papanicolaou smears, 62.8% of the patients were positive for HPV DNA. Amongst these patients, 59% demonstrated a high-risk HPV genotype, suggesting higher aggressiveness in immunosuppressed patients [182]. In light of this, adolescent female transplant candidates and recipients should receive the HPV vaccine [151]. The recommended age for the quadrivalent HPV vaccine is 11 to 12 years, but it can be administered to girls as young as nine years of age.

Cardiovascular Disease Post-Renal Transplantation

As a result of the excellent outcomes in pediatric renal transplantation, patients who received a renal transplant in childhood now routinely survive to adulthood. However, the life expectancy of these patients remains lower than the general population, with the main cause of mortality being premature cardiovascular disease [183-185]. Indeed, cardiovascular disease is the most common cause of death in young adults who developed ESRD during childhood [183, 185]. These young adults have a ten-fold increased risk of cardiovascular disease compared to their peers [186]. This risk, though much lower than dialysis patients, remains unacceptably high. This may not be unexpected given that children after transplantation have a high prevalence of traditional cardiovascular risk factors, contributed partly by immunosuppressive medications like steroids and CNIs. For example, the prevalence of obesity increased from 12% at time of transplantation to 29% at one year after transplantation [187]. In addition, 65 to 73% of transplant recipients needed anti-hypertensive medications at two years post-transplant [15] and 40 to 60% of children have dyslipidemia after transplant [188]. New-onset insulin resistance or diabetes mellitus is not uncommon post-transplantation, contributed by obesity and immunosuppressive drugs like tacrolimus. The co-existence of these interrelated cardiovascular risk factors points towards the diagnosis of metabolic syndrome, which is associated with a higher risk for cardiovascular-associated morbidity and mortality in adults. In addition to traditional risk factors, chronic kidney disease can also contribute to cardiovascular morbidity *via* non-traditional risk factors like increased oxidative stress, chronic inflammation, alterations in calcium and phosphate homeostasis and anemia. Several new biomarkers such as asymmetric dimethylarginine (ADMA) and Fetuin-A have emerged as potential markers of early cardiovascular disease in children with chronic kidney disease [189].

Left ventricular hypertrophy (LVH) is the most studied and reported marker of cardiovascular disease in pediatric renal patients. Its prevalence in the pediatric population after transplantation is high at 48 to 75% [190-192] and this may be associated with early subclinical systolic dysfunction [190, 193]. Results are mixed in terms of whether LVH improves with renal transplantation. Elevated aortic stiffness, shown to be a better predictive factor of cardiovascular morbidity in adults [194], often appears earlier than LVH. Aortic stiffness has been shown to remain stable before and six months after renal transplantation in children [195].

CONCLUSIONS

Advances in both immunosuppression protocols and surgical techniques have resulted in excellent short and medium-term patient and graft survival outcomes in pediatric renal transplantation. Long-term graft survival, however, remains suboptimal, due to factors such as CNI toxicity, cardiovascular disease, infections and non-adherence. Other adverse effects of immunosuppressive drugs such as growth retardation and malignancy also remain a problem. Therefore the current challenge in pediatric renal transplantation will be to improve long-term graft survival by minimizing the side effects of immunosuppression while preventing rejections.

As more adolescent renal transplant recipients survive into adulthood, one of the challenges will also be their social rehabilitation and quality of life. Issues pertaining to their adjustment into schools and workplace, involvement in romantic and sexual relationships and reproductive health care needs will have to be addressed. The transition from pediatric-oriented to adult-oriented health care systems will be an important milestone for the graduate of the pediatric renal transplant program. This should be carefully planned and carried out so as to ensure ongoing engagement of the young adults with the health care system.

REFERENCES

[1] Fine RN. Renal transplantation for children--the only realistic choice. Kidney Int Suppl. 1985;17:S15-17.

[2] Horslen S, Barr ML, Christensen LL, *et al.* Pediatric transplantation in the United States, 1996-2005. Am J Transplant 2007;7:1339-1358.

[3] Wolfe RA, Ashby VB, Milford EL, *et al.* Comparison of mortality in all patients on dialysis, patients on dialysis awaiting transplantation, and recipients of a first cadaveric transplant. N Engl J Med 1999;341:1725-1730.

[4] Dudley CR, Johnson RJ, Thomas HL, *et al.* Factors that influence access to the national renal transplant waiting list. Transplantation 2009;88:96-102.

[5] Sequist TD, Narva AS, Stiles SK, *et al.* Access to renal transplantation among American Indians and Hispanics. Am J Kidney Dis 2004;44:344-352.

[6] Ayanian JZ, Cleary PD, Weissman JS, Epstein AM. The effect of patients' preferences on racial differences in access to renal transplantation. N Engl J Med 1999;341:1661-1669.

[7] Navaneethan SD, Singh S. A systematic review of barriers in access to renal transplantation among African Americans in the United States. Clin Transplant 2006;20:769-775.

[8] Mathur AK, Ashby VB, Sands RL, Wolfe RA. Geographic variation in end-stage renal disease incidence and access to deceased donor kidney transplantation. Am J Transplant 2010;10:1069-1080.

[9] Tonelli M, Klarenbach S, Rose C, *et al.* Access to kidney transplantation among remote- and rural-dwelling patients with kidney failure in the United States. JAMA. 2009;301:1681-1690.

[10] Axelrod DA, Guidinger MK, Finlayson S, *et al.* Rates of solid-organ wait-listing, transplantation, and survival among residents of rural and urban areas. JAMA 2008;299:202-207.

[11] Lee G. End-stage renal disease in the Asian-Pacific region. Semin Nephrol 2003;23:107-114.

[12] Shapiro R, Sarwal MM. Pediatric kidney transplantation. Pediatr Clin North Am. 2010;57:393-400.

[13] Salvatierra O, Jr., Alexander SR, Krensky AM. Pediatric Transplant Grand Rounds. Pediatric kidney transplantation at Stanford. Pediatr Transplant. 1998;2:165-176.

[14] United States Renal Data System, USRDS 2009 Annual Data Report: Atlas of Chronic Kidney Disease and End-Stage Renal Disease in the United States, National Institutes of Health, National Institute of Diabetes and Digestive and Kidney Diseases, Bethesda, MD.

[15] North American Pediatric Renal Trials and Collaborative Studies, 2008 Annual Report. Available from: https://www.naprtcs.org.

[16] Renal Association. Report of the Paediatric Renal Registry. Renal Association UK Renal Registry, 7th Annu Rep 2004, No. 13, pp 187-202.

[17] van Stralen KJ, Tizard EJ, Verrina E, *et al.* Demographics of paediatric renal replacement therapy in Europe: 2007 annual report of the ESPN/ERA-EDTA registry. Pediatr Nephrol 2010;25:1379-1382.

[18] Rizvi SA, Naqvi SA, Hussain Z, *et al.* Living-related pediatric renal transplants: a single-center experience from a developing country. Pediatr Transplant 2002;6:101-110.

[19] Abeysekera CK, Gunasekara WD, Abegunawardena A, *et al.* First experiences of pediatric kidney transplantation in Sri Lanka. Pediatr Transplant 2007;11:408-413.

[20] Mong Hiep TT, Janssen F, Ismaili K, *et al.* Etiology and outcome of chronic renal failure in hospitalized children in Ho Chi Minh City, Vietnam. Pediatr Nephrol 2008;23:965-970.

[21] Pitcher GJ, Beale PG, Bowley DM, *et al.* Pediatric renal transplantation in a South African teaching hospital: a 20-year perspective. Pediatr Transplant. 2006;10:441-448.

[22] Rizvi SA, Zafar MN, Lanewala AA, Naqvi SA. Challenges in pediatric renal transplantation in developing countries. Curr Opin Organ Transplant 2009;14:533-539.

[23] Chacko B, Rajamanickam T, Neelakantan N, *et al.* Pediatric renal transplantation--a single center experience of 15 yr from India. Pediatr Transplant 2007;11:844-849.

[24] El-Husseini AA, Foda MA, Bakr MA, *et al.*Pediatric live-donor kidney transplantation in Mansoura Urology & Nephrology Center: a 28-year perspective. Pediatr Nephrol 2006;21:1464-1470.

[25] Delucchi A, Ferrario M, Varela M, *et al.* Pediatric renal transplantation: a single center experience over 14 years. Pediatr Transplant 2006;10:193-197.

[26] Sumboonnanonda A, Lumpaopong A, Kingwatanakul P, *et al.* Pediatric kidney transplantation in Thailand: experience in a developing country. Transplant Proc. 2008;40:2271-2273.

[27] Otukesh H, Basiri A, Simfrosh N, *et al.* Outcome of pediatric renal transplantation in Labfi Nejad Hospital, Tehran, Iran. Pediatr Nephrol 2006;21:1459-1463.

[28] Emiroglu R, Moray G, Sevmis S, *et al.* Long-term results of pediatric kidney transplantation at one center in Turkey. Transplant Proc 2005;37:2951-2953.

[29] Ardissino G, Dacco V, Testa S, *et al.* Epidemiology of chronic renal failure in children: data from the ItalKid project. Pediatrics. 2003;111:e382-387.

[30] Finnish Registry for Kidney Diseases (1999) Report 1998, Helsinki, p 7.

[31] Hattori S, Yosioka K, Honda M, Ito H. The 1998 report of the Japanese National Registry data on pediatric end-stage renal disease patients. Pediatr Nephrol 2002;17:456-461.

[32] Australia and New Zealand Dialysis and Transplant Registry. The 28th annual report. 2005 report-data to 2004. http://www.anzdata.org.

[33] Warady BA, Chadha V. Chronic kidney disease in children: the global perspective. Pediatr Nephrol 2007;22:1999-2009.

[34] Barsoum RS. Chronic kidney disease in the developing world. N Engl J Med 2006;354:997-999.

[35] Churchill BM, Jayanthi RV, McLorie GA, Khoury AE. Pediatric renal transplantation into the abnormal urinary tract. Pediatr Nephrol 1996;10:113-120.

[36] Krieger JN, Stubenbord WT, Vaughan ED, Jr. Transplantation in children with end stage renal disease of urologic origin. J Urol 1980;124:508-512.

[37] Warshaw BL, Edelbrock HH, Ettenger RB, *et al.* Renal transplantation in children with obstructive uropathy. J Urol 1980;123:737-741.

[38] Cochat P, Fargue S, Mestrallet G, *et al.* Disease recurrence in paediatric renal transplantation. Pediatr Nephrol 2009;24:2097-2108.

[39] Baqi N, Tejani A. Recurrence of the original disease in pediatric renal transplantation. J Nephrol 1997;10:85-92.

[40] Mathew TH. Recurrence of disease following renal transplantation. Am J Kidney Dis 1988;12:85-96.

[41] Habib R, Antignac C, Hinglais N, *et al.* Glomerular lesions in the transplanted kidney in children. Am J Kidney Dis 1987;10:198-207.

[42] Andresdottir MB, Assmann KJ, Hoitsma AJ, *et al.* Renal transplantation in patients with dense deposit disease: morphological characteristics of recurrent disease and clinical outcome. Nephrol Dial Transplant 1999;14:1723-1731.

[43] Eddy A, Sibley R, Mauer SM, Kim Y. Renal allograft failure due to recurrent dense intramembranous deposit disease. Clin Nephrol 1984;21:305-313.

[44] Miller RB, Burke BA, Schmidt WJ, *et al.* Recurrence of haemolytic-uraemic syndrome in renal transplants: a single-centre report. Nephrol Dial Transplant 1997;12:1425-1430.

[45] Loirat C, Niaudet P. The risk of recurrence of hemolytic uremic syndrome after renal transplantation in children. Pediatr Nephrol 2003;18:1095-1101.

[46] Lemire J, Kaplan BS. The various renal manifestations of the nephropathic form of cystinosis. Am J Nephrol 1984;4:81-85.

[47] Gahl WA. Cystinosis coming of age. Adv Pediatr 1986;33:95-126.

[48] Sutherland SM, Alexander SR, Sarwal MM, *et al.* Combined liver-kidney transplantation in children: indications and outcome. Pediatr Transplant 2008;12:835-846.

[49] Chava SP, Singh B, Pal S, *et al.* Indications for combined liver and kidney transplantation in children. Pediatr Transplant 2009;13:661-669.

[50] Cochat P, Liutkus A, Fargue S, *et al.* Primary hyperoxaluria type 1: still challenging! Pediatr Nephrol 2006;21:1075-1081.

[51] Hoppe B, Langman CB. A United States survey on diagnosis, treatment, and outcome of primary hyperoxaluria. Pediatr Nephrol 2003;18:986-991.

[52] Jamieson NV. A 20-year experience of combined liver/kidney transplantation for primary hyperoxaluria (PH1): the European PH1 transplant registry experience 1984-2004. Am J Nephrol 2005;25:282-289.

[53] Grewal HP, Brady L, Cronin DC, *et al.* Combined liver and kidney transplantation in children. Transplantation. 2000;70:100-105.

[54] De Kerckhove L, De Meyer M, Verbaandert C, *et al.* The place of liver transplantation in Caroli's disease and syndrome. Transpl Int 2006;19:381-388.

[55] Salvatierra O, Jr., Millan M, Concepcion W. Pediatric renal transplantation with considerations for successful outcomes. Semin Pediatr Surg 2006;15:208-217.

[56] van Heurn E, de Vries EE. Kidney transplantation and donation in children. Pediatr Surg Int 2009;25:385-393.

[57] Harmon WE, McDonald RA, Reyes JD, *et al.* Pediatric transplantation, 1994-2003. Am J Transplant 2005;5:887-903.

[58] Najarian JS, Frey DJ, Matas AJ, *et al.* Renal transplantation in infants. Ann Surg 1990;212:353-365.

[59] Offner G, Hoyer PF, Ehrich JH, *et al.* Paediatric aspects of renal transplantation: experience of a single centre. Eur J Pediatr 1992;151 Suppl 1:S16-22.

[60] Salvatierra O, Jr., Concepcion W, Sarwal MM. Renal transplantation in children with thrombosis of the inferior vena cava requires careful assessment and planning. Pediatr Nephrol 2008;23:2107-2109.

[61] Snoeijs MG, Wiermans B, Christiaans MH, *et al.* Recipient hemodynamics during non-heart-beating donor kidney transplantation are major predictors of primary nonfunction. Am J Transplant 2007;7:1158-1166.

[62] Humar A, Arrazola L, Mauer M, *et al.* Kidney transplantation in young children: should there be a minimum age? Pediatr Nephrol 2001;16:941-945.

[63] Sarwal MM, Cecka JM, Millan MT, Salvatierra O, Jr. Adult-size kidneys without acute tubular necrosis provide exceedingly superior long-term graft outcomes for infants and small children: a single center and UNOS analysis. United Network for Organ Sharing. Transplantation 2000;70:1728-1736.

[64] Sarwal MM. Out with the old, in with the new: immunosuppression minimization in children. Curr Opin Organ Transplant 2008;13:513-521.

[65] Levey AS, Schmid CH, Lau J. Antilymphocyte antibodies, renal transplantation, and meta-analysis. Ann Intern Med 1998;128:863-865.

[66] Olaitan OK, Zimmermann JA, Shields WP, *et al.* Long-term outcome of intensive initial immunosuppression protocol in pediatric deceased donor renal transplantation. Pediatr Transplant 2010;14:87-92.

[67] Waldmann H, Hale G. CAMPATH: from concept to clinic. Philos Trans R Soc Lond B Biol Sci 2005;360:1707-1711.

[68] Calne R, Friend P, Moffatt S, *et al.* Prope tolerance, perioperative campath 1H, and low-dose cyclosporin monotherapy in renal allograft recipients. Lancet 1998;351:1701-1702.

[69] Watson CJ, Bradley JA, Friend PJ, *et al.* Alemtuzumab (CAMPATH 1H) induction therapy in cadaveric kidney transplantation--efficacy and safety at five years. Am J Transplant 2005;5:1347-1353.

[70] Tan HP, Donaldson J, Ellis D, *et al.* Pediatric living donor kidney transplantation under alemtuzumab pretreatment and tacrolimus monotherapy: 4-year experience. Transplantation 2008;86:1725-1731.

[71] McLaughlin P, Grillo-Lopez AJ, Link BK, *et al.* Rituximab chimeric anti-CD20 monoclonal antibody therapy for relapsed indolent lymphoma: half of patients respond to a four-dose treatment program. J Clin Oncol 1998;16:2825-2833.

[72] Becker YT, Samaniego-Picota M, Sollinger HW. The emerging role of rituximab in organ transplantation. Transpl Int 2006;19:621-628.

[73] Webster AC, Ruster LP, McGee R, *et al.* Interleukin 2 receptor antagonists for kidney transplant recipients. Cochrane Database Syst Rev. 2010(1):CD003897.

[74] Li L, Chang A, Naesens M, *et al.* Steroid-free immunosuppression since 1999: 129 pediatric renal transplants with sustained graft and patient benefits. Am J Transplant 2009;9:1362-1372.

[75] Sarwal MM BM, Ettenger R, Dharnidharka V, *et al.* One year results of a prospective, randomized, multicenter trial of steroid avoidance in pediatric renal transplantation (IPTA abstract LB2). Pediatr Transplant 2009;13(S1):63.

[76] Grenda R WA, Trompeter R, Tönshoff B (TWIST Study Group). Early steroid withdrawal in paediatric kidney recipients after two-doses of daclizumab induction, tacrolimus and MMF *versus* tacrolimus, MMF and steroids—TWIST Study (IPTA abstract 453). Pediatr Transplant. 2009;13(S1):154-5.

[77] Elion GB. The George Hitchings and Gertrude Elion Lecture. The pharmacology of azathioprine. Ann N Y Acad Sci 1993;685:400-407.

[78] Neipp M, Offner G, Luck R, *et al.* Kidney transplant in children weighing less than 15 kg: donor selection and technical considerations. Transplantation 2002;73:409-416.

[79] Mir S, Erdogan H, Serdaroglu E, Kabasakal C, *et al.* Pediatric renal transplantation: single center experience. Pediatr Transplant 2005;9:56-61.

[80] Magee JC, Krishnan SM, Benfield MR, *et al.* Pediatric transplantation in the United States, 1997-2006. Am J Transplant 2008;8:935-945.

[81] Knight SR, Russell NK, Barcena L, Morris PJ. Mycophenolate mofetil decreases acute rejection and may improve graft survival in renal transplant recipients when compared with azathioprine: a systematic review. Transplantation 2009;87:785-794.

[82] Butani L, Palmer J, Baluarte HJ, Polinsky MS. Adverse effects of mycophenolate mofetil in pediatric renal transplant recipients with presumed chronic rejection. Transplantation 1999;68:83-86.

[83] Zhao W, Fakhoury M, Deschenes G, *et al.* Population Pharmacokinetics and Pharmacogenetics of Mycophenolic Acid Following Administration of Mycophenolate Mofetil in *de novo* Pediatric Renal-Transplant Patients. J Clin Pharmacol. 2010 Feb 10 [Epub head of print].

[84] Moore J, Middleton L, Cockwell P, *et al.* Calcineurin inhibitor sparing with mycophenolate in kidney transplantation: a systematic review and meta-analysis. Transplantation 2009;87:591-605.

[85] Ferraris JR, Tambutti ML, Redal MA, *et al.* Conversion from azathioprine [correction of azathioprina] to mycophenolate mofetil in pediatric renal transplant recipients with chronic rejection. Transplantation 2000;70:297-301.

[86] Calne R. Cyclosporine as a milestone in immunosuppression. Transplant Proc 2004;36:13S-15S.

[87] Trompeter R, Filler G, Webb NJ, *et al.* Randomized trial of tacrolimus *versus* cyclosporin microemulsion in renal transplantation. Pediatr Nephrol 2002;17:141-149.

[88] Webster A, Woodroffe RC, Taylor RS, *et al.* Tacrolimus *versus* cyclosporin as primary immunosuppression for kidney transplant recipients. Cochrane Database Syst Rev. 2005(4):CD003961.

[89] Habwe VQ. Posttransplantation quality of life: more than graft function. Am J Kidney Dis 2006;47:S98-110.

[90] Ekberg H. Calcineurin inhibitor sparing in renal transplantation. Transplantation. 2008;86:761-767.

[91] Alexander SI, Fletcher JT, Nankivell B. Chronic allograft nephropathy in paediatric renal transplantation. Pediatr Nephrol 2007;22:17-23.

[92] Brook NR, Waller JR, Bicknell GR, Nicholson ML. The novel antifibrotic agent pirfenidone attenuates the profibrotic environment generated by calcineurin inhibitors in the rat salt-depletion model. Transplant Proc 2005;37:130-133.

[93] Tredger JM, Brown NW, Dhawan A. Calcineurin inhibitor sparing in paediatric solid organ transplantation : managing the efficacy/toxicity conundrum. Drugs 2008;68:1385-1414.

[94] Ellis D, Shapiro R, Moritz M, *et al.* Renal transplantation in children managed with lymphocyte depleting agents and low-dose maintenance tacrolimus monotherapy. Transplantation 2007;83:1563-1570.

[95] Shapiro R, Zeevi A, Basu A, *et al.* Alemtuzumab preconditioning with tacrolimus monotherapy-the impact of serial monitoring for donor-specific antibody. Transplantation. 2008;85:1125-1132.

[96] Shapiro R, Ellis D, Tan HP, *et al.* Antilymphoid antibody preconditioning and tacrolimus monotherapy for pediatric kidney transplantation. J Pediatr 2006;148:813-818.

[97] Harmon W, Meyers K, Ingelfinger J, *et al.* Safety and efficacy of a calcineurin inhibitor avoidance regimen in pediatric renal transplantation. J Am Soc Nephrol. 2006;17:1735-1745.

[98] Kahan BD, Camardo JS. Rapamycin: clinical results and future opportunities. Transplantation 2001;72:1181-1193.

[99] Hocker B, Feneberg R, Kopf S, *et al.* SRL-based immunosuppression *vs.* CNI minimization in pediatric renal transplant recipients with chronic CNI nephrotoxicity. Pediatr Transplant 2006;10:593-601.

[100] Rees L, Shroff R, Hutchinson C, *et al.* Long-term outcome of paediatric renal transplantation: follow-up of 300 children from 1973 to 2000. Nephron Clin Pract. 2007;105:c68-76.

[101] Levey AS. Controlling the epidemic of cardiovascular disease in chronic renal disease: where do we start? Am J Kidney Dis 1998;32:S5-13.

[102] United States Renal Data System (USRDS) The 2005 Annual Data Report. Bethesda, MD: National Institutes of Health, National Institute of Diabetes and Digestive and Kidney Diseases, 2005.

[103] Gillen DL, Stehman-Breen CO, Smith JM, *et al.* Survival advantage of pediatric recipients of a first kidney transplant among children awaiting kidney transplantation. Am J Transplant 2008;8:2600-2606.

[104] Offner G, Latta K, Hoyer PF, *et al.* Kidney transplanted children come of age. Kidney Int 1999;55:1509-1517.

[105] Englund M, Berg U, Tyden G. A longitudinal study of children who received renal transplants 10-20 years ago. Transplantation 2003;76:311-318.

[106] Mehrabi A, Kashfi A, Tonshoff B, *et al.* Long-term results of paediatric kidney transplantation at the University of Heidelberg: a 35 year single-centre experience. Nephrol Dial Transplant 2004;19 Suppl 4:iv69-74.

[107] Rosati P, Pinto V, Delucchi A, Salas P, *et al.* Pediatric renal transplantation: 13 years of experience--report from the Chilean Cooperative Multicenter Group. Transplant Proc 2005;37:1569-1573.

[108] Renal Association. Report of the paediatric renal registry. Renal Association UK Renal Registry, 7th Annual Report 2004;13:187-202.

[109] Cransberg K, Smits JM, Offner G, *et al.* Kidney transplantation without prior dialysis in children: the Eurotransplant experience. Am J Transplant 2006;6:1858-1864.

[110] Johnson RJ, Armstrong S, Belger MA, *et al.* The outcome of pediatric cadaveric renal transplantation in the UK and Eire. Pediatr Transplant 2002;6:367-377.

[111] Hiramoto JS, Freise CE, Randall HR, *et al.* Successful long-term outcomes using pediatric en bloc kidneys for transplantation. Am J Transplant 2002;2:337-342.

[112] Ruff T, Reddy KS, Johnston TD, *et al.* Transplantation of pediatric en bloc cadaver kidneys into adult recipients: a single-center experience. Am Surg. 2002;68:857-859.

[113] Cecka JM, Gjertson DW, Terasaki PI. Pediatric renal transplantation: a review of the UNOS data. United Network for Organ Sharing. Pediatr Transplant 1997;1:55-64.

[114] Kari JA, Romagnoli J, Duffy P, *et al.* Renal transplantation in children under 5 years of age. Pediatr Nephrol 1999;13:730-736.

[115] Hwang AH, Cho YW, Cicciarelli J, *et al.* Risk factors for short- and long-term survival of primary cadaveric renal allografts in pediatric recipients: a UNOS analysis. Transplantation 2005;80:466-470.

[116] Smith JM, Ho PL, McDonald RA. Renal transplant outcomes in adolescents: a report of the North American Pediatric Renal Transplant Cooperative Study. Pediatr Transplant 2002;6:493-499.

[117] Baum MA, Ho M, Stablein D, Alexander SR. Outcome of renal transplantation in adolescents with focal segmental glomerulosclerosis. Pediatr Transplant 2002;6:488-492.

[118] Gjertson DW, Cecka JM. Determinants of long-term survival of pediatric kidney grafts reported to the United Network for Organ Sharing kidney transplant registry. Pediatr Transplant 2001;5:5-15.

[119] Shapiro R. Living donor kidney transplantation in pediatric recipients. Pediatr Transplant 2006;10:844-850.

[120] Tejani A, Sullivan EK. Do six-antigen-matched cadaver donor kidneys provide better graft survival to children compared with one-haploidentical living-related donor transplants? A report of the North American Pediatric Renal Transplant Cooperative Study. Pediatr Transplant 2000;4:140-145.

[121] Ferraris JR, Tambutti M, Prigoshin N. Improved long-term graft function in kidney transplant recipients with donor antigen-specific hyporeactivity. Pediatr Transplant. 2007;11:139-144.
[122] Ettenger RB. Age and the immune response in pediatric renal transplantation. Eur J Pediatr 1992;151 Suppl 1:S7-8.
[123] Tejani AH, Stablein DM, Sullivan EK, *et al.* The impact of donor source, recipient age, pre-operative immunotherapy and induction therapy on early and late acute rejections in children: a report of the North American Pediatric Renal Transplant Cooperative Study (NAPRTCS). Pediatr Transplant 1998;2:318-324.
[124] Scornik JC, Pfaff WW, Howard RJ, *et al.* Increased antibody responsiveness to blood transfusions in pediatric patients. Transplantation 1994;58:1361-1365.
[125] Humar A, Hassoun A, Kandaswamy R, *et al.* Immunologic factors: the major risk for decreased long-term renal allograft survival. Transplantation 1999;68:1842-1846.
[126] Singh A, Stablein D, Tejani A. Risk factors for vascular thrombosis in pediatric renal transplantation: a special report of the North American Pediatric Renal Transplant Cooperative Study. Transplantation 1997;63:1263-1267.
[127] Dharnidharka VR, Stevens G, Howard RJ. En-bloc kidney transplantation in the United states: an analysis of united network of organ sharing (UNOS) data from 1987 to 2003. Am J Transplant 2005;5:1513-1517.
[128] Bresnahan BA, McBride MA, Cherikh WS, Hariharan S. Risk factors for renal allograft survival from pediatric cadaver donors: an analysis of united network for organ sharing data. Transplantation 2001;72:256-261.
[129] Sureshkumar KK, Reddy CS, Nghiem DD, *et al.* Superiority of pediatric en bloc renal allografts over living donor kidneys: a long-term functional study. Transplantation. 2006;82:348-353.
[130] Sanchez-Fructuoso AI, Prats D, Perez-Contin MJ, *et al.* Increasing the donor pool using en bloc pediatric kidneys for transplant. Transplantation 2003;76:1180-1184.
[131] McDonald RA, Smith JM, Stablein D, Harmon WE. Pretransplant peritoneal dialysis and graft thrombosis following pediatric kidney transplantation: a NAPRTCS report. Pediatr Transplant 2003;7:204-208.
[132] Kelly DA. Current issues in pediatric transplantation. Pediatr Transplant 2006;10:712-720.
[133] Kaufman M, Shemesh E, Benton T. The adolescent transplant recipient. Pediatr Clin North Am 2010;57:575-592.
[134] Dobbels F, Ruppar T, De Geest S, *et al.* Adherence to the immunosuppressive regimen in pediatric kidney transplant recipients: A systematic review. Pediatr Transplant 2010;14:603-613.
[135] Bell LE, Bartosh SM, Davis CL, *et al.* Adolescent Transition to Adult Care in Solid Organ Transplantation: a consensus conference report. Am J Transplant 2008;8:2230-2242.
[136] Remorino R, Taylor J. Smoothing things over: the transition from pediatric to adult care for kidney transplant recipients. Prog Transplant 2006;16:303-308.
[137] Watson AR. Non-compliance and transfer from paediatric to adult transplant unit. Pediatr Nephrol 2000;14:469-472.
[138] Ng KH, Shrestha P, Aragon E, *et al.* Nineteen-year experience of paediatric renal transplantation in Singapore. Ann Acad Med Singapore 2009;38:300-309.
[139] Nankivell BJ, Chapman JR. Chronic allograft nephropathy: current concepts and future directions. Transplantation 2006;81:643-654.
[140] Gulati S, Kumar A, Sharma RK, *et al.* Outcome of pediatric renal transplants in a developing country. Pediatr Nephrol 2004;19:96-100.
[141] Berber I, Tellioglu G, Yigit B, *et al.* Pediatric renal transplantation: Clinical analysis of 28 cases. Transplant Proc 2006;38:430-431.
[142] Vlaminck H, Maes B, Evers G, *et al.* Prospective study on late consequences of subclinical non-compliance with immunosuppressive therapy in renal transplant patients. Am J Transplant 2004;4:1509-1513.
[143] Gerson AC, Furth SL, Neu AM, Fivush BA. Assessing associations between medication adherence and potentially modifiable psychosocial variables in pediatric kidney transplant recipients and their families. Pediatr Transplant 2004;8:543-550.
[144] Kahana S, Drotar D, Frazier T. Meta-analysis of psychological interventions to promote adherence to treatment in pediatric chronic health conditions. J Pediatr Psychol 2008;33:590-611.
[145] Graves MM, Roberts MC, Rapoff M, Boyer A. The efficacy of adherence interventions for chronically ill children: a meta-analytic review. J Pediatr Psychol. 2010;35:368-382.
[146] Fredericks EM, Dore-Stites D. Adherence to immunosuppressants: how can it be improved in adolescent organ transplant recipients? Curr Opin Organ Transplant. 2010;15:614-620.
[147] Ulinski T, Cochat P. Longitudinal growth in children following kidney transplantation: from conservative to pharmacological strategies. Pediatr Nephrol. 2006;21:903-909.
[148] Fine RN. Management of growth retardation in pediatric recipients of renal allografts. Nat Clin Pract Nephrol 2007;3:318-324.

[149] Neu AM. Special issues in pediatric kidney transplantation. Adv Chronic Kidney Dis 2006;13:62-69.
[150] Fuqua JS. Growth after organ transplantation. Semin Pediatr Surg. 2006;15:162-169.
[151] Allen U, Green M. Prevention and treatment of infectious complications after solid organ transplantation in children. Pediatr Clin North Am 2010;57:459-479.
[152] Gulati A, Sarwal MM. Pediatric renal transplantation: an overview and update. Curr Opin Pediatr 2010;22:189-196.
[153] Fonseca-Aten M, Michaels MG. Infections in pediatric solid organ transplant recipients. Semin Pediatr Surg 2006;15:153-161.
[154] Ballardie FW, Winearls CG, Cohen J, *et al.* Pneumocystis carinii pneumonia in renal transplant recipients--clinical and radiographic features, diagnosis and complications of treatment. Q J Med 1985;57:729-747.
[155] Talseth T, Holdaas H, Albrechtsen D, *et al.* Increasing incidence of Pneumocystis carinii pneumonia in renal transplant patients. Transplant Proc 1988;20:400-401.
[156] Franson TR, Kauffman HM, Jr., Adams MB, *et al.* Cyclosporine therapy and refractory Pneumocystis carinii pneumonia. A potential association. Arch Surg 1987;122:1034-1035.
[157] Neff RT, Jindal RM, Yoo DY, *et al.* Analysis of USRDS: incidence and risk factors for Pneumocystis jiroveci pneumonia. Transplantation 2009;88:135-141.
[158] Li L, Chaudhuri A, Weintraub LA, *et al.* Subclinical cytomegalovirus and Epstein-Barr virus viremia are associated with adverse outcomes in pediatric renal transplantation. Pediatr Transplant 2007;11:187-195.
[159] Sato T, Fujieda M, Tanaka E, *et al.* Monitoring of Epstein-Barr virus load and antibody in pediatric renal transplant patients. Pediatr Int 2008;50:454-458.
[160] Kotton CN, Kumar D, Caliendo AM, *et al.* International consensus guidelines on the management of cytomegalovirus in solid organ transplantation. Transplantation 2010;89:779-795.
[161] Rubin RH. Cytomegalovirus in solid organ transplantation. Transpl Infect Dis 2001;3 Suppl 2:1-5.
[162] Humar A, Uknis M, Carlone-Jambor C, *et al.* Cytomegalovirus disease recurrence after ganciclovir treatment in kidney and kidney-pancreas transplant recipients. Transplantation 1999;67:94-97.
[163] Cytomegalovirus. Am J Transplant. 2004 Nov;4 Suppl 10:51-58.
[164] Fishman JA, Rubin RH. Infection in organ-transplant recipients. N Engl J Med 1998;338:1741-1751.
[165] Preiksaitis JK, Brennan DC, Fishman J, Allen U. Canadian society of transplantation consensus workshop on cytomegalovirus management in solid organ transplantation final report. Am J Transplant 2005;5:218-227.
[166] Asberg A, Humar A, Jardine AG, *et al.* Long-term outcomes of CMV disease treatment with valganciclovir *versus* IV ganciclovir in solid organ transplant recipients. Am J Transplant 2009;9:1205-1213.
[167] Vaudry W, Ettenger R, Jara P, *et al.* Valganciclovir dosing according to body surface area and renal function in pediatric solid organ transplant recipients. Am J Transplant 2009;9:636-643.
[168] Cockfield SM. Identifying the patient at risk for post-transplant lymphoproliferative disorder. Transpl Infect Dis 2001;3:70-78.
[169] Smets F, Sokal EM. Epstein-Barr virus-related lymphoproliferation in children after liver transplant: role of immunity, diagnosis, and management. Pediatr Transplant 2002;6:280-287.
[170] Epstein-Barr virus and lymphoproliferative disorders after transplantation. Am J Transplant. 2004 Nov;4 Suppl 10:59-65.
[171] Hariharan S, Johnson CP, Bresnahan BA, *et al.* Improved graft survival after renal transplantation in the United States, 1988 to 1996. N Engl J Med. 2000;342:605-612.
[172] Hirsch HH. Polyomavirus BK nephropathy: a (re-)emerging complication in renal transplantation. Am J Transplant 2002;2:25-30.
[173] Ramos E, Drachenberg CB, Portocarrero M, *et al.* BK virus nephropathy diagnosis and treatment: experience at the University of Maryland Renal Transplant Program. Clin Transpl 2002:143-53.
[174] Ramos E, Hirsch HH. Polyomavirus-associated nephropathy: updates on a persisting challenge. Transpl Infect Dis 2006;8:59-61.
[175] Smith JM, McDonald RA, Finn LS, *et al.* Polyomavirus nephropathy in pediatric kidney transplant recipients. Am J Transplant 2004;4:2109-2117.
[176] Chen CH, Wen MC, Wang M, *et al.* High incidence of malignancy in polyomavirus-associated nephropathy in renal transplant recipients. Transplant Proc 2010;42:817-818.
[177] Vats A, Shapiro R, Singh Randhawa P, *et al.* Quantitative viral load monitoring and cidofovir therapy for the management of BK virus-associated nephropathy in children and adults. Transplantation 2003;75:105-112.
[178] Danzinger-Isakov L, Kumar D. Guidelines for vaccination of solid organ transplant candidates and recipients. Am J Transplant 2009;9 Suppl 4:S258-262.

[179] Kumar D, Morris MI, Kotton CN, *et al.* Guidance on novel influenza A/H1N1 in solid organ transplant recipients. Am J Transplant 2010;10:18-25.
[180] Kiberd BA, Rose C, Gill JS. Cancer mortality in kidney transplantation. Am J Transplant 2009;9:1868-1875.
[181] Ju MK, Joo DJ, Kim SJ, *et al.* Chronologically different incidences of post-transplant malignancies in renal transplant recipients: single center experience. Transpl Int 2009;22:644-653.
[182] Veroux M, Corona D, Scalia G, *et al.* Surveillance of human papilloma virus infection and cervical cancer in kidney transplant recipients: preliminary data. Transplant Proc 2009;41:1191-1194.
[183] McDonald SP, Craig JC. Long-term survival of children with end-stage renal disease. N Engl J Med 2004;350:2654-2662.
[184] Parekh RS, Carroll CE, Wolfe RA, Port FK. Cardiovascular mortality in children and young adults with end-stage kidney disease. J Pediatr 2002;141:191-197.
[185] Oh J, Wunsch R, Turzer M, *et al.* Advanced coronary and carotid arteriopathy in young adults with childhood-onset chronic renal failure. Circulation 2002;106:100-105.
[186] Becker-Cohen R, Nir A, Rinat C, *et al.* Risk factors for cardiovascular disease in children and young adults after renal transplantation. Clin J Am Soc Nephrol 2006;1:1284-1292.
[187] Mitsnefes MM, Khoury P, McEnery PT. Body mass index and allograft function in pediatric renal transplantation. Pediatr Nephrol 2002;17:535-539.
[188] Kasiske B, Cosio FG, Beto J, *et al.* Clinical practice guidelines for managing dyslipidemias in kidney transplant patients: a report from the Managing Dyslipidemias in Chronic Kidney Disease Work Group of the National Kidney Foundation Kidney Disease Outcomes Quality Initiative. Am J Transplant 2004;4 Suppl 7:13-53.
[189] Patel HP. Early origins of cardiovascular disease in pediatric chronic kidney disease. Ren Fail 2010;32:1-9.
[190] El-Husseini AA, Sheashaa HA, Hassan NA, *et al.* Echocardiographic changes and risk factors for left ventricular hypertrophy in children and adolescents after renal transplantation. Pediatr Transplant 2004;8:249-254.
[191] Kitzmueller E, Vecsei A, Pichler J, *et al.* Changes of blood pressure and left ventricular mass in pediatric renal transplantation. Pediatr Nephrol 2004;19:1385-1389.
[192] Morgan H, Khan I, Hashmi A, *et al.* Ambulatory blood pressure monitoring after renal transplantation in children. Pediatr Nephrol 2001;16:843-847.
[193] Weaver DJ, Jr., Kimball T, Witt SA, *et al.* Subclinical systolic dysfunction in pediatric patients with chronic kidney disease. J Pediatr 2008;153:565-569.
[194] Zoungas S, Asmar RP. Arterial stiffness and cardiovascular outcome. Clin Exp Pharmacol Physiol 2007;34:647-651.
[195] Aoun B, Lorton F, Wannous H, *et al.* Aortic stiffness in ESRD children before and after renal transplantation. Pediatr Nephrol 2010;25:1331-1336.

CHAPTER 12

Diagnostic Challenges in Kidney Transplantation

Kevin Herman, Abid Irshad*, Susan Ackerman and Mehwish Shazly

Medical University of South Carolina, Charleston, South Carolina, USA

Abstract: The growing success of renal transplantation around the world in the treatment of chronic renal failure has increased the significance of imaging in evaluating the transplanted kidney. Accurate interpretation of imaging studies plays a crucial role in the evaluation of renal grafts, the monitoring of developing pathology and the treatment of complications. Ultrasound, in particular, has proven to be an integral part of the burgeoning success of renal transplantation and subsequent monitoring. The role of imaging, especially ultrasound in detecting and evaluating complications of the parenchyma, vasculature, collecting system and ureter are discussed here with special attention to percutaneous transplant biopsy.

Keywords: Ultrasound, Renal Transplantation, Transplant Rejection, Transplant Complications, Lymphocele, Fluid Collection, Renal Vein Thrombosis, Renal Artery Thrombosis, Delayed Graft Function, Renal Cyst.

INTRODUCTION

The use of renal transplantation has significantly increased in developed and developing countries for treatment of chronic renal failure. Consequently, the understanding of the normal and abnormal imaging features of the transplanted kidney has become even more important for the radiologists and technologists around the world. Many healthcare providers who do not deal with these patients on regular basis will not have enough experience in this regard. Hence it is important to familiarize ourselves with the appropriate imaging studies that may help to evaluate a renal graft at various stages and to identify the imaging findings which suggest an abnormality of the renal graft. Imaging plays a critical role in monitoring the health of a renal graft, as well as in making appropriate treatment decisions in cases of postoperative complications. Ultrasound is particularly useful for detecting such complications in the transplanted kidney. Advances in imaging techniques have been an integral part of the growing efficacy of renal transplantation. These advances have led to early detection and management of the anatomic and functional graft abnormalities in both the early and late post-transplant period. This, in turn, has led to the improved treatment of such complications and better long-term graft survival.

Familiarity with the usual and variant anatomy of renal transplant, as well as the surgical technique involved, is essential in the imaging evaluation of renal transplant. Usually, the transplanted kidney is placed extraperitoneally in the right or left iliac fossa. Because of a simpler technical approach to vascular anastomosis, the right side is preferred. In both cadaveric and living donor transplants, vascular anastomosis is achieved with the external iliac vessels, but through differing techniques. Anastomosis of the ureters is achieved through creation of a new ureterocystostomy. Most commonly, the donor ureter is tunneled through dome of the bladder wall to create a new ureteral orifice that is anatomically higher than the native orifices. Alternative techniques include uretero-ureterostomy and pyelo-ureterostomy. In pediatric recipients, the kidney may need to be placed in a more cephalad abdominal position, in which case vascular anastomosis may be created with the distal aorta and inferior vena cava (IVC).

ROLE OF IMAGING

In the early post-operative period, ultrasound (US), especially Doppler US and radionuclide imaging are the two most commonly used imaging modalities for evaluating the transplanted kidney. While Gray scale US

***Address correspondence to Abid Irshad:** Medical University of South Carolina, 169 Ashley Avenue, Charleston, South Carolina 29425, USA; Tel: (843) 792-1957; Fax: (843) 792-9503; E-mail: irshada@musc.edu helps in evaluating the anatomic abnormalities of the graft or adjacent areas, the Doppler US helps to detect any vascular abnormalities. Nuclear medicine (MAG-3) scan, on the other hand helps in evaluating the function of the graft by evaluating the renal parenchymal perfusion, uptake and excretion. It also helps to rule out a urine leak in early post-operative period.

Other, less frequently used modalities include computed tomography (CT) scan, magnetic resonance imaging (MRI) and angiography (MRA), as well as conventional angiography.

Ultrasound is the most frequently used imaging modality for evaluating renal transplant. Typically, a baseline examination may be obtained within the first 24-48 hours using both gray-scale and Doppler imaging. These baseline images establish the renal size and echogenicity, the status of the collecting system and ureter and the size and location of any postoperative peri-nephric fluid collections. Additionally, any pre-existing renal parenchymal lesions can be noted on this baseline scan. Interventional procedures are also aided by the use of US. Real-time US guidance is helpful in directing the renal biopsy; not only does US guidance aid in avoiding the main vessels, but it also effects preferable sampling of the glomeruli through angling of the needle tangentially toward the renal cortex. US is also helpful in the management of postoperative complications, such as draining peri-nephric fluid collections or placing a percutaneous nephrostomy tube.

Radionuclide imaging is frequently used in early post-transplant period. Renal function, radiotracer excretion and urological abnormalities (including ureteral obstruction or urine leak) can be assessed using Tc-99 MAG3 scanning. For example, US may not differentiate obstructive hydronephrosis from a dilated, non-obstructed collecting system. In such cases, a Tc-99 MAG3 renal scan with a diuretic such as Furosemide may be helpful in differentiating between the two conditions. Tc-99 DMSA is considered a parenchymal agent and can be used to evaluate perfusion defects or small infarcts.

The use of CT scan in evaluating renal transplants is limited because of the nephrotoxic effects of iodinated contrast. However, a non-contrast CT may be used to assess the size of a perinephric fluid collection and its spatial relationship to the kidney. Additionally, CT guidance may be used in interventional management, such as drain placement or performing a percutaneous nephrostomy.

The multiplanar imaging capability of MRI allows for excellent anatomic orientation of the kidney and its associated vessels. Furthermore, renal parenchymal abnormalities including perfusion defects, post-transplant lymphoproliferative disorders and renal tumors are well-visualized with MRI. In cases of renal artery stenosis, magnetic resonance angiography (MRA) may be used to evaluate the renal vessels. However, caution must be exercised in the administration of gadolinium contrast in patients with impaired renal function and low glomerular filtration rate due to the risk of nephrogenic systemic fibrosis.

In select instances of a suspected vascular abnormality when US shows no or equivocal findings; or conversely, in situations where US suggest an abnormality that is not supported by the clinical impression, conventional angiography may be used. More important, however, are the interventional vascular management techniques that may pre-empt the necessity of open surgery. For example, the first line treatment of RAS is currently considered to be percutaneous transluminal angioplasty (PTA), with or without stent placement. Vascular thrombi may be treated with thrombolytic therapy, and coiling may be employed in cases of arteriovenous fistulas and pseudoaneurysms.

NORMAL POST-SURGICAL FINDINGS

Due to its more superficial location, the normal transplant kidney may appear slightly different from the normal native kidney. Being closer to the transducer, the renal cortex may appear relatively bright or echogenic. In transplants, there is improved corticomedullary differentiation with the medullary pyramids appearing relatively hypoechoic and the cortex appearing relatively brighter (Fig. **1**).

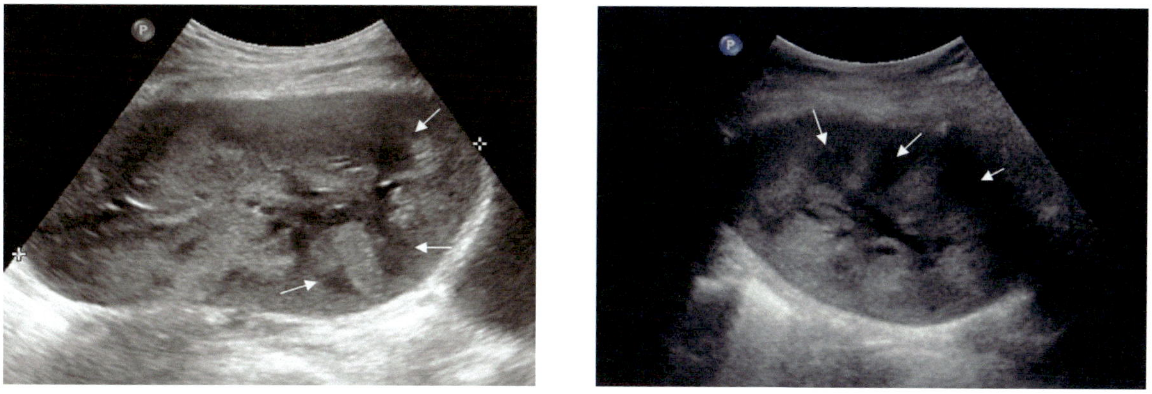

Figure 1A and B: Normal transplant kidney Sagittal and transverse images of the transplant kidney show relatively bright renal cortex with hypoechoic medullary pyramids (arrows) seen relatively clearly.

The normal ureter is more anteriorly placed and is visualized relatively easily (Fig. **2A**). The uretero-vesical junction is seen more superiorly along the dome of the bladder (Fig. **2B**).

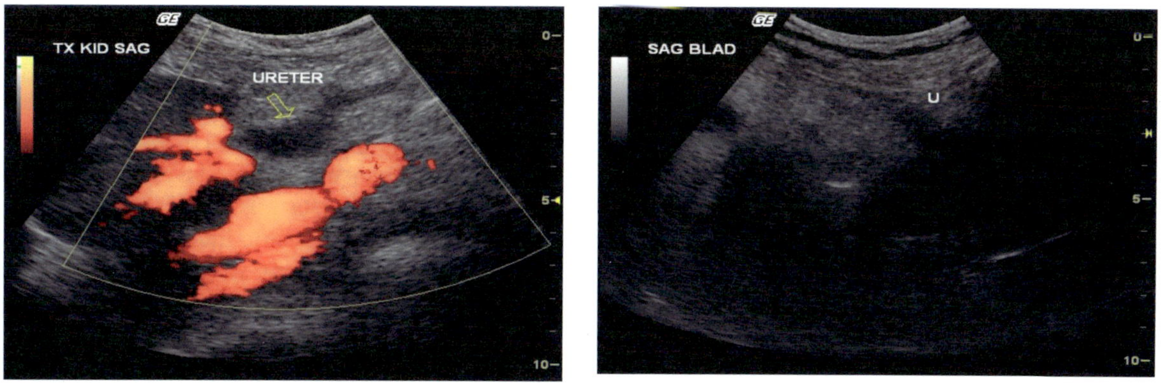

Figure 2 A and B: Normal transplant ureter. Image A, a Doppler image through the transplant kidney shows prominent proximal ureter (arrow) located relatively anteriorly. Image B, an US image through the bladder (B) shows transplant ureter (U), implanted high towards the bladder dome.

The collecting system and ureter may show some fullness due to absent peristalsis secondary to denervation. Small hematomas or collections around the kidney are considered to be an expected finding in early post-transplant period.

On Doppler exam, a normal renal arterial flow is antegrade throughout the cardiac cycle (Fig. **3**).

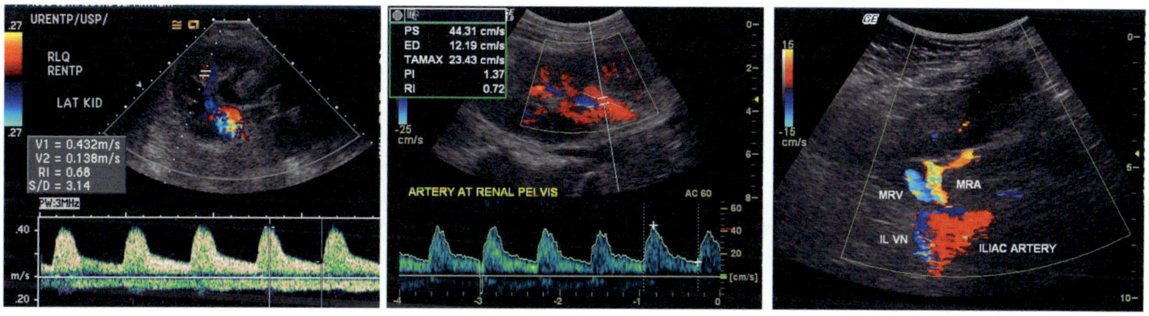

Figure 3 A, B and C: Normal arterial waveform. Image A, a Doppler image through the intrarenal arcuate artery in lateral part of the transplant kidney and image B, though the renal artery at the hilum show normal antegrade flow with sharp systolic upstroke and pan-diastolic antegrade flow. The resistive indices (about 0.7) are within the normal range. Image C, a color Doppler image through the anastomotic site shows normal renal artery and vein anastomosing with the iliac vessels.

The resistive index may be slightly high due to early post-op changes. However, absence or reversal of the diastolic flow should be interpreted with suspicion. Isolated finding of high velocity with the renal artery may sometimes be seen secondary to anastomotic edema, vessel tortuosity or compression. Any increase or decrease in renal arterial velocities should be compared to any similar changes in the adjacent iliac artery to differentiate local causes from systemic causes.

A baseline Doppler examination evaluates vascular flow in the renal and iliac vessels and helps to correctly interpret any subsequent changes in the flow velocities or pattern.

IMAGING EVALUATION OF TRANSPLANT COMPLICATIONS

These complications can be classified as parenchymal complications, perinephric fluid collections, vascular complications and urologic complications.

Parenchymal complications

Complications having diffuse parenchymal involvement include acute tubular necrosis (ATN), rejection and drug nephrotoxicity. These can lead to graft dysfunction and are difficult to differentiate on imaging. Neither gray-scale nor duplex US is considered sensitive or specific in diagnosing these conditions. Generally, a core needle biopsy is required to differentiate between these processes.

Acute Tubular Necrosis (ATN)

ATN is a common cause of impaired renal function in the early post-transplant period. It is caused by ischemia of the donor kidney during transplantation and occurs more frequently with cadaveric donors than with living donors. ATN usually causes renal dysfunction in the immediate postoperative period and resolves within 2 weeks. US exam will usually be normal or demonstrate nonspecific findings such as renal enlargement, increased resistive indexes (Fig. **4**) or changes in the echogenicity of the parenchyma or pyramids. Functional imaging, such as renal scintigraphy, typically demonstrates a delayed time to peak, a persistent parenchymal activity with delayed excretion [1]. While ATN is usually a self-limiting condition, severe cases may require dialysis.

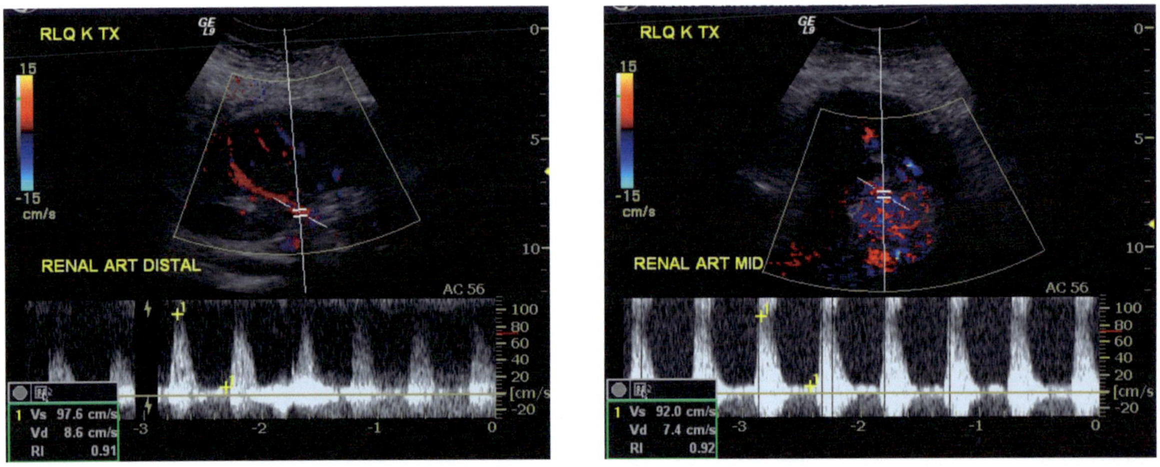

Figure 4 A and B: High resistive index secondary to Acute Tubular necrosis (ATN). Image A, a color and spectral Doppler through the distal transplant renal artery shows normal systolic and low diastolic velocity and an increased resistive index of 0.91. Image B, through the mid renal artery shows similar waveform with a high resistive index.

Hyperacute Rejection

Depending on the time interval after transplantation, rejection can be classified as hyperacute, acute or chronic. Hyperacute rejection, the least common of the three, is caused by preformed antibodies present in the recipient. This type of rejection is typically recognized in the operating room as it happens immediately after transplantation. Therefore, the kidneys are not often imaged.

Acute Rejection

The most common type of rejection in renal transplant is acute rejection. This happens in about10% of renal transplants [2], usually occurring 1-3 weeks after transplantation [3]. Fever, tenderness over the graft, proteinuria and oliguria are all symptoms associated with acute rejection. When acute rejection is suspected, current guidelines recommend biopsy before beginning treatment, except in such cases where this may cause significant delay of treatment [4]. Acute cellular rejection is an acute T-cell-mediated process characterized by a decline in kidney function along with the presence of well-established diagnostic features on biopsy. These same biopsy findings in the absence of clinical manifestations lead to a classification of subclinical acute rejection. Furthermore, borderline acute rejection is defined by histopathological findings "suspicious for acute rejection" according to the guidelines set forth in the Banff classification [5]. Current recommendations call for the treatment of subclinical and borderline acute rejection, most commonly with corticosteroids [6]. In cases resistant to treatment with corticosteroids, anti-T-cell antibodies such as muromonab, anti-thymocyte globulin or anti-lymphocyte globulin can be used [7]. Further, there are studies to suggest that polyclonal or monoclonal anti-T-cell antibodies are useful for treating steroid-resistant or recurrent T-cell-mediated rejection [8]. Following the rejection episode, changes to the maintenance immunosuppressive medication regimen include addition of mycophenolate mofetil, or replacement of azathioprine with mycophenolate mofetil [7, 9].

US may show renal enlargement, increased or decreased parenchymal echogenicity, or it may be completely normal. Doppler US usually shows high resistive and pulsatility indexes (>0.9). Reversal of diastolic flow in the renal artery may be seen in severe cases of acute rejection (Fig. **5**); however, this finding is more commonly seen in renal vein thrombosis [10]. In such cases, demonstration of a patent renal vein is helpful in ruling out venous thrombus. Ultrasound detection of parenchymal edema of the transplant kidney is a reliable indicator both of manifested and subclinical rejection changes [11]. On radionuclide imaging, flow is diminished, which is sometimes also seen with ATN.

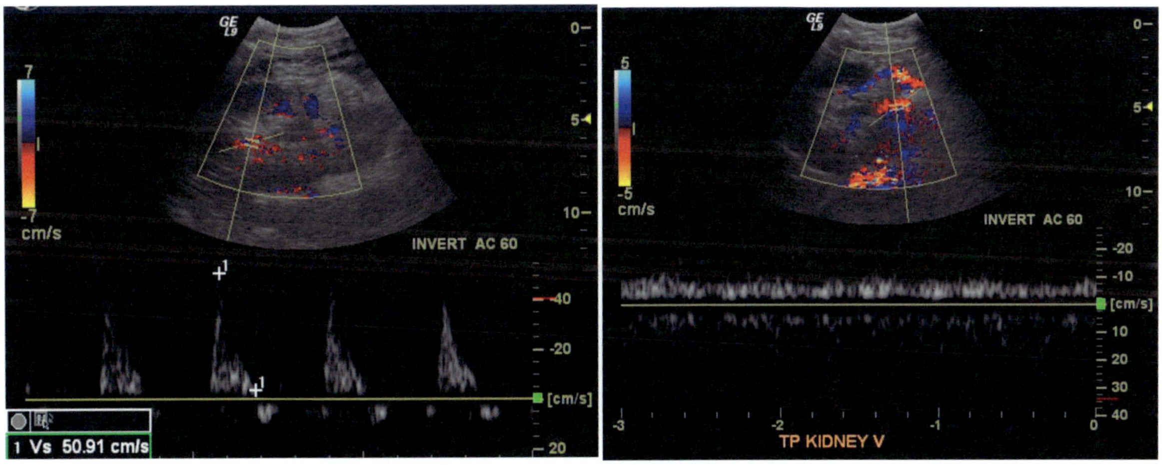

Figure 5 A and B: Severe acute rejection. Image A, a color Doppler and spectral waveform US image through the intrarenal artery close to the hilum demonstrates early diastolic flow reversal suggestive of severely increased resistance. Image B, a Doppler image through the renal vein shows a patent renal vein.

Chronic Allograft Injury

Chronic allograft injury (CAI) – traditionally known as chronic rejection – is the most common cause of late graft failure; it leads to interstitial fibrosis and sclerosing vasculitis. By definition, CAI occurs more than 3 months after transplantation [10]. Renal biopsy is required for the diagnosis. Histologically, CAI is defined by interstitial fibrosis and tubular atrophy [12, 13]. US may be normal or show increased parenchymal echogenicity, cortical thinning, and mild hydronephrosis. Radionuclide scintigraphy shows decreased radiotracer uptake.

Drug Toxicity

Immunosuppressive drugs are commonly employed to protect the transplanted kidney from acute rejection; however, most of these drugs are nephrotoxic. The most commonly used drugs in current practice include cyclosporin A, tacrolimus/FK-506, sirolimus/everolimus, azathioprine, prednisone, mycophenolate mofetil and T-cell antibodies. Correlated cyclosporine levels are used to rule out cyclosporine nephrotoxicity. US findings are generally normal or nonspecific. Radionuclide scan of cases of acute cyclosporine toxicity are similar to the findings of acute rejection.

Focal Renal Parenchymal Lesions

Focal lesions are a less common occurrence in the transplanted kidney. Hematoma, focal contusion or scar (Fig. **6**) may occur as a result of surgery or biopsy.

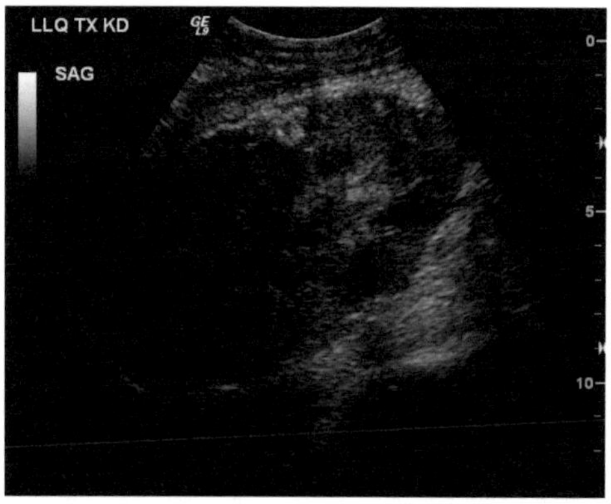

Figure 6: Renal scar after a renal biopsy Sagittal US image through the transplant kidney shows an echogenic peripheral area at the lower pole cortex suggesting a renal scar in the area of a previous biopsy.

Additionally, stones or small tumors may incidentally be carried from a donor kidney during the transplant process. Long term dialysis may lead to acquired cystic changes (Fig. **7**). Other parenchymal lesions that may develop in the graft include renal carcinoma, transitional cell cancer, lymphoproliferative disorders, simple or complex cysts and infective lesions. While needle biopsy may occasionally be required for diagnosis, anatomic imaging modalities such as US, CT, or MRI are often helpful in evaluating these lesions.

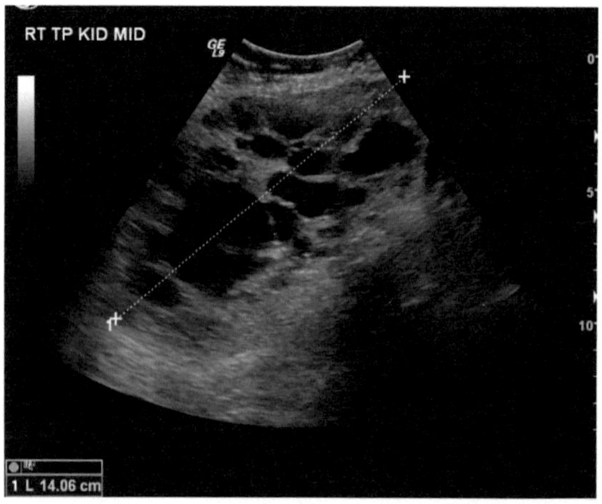

Figure 7: Acquired cystic disease of the transplant kidney. US image through the transplant kidney shows slightly enlarged kidney with numerous cystic changes scattered throughout the parenchyma replacing the normal parenchymal tissue.

Perinephric Fluid Collections

Perinephric fluid collections occur during the early post-transplant period of up to 50% of renal transplants [14-16]. These fluid collections include hematomas, lymphoceles, urinomas and abscesses. US is not specific in differentiating between the various types of perinephric fluid collections. Correlation with the postoperative time interval, however, may suggest etiology. Hematomas and urinomas are usually seen in the early postoperative period, whereas lymphoceles typically are not present until 4-8 weeks after transplantation. To confirm diagnosis, aspiration of the fluid and analysis is necessary.

Urinoma or Urinary Leak

Urinomas occur in 1-5% [17] of transplant cases, most commonly in the first 2 weeks. Urinomas are extraperitoneal collections that are typically seen between the bladder and kidney and may occasionally rupture intraperitoneally. Leaks are most often found at the distal ureter or at the site of ureterocystostomy; they are caused by ureteric ischemia or surgical technique. US demonstrates anechoic fluid collections that may rapidly increase in size (Fig. **8**).

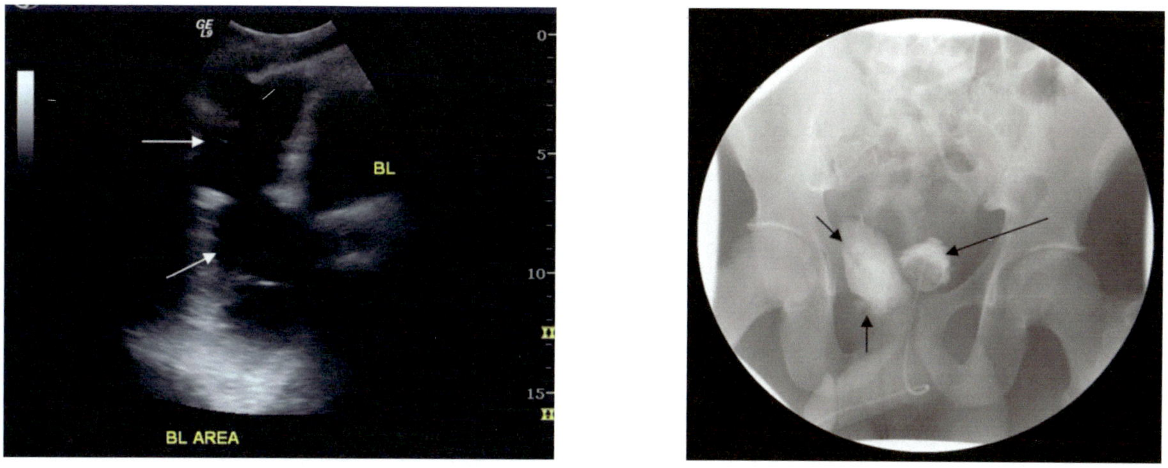

Figure 8: Urinoma. (A), a transverse US image through the pelvis shows an irregular fluid collection (arrows) towards the right side of the bladder (BL). (B), an antegrade cystogram shows extravasated contrast material on the right side of the bladder (small arrows). The bladder shows Foley's catheter in place (long arrow).

Care must be taken to differentiate urinomas from other cystic collections, including adnexal cysts in females or prosthetic reservoir in males. Intraperitoneal leaks appear as simple ascites on US with fluid around the bowel loops (Fig. **9**).

Radionuclide scintigrams demonstrate radiotracer activity outside the borders of the urinary system and are useful in differentiating urinomas from other collections. Drainage under US or CT guidance shows a high creatinine level and provides a more definitive diagnosis. While surgical repair is occasionally necessary, most leaks are managed conservatively by percutaneous nephrostomy and stent placement. Other studies occasionally helpful in diagnosing and localizing leaks are antegrade nephrostogram and cystogram (Fig. **8B**).

Hematoma

Hematomas are a common complication of the early post-operative period; the incidence of significant post-transplant hematomas is 4-8% [18-20]. They frequently appear on US as complex crescentic collections around the kidney (Fig. **10**). Measurement of hematomas on baseline scans is important, as they normally will gradually decrease in size over time. A hematoma that increases in size should raise suspicion of an active or repeat bleed. Acute hematomas are complex and echogenic on US, while chronic hematomas are usually more hypoechoic in appearance [21]. CT scan shows acute hematomas as hyperattenuating areas not enhanced with contrast medium administration, whereas older hematomas will appear as heterogeneous fluid collections [22]. MRI is particularly sensitive for detecting the blood products at various stages of hematoma.

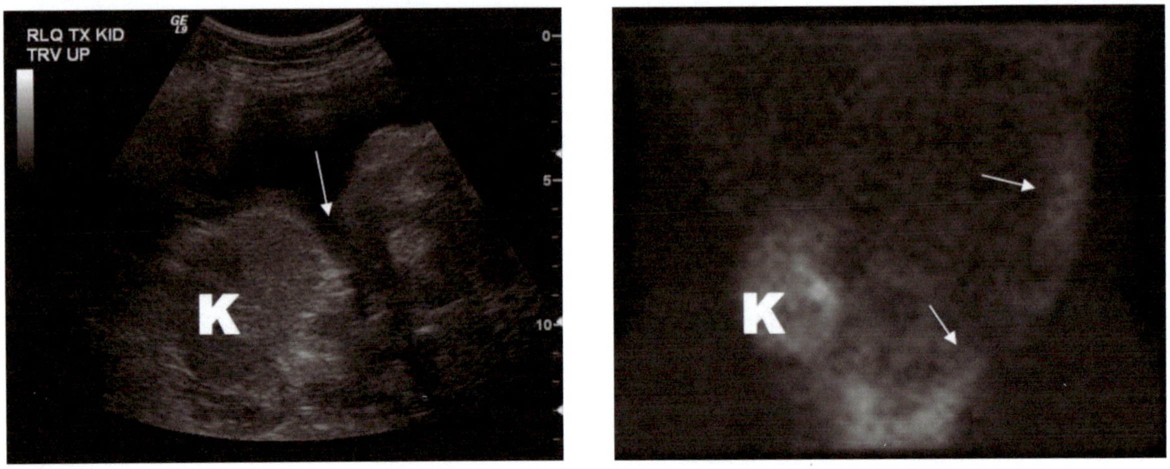

Figure 9: Intraperitoneal urine leak. (A), a transverse US image through the transplant kidney (K) shows moderate amount of fluid collection around the kidney that extend into the bowel recesses (arrow). (B), a nuclear medicine MAG 3 scan shows transplant kidney in the right lower quadrant with free radiotracer within the peritoneal cavity (arrows).

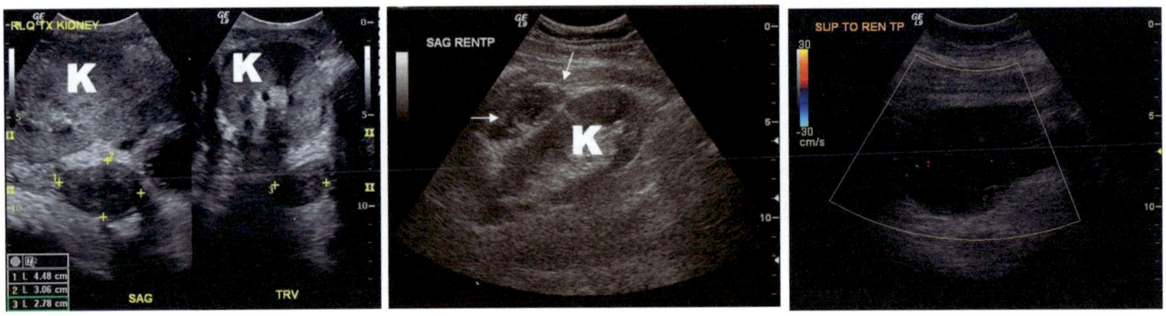

Figure 10: Post-surgical hematomas. (A), a dual image (sagittal and transverse) through the transplant kidney shows a well circumscribed solid appearing hematoma (calipers) posterior to the kidney (K). (B) shows a hematoma (arrows) seen as complex fluid collection anterior to the kidney (K). (C), a color Doppler image through a large hematoma which is mostly avascular.

Lymphoceles

The reported incidence of lymphocele is as high as 18% of transplants. They usually occur 4-8 weeks after transplant, secondary to post-surgical disruption of the lymphatics. While lymphoceles are usually asymptomatic, larger ones may cause a mass effect and compression of the ureter or adjacent structures. Such collections will be seen as cold defects on radionuclide scintigrams. US typically shows lymphoceles as anechoic collections without much complexity. Treatment include US- or CT-guided percutaneous needle aspiration, drain placement, sclerotherapy with absolute alcohol [23], bleomycin [24], or doxycycline [25].

Perinephric Abscesses

Infection is not altogether unusual after transplant, but the formation of a perinephric abscess is relatively uncommon. The abscess may develop by either infection of a perinepheric collection or extension of renal abscess into perinephric space (Fig. **11**). Pain and fever are typical of the clinical presentation. US is non-specific in differentiating the abscess from other collections; however, presence of air (seen as echogenic interface with ring down artifacts) is suggestive of an abscess. CT exam demonstrates presence of air and strong rim enhancement of the collection wall. Treatment includes antibiotic therapy and drainage under CT or US guidance (Fig. **11D**).

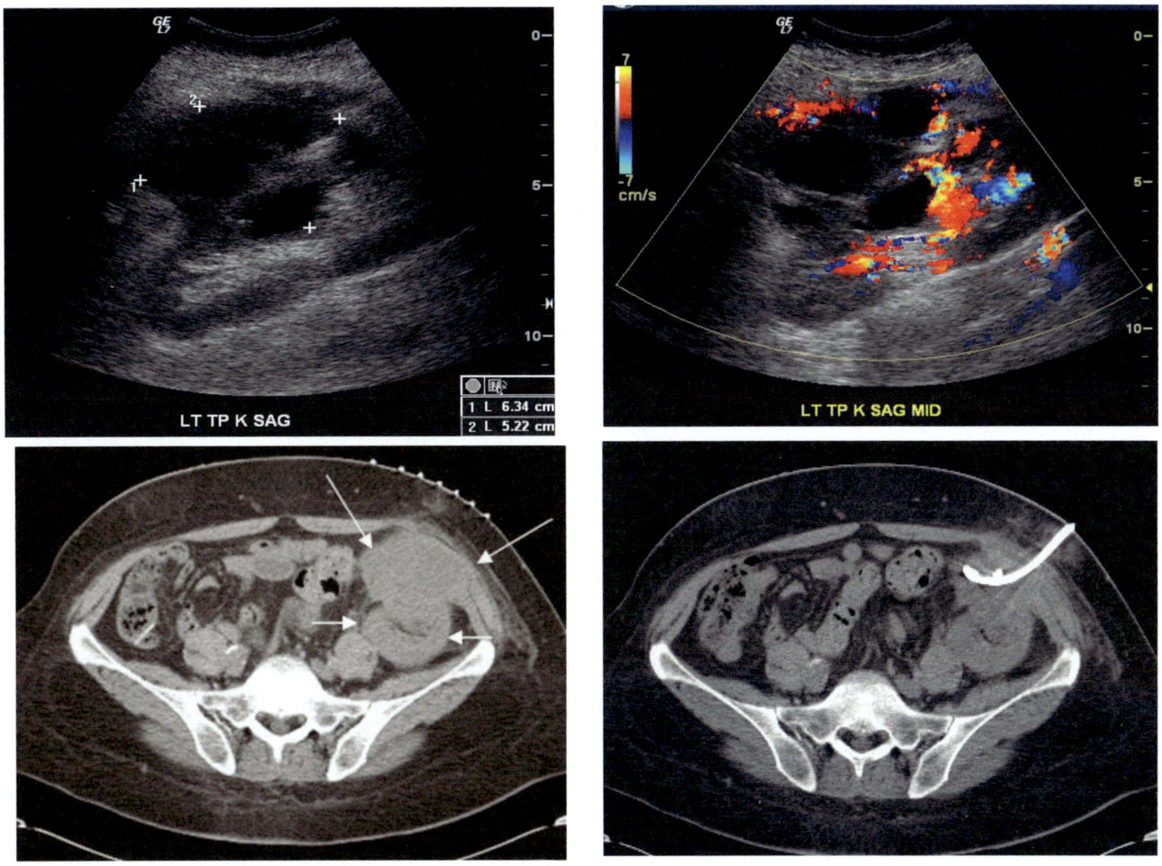

Figure 11: Renal Abscess. (A) is a gray scale sagittal image through the transplant kidney that shows an exophytic multi-septated abscess (calipers). (B), a color Doppler image of the same area shows peripheral vascularity without any significant internal flow. (C), an axial CT scan image through the pelvis shows transplant kidney (short arrows) with the abscess protruding anteriorly (long arrows). (D) shows a drain placed in the abscess.

VASCULAR COMPLICATIONS

Vascular complications are associated with significant morbidity in renal transplants and may even lead to graft loss. Early identification and intervention in cases of vascular complication may save the graft. Color Doppler US and duplex waveform are the preferred methods of initial evaluation of early vascular complications. While MRA has some diagnostic use, conventional angiography is still considered the gold standard for the diagnosis and management of vascular complications.

Renal Artery Stenosis (RAS)

RAS is the most commonly encountered vascular complication in renal transplants [1, 26-28]. It occurs in up to 10% of cases and is responsible for roughly 1-5% of cases of post-transplant hypertension [29]. Most commonly, it presents within the first 3 months following transplant, but it may develop early or late. A stricture may occur near the anastomotic site, at the distal donor artery or at the recipient artery [1]. The anastomotic site and the proximal renal artery are the most commonly affected locations, usually occurring in cases of end-to-end vascular anastomoses. There is a 3 times greater risk of stenosis in end-to-end anastomosis *versus* end-to-side anastomosis [30-31]. Proposed causes of RAS include sutural technique, infection, kinking of the vessel, arterial trauma during surgery, atherosclerosis and rejection.

Color Doppler ultrasound has been used for many years in screening for transplant renal artery stenosis [32-34]. Its non-invasive nature, portability, low cost and lack of iodine contrast makes it very useful for detecting RAS and monitoring for recurrence after interventional or surgical correction [35].

Characteristic US findings in cases of RAS include focal areas of color aliasing, turbulence and spectral broadening. A peak systolic velocity of >200 cm/s or a Doppler frequency shift of greater than 7.5 kHz when a 3-MHz transducer is used are expected findings [13, 36] (Fig. **12**). A velocity ratio of stenotic to prestenotic segment greater than 2:1 is another supportive finding. An additional helpful finding is a tardus-parvus waveform (delayed systolic upstroke) distal to the stenosis and in the intrarenal arcuate arteries (Fig. **12**). Conservative management is recommended for patients without clinical symptoms but with abnormal Doppler findings [13].

Gadolinium-enhanced MRA not only allows accurate assessment of the vascular anatomy, it also has the potential of providing important hemodynamic flow information. It is less operator-dependent than Doppler sonography [37]. However, in patients with renal impairment, gadolinium must be used cautiously; as nephrogenic systemic fibrosis has been correlated with exposure to gadolinium-containing MRI contrast agents [38].

The gold standard for the management and diagnosis of RAS continues to be contrast angiography. Luminal narrowing of >50% suggests hemodynamically significant RAS. This may be managed by PTA with or without stent placement. The clinical success rate of stent placement, as measured by improvement in blood pressure control, is about 82% [39]. Still, restenosis will occur in 5-30% of cases within 6-8 months [40].

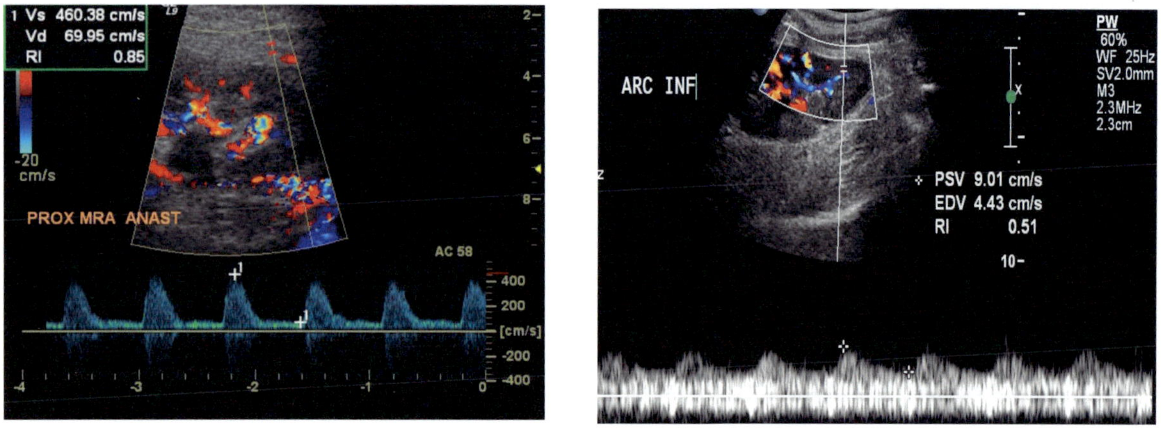

Figure 12: Renal artery stenosis. (A), a color Doppler and spectral waveform image through the anastomotic region of the transplant renal artery shows increased velocity (460 cm/s) through the anastomotic area. (B), a color Doppler and waveform through the intrarenal arcuate artery shows a delayed and slow upstroke with a 'tardus-parvus' waveform.

Renal Artery Thrombosis

Renal Artery Thrombosis is a less common complication of transplant, occurring in less than 1% of cases [1]. Surgical technique leading to kinking or torsion of the artery or dissection of the arterial wall is often the cause. Other precipitating factors include acute or hyperacute rejection, acute tubular necrosis and hypercoagulable states. Often, it results in transplant loss [1]. Clinical manifestations include absent urinary output and tenderness and swelling in the graft area.

The most common US finding is the absence of arterial and venous flow distal to the thrombus and in the intrarenal vessels (Fig. **13**). The absence of flow on US is a rare finding in severe cases of acute rejection [1]. It is important to adjust technical parameters to avoid a false-positive result. Power Doppler US may help to demonstrate flow in a technically difficult patient.

Renal artery thrombosis will present on radionuclide scan as a photopenic graft area without perfusion. Immediate surgery is often the intervention of choice in patients with acute graft dysfunction accompanied by US findings of renal artery thrombosis. Catheter-directed thrombolysis is another therapeutic option.

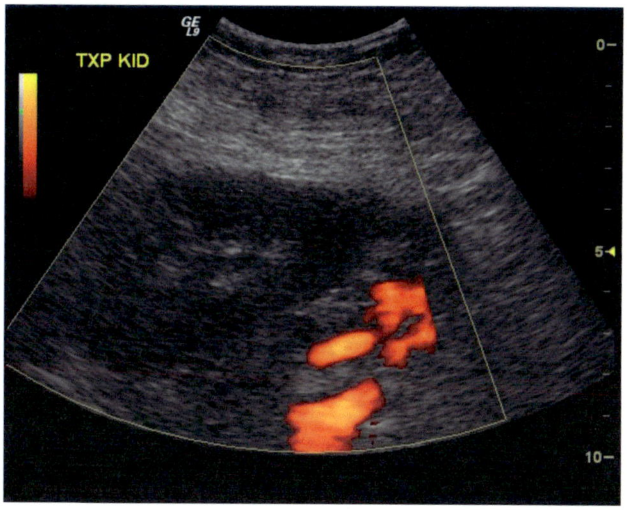

Figure 13: Renal artery thrombosis. Doppler US image through the transplant kidney shows no flow through the kidney or in the main renal vessels. Iliac vessels adjacent to the kidney show normal color flow.

Renal Vein Thrombosis

Thrombosis of the renal vein is a rare cause of transplant dysfunction, occurring in <4% of cases [1]. Usually, it occurs in the early post-transplant period and is clinically manifested by abrupt onset of graft tenderness accompanied by swelling, oliguria, proteinuria and impaired renal function [41]. Renal vein thrombosis may be caused by surgical complications, hypovolemia, acute rejection, hypercoagulable states and venous compression. On gray scale US, echogenic material may be seen within the renal vein. Duplex US studies demonstrate findings of absent venous flow in the main renal vein and diastolic reversal of the arterial flow in the main artery and/or intrarenal arteries [13, 42, 43] (Fig. **14**).

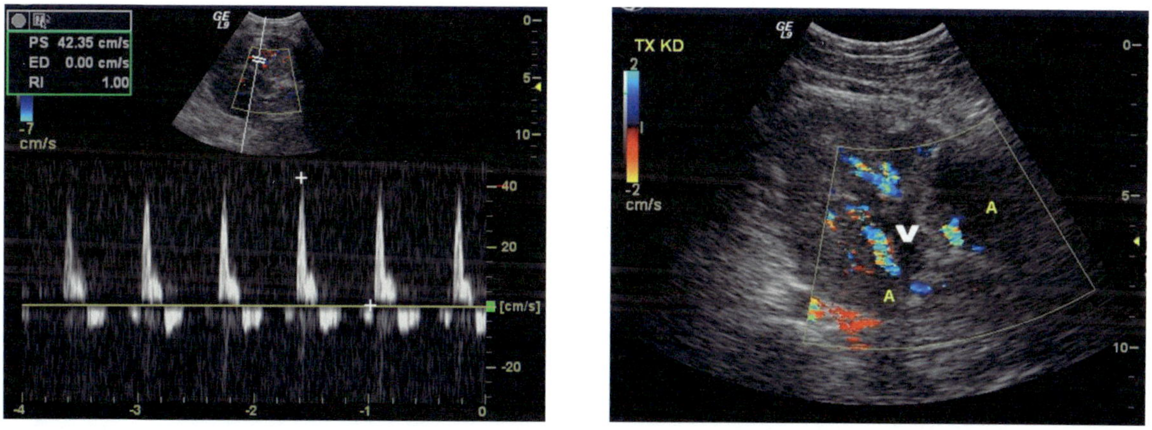

Figure 14: Renal vein thrombosis. (A), Doppler US of an intrarenal arcuate artery shows reversal of the diastolic flow below the baseline. (B), color Doppler image through the renal hilum shows two renal arteries (A) with no flow in the central renal vein (V) consistent with renal vein thrombosis.

A high resistive index may accompany partial venous thrombosis. In some cases, an increase in segmental venous velocity may be seen in partial thrombus, kinking of the vein or extrinsic pressure by a fluid collection (Fig. **15**). The kidney may be enlarged and hypoechoic on gray-scale imaging and may demonstrate effacement of the renal sinus.

Renal perfusion may appear abnormal on radionuclide renal scan [44]. Diagnosis of renal vein thrombosis may also be made with magnetic resonance venography or conventional angiography.

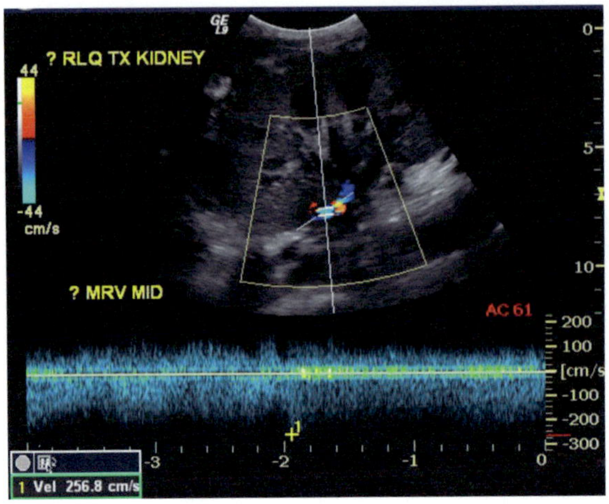

Figure 15: Venous stenosis. Doppler image through the transplant renal vein shows extremely high velocity within the renal vein suggesting stenosis.

Segmental Infarction

Thrombosis of the intrarenal arterial branches causes segmental infarction. Infarcts may be seen as focal hypoechoic areas on gray-scale US imaging. They may have echogenic borders. Radionuclide renal scan, especially with Tc-99 DMSA, and color Doppler imaging are also useful for noting focal perfusion defects.

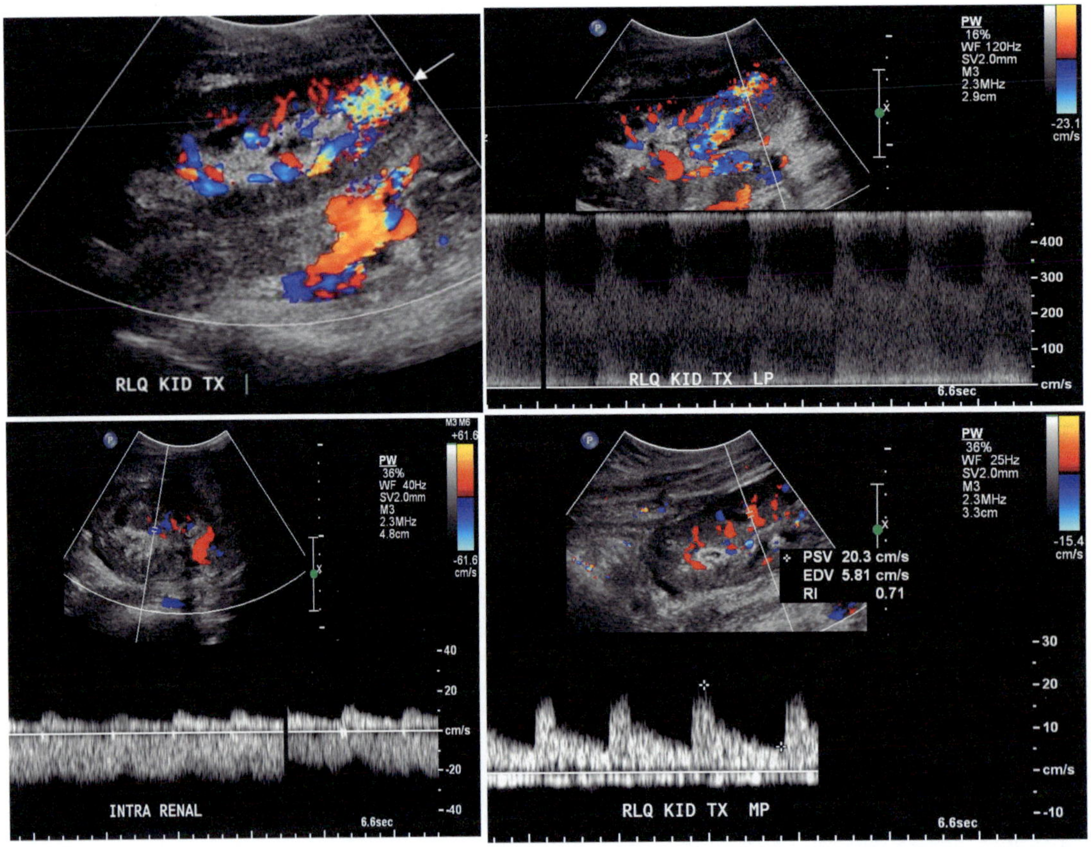

Figure 16: Arteriovenous fistula at the lower pole in the area of previous biopsy. (A) is a color Doppler image through the transplant kidney that shows color aliasing and turbulence at the lower pole suggestive of high velocity (arrow). (B), spectral waveform through the lower pole artery shows very high velocity (up to 400 cm/s) with increased diastolic flow. (C), spectral waveform through a mid pole vein shows slightly pulsatile waveform due to AV fistula. (D), through a mid pole vessel shows normal arterial velocity and wave form.

Arteriovenous Fistulas and Pseudoaneurysms

Percutaneous biopsy of renal transplants is crucial in determining the cause of transplant dysfunction and making the correct treatment decisions. However, renal biopsy may lead to vascular complications such as arteriovenous fistula (AVF) or pseudoaneurysm formation in 1-18% of cases [45]. Both usually are self-limiting and resolve spontaneously. Predisposing factors include arterial hypertension, renal medullary disease, central renal biopsies, and multiple needle passes [46, 47]. US of an AVF shows a focal area of turbulent flow and aliasing on color Doppler (Fig. **16**). Duplex US shows high velocity with a low resistive index in the feeding artery [9] along with arterialization of the flow in the draining vein (Fig. **16C**). Approximately 70% of AVFs will resolve spontaneously within 2 years. Large AVFs may cause renal ischemia through the "steal phenomenon." In such cases, angiography and coiling may be necessary for treatment. Superselective embolization with coaxial or single-catheter techniques and metallic coils usually results in little loss of parenchyma, thereby preserving renal function [7].

Pseudoaneurysm (PA) appears as a simple or minimally complex cystic structure on gray-scale US. Color Doppler imaging shows turbulent, swirling flow pattern within the PA. Both AVF and PA are usually self-limiting and resolve spontaneously

Extrarenal PA is very uncommon [48] and has a high mortality rate when it ruptures. Surgical technique or infection are the usual etiologies for these lesions. Coil embolization [49] and thrombin injection [50] have been tried to treat these lesions. Other useful embolic agents include N-butyl-cyanoacrylate, gelfoam, and detachable balloons [51]. Technical success rates for percutaneous embolotherapy are high and adverse effects, such as major parenchymal infarction are uncommon [52, 53]; however, transplant nephrectomy may be required.

COMPLICATIONS OF THE COLLECTING SYSTEM AND URETER

Most urological complications occur during the first month post-transplant. Ureteric obstruction and urine leak are the most common of these. Because of its limited blood supply, the transplanted ureter is relatively prone to ischemia.

Ureteral Obstruction

While mild fullness of the collecting system and ureter is a common finding on US due to loss of tonicity secondary to denervation, true ureteral obstruction occurs in about 2% of cases [13]. Ureteral obstruction is caused by ureteral ischemia, infection, ureteral kinking, edema at the anastomosis and extrinsic compression of the ureters by fluid collections. Most commonly, the distal third of the ureter is affected.

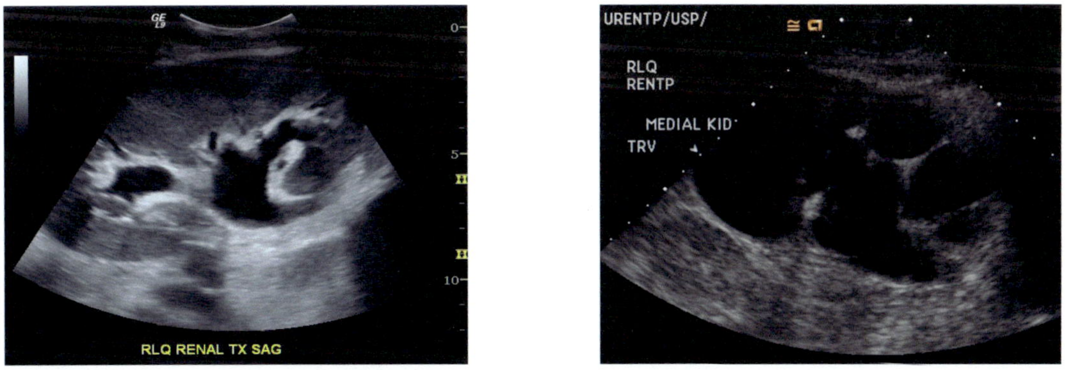

Figure 17: Hydronephrosis. (A), through a transplant kidney shows mild hydronephrosis and proximal hydroureter. The renal parenchymal thickness is preserved. (B) is transplant kidney of a different patient that shows marked hydronephrosis and proximal hydroureter. There is loss of parenchyma due to pressure atrophy.

Gray-scale US shows dilation of the renal pelvis and calyces (Fig. **17**). The transplant ureter is actually easier to evaluate compared to the native ureters because of its relatively anterior position, allowing for visualization of the site of obstruction on US examination.

Chronic rejection may demonstrate a sonographic appearance similar to that of obstruction since both complications are associated with a rising creatinine and dilated collecting system. Internal echoes within the dilated collecting system are suggestive of pyelonephrosis, fungal infections, clots or tumor (Fig. **18**).

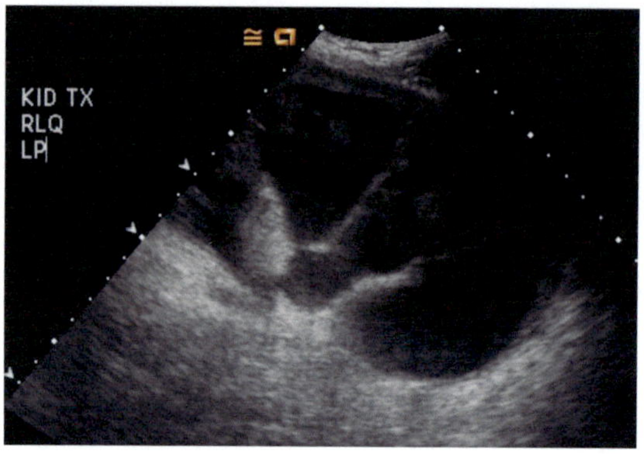

Figure 18: Fungal infection. Sagittal US image through the transplant kidney shows marked hydronephrosis. The calyces show internal debris and soft tissue material consistent with fungal infection.

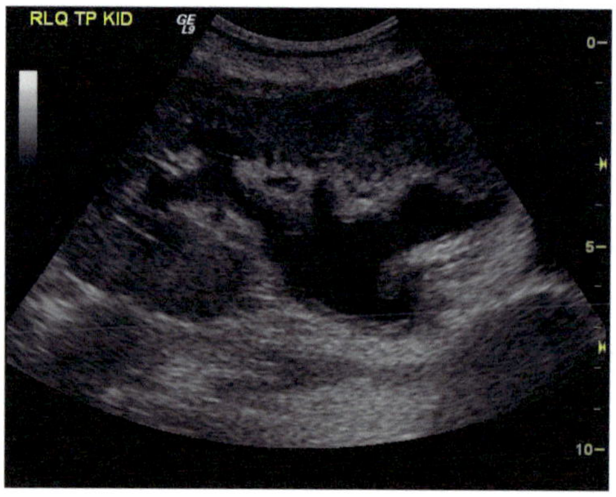

Figure 19: Pyelonephritis. US image through the transplant kidney shows thickened urothelium along the renal pelvis and calyces suggesting reactive hypertrophy secondary to inflammation.

In cases of dilated collecting systems, urinary obstruction may be differentiated from non-obstruction by scintigraphy. Obstruction may also be ruled out by delayed radionuclide imaging or diuretic administration. Antegrade urography is helpful for identifying the site of obstruction prior to therapy, which is often by percutaneous nephrostomy, ureteral stenting or balloon dilatation.

US may also detect pyelonephritis, clots, fungus, tumors and stones. Pyelonephritis appears as a thickening of the urothelium (Fig. **19**), a finding that may also be seen in chronic rejection. Renal stones may form in the transplant kidney or be carried from the donor kidney; however, due to the denervation of the kidney and ureter, presentation does not feature typical colicky pain.

PERCUTANEOUS TRANSPLANT BIOPSY

Histological evaluation of allograft biopsies is the gold standard for assessing the type and grade of renal allograft rejection [6]. Percutaneous renal biopsy often yields important diagnostic information that cannot be obtained through imaging alone. In addition to a protocol biopsy to evaluate baseline renal status, current recommendations call for biopsy of all patients meeting any of the following criteria:

1. Declining kidney function of unclear cause.

2. Persistent, unexplained increase in serum creatinine.

3. Failure of serum creatinine to return to baseline following treatment.

4. Failure to reach expected kidney function within 1-2 months after transplantation.

5. New onset of proteinuria.

6. Unexplained proteinuria $\geq$ 3.0 g/g creatinine or $\geq$ 3.0 g per 24 hours [47].

Traditionally, the Banff Classification has been the mainstay of classifying renal allograft rejection. In its initial incarnation in 1991, it categorized rejection episodes based largely on the extent and location of immune cell infiltration [6]. It has subsequently been revised to include defined diagnostic criteria addressing the underlying pathogenesis of rejection, including chronic active T-cell-mediated and chronic active antibody-mediated modes of rejection [12]. Histopathologic diagnosis correlates well with graft outcome [54-56]; for example, the persistence of inflammation in sequential biopsies has been shown to predict creatinine clearance at 1 and 2 years, regardless of the severity or cellular composition of the inflammation [57]. Still, others argue that there exists little evidence to validate the accuracy of histopathology, as there is no independent system for assessing rejection [58].

There are a number or recent studies linking the poor long-term graft outcomes with the presence of circulating anti-HLA antibodies [59-64]; however, others suggest that this evidence is circumstantial and that a lack of standardization between studies in the methods of detecting circulating antibodies makes the studies difficult to compare and positive results somewhat arbitrarily defined [6]. Potentially, more accurate risk assessment might be obtained by staining protocol biopsies for C4d, the split product of C4 of the classical complement pathway [65]. In cases of acute allograft dysfunction, C4d seems to a reliable marker of antibody-mediated rejection, suggesting that complement activation may be a crucial component of its pathogenesis [6].

In obtaining the biopsy sample, US is used to guide the needle into the renal cortex to obtain glomeruli, improving the diagnostic yield and decreasing the potential for complications. Pre-biopsy color Doppler imaging allows for identification of the intrarenal and extrarenal major vessels, which may then be avoided by angling the needle towards upper or lower poles and away from the major or central vessels. The anterior, superficial extraperitoneal position of the transplanted kidney makes percutaneous biopsy easier than with native kidneys. Before biopsy, assessment of the renal hilum and major vessels is crucial. The hilum may rotate around its axis, causing the vessels to cross the lower pole, in which case upper pole biopsy becomes preferable. Most biopsies are performed with an automatic spring-loaded device with a 14- to 18-gauge needle. The Banff Classification delineates the criterion for adequate biopsy as the presence of 7 glomeruli and 1 artery [1]. Post-biopsy US is routinely used to evaluate for any immediate complications, including active bleeding or hematoma.

Most institutions report a lower complication rate with renal transplant biopsy *versus* native kidney biopsy [65, 66]. Post-biopsy complications include major and minor bleeding, pseudoaneurysm, graft loss infection, arteriovenous fistula or, possibly, death. Generally, however, US-guided renal biopsy is very safe and major complications are rare when real-time guidance is used properly.

REFERENCES

[1] Taylor KJ, Morse SS, Rigsby CM, *et al.* Vascular complications in renal allografts: Detection with duplex Doppler US. Radiology 1987;162:31-38.

[2] U.S. Renal Data System, USRDS 2009 Annual Data Report: Atlas of Chronic Kidney Disease and End-Stage Renal Disease in the United States, National Institutes of Health, National Institute of Diabetes and Digestive and Kidney Diseases, Bethesda, MD, 2009.

[3] Rumack CM, Wilson SF, Charboneau JW. Diagnostic Ultrasound, vol 1. St. Louis, MO, Elsevier Mosby, 2005.

[4] Kidney Disease: Improving Global Outcomes (KDIGO) Transplant Work Group. KDIGO clinical practice guideline for the care of kidney transplant recipients. American Journal of Transplantation 2009; 9(Suppl 3): S1–S157.

[5] Solez K, Colvin RB, Racusen LC, *et al.* Banff 07 classification of renal allograft pathology: Updates and future directions. Am J Transplant 2008; 8: 753–760.

[6] Kozakowski N, Regele H. Biopsy diagnostics in renal allograft rejection: from histomorphology to biological function. European Society for Organ Transplantation 2009; 22: 945–953.

[7] Loffroy R, Guiu B, Lambert A, *et al.* Management of post-biopsy renal allograft arteriovenous fistulas with selective arterial embolization: immediate and long-term outcomes. Clinical Radiology 2008; 63: 657-665.

[8] Webster AC, Pankhurst T, Rinaldi F, *et al.* Monoclonal and polyclonal antibody therapy for treating acute rejection in kidney transplant recipients: A systematic review of randomized trial data. Transplantation 2006; 81: 953–965.

[9] Mycophenolate mofetil for the treatment of a first acute renal allograft rejection: Three-year follow-up. The Mycophenolate Mofetil Acute Renal Rejection Study Group. Transplantation 2001; 71: 1091–1097.

[10] Irshad A, Ackerman S, Sosnouski D, *et al*: A review of sonographic evaluation of renal transplant complications. Curr Probl Diagn Radiol 2008;37:67-79.

[11] Krejci K, Zadrazil J, Tichy T, *et al.* Sonographic findings in borderline changes and subclinical acute renal allograft rejection. Eur J Radiol 2009;71: 288–295.

[12] Solez K, Colvin RB, Racusen LC, *et al.* Banff '05 Meeting Report: Differential diagnosis of chronic allograft injury and elimination of chronic allograft nephropathy ('CAN'). Am J Transplant 2007; 7: 518–526.

[13] Nankivell BJ, Chapman JR. Chronic allograft nephropathy: Current concepts and future directions. Transplantation 2006; 81: 643–654.

[14] Tublin ME, Dodd GD III: Sonography of renal transplantation. Radiol Clin North Am 1995;33:447-459.

[15] Pozniak MA, Dodd GD, Kelcz F. Ultrasonographic evaluation of renal transplantation. Radiol Clin North Am 1992;30:1053-1066.

[16] Irving HC, Kashi SH: Complications of renal transplantation and the role of interventional radiology. J Clin Ultrasound 1992;20:545-552.

[17] Bennett LN, Voegeli DR, Crummy AB, *et al.* Urologic complications following renal transplantation: Role of interventional radiologic procedures. Radiology 1986;160:531-536.

[18] Borrego J, Burgos FJ, Galmes I, *et al.* Surgical complications in 479 renal transplantations. Actas Urol Esp 1994;18:253-257.

[19] Yap R, Madrazo B, Oh HK, *et al.* Perirenal fluid collection after renal transplant. Am Surg 1981;47:287-290.

[20] Silver TM, Campbell D, Wicks JD, *et al.* Peritransplant fluid collections. Ultrasound evaluation and clinical significance. Radiology 1981;138:145- 151.

[21] Dimitroulis D, Bokos J, Zavos G. Vascular Complications in Renal Transplantation: A Single-Center Experience in 1367 Renal Transplantations and Review of the Literature. Transplant Proc 2009;41:1609–1614.

[22] Sebastià C, Quiroga S, Boyé R, *et al.* Helical CT in renal transplantation: normal findings and early and late complications. Radiographics 2001;21:1103.

[23] Zuckerman DA, Yeager TD. Percutaneous ethanol sclerotherapy of postoperative lymphoceles. AJR Am J Roentgenol 1997;169:433-437.

[24] Kerlan RK Jr, LaBerge JM, Gordon RL, *et al.* Bleomycin sclerosis of pelvic lymphoceles. J Vasc Interv Radiol 1997;8:885-887.

[25] Caliendo MV, Lee DE, Queiroz R, *et al.* Sclerotherapy with use of doxycycline after percutaneous drainage of postoperative lymphoceles. J Vasc Interv Radiol 2001;12:73-77.

[26] Dodd GD, Tublin AS, Sajko AB. Imaging of vascular complications associated with renal transplants. Am J Roentgenol 1991;157:449-459.

[27] Brown ED, Chen MY, Wolfman NT. Complications of renal transplantation: Evaluation with US and radionuclide imaging. Radiographics 2000;20:607-622.

[28] Hohnke C, Abendroth D, Schleibner S, *et al.* Vascular complications in 1200 kidney transplantations. Transplant Proc 1987;19:3691-3692.

[29] Luke RG, Curtus J. Biology and treatment of transplant hypertension, in Laragh JH, Brenner BM (eds): Hypertension: Pathophysiology, Diagnosis, and Management (ed 2). New York, NY, Raven, 1995, pp 2471- 2483.

[30] Akbar SA, Jafri SZ, Amendola MA, *et al.* Complications of renal transplantation. RadioGraphics 2005;25:1335-1356.

[31] Jordan ML, Cook GT, Ten Cardell CJ. Years of experience with vascular complications in renal transplantation. J Urol 1982;128:689-692.

[32] De Morais RH, Muglia VF, Mamere AE. Duplex Doppler sonography in transplant renal artery stenosis. J Clin Ultrasound 2003:135–141.

[33] Fervenza FC, Lafayette RA, Alfrey EJ, Petersen J. Renal artery stenosis in kidney transplants. Am J Kidney Dis 1998;31:142–148.

[34] Clerbaux G, Goffette P, Pirson Y, Goffin E. Two kidney tra1nsplant women with therapy-resistant hypertension: diagnostic error of a renal artery stenosis. Nephrol Dial Transplant 2003;18:1401–1404.

[35] Gao J, Li J, Meng-Su X, *et al.* Color duplex sonography in severe transplant renal artery stenosis: a comparison of end-to-end and end-to-side arterial anastomoses. Clinical Imaging 2009,33:116–122.

[36] Snider JF, Hunter DW, Moradian GP, *et al.* Transplant renal artery stenosis: Evaluation with duplex sonography. Radiology 1989;172:1027- 1030.

[37] Law Y, Tay K, Gan Y, *et al.* Gadolinium-enhanced magnetic resonance angiography in renal artery stenosis: comparison with digital subtraction angiography. Hong Kong Med J 2008; 14: 136-141.

[38] Public health advisory on gadolinium containing contrast agents for magnetic resonance imaging (MRI). FDA website: http://www.fda.gov/Drugs/DrugSafety/PublicHealthAdvisories/ucm053112.htm. Accessed Feb 2010.

[39] Sandhu C, Patel U. Renal transplantation dysfunction: the role of interventional radiology. Clin Radiol 2002; 57:772-783.

[40] Sierre SD, Raynaud AC, Carreres T, *et al.* Treatment of recurrent transplant renal artery stenosis with metallic stents. J Vasc Interv Radiol 1998;9:639-644.

[41] Vollmer WM, Wahl PW, Blagg CR. Survival with dialysis and transplantation in patients with end-stage renal disease. N Engl J Med 1983;308: 1553-1558.

[42] Reuther G, Wanjura D, Bauer H. Acute renal vein thrombosis in renal allografts: Detection with duplex Doppler US. Radiology 1989;170:557-558.

[43] Surlan M, Popovic P: The role of interventional radiology in management of patients with end-stage renal disease. Eur J Radiol 2003;46:96-114.

[44] Kahan BD: Surgical complications, in Kahan BD, Ponticelli C (eds): Principles and Practice of Renal Transplantation. London, England, Martin Dunitz, 2000, pp 219-250.

[45] Grenier N, Claudon M, Trillaud H, *et al.* Noninvasive radiology of vascular complications in renal transplantation. Eur Radiol 1997;7:385-391.

[46] Martinez T, Palomares M, Bravo JA, *et al.* Biopsy-induced arteriovenous fistula and venous aneurysm in a renal transplant. Nephrol Dial Transplant 1998;13:2937-2939.

[47] Barley FL, Kessel D, Nicholson T, *et al.* Selective embolization of large symptomatic iatrogenic renal transplant arteriovenous fistula. Cardiovasc Interv Radiol 2006;29:1084-1087.

[48] Donckier V, De Pauw L, Ferreira J, *et al.* False aneurysm after transplant nephrectomy: Report of two cases. Transplantation 1995;60:303-304.

[49] Koo CK, Rodger S, Baxter GM: Extrarenal pseudoaneurysm: An uncommon complication following renal transplantation. Clin Radiol 1999;54: 755-758.

[50] Reus M, Morales D, Vazquez V, *et al.* Ultrasound-guided percutaneous thrombin injection for treatment of extrarenal pseudoaneurysm after renal transplantation. Transplantation 2002;74:882-884.

[51] Yagci A, Parildar M, Oran I, Memis A. Interventional radiological management of vascular complications following renal transplantation. Diagn Interv Radiol 2006;12:206-210.

[52] Maleux G, Messiaen T, Stockx L, *et al.* Transcatheter embolization of biopsy-related vascular injuries in renal allografts. Long-term technical, clinical and biochemical results. Acta Radiol 2003;44:13-17.

[53] Perini S, Gordon RL, LaBerge JM, *et al.* Transcatheter embolization of biopsy-related vascular injury in the transplant kidney: immediate and long-term outcome. J Vasc Interv Radiol 1998;9:1011-1019.

[54] Gaber LW,Moore LW, Alloway RR, *et al.* Correlation between Banff classification, acute renal rejection scores and reversal of rejection. Kidney Int 1996; 49: 481–487.

[55] Colvin RB, Cohen AH, Saiontz C, *et al.* Evaluation of pathologic criteria for acute renal allograft rejection: Reproducibility, sensitivity, and clinical correlation. J Am Soc Nephrol 1997; 8: 1930–1941.

[56] Haas M, Kraus ES, Samaniego-Picota M, Racusen LC, Ni W, Eustace JA. Acute renal allograft rejection with intimal arteritis: Histologic predictors of response to therapy and graft survival. Kidney Int 2002; 61: 1516–1526.

[57] Mengel M, Gwinner W, Schwarz A, *et al.* Infiltrates in protocol biopsies from renal allografts. Am J Transplant 2007; 7: 356.

[58] Reeve J, Einecke G, Mengel M, Sis B, Kayser N, Kaplan B, Halloran PF. Diagnosing Rejection in Renal Transplants: A Comparison of Molecular- and Histopathology-Based Approaches. Am J Transplant 2009; 9: 1802–1810.

[59] Piazza A, Poggi E, Borrelli L, *et al.* Impact of donor-specific antibodies on chronic rejection occurrence and graft loss in renal transplantation: posttransplant analysis using flow cytometric techniques. Transplantation 2001;71: 1106-1112.

[60] Terasaki PI. Humoral theory of transplantation. Am J Transplant 2003; 3: 665-673.

[61] Worthington JE, Martin S, Al-Husseini DM, Dyer PA, Johnson RW. Posttransplantation production of donor HLA-specific antibodies as a predictor of renal transplant outcome. Transplantation 2003; 75: 1034-1040.

[62] Terasaki PI, Ozawa M. Predictive value of HLA antibodies and serum creatinine in chronic rejection: results of a 2-year prospective trial. Transplantation 2005; 80: 1194-1197.

[63] Piazza A, Poggi E, Ozzella G, *et al.* Post-transplant donor-specific antibody production and graft outcome in kidney transplantation: results of sixteen-year monitoring by flow cytometry. Clin Transpl 2006: 323-326.

[64] Racusen LC, Colvin RB, Solez K, *et al.* Antibody-mediated rejection criteria – an addition to the Banff 97 classification of renal allograft rejection. Am J Transplant 2003; 3: 708.

[65] Preda A, Van Dijk L, Van Oostaijen J, *et al.* Complication rate and diagnostic yield of 515 consecutive ultrasound guided biopsies of renal allografts and native kidneys using a 14 gauge Biopsy gun. Eur Radiol 2003;13:527-530.

[66] Riehl J, Maigatter S, Kierdorf H, *et al*: Percutaneous renal biopsy: Comparison of manual and automated puncture techniques with native and transplanted kidneys. Nephrol Dial Transplant 1994;9:1568-1574.

CHAPTER 13

Immunosuppression in Kidney Transplantation

Giuseppe Grandaliano*, Vincenzo Losappio and Annamaria Maiorano

Nephrology, Dialysis and Transplantation Unit, Department of Emergency and Organ Transplantation, University of Bari, Italy

Abstract: One-year graft survival of renal grafts increased progressively in the last two decades and can be now considered excellent, but long-term outcomes has not improved proportionally in the last years. Indeed, chronic allograft dysfunction is a growing problem among renal transplant recipients and together with death from cardiovascular disease, infection and malignancy is the leading cause of graft failure.

The goal of immunosuppressive therapy is to balance the beneficial effects of reducing acute rejection while minimizing adverse effects from over-immunosuppression such as infections, malignancy, and cardiovascular disease. Current immunosuppressive protocols use combinations of immunosuppressive drugs with different mechanisms of action to maximize efficacy and minimize the toxicity of each drug. During the past decade, there has been a increasing interest in identifying regimens that may allow the minimization of immunosuppressive drugs characterized by significant side effects, including nephrotoxicity and metabolic dysregulation. The emergence of new immunosuppressive agents and tolerance protocols appears promising as a means to deliver immunosuppression without long-term toxicity. Ultimately, the goal of "future" immunosuppression is to move from an empiric therapy to a personalized treatment.

Keywords: Kidney Transplantation, Calcineurin Inhibitors, Mtor Inhibitors, Mycophenolate, Biological Agents.

INTRODUCTION

The current era of kidney transplantation was pioneered in Boston by Murray in 1954 with the first kidney transplantation between identical twins. Since then our knowledge about transplantation immunology developed and a growing number of powerful immunosuppressive drugs has been introduced in the clinical practice. Over time, the strength and specificity of immunosuppressive drugs increased and allowed us to control alloimmune response and reduce the number of graft loss due to immunological events. Thus, to date, kidney transplantation is considered worldwide the treatment of choice for the patients with end-stage renal disease, by offering an increased survival and a better quality of life compared to hemodialysis and peritoneal dialysis. However, although one-year graft survival increased progressively in the last two decades and can be now considered excellent, long-term outcomes has not improved proportionally in the last years. Indeed, chronic allograft dysfunction is a growing problem among renal transplant recipients and together with death from cardiovascular disease, infection and malignancy is the leading cause of graft failure.

The goal of immunosuppressive therapy is to balance the beneficial effects of reducing acute rejection while minimizing adverse effects from over-immunosuppression such as infections, malignancy, and cardiovascular disease. Current immunosuppressive protocols use combinations of immunosuppressive drugs with different mechanisms of action to maximize efficacy and minimize the toxicity of each drug. During the past decade, there has been a increasing interest in identifying regimens that may allow the minimization of immunosuppressive drugs characterized by significant side effects, including nephrotoxicity and metabolic dysregulation. The emergence of new immunosuppressive agents and tolerance protocols appears promising as a means to deliver immunosuppression without long-term toxicity. Ultimately, the goal of "future" immunosuppression is to move from an empiric therapy to a personalized treatment.

***Address correspondence to Giuseppe Grandaliano:** Nephrology, Dialysis and Transplantation Unit, Department of Emergency and Organ Transplantation, University of Bari, Italy; Tel: +39 0805478868; E-mail: g.grandaliano@nephro.uniba.it

Massimiliano Veroux and Pierfrancesco Veroux (Eds)

The immunosuppressive agent 5-mercaptopurine/azathioprine in combination with corticosteroids represented the first "immunological" breakthrough in the 1960. In the late 1970s the introduction of the calcineurin inhibitor cyclosporine represented a real milestone in the history of clinical organ transplantation. Since then, every step beyond, in solid organ transplantation, has been directly linked to the discovery of a new and more potent immunosuppressive agent. During the 1990s, the continue evolution of pharmacological searches led to a wide range of new immunosuppressants that expanded our possibilities to prevent and treat allograft rejection. The result gained with these new drugs was an excellent short-term outcome and an acceptable long-term one.

If surgical transplant procedures are standardized, the variety of immunosuppressive agents are not and offer many different combinations, generally resulting in mostly centre-specific protocols. The most commonly accepted immunosuppressive protocols adopted are based on an higher immunosuppressive load in the early transplant phase (induction phase), frequently including an induction-antibody therapy combined with a cornerstone immunosuppressant (usually a calcineurin inhibitor), corticosteroids and an anti-proliferative agent (*e.g.,* mycophenolate or azathioprine). The following maintenance phase contains the cornerstone immunosuppressant [calcineurin ihibitor or, eventually, a mammalian-target-of-rapamycin (mTOR) inhibitor] with lower blood levels combined with corticosteroids and/or one anti-proliferative agent. The features of the immunosuppressive regimen are based on the transplanted organ, the time-span after transplantation and by patient's risk profile. Obviously, immunosuppressive agents have side effects including bacterial infections, virus-triggered infections, nephrotoxicity with chronic renal failure, *de novo* diabetes mellitus (NODM), hyperlipidaemia, hypertension, cardiovascular disease, osteoporosis, neurotoxicity, haematological toxicity like anaemia, leucopenia and/or thrombocytopenia, malignancies.

The combination of synergistic immunosuppressive drugs may maximize efficacy and reduce, as far as it is possible, toxicity. This knowledge led to the concept of "tailored immunosuppressive" protocols, seized to determine the most effective protocol with no/little acute rejection, few toxicities/side effects and few long-term drug-related morbidity and mortality based on the main clinical features of the recipients and on the quality of the graft. This approach relies on the knowledge of the potential beneficial effects of any specific immunosuppressive agent along with its safety profile

CALCINEURIN INHIBITORS

Cyclosporine is a small cyclic polypeptide of 11 amino acids of fungal origin, neutral and insoluble in water but soluble in organic solvents and lipids while tacrolimus is a macrolid isolated by *Streptomyces tsukubaensis.* Calcineurin inhibitors create a complex with their cytoplasmic receptors, Cyclophilin for cyclosporine and FK-Binding Protein 12 (FKBP-12) for tacrolimus. Each complex binds to and inhibits calcineurin, which is a phosphatase that dephosphorylates nuclear regulatory proteins and eases their passage through the nuclear membrane. Calcineurin inhibition also reduces the expression of critical cytokine genes that promote T-cell activation, including IL-2, IL-4, IFN-gamma and TNF-alfa. Finally, calcineurin inhibitors enhance the expression of TGF-beta that inhibits IL-2 and the generation of cytotoxic T lymphocytes and has been suggested to play a key role in the development and progression of interstitial fibrosis.

The introduction in 1983 of cyclosporine in clinical practice represented a milestone in the history of immunosuppressive therapy in transplantation. Indeed, cyclosporine dramatically improved graft survival when compared with previous immunosoppressive drugs and resulted in a significantly lower acute rejection rate [1].

The administration of cyclosporine is characterized by two different moments: the absorption and the elimination phases. The absorption phase presents the peak level (Cmax), generally during the first 2 to 3 hours after administration, that represents the time of maximal calcineurin inhibition [2, 3]. During the elimination phase, drugs levels fall to the lowest, or trough, level (C0) just before the next dose. The cytochrome P450 3A enzyme system in the liver, the intestinal cytochrome P450 3A4 and the P-glycoprotein counter-transport in the intestinal mucosa are involved in the metabolism of calcineurin inhibitors and it's important to underline that both tacrolimus and cyclosporine present a great inter and intra patient variability in their blood levels for the events occurring in the absorption phase rather than in the elimination one [4].

The first formulation of cyclosporine was a corn oil-based preparation that presented a great inter and intra-patient variability because its absorption required the solubilization of the drug in the bile. Moreover, the presence or absence of food, gastrointestinal transit time, time of the day and even race and renal function had a great influence on its absorption and bioavailability [5, 6]. The following preparation of cyclosporine was a microemulsion, specifically developed to reduce this variability. Several randomized studies confirmed that this formulation was as safe as the previous one in stable and *de novo* kidney transplant recipients [7, 8].

The next generation of calcineurin inhibitors is represented by Tacrolimus, that was first used in transplantation in 1989 and it has been used world-wide since the mid-1990s in kidney transplantation for graft rejection prophylaxis and 'rescue' therapy (treatment of refractory or chronic graft rejection or for those not tolerating cyclosporine).

Tacrolimus presents a rapid absorption and a peak level in the first 3 hours after administration [9]. Its metabolism absorption depends on the gastrointestinal transit time and for this reason is affected by presence of food, in particular by its lipid content. Moreover, tacrolimus blood levels may be influenced by serum albumin, hematocrit and the presence of liver diseases [10]. Recently, a once-daily formulation was introduced with an equivalent pharmacokinetic profile [11, 12].

The most important challenge for physicians has always been the modulation of calcineurin inhibitors dosage to guarantee an optimal immunosuppression, protecting the graft from acute rejection episodes, while avoiding the calcineurin inhibitors-related adverse events. The inter and intra-patients variability in drug adsorption and disposition of this class of drug and the limited therapeutic windows of calcineurin inhibitors clearly requires a therapeutic drug monitoring.

Before the introduction of drug monitoring, cyclosporine administration was associated with a low rejection rate but with a high incidence of adverse events, including nephrotoxicity and subsequent renal failure [13]. These observations induced clinicians to start a therapeutic monitoring of the drug based on its through levels on whole blood. When the microemulsion formulation was introduced, many clinical trials aimed to evaluate its pharmacokinetics. These studies demonstrated that cyclosporine exposure during a time lapse of 12 hours might be accurately predicted by monitoring the drug levels two hours after administration, at its Cmax [14, 15]. According to these observations, the CONCERT group published a consensus statement on cyclosporine microemulsion monitoring in transplant recipients assuming that C2 monitoring was the best method to estimate Neoral bioavailibity and that the blood drawn had to be executed within 15 minutes before or after the 2 hours endpoint. For patients defined low absorbers, with a low Cmax, or slow absorbers, with a delayed Cmax, the CONCERT group suggested a limited sampling strategy to calculate directly the area under the curve of drug blood levels [3].

According to the time after transplantation, without induction therapy or concomitant mTOR inhibition therapy, CsA C2 levels are suggested to be higher than 1700 ng/ml by day 5, between 1600 and 2000 ng/ml up to month 1, between 1400 and 1600 ng/ml until month 2 and 1200-1400 until month 3. From month 3 to the end of the first year after transplantation there should be a progressive reduction of C2 levels from 800-1000 ng/ml to 600-800 ng/ml. After the first year C2 is approximately should be kept 800 ng/ml [16]. However, kidney transplant recipients receiving induction therapy with anti-CD25 antibodies or ATG or concomitant mTOR inhibitors should aim at significantly lower targets. This reduction is particularly relevant when cyclosporine is associated with mTOR inhibitors, since this association may amplify the nephrotoxic effects of CNIs [16].

Monitoring blood levels is a standard also for tacrolimus-based immunosuppressive therapies. Tacrolimus through levels or C0 is actually considered the best approach to evaluate tacrolimus exposure. Target tacrolimus through levels in kidney transplantation have been defined by several trials and need to be adjusted in the presence of induction therapy with anti-CD25 antibodies or ATG or concomitant mTOR inhibition, as previously observed for cyclosporine. The target ranges suggested for patients receiving tacrolimus in the absence of induction therapy are between 10 and 15 ng/ml up to month 3, from 5 to 15 ng/ml until the first year after transplantation and from 5 to 10 ng/ml for the following period [16].

According to these trough levels, the recommended initial oral dose of cyclosporine in kidney transplantation is reported to be of 5-7 mg/Kg, twice daily, widely different for the different immunosoppressive protocols [17] and the recommended starting oral dose of tacrolimus for adult kidney transplant recipients is 0.2 mg/Kg/d administered twice in the day [18]. Several data based on clinical practice, suggest a lower initial oral dose of 0.15-0.10 mg/Kg/d followed by a maintenance dose of 0.07-0.1 mg/Kg/d.

Several trials compared cyclosporine and tacrolimus. According to the existing literature neither tacrolimus or cyclosporine showed a significant benefit in terms of patient or graft survival, although a 2005 meta-analysis [19] suggested fewer acute rejection episodes and graft losses in tacrolimus-treated patients and a 2005 retrospective study showed a more rapid decline in GFR in the kidney transplant recipients treated with cyclosporine [20]. In the US phase 3 study, transplant recipients were randomly assigned to treatment with tacrolimus or cyclosporine, with crossovers allowed only for treatment failure. A first interpretation of the data, 5 years after transplantation, revealed the same outcomes in the two groups in terms of patients and graft survival. A further analysis, based on the last treatment given to the patients, showed a better graft survival in the tacrolimus group at 3 and 5 years after transplantation [21].

A retrospective study based on data of the Scientific Registry of Transplant Recipients (SRTR), [22] evaluated donor variables using a paired-kidney analysis of deceased-donor kidneys. Results showed similar 5 years graft and patient survival rates for the two calcineurin inhibitors. However, many recent head-to-head clinical trials underlined a better preservation of renal function in tacrolimus compared to cyclosporine-treated patients [23-25]. Even Kaplan with his paired kidney study, showed that tacrolimus-treated patients had a better renal function during the 5 years follow-up compared to patients receiving cyclosporine [22].

According to these perceptions, tacrolimus based protocols are spread worldwide: in the USA, in last decade there was an inversion in tacrolimus usage, passing from about 20% in latest 1990s to more than 70% to date [26].

Calcineurin inhibitors represented a significant step forward in the history of immunosuppression and still represent the main actor in most of the immunosuppressive regimen nowadays. However, this class of drug present a significant number of side effects, including the development of hypertension, nephrotoxicity, hyperlipidemia, new-onset diabetes mellitus (NODM) and cosmetic changes, that may significantly influence not only the quality of life of transplant recipients but also graft and patient survival.

NODM

NODM develops in response to a relative insulin deficiency resulting from increased insulin resistance or impaired insulin production, or a combination of both according to Van Hooff's definition [28]. This condition is one of the most common adverse event related to kidney transplantation and has a great importance for physicians because recipients developing NODM are exposed to higher risk of cardiovascular diseases, particularly ischemic heart disease [29], infections/sepsis and malignancies. In the long term different studies showed a worst profile, for these patients, in terms of graft and patient survival [30-32].

Different studies underlined the presence of non modifiable risk factors such as older age, race, genetic background, family history of diabetes, pre-transplant impaired glucose tolerance, metabolic syndrome and male gender along with modifiable risk factors including obesity, weight gain, HCV infection, CMV infection and immunosuppressive drugs. Among the different immunosoppressive agents, calcineurin inhibitors are frequently related to the development of NODM. Particularly, cyclosporine has been proved to be toxic for pancreatic Beta-cells [33, 34] and able to inhibit insulin release [35, 36] creating a mechanism of insulin resistance. Other studies, focusing on tacrolimus effects on Beta-cells, showed a reduced insulin secretion, which is significantly more intense than the one observed with cyclosporine. This evidence was confirmed by a study based on the evaluation of insulin secretion in kidney transplant recipients treated with calcineurin inhibitors. Vincenti *et al.* showed that insulin secretion is reduced for both cyclosporine and tacrolimus-treated patients, but this condition was more evident in the tacrolimus-treated population, while insulin sensitivity was equally reduced in both patients groups [37]. Moreover, there are new evidences that both cyclosporine and tacrolimus may negatively influence insulin gene expression [33, 34, 38, 39].

Other studies investigated the effects of cyclosporine and tacrolimus on peripheral insulin sensitivity [36, 40, 41]. A substudy of a published randomized trial developed by Asberg *et al.* [42] showed an higher sensitivity in patients never treated with calcineurin inhibitors, suggesting another mechanism for the development of NODM. On the basis of previous publications suggesting, in the early post-transplant period, a possible "irritative effect" of calcineurin inhibitors on the endothelium, Asberg hypothesized that the observed impaired insulin sensitivity might be due to a reduced glucose delivery to skeletal muscles [43].

Although cyclosporine and tacrolimus seem quite similar in developing NODM. Vincenti *et al.* tried to verify which one of the two calcineurin inhibitors present the better safety profile with a 6 month, open label, randomized multicentre study [37]. Their results showed that NODM or impaired fasting glucose occurred more frequently in the tacrolimus-treated population. These results led to the conclusion that, in the first 6 months after kidney transplantation, there seem to be a better performance of cyclosporine compared to tacrolimus. Recent observations on the long term showed that CsA reduces the prevalence of NODM at 1 and 3 years after transplantation when compared to tacrolimus even in the presence of higher corticosteroids doses. Moreover, NODM rate was higher for the tacrolimus-treated patients even with the lowest doses of the drug [44].

Nephrotoxicity

Nephrotoxicity is one of the most important calcineurin inhibitors-related side effects. The clinical pattern of nephrotoxicity is characterized by mild/severe graft dysfunction in the early post-transplant, acute microvascular disease, hypertension and electrolyte abnormalities, including hyperkalemia, sodium retention, hyperchloremia and hyperuricemia. This chain of events is all related to the renal vasocostrinction induced by calcineurin inhibitors, particularly on the afferent arteriole, and to tubular damage induced by this class of drugs, particularly on proximal tubular cells [45]. The loss in GFR rate may be related also to an increased release of endothelin and to the subsequent increased mesangial cell contractility. This early functional events may, in the long term, cause significant structural changes within the vascular, glomerular and tubulointerstitial compartments including arteriolar hyalinosis, glomerular sclerosis and striped interstitial fibrosis, respectively. The chronic, structural nephrotoxicity of calcineurin inhibitors represent the main pathogenic factor in the progressive renal failure observed in an increasing number of extra-renal solid organ transplant recipients [46].

In order to reduce the impact of calcineurin inhibitors side nephrotoxicity, different studies focused on the opportunity to reduce or withdraw cyclosporine or tacrolimus administration in kidney transplant recipients. A reduced dose of calcineurin inhibitors may improve graft function in the long term, but clearly exposes kidney recipients to an higher risk of acute rejection. Additionally, the decreased levels of immunosoppression may manifest many months later as overt rejection or, even worse, as subclinical rejection not readily apparent during a serum creatinine based follow-up [47]. However, the concomitant use of other immunosuppressive drugs may allow to safely reduce the long-term exposure to the nephrotoxic effects of calcineurin inhibitors [48]. Indeed, Nankivell *et al.* [27] showed that calcineurin inhibitors-induced morfological alterations are less common in patients treated with cyclosporine associated to mycophenolate mofetil.

Hypertension

Calcineurin inhibitors-treated patients show higher blood pressure levels and fluid retention. Several studies demonstrated that cyclosporine induces a reduction in atrial natriuretic factor availability for the activation of the renin-angiotensin-aldosteron pathway and of the symphatetic nervous system [49]. This mechanism could cause an overload of fluids and a consequent systemic hypertension. Tacrolimus has been shown to present a less potent peripheral vasoconstrictive action and a subsequent lower incidence of hypertension [50].

Hepatic Toxicity

Hyperbilirubinemia, elevation of serum aminotransferase levels and general hepatic dysfunction are more frequently related to tacrolimus. However, there is no evidence of hepatic hystological lesions and hyperbirilubinemia seems to be related to an alterate bile secretion in absence of a documented and direct hepatocellular damage. Cyclosporine-treated patients, instead, show a higher incidence of cholelitiasis due to the well-known lythogenic activity of this calcineurin inhibitor [45]. Other side effects like anorexia, diarrhea, vomiting and nausea are more common in the tacrolimus-treated population.

Neurotoxicity

The wide range of neurological side effects of calcineurin inhibitors is more evident in the tacrolimus-treated patients, presenting tremors, headache, dysestesia and insomnia. These effects are almost invariably dose-related. An appropriate monitoring of trough whole blood levels and the reduction of drug doses usually lead to a complete recovery [51, 52].

Cosmetic Side Effects

Hypertrichosis is one of the most common side effects of the cyclosporine-based immunosoppressive regimen while alopecia is more frequently observed in the tacrolimus-treated patients. Gingival hyperplasia is often observed in the cyclosporine-treated population and is more frequent and severe if associated to poor dental hygiene. This particular side effect benefit from short term antibiotics therapy [53].

MYCOPHENOLIC ACID (MPA)

MPA is currently available in two different formulation: mycophenolate mofetil (MMF) and Enteric-Coated Mycophenolate Sodium (EC-MPS). MMF, the first formulation introduced in the market of immunosuppression in kidney transplantation, is the most prescribed immunosoppressant in the U.S. for new kidney transplant recipients. Currently, the use of tacrolimus/MMF associated immunosoppression is considered the gold standard in most of the U.S.-based transplant programs [54].

T-cells are well-known to play a key role in the immune response and most current immunosuppressive drugs target T-cell activation. Alloantigens activate T-cells by T-cell receptor- (TCR) mediated interaction. In this way the calcium-calcineurin pathway is activated, leading to the expression of survival and pro-inflammatory cytokines and their receptors. The engagement of the IL-2 receptor delivers growth and proliferation signals priming the cell cycle. MMF inhibits T- and B-cell proliferation in a calcineurin-indipendent pathway [55]. MPA, originally obtained from a *Penicillium* fungus and shown to have pleiotropic effects (anti-neoplastic, anti-viral, anti-fungal and immunosuppressive) selectively and reversibly blocks a critical step in the *de novo* synthesis of purine. This drug inhibits inosine monophosphate dehydrogenase (IMPDH), an enzyme that allows the conversion of IMP to xanthosine monophosphate, the precursor of guanosine nucleotides required for DNA synthesis [56]. MPA does not affect the *salvage pathway* of purine nucleotide synthesis which is not present in lymphocytes. Thus, lymphocytes depend primarily on the *de novo* purine synthesis pathway and may be more specifically targeted by MPA. In addition, different isoforms of IMP dehydrogenase exist. The type II isoform is upregulated in activated lymphocytes and MPA shows a higher binding affinity for this isoform. In this light, MPA-based therapy should be considered a sort of selective immunosuppression despite of Azathioprine (AZA), a non selective antimetabolitic immunosuppressive drug [56]. *In vitro* and *in vivo* studies have shown that MPA is able to prevent antibody production by B cells inhibiting the generation of cytotoxic T cells but has no direct effect on the production of cytokines [57]. MPA also downregulates the synthesis of leukocyte surface adhesion molecules (selectins and integrins) which is closely dependant on guanosine nucleotides. MPA treatment may thus also interfere with the recruitment of lymphocytes to sites of inflammation and their interaction with the endothelium of a vascularized allograft [58].

The immunosoppressive regimen for kidney transplantation is based on a recommended oral dosage of MMF of 1 g b.i.d. associated either with cyclosporine or tacrolimus. This dosage was suggested after an empiric phase 1 trial performed in 2 transplant centers in the United States which showed that 2000 mg/d treated patients had fewer episodes of acute rejection and adverse events than the one treated with lower doses of the drug [59]. Moreover, 2000 mg/d-treated patients presented less adverse events than the patients receiving 3000 mg/d [59, 60]. Subsequent studies, based on register analysis and single transplant center experiences, demonstrated a significant better outcomes for MMF-based regimens in terms of graft and patients survival compared to previous immunosuppressive protocols [61].

MMF should be assumed on an empty stomach in consideration of the food-related decrease in drug bioavailability, which may be responsible of a decrease up to 40% of the drug blood levels [60]. Bioavailability of MMF increase over time and is deeply influenced by the other immunosoppressive agents: MPA exposure is greater in patients assuming tacrolimus and sirolimus then in those treated with cyclosporine. MMF/tacrolimus-treated patients presented an increase in MPA serum through levels when compared to patients assuming MMF/cyclosporine [62]. MPA through levels has been also compared in cyclosporine and sirolimus-associated therapy in a prospective study conducted upon 61 kidney transplant recipients. Patients were randomly assigned either to MMF and cyclosporine (n=30; 6 to 8 mg/kg/d in divided dose) or MMF and sirolimus (n=31; 5 mg/d after a 15 mg loading dose) treatment, all 61 with a base regimen of corticosteroid and a 2 g/day of MMF. The sirolimus group had greater MPA serum levels compared with the cyclosporine group (4.16 *vs.* 1.93 ng/mL; P=0.001) [63] even if the maintenance dose of MMF tends to be lower than 2 g/d in sirolimus-treated patients. These differences are due to the differential impact of tacrolimus, sirolimus and cyclosporine on the enterohepatic recirculation of MPA [64, 65].

Several studies were also focused on the second formulation of MPA, the EC-MPS, showing that 720 mg of this formulation administered twice daily are therapeutically equivalent to the 1000 mg twice daily dose of MMF with a similar safety profile [66, 67]. Multicenter trials comparing EC-MPS with MMF show no differences in outcomes like rejection, graft and patient survival or significant adverse events between the 2 formulations [66].

mTOR INHIBITORS

The *mammalian target of rapamycin* (mTOR), also known as *FK506-binding protein 12-rapamycin associated protein 1* (FRAP1), is a serine-threonine kinase of the phosphatidylinositol-3-kinase pathway that regulates cell growth, cell proliferation, motility, survival, protein synthesis and transcription [68, 69]. Current research indicates that mTOR represents a crossroad for multiple metabolic pathways, including insulin, growth factors (such as IGF-1 and IGF-2) and mitogens [68]. mTOR also functions as a sensor of cellular nutrient, energy levels and redox status [69]. The disregulation of the mTOR pathway is implicated as a contributing factor to various human diseases, especially various types of cancer [70]. The term *mTOR inhibitors* refers to two similar immunosuppressive drugs, sirolimus and everolimus, with the same mechanism of action but different pharmacokinetic profiles.

Sirolimus is a lipophilic microcyclic lactone isolated from a strain of fungus called *Streptomyces hygroscopicus* first isolated in a soil sample from Easter Island (Rapa Nui). Sirolimus was found to have potent immunosuppressive activity with a mechanism of action distinct from calcineurin inhibitors. Interestingly, sirolimus structurally resembles tacrolimus and binds the same binding protein, FKBP-12. In this way, it forms an immunophilin complex targeting mTOR. This serine-threonine kinase is usually associated with two different proteins rictor and raptor constituting two complexes, mTORC1 and mTORC2, respectively, with different cell functions. Sirolimus prefentially binds and inhibits the activity of mTOR within TORC1. More recently, a 40-O-(2-hydroxyethyl)-derivative of sirolimus, everolimus, was developed. Like sirolimus, everolimus forms a complex with FKBP-12 and blocks mTOR activity. The affinity of everolimus for FKBP-12 is lower and its half-life is shorter then sirolimus.

The sirolimus/everolimus-FKBP-12 complex inhibits mTOR-mediated signal transduction pathways, blocking post-receptor immune responses to co-stimulatory signal 2 during G0 to G1 transition and to cytokine signal 3 during G1 progression. It also inhibits the IL-2- and IL-4-dependent proliferation of T- and B-cells leading to suppression of new ribosomal protein synthesis and arrest of the G1-S phase of the cell cycle [71-74]. Proliferation of non-immune cells, such as fibroblasts, endothelial cells, hepatocytes and smooth muscles is also impaired by inhibition of the growth-factor mediated responses [75]. Additionally, it has been shown that mTOR takes part in several protein synthesis pathways that could be involved in oncogenesis [75, 76].

Sirolimus

Originally investigated as anti-fungal and anti-neoplastic agent, sirolimus showed immediately immunosuppressive properties. The first *in vivo* studies documenting the immunosuppressive power of sirolimus in heterotopic cardiac allograft in rats were published in 1989 [77, 78]. Sirolimus demonstrated to be 20 to 100 times more potent than cyclosporine and acted in a dose-dependent manner to prevent acute allograft rejection [79, 80]. Moreover, several *in vivo* studies suggested the synergy between sirolimus and cyclosporine observed *in vitro* [81-83]. On the other hand, the similarity in structure and the potential competitivity for the same binding protein suggested a non synergistic effect between tacrolimus and sirolimus, although *in vivo* investigation contradicted this postulation, showing a potential synergism and the absence of any competition for FKBP12 [84].

In the first human studies sirolimus was investigated in association with cyclosporine and showed a reduction of acute rejection incidence [85, 86]. Based on this evidence, sirolimus was approved by the FDA for human use in the prevention of acute rejection in renal transplantation in 1999. However, different clinical trial suggested that concomitant sirolimus treatment significantly increased the incidence of cyclosporine-related side effects, in particular nephrotoxicity, and because of these observations its approval in Europe was delayed to 2000. The success of initial studies on combining full-dose of cyclosporine and sirolimus encouraged the introduction of regimens that maintained the synergy between these drugs yet minimized nephrotoxicity and side effects. Several post-approval studies investigated the safety of minimization or withdrawal of calcineurin inhibitors in sirolimus-based immunosuppressive regimens. The SMR study [87] clearly demonstrated that early (three months) planned withdraw of cyclosporine in low- to moderate-risk patients can be safely accomplished with reasonable tolerability and a low incidence of acute rejection episodes in the majority of patients. Early conversion is associated with better one year graft function, which may prove to be important for the long-term preservation of kidney function [88]. Indeed, 3 and 5 years results confirmed that cyclosporine withdrawal was associated with an improved graft survival and with a significant reduction in chronic graft changes [89, 90].

Indeed, recently, several data suggest that sirolimus may beneficially modulate the balance between pro- and anti-fibrotic molecules and it has been suggested the possibility that sirolimus could improve interstitial fibrosis in chronic allograft nephropathy and ameliorating graft survival [91, 92]. These observation led to hypothesize the possibility of a late conversion from calcineurin inhibitors to sirolimus as prevention or treatment of chronic allograft nephropathy. Stallone *et al.* demonstrated that two years after conversion graft histology and survival was significantly better in patients converted compared to patients continuing on calcineurin inhibitor-based therapy [92]. This observation was confirmed by an international multicenter trial (CONVERT) which demonstrated a significant advantage in term of graft survival and function in patients converted to sirolimus between 6 months and 10 years after transplantation [93].

Several groups also suggested the use of sirolimus as primary immunosuppressive drugs in *de novo* transplant recipients. Flechner *et al.* [94] clearly demonstrated that this approach may significantly improve long term outcomes. However, the beneficial effects of this sirolimus use has been not confirmed by multicenter randomized trials.

Interestingly, mTOR dependent signaling within endothelial cells is induced by vascular endothelial growth factor (VEGF) and play a key role in the angiogenic effects of this growth factor. Indeed, mTOR inhibitors have been shown *in vitro* and *in vivo* to be potent blockers of angiogenesis. This peculiar characteristic of sirolimus may explain its potential role both in vascular modification occurring in chronic allograft nephropathy and malignancy growth. On the basis of these observation Guba *et al.* [77] demonstrated that sirolimus exerts a powerful anti-neoplastic effect in an experimental model of colon cancer. Stallone *et al.* showed that this effect may be of clinical relevance, since conversion to sirolimus was able to induce a complete remission of cutaneous Kaposi sarcoma in a series of 15 cases [95]. Campistol *et al.* suggested that the anti-neoplastic effect of sirolimus was evident also on other post-transplant neoplastic diseases [96]. This observation, was further confirmed by retrospective analysis of registry-based data [97] and in prospective randomized clinical trials [93].

The original formulation of sirolimus was an oral solution with a concentration of 1 mg/ml to be dispensed in water or orange-juice. This formulation has been largely replaced by the more practical 1 or 2 mg capsules. Sirolimus is rapidly adsorbed from the gastro-intestinal tract, reaches a peak concentration in 1-2 hours and has an half-life of 62 hours. The steady-state through concentration can be achieved in 24 hours from the first administration with a substantial stability of blood levels. The target through level could change by center or clinical use. Usually, it ranges between 5-15 ng/ml. Because of its long half-life, levels should be checked several days after a dose adjustment. It has been demonstrated a pharmacokinetic interaction between sirolimus and cyclosporine. In fact, concomitant administration of both could increase the AUC for sirolimus by 230%. Administration 4 hours after cyclosporine increase the sirolimus AUC only of the 80%, significantly reducing the potential toxicity. Thus, in cyclosporine/sirolimus association protocols, it is recommended to delay the sirolimus administration of 4 hours after the morning dose of CsA.

The introduction of mTOR inhibitors in the immunosuppressive regimen of kidney transplant recipients has been shown to improve significantly graft function and survival along with the possible influence of this class of drug on the development of post-transplant malignancies. However, the use sirolimus is still complicated by several side effects.

Impaired Wound Healing

The presence of factors such as diabetes, malnourishment, obesity or corticosteroids treatment are well known to negatively affect wound-healing [98]. The use of sirolimus in the presence of one or several of these factors may exacerbate the wound-healing process, and its use should be carefully considered. However, sirolimus itself is associated with impaired wound healing in a dose-dependent manner [99]. This effect is due to the ability of sirolimus to reduce VEGF expression, nitric oxide (NO) release [100], smooth muscle cells and fibroblast proliferation [101] and matrix deposition [102]. Many clinicians avoid using sirolimus during the first week post-transplantation in an effort to avoid impaired wound-healing.

Lymphoceles

The use of SRL is associated with an increase in lymphocele development [103]. Sirolimus could inhibits the post-surgical adhesion and has been recently demonstrated to significantly reduce lymphangiogenesis [104].

Hyperlipidemia

mTOR is involved in several metabolic pathways and its inhibition could cause metabolic disorders. Indeed, hyperlipidemia, with an increase of both cholesterol and tryglicerides, represent the most common side effects of sirolimus. Hypercholesterolemia is likely due to increases in LDL, VLDL and non-HDL cholesterol. The effects of mTOR inhibitors on dyslipidemias have been suggested to be different when they are combined with cyclosporine compared with tacrolimus but no data are available to define the exact interaction. The pathogenesis of mTOR inhibitor dyslipidemia is unclear. Increased plasma levels of apolipoprotein B100 (apo B100; a major component of VLDL and LDL, and a ligand for the LDL receptor) have been demonstrated in sirolimus-treated kidney transplant recipients, resulting in elevated VLDL (triglycerides) and LDL (cholesterol) levels [105]. These alterations could be ascribed to a decreased catabolism rather than increased synthesis of apoB100. However, there is a paucity of studies investigating the pathophysiology of mTOR inhibitor dyslipidemia. To date, there are no clinical data to determine the effects of mTOR inhibitor dyslipidemia on cardiovascular disease in kidney transplant recipients. There are some experimental data that suggest that atheromatous changes in the vascular wall may be directly inhibited by mTOR inhibitors *via* interference with pro-inflammatory cytokines and cell proliferation mechanisms. In an atherosclerosis-prone mouse model (apo E knockout), animals treated with sirolimus were protected from atherosclerotic changes of the aorta, despite the increased cholesterol (due to increased LDL) levels [106]. This paradox could be explained by the blockade of the local inflammatory cytokines [106, 107], pro-atherogenic factors (monocyte chemotactic protein-1) [29] and modulation of T-cell response [108] exerted by sirolimus. Varghese *et al.* have shown that sirolimus reduced lipid accumulation in human glomerular mesangial cells suppressing the expression of LDL and VLDL receptors and CD36 (a receptor for oxidized LDL), inhibiting pro-inflammatory cytokine expression, and increasing the efflux of cholesterol [107]. The same group also showed that sirolimus reduced intra-cellular lipid accumulation caused by inflammatory mediators in vascular smooth muscle cells, possibly due to reduced LDL and VLDL receptors [109]. However, whether these findings in cell models will translate into reduced cardiovascular events in humans can only be determined in adequately powered, randomized, controlled trials. Clearly, an adequately designed, large RCT is needed to determine the effect of mTOR inhibitors on CVD in kidney transplant recipients. In most of the patients hyperlipidemia could be manageable with statins following the KDOQI and NCEP guidelines.

Diabetes

Recently, several reports suggested that sirolimus treatment may worsen insulin resistance and is associated with an increased incidence of NODM after transplantation. However, this effect was significant only when sirolimus was associate with calcineurin inhibitors and in particular with tacrolimus. The mechanism underlying the interference of sirolimus on insulin sensitivity is still largely unclear, although Teutonico *et al.* [110] suggested a role for hypertrigliceridemia.

Pneumonia

Sirolimus-associated pneumonitis has been described after renal, liver, heart, and heart–lung transplantation [111, 112]. It is defined as a non-infectious interstitial pneumonia, typically presenting as a bilateral lower-lobe interstitial pneumonia with a possible fatal evolution. Pathologic features are similar to bronchiolitis obliterans organizing pneumonia, with alveolar hemorrhage and lymphocytic infiltration. Sirolimus-associated pneumonitis remains ill-defined because of the absence of specific diagnostic criteria. Sirolimus-induced lung toxicity is dose-dependent [112, 113] and there are some reports of recovery with 2-3 weeks of sirolimus discontinuation and/or dose reduction. The exact mechanism underlying this severe complication is still unknown and it seems to be more dramatic in patients converted from calcineurin inhibitors to sirolimus with a poor graft function (GFR<40ml/min).

Proteinuria

The development of overt proteinuria was reported in several studies evaluating the effect of conversion from calcineurin inhibitors to sirolimus in patients with chronic allograft dysfunction [114]. This nephrotoxic effects of sirolimus has been suggested to be due to a direct effect of the drug on podocytes integrity and functions. Indeed, several authors demonstrated a direct effect of sirolimus on the expression of slit-diaphragm-associated proteins. Letavernier *et al.* [115] also suggested that this effect may lead to a FSGS-like picture and that are most likely dose-related, since the morphological changes were observed only in patients exposed to high sirolimus blood levels. The Campistol group [116] clearly demonstrated that this adverse effect of sirolimus may be predicted, in patients converted from calcineurin inhibitors-based therapy, by renal function and baseline urine protein excretion levels. According to their observation to avoid a significant post-conversion proteinuria this therapeutic maneuver should be avoided in patients with a GFR<40 ml/min and a baseline daily proteinuria >800mg.

Everolimus

The use of Everolimus is indicated in combination with cyclosporine for the prevention of organ rejection in renal and hearth transplant patients. Preclinical studies demonstrated a powerful synergistic interaction between everolimus and cyclosporine, suggesting that everolimus may allow for a significant calcineurin inhibitors dose reduction [117]. Indeed, a 3-year Phase II trial [118] has confirmed that everolimus in combination with reduced-exposure to calcineurin inhibitors results in improved renal function. Therapeutic drug monitoring of everolimus was found to improve outcomes in renal transplant patients by providing an optimal dosing strategy. A target range for everolimus through blood levels of 3–8 ng/ml has been identified as being efficacious while minimizing the risk of adverse events. Two large-scale studies demonstrated the efficacy of concentration-controlled everolimus with reduced-exposure cyclosporine in *de novo* renal transplant patients [119, 120]. This approach was shown to result in good long term renal function. The ability to minimize doses of cyclosporine may be of particular value for patients at increased risk of renal dysfunction from full-dose cyclosporine (*e.g.*, recipients of marginal kidneys, such as those from elderly donors). Indeed, the inclusion of everolimus in the immunosuppressant regimen of *de novo* "old-for-old" renal transplant recipients allows cyclosporine dose reduction and discontinuation, thus minimizing the risk of nephrotoxicity in the older renal graft. In addition, reduced-exposure cyclosporine may be beneficial for young recipients for whom prolonged graft function and survival are particularly important. Everolimus in combination with reduced-exposure cyclosporine is generally well tolerated, although the mTOR inhibitor has the same risk profile described for sirolimus. Everolimus has the potential to reduce chronic allograft vasculopathy and improve long-term survival [121].

BIOLOGIC AGENTS

Administration of antibody preparations for therapeutic purposes originated in the early 1960s. When administered in the peri-operative period, these agents are thought to decrease the incidence of early acute rejection offering added benefits in terms of avoiding nephrotoxicity and other nonspecific immunologic effects [122]. After declining in the 1990s, popularity of antibody induction therapy has increased in recent years. There was a gradual increase in use of antibody induction therapy from 1994 (25%) to 2003 (70%) in patients who underwent kidney transplantation [123].

In 1995, muromonab-CD3 was the primary antibody agent for 25% of kidney transplant recipients; however, by 2002, only 1% of kidney transplant recipients were administered this drug. The most commonly used agents in 2002 were rabbit anti-thymocyte globulins and the anti-CD25 antibodies basiliximab and daclizumab; none of these drugs was available a decade earlier [124].

Beginning with publication of the registration trials of basiliximab and daclizumab, strong data now support both the immunologic and non-immunologic benefits of antibody induction [125, 126]. Analysis of more than 60, 000 patients who received kidney transplants between 1996 and 2000 (using data from United Network for Organ Sharing/SRTR) showed that antibody induction increased graft survival in unsensitized transplant recipients [127].

Antithymocyte Globulins (ATG)

ATG is a polyclonal antibody with a wide range of depleting peripheral effects against blood mononuclear cell epitopes, primarily targeting T cell, which has been introduced in kidney transplantation as an induction therapy to prevent early acute graft rejection, delay the introduction of potentially nephrotoxic drugs (calcineurin inhibitors) and minimize maintenance calcineurin inhibitors dosage [128]. ATG induction therapy is often used in graft recipients at high immunological risk and there are many reports of its efficacy from several multicenter studies [128, 129].

Mourad *et al.* [128] in a 12-month open-label multicenter study on kidney transplant recipients confronted patients with tacrolimus-based immunosuppression therapy with and without rabbit ATG induction. They noticed that patient and graft survival were similar between the two groups but patients on rabbit ATG induction therapy, even experiencing significantly fewer biopsy-confirmed acute rejection episodes, had an increased occurrence of adverse events, specifically cytomegalovirus (CMV) infection.

A randomized trial compared three different induction protocols based on the administration of ATG *vs.* Alemtuzumab *vs.* Daclizumab [130] in kidney transplant recipient evaluating as endpoint acute rejection, delayed graft function, incidence of chronic allograft nephropathy, patient and graft survival. Acute rejection rate was similar among the three groups, Alemtuzumab had a worst profile in terms of chronic allograft nephropathy and the best result in terms of renal function after two years were obtained in the ATG and daclizumab-treated groups.

Anti-CD25 Antibodies (IL2Ra)

IL2Ra are humanised or chimeric (murine/human) IgG monoclonal antibodies directed to the alpha subunit of the IL2 receptor expressed only on activated T lymphocytes. There are two different IL2Ra: Basiliximab that is a chimeric immunoglobulin G monoclonal antibody and Daclizumab, that is a humanized immunoglobulin G1 monoclonal antibody that binds to the CD25 molecule. The IL2-receptor complex induces second messenger signals that stimulates the T cell to start the cell cycle and proliferate, resulting in clonal expansion and activation. IL2Ra inhibits this IL2-mediated activation. IL2Ra has been considered, for this reason, a useful induction agents in combination with standard immunosuppression to prevent acute rejection or reduce exposure the to the calcineurin inhibitors, particularly in recipients considered at high risk of delayed graft function, trying to ameliorate their short and long-term nephrotoxic side effects [131]. However there is no direct proof that a decrease in early rejection rates translates into a uniform increase in long-term graft survival [132]. Several studies compared the efficacy of the induction with IL2Ra with the administration of placebo or the absence of an induction therapy. The Cochrane review shows many interesting results [133]. The comparison between patients treated with IL2Ra, placebo or no treatment shows no differences between the different IL2Ra used and the differing combinations of additional immunosuppressive drugs. Graft loss favored the use of IL2Ra, although the differences did not achieve the statistical significance either at one year or three years after transplantation. The incidence of clinically diagnosed acute rejection within six months of transplantation was reduced by 34% for those treated with an IL2Ra. This advantage was similar for biopsy proven rejection, showing a 36% reduction. Treatment with an IL2Ra showed a substantial effect in preventing steroid-resistant rejection, reducing its incidence at six months by 49%. CMV infection was reduced in IL2Ra treated patients, but the difference was not statistically significant at one year.

The comparison between IL2Ra and other mono and polyclonal antibodies in preventing acute rejection shows no statistically significant differences in treatment effects, considering graft loss, mortality, CMV infection or the incidence of malignancies. IL2Ra presented, although without a statistically significance, fewer adverse events including fever, leucopaenia and thrombocytopaenia.

The use of an IL2Ra in addition to standard dual or triple therapy significantly reduced acute rejection within the first year post-transplantation with no evidence that the effects of basiliximab and daclizumab are different. Attending to Cochrane review there is no significant effect on graft survival adding IL2Ra to the standard therapy and there is no demonstrable difference in acute rejection rates or graft loss among IL2Ra and other mono or polyclonal antibody preparations used in this context. ILRa has, indeed, a more safely adverse risk profile than other antibody preparations and presents a potential reduction of the CMV infection risk profile but with no statistical significance. On the long term, few data were available to determine the effect on developing malignancies or chronic allograft nephropathy [133].

Actually the use of antibody induction regard 63% of kidney transplant and in almost 50% of graft recipients receiving an induction therapy are treated with IL2Ra [134]. Administering IL2Ra to standard-low risk recipients made possible, with a low risk of rejection, an early tapering of the steroid with calcineurin inhibitors-based immunosoppressive regimens. Calcineurin inhibitors withdrawal, instead, even presenting a better graft function is more frequently associated with acute rejection episodes [134].

Alemtuzumab (Campath-1H)

Alemtuzumab is a humanized monoclonal antibody directed against the CD52 antigen, which is expressed on all blood mononuclear cells and also on cells lining the male reproductive tract. It is a powerful depleting agent and has been used, in the past, in bone marrow transplantation and several autoimmune disease [135]. This monoclonal antibody is approved by FDA for chronic B-cell lymphocytic leukemia and is a cheaper alternative to other induction agents [136].

Alemtuzumab produces a deep and long lasting lymphopenia, especially of T lymphocytes and its use in kidney transplant shows a low rate of rejection if compared with other monoclonal antibodies [137, 138]. Alemtuzumab can be used in steroid free protocols [137] and it is also able to reverse steroid resistant acute rejection, although with a significant high risk of infection [139, 140]. Graft survival is better for Campath-treated patients compared to other monoclonal antibodies inductions [137] at 3 years after transplantation. A steroid free protocol based on Alemtuzumab induction and tacrolimus-based maintenance therapy in living donors compared to a typical steroid-MMF-tacrolimus-based immunosuppression showed a better graft survival.

Alemtuzumab may also allow the use of protocols that avoid the use of steroids or try to reduce the use of calcineurin inhibitors for their nephrotoxicity. At Cambridge [135], alemtuzumab administered with low-dose cyclosporine, promoted a graft and patient survival similar to the one related to much more intense maintenance therapy while avoiding corticosteroid therapy.

Induction with Alemtuzumab could allow therapies based on low doses tacrolimus and MMF [141] or even tacrolimus solo therapies in living recipients with patients and graft survival at 1 year after transplantation of 99% and 98% respectively. A more recent prospective randomized trial reached the same conclusion, suggesting that alemtuzumab induction with a tacrolimus monotherapy is at least as efficient in renal transplantation as a tacrolimus-based triple drug regimen with a similar safety profile but more CMV infections [142].

Rituximab

Rituximab is an engineered chimeric monoclonal antibody presenting a murine heavy and light chains, directed against CD20 plus a human IgG1 constant region. It is well known that CD20 mediates B cells proliferation and differentiation, thus B cells treated with Rituximab have a reduced replication rate. The elimination of B cells is based on three possible mechanism: antibody dependent cell mediated cytotoxicity, complement dependent citotoxicity and apoptosis. Rituximab depletes pre-B and mature B cells, preserving plasma cells, and suppresses antibody production: B cells depletion generally persist for 6-9 months in over 80% of patients even if the depletion rate is highly variable. According to these characteristic, Rituximab has been used in kidney transplantation in refractory humoral rejections and for the treatment of post transplantation lymphoproliferative disorders.

In kidney transplant recipients, a biopsy proven presence of CD20+ B cells infiltration, is associated with poorer outcome and less steroid responsiveness. These cases have been shown to respond to a Rituximab-based therapy. Its efficacy is also reported for rejection episodes related to a predominant role of alloantibodies resistant to conventional treatment with pulse steroids, plasmapheresis, intravenous immunoglobulins and anti-lymphocyte globulins [143, 144].

Several experiences with rituximab induction showed a reduction in the preformed alloantibodies titers in highly sensitized kidney transplant recipients and in ABO-incompatible recipients. These patients, treated even with a single dose of Rituximab, often along with splenectomy and plasmapheresis, presented a better outcome in terms of acute rejection, suggesting that the use of anti-CD20 monoclonal antibodies could be a promising choice in desensitization or induction strategies for transplant recipients [145-148].

Vo *et al.* in 2008, suggested for highly sensitized patients waiting for a kidney transplant, a desensitization regimen based on the combination of intravenous immune globulin and Rituximab in order to reduce their time on the waiting list. Their results showed, at 1 year, a reduced waiting time after the desensitization treatment, good patient and graft survival and no adverse events due to drugs infusion. However, acute rejection episodes occurred in 50% of the patients and a long term monitoring was necessary to evaluate the incidence of infections and long term side effects [149].

Several adverse side effects are related to Rituximab infusion, even if the large part of these studies are based on the administration of anti-CD20 monoclonal antibodies for the treatment of hematological disorders. The side effects could be distinguished by time of manifestation in infusion-related side effects, such as hypotension, broncospasm, dyspnea, fever, rigors, angioedema and rush. Short term side effects, within 6 months from the infusion, include viral infections, like herpes zoster or influenza, upper respiratory tract infections, abdominal pain, purpura, mialgia, neutropenia and thrombocytopenia. On the long term, up to 6 months, there are evidences of an increased incidence of neoplastic diseases.

In order to reduce the incidence of these side effects, recent trials are based on the administration of reduced Rituximab doses. Tyden in 2009 proposed the administration of a single dose of Rituximab as induction in kidney transplantation, showing a good safety profile of this drug with no increase in the incidence of infections or leucopenia. There is agreement in literature that more randomized controlled studies are necessary for a better evaluation on the long term effects of Rituximab in kidney transplantation [150].

Belatacept

This drug derived from Abatacept (CTLA4-Ig), a dimeric fusion protein that was developed in order to block the interaction between CD28 and CD80- CD86, by adding an IgG1 domain that solubilizes the CTLA4 domain. Belatacept belongs to a new family of drugs, inhibiting co-stimulation signals.

T cell is activated when recognizes two signals. The first one is represented by the allopeptide linked to the MHC of the antigen presenting cell and recognized by the T-cell receptor (TCR). The second signal or co-stimulation signal is provided by the binding of co-stimulatory molecules present on the surface of T cells and antigen-presenting cells. The best characterized co-stimulatory signal is represented by the binding of CD28 present on T cells and CD80 and CD86 on antigen-presenting cells. Only when these two signals are presented, T-cells are activated and proliferate [151].

After T-cell activation a second receptor, CTLA4, is upregulated. This receptor is structurally homologous to CD28, with an higher avidity for CD80 and CD86, but with a negative effect of T cells in order to switch off T cells activation. Thus, CD28 and CTLA4 present similar structures but opposite functions, because CD28 activates T cells while CTLA4 inhibits them [151].

In 1998 Biancone *et al.* demonstrated that in acute rejections there was a focal and intense infiltration of CD80+, CD86+ and CTLA4+ T lymphocytes while in chronic rejection there were only few CD80+, CD86+ and CTLA4+ T lymphocyte. In patients with cyclosporine nephrotoxicity there were no evidence of CD80+, CD86+, CTLA4+ cells.

According to these results, the previously described involvement of the costimulatory pathways in experimental animal transplant models, was confirmed in human suggesting a role for Belatacept as immunosoppressive agent in kidney transplantation [152].

A clinical trial developed by Vincenti *et al.* [153] in order to evaluate the efficacy of Belatacept compared to calcineurin inhibitors in kidney transplant recipients, demonstrated the great potentiality of this drug. The acute rejection rate profile of Belatacept was similar to the one obtained with a cyclosporine-based immunosuppressive therapy, but the graft function was better in the population treated with Belatacept and the risk profile was significantly better than in the cyclosporine group. Moreover, the incidence of infections was similar between the two groups and the higher incidence of malignancies observed after the infusion of Belatacept was related to its higher dosage in one arm of the study.

In order to evaluate its pharmacodynamic effects, a 2009 study observed that Belatacept-mediated inhibition of alloresponses involved in transplant rejection correlates with CD86 saturation, indicating that CD86 receptor occupancy may be an affordable pharmacodynamic measure of costimulation blockade and provides the first clinical evidence that Belatacept binds to one of its target. However, more studies are undergoing to evaluate its safety, especially on the long term, and its efficacy in kidney transplantation [154].

TOLERANCE AND TOLEROGENIC IMMUNOSUPPRESSIVE PROTOCOLS

Tolerance is defined as the absence of immune response to different antigens or, in transplantation, as the maintenance of a stable allograft function without clinically evident immunosuppression. This fascinating process could be explained by several immunologic mechanisms that may act simultaneously. It is now recognized that immunological tolerance involves both *central* and *peripheral* mechanisms. *Central tolerance* results from intrathymic deletion of T cells with high avidity for thymically expressed self antigens. *Peripheral tolerance* to non-self molecules can be achieved by various mechanisms including deletion of activated/effector T cells, anergy induction and active regulation of effector T cells.

Central Tolerance

Over recent years experimental models have shown that it is possible to exploit the mechanisms that normally maintain immune homeostasis and tolerance to self-antigens to induce tolerance to alloantigens [155, 156]. *Central tolerance* could be exploited in transplantation by the delivery of donor antigens to the thymus of adult recipients leading to the central elimination of detrimental alloreactive T-cell clones, resulting in specific tolerance to donor organs. This could either be performed experimentally by direct intrathymic injections of donor-derived allopeptides or by the induction in the recipient of haematopoietic mixed chimerism leading to the co-existence of cells from both recipient and donor origin. First evidence of the importance of donor chimerism on immune tolerance came from studies in newborn mice in which the infusion of donor's allogenic cells determined in an immature immune system a full tolerance of skin engraftment. In these mice the engraftment of donor cells and the migration of donor antigen presenting cells to the recipient thymus induced negative selection of donor-reactive T cells, prior to release into the circulation. Encouraged by these evidences, further studies were conducted about the availability of tolerance induction in humans. An increasing body of evidence suggest that bone marrow transplant before kidney transplantation may induce, in kidney transplant recipients, a significant donor chimerism with long-term acceptance of their renal allograft in the absence of ongoing immunosuppression. However, more studies are needed to confirm the efficacy and the safety of this approach.

Peripheral Tolerance

In the transplant setting, circulating alloreactive T cells are crucial in the initiation and the coordination of the rejection response and, to promote tolerance, it is basic to deplete or minimize the alloreactive effector T-cell pool while enhancing the regulatory mechanisms. Various strategies have been explored to achieve *peripheral tolerance.*

The advent of monoclonal antibodies has allowed the development of various cell-depleting protocols. Cell-depleting approaches result in a profound reduction of circulating leucocytes capable of mounting an alloresponse. However, effector memory T cells seem to be relatively resistant to depletion and, in addition, remaining T cells after depletion undergo homeostatic repopulation and will gradually repopulate the host weeks to months later when the innate immune response has resumed and the allograft is more quiescent. In this light, at the present, the tolerance induction strategies should be read as a mean to minimizing the weight of maintenance immunosuppression, a condition described as "*prope*" or "*almost*" tolerance.

Depletion strategies have been extensively studied in non-human primates transplantation models. In these studies, encouraging results were obtained using rabbit ATG or anti-CD3-immunotoxin (monoclonal anti-Rhesus CD3 antibody with a modified diphtheria toxin) alone or in combination with sirolimus. Indeed in these models, despite profound peritransplant T-cell depletion, consistent transplantation tolerance was not achieved with monotherapy since most of the treated animals eventually lost their grafts through chronic rejection. In humans, other T-cell depleting antibodies have been used, such as alemtuzumab. This immunosuppressive drug is demonstrated facilitating the peripheral deletion of effector T cells by promoting activation-induced cell death, while inducing Tregs in the periphery. In addition, it has been shown that the addition of sirolimus as the maintenance therapy may further promote the development of peripheral Tregs. More studies are warranted to confirm these initial promises

It is clear that the future of immunosuppression is mainly represented by the search for less toxic protocols allowing adequate graft survival while avoiding the long-term side effects of current immunosuppression. In this scenario the research for tolerogenic protocols represent one of the main target for transplant physician in the next decade.

REFERENCES

[1] Danovitch GM. Choice of immunosuppressive drugs and individualization of immunosuppressive therapy for kidney transplant patients. Transplant Proc 1999; 31:S2-6.

[2] Halloran FP, Helms LM, Kung L, *et al.* The temporal profile of calcineurin inhibition by cyclosporine *in vivo*. Transplantation 1999; 68: 1356-1361.

[3] Levy G, Thervet E, Lake J, *et al.* Patient management by Neoral C2 monitoring: an international consensus statement. Transplantation 2002; 73: S12-S18.

[4] Dunn CJ, Wagstaff AJ, Perry CM, *et al.* Cyclosporin: an update review of the pharmacokinetic properties, clinical efficacy and tolerability of a microemulsion-based formulation (Neoral) in organ transplantation. Drugs 2001; 61: 1957-2016.

[5] Kahan BD, Welsh M., Schoenberg L, *et al.* Variable oral absorption of cyclosporine. A biopharmaceutical risk factor for chronic renal allograft rejection. Transplantation 1996; 62: 599-606.

[6] Ptachcinski RJ, Venkataramanan R, Rosenthal JT, *et al.* The effect of food on cyclosporine absorption. Transplantation 1985; 40: 174-176.

[7] Keown P, Niese D. Cyclosporine microemulsion increases drug exposure and reduce acute rejection without incremental toxicity in *de novo* renal transplantation. International Sandimmune Neoral Study Group. Kidney Int 1998; 54: 938-44.

[8] Barone G, Bunke GM, Choc MG, *et al.* The safety and tolerability of cyclosporine emulsion versus cyclosporine in a randomized, double-blind comparison in primary allograft recipients. The Neoral Study Group. Transplantation 1996; 61:968-970.

[9] Scott LJ, McKeage K, Keam SJ, *et al.* Tacrolimus: a further update of its use in the management of organ transplantation. Drugs 2003; 63: 1247-1297.

[10] Hu RH, Lee PH, Tsai MK, *et al.* Clinical influencing factors for daily dose, trough level, and relative clearance of tacrolimus in renal transplant recipients. Transplant Proc 2000; 32: 1689-1692.

[11] Wlodarczyk Z, Squifflet JT, Ostrowski M, *et al.* Pharmacokinetics for once versus twice daily tacrolimus formulations in *de novo* kidney transplantation: a randomized open-label trial. Am J Transplant 2009; 9: 2505-2513.

[12] Alloway R, Steinberg S, Khalil K, *et al.* Two years post conversion from a Prograf-based regimen to a once daily Tacrolimus extended-release formulation in stable kidney transplant recipients. Transplantation 2007; 83: 1648-1651.

[13] Calne RY, Rolles K, White DJ, *et al.* Cyclosporin A initially as the only immunosuppressant in 34 recipients of cadaveric organs: 32 kidneys, 2 pancreases and 2 livers. Lancet 1979; 2: 1033-1036.

[14] Cantarovich M, Barkum JS, Tchervenkov JI, *et al.* Comparison of Neoral dose monitoring with cyclosporine throught levels versus 2-hr postdose levels in stable liver transplant patients. Transplantation 1998; 66: 1621-1627.

[15] Caforio AL, Tona F, Piaserio S, *et al.* C2 is superior to C0 as predictor of renla toxicity and rejection risk profile in stable heart transplant recipients. Transplant Int 2005; 18: 116-124.

[16] Schiff J, Cole E, Cantarovich M. Therapeutic monitoring of calcineurin inhibitors for the nephrologist. Clin J Am Soc Nephrol 2007; 2: 374-384.

[17] Novartis Pharmaceuticals Corp: Neoral package insert. East Hanover, NJ, Novartis Pharmaceutical Corp, 2004.

[18] Astellas Pharma US Inc: Prograf Pacjage Insert. Deerfield, IL, Astellas Pharma US Inc, 2005.

[19] Webster AC, Woodroffe RC, Taylor RS, *et al.* Tacrolimus versus cyclosporine as primary immunosuppression for kidney transplant recipients. Cochrane Database Syst Rev; 2005; 4 CD003961.

[20] Morales JM, Andrés A, Dominguez-Gil B, *et al.* Ten years of treatment with tacrolimus is related to an excellent renal function, allowing monotherapy in a large proportion of cases: unicentric results of the tacrolimus versus cyclosporine A European Multicentric Study in kidney transplant patients. Transplant Proc 2005 37:3738-3742.

[21] Vincenti F, Jensik SC, Filo RS, *et al.* A long term comparison of tacrolimus (FK506) and cyclosporine in kidney transplantation: evidence for improve allograft survival at 5 years. Transplantation 2002; 73: 775-782.

[22] Kaplan B, Schold JD, Meier-Kriesche HU. Long-term graft survival with Neoral and Tacrolimus: a paired kidney analysis. J Am Soc Nephrol 2003; 14: 2980-2984.

[23] Johnson C, Ahsan N, Gonwa T, *et al.* Randomized trial of tacrolimus (Prograf) in combination with azathioprine or mycophenolate mofetil versus cyclosporine (Neoral) with mycophenolate mofetil after cadaveric kidney transplantation. Transplantation 2000; 69: 834-841.

[24] Gonwa T, Johnson C, Ahsan N, *et al.* Randomized trial of tacrolimus+mycophenolate mofetil or azathioprine versus cyclosporine+mycophenolate mofetil after cadaveric kidney transplantation: results at three years. Transplantation 2003; 75: 2048-2053.

[25] Ciancio G, Burke GW, Gaynor JJ, *et al.* A randomized long-term trial of tacrolimus/sirolimus versus tacrolimus/mycophenolate mofetil versus cyclosporine (NEORAL)/sirolimus in renal transplantation. II. Survival, function, and protocol compliance at 1 year. Transplantation 2004; 77: 252-258.

[26] OPTN/SRTR 2008 Annual Report.

[27] Nankivell BJ, Wavamunno MD, Borrows RJ, *et al.* Mycophenolate mofetil is associated with altered expression of chronic renal transplant histology. Am J Transplant 2007; 7: 366-376.

[28] Van Hooff JP, Christiaans MHL, Van Duijnhoven EM. Evaluating mechanism of post-transplant diabetes mellitus. Nephrol Dial Transplant 2004; S6: vi8-vi12.

[29] Lindholm A, Albrechtsen D, Frodin L, *et al.* Ischemic heart disease-Mayor cause of death and graft loss after renal transplantation in Scandinavia. Transplantation 1995; 60: 451-457.

[30] Boudreaux JP, McHugh L, Canafax DM, *et al.* The impact of cyclosporine and combination immunosuppression on the incidence of posttransplant diabetes in renal allograft recipients. Transplantation 1987; 44: 376-381.

[31] Cosio FG, Pesavento TE, Kim S, *et al.* Patient survival after renal transplantation: IV. Impact of post-transplant diabetes. Kidney Int 2002; 1440-1446.

[32] Meier-Kriesche HU, Kaplan B. Cyclosporine microemulsion and tacrolimus are associated with decreased chronic allograft failure and improved long-term graft survival as compared with Sandimmune. Am J Transplant 2002; 2: 100-104.

[33] Weir MR, Fink JC. Risk for posttransplant diabetes mellitus with current immunosuppressive medications. Am J Kidney Dis 1999; 34: 1-13.

[34] Markell MS. Post transplant diabetes: incidence, relationship to choice of immunosuppressive drugs and treatment protocol. Adv Ren Replace Ther 2001; 8:64-69.

[35] Gillison SL, Bartlett ST, Curry DL. Inhibition by cyclosporine of insulin secretion-A beta cell-specific alteration of islet tissue function. Transplantation 1991; 52: 890-895.

[36] Menegazzo LA, Ursich MJ, Fukui RT, *et al.* Mechanism of the diabetogenic action of cyclosporin A. Horm Metab Res 1998; 30:663.

[37] Vincenti F, Friman S, Scheuermann E, *et al.* Result of an international, randomized trial comparing glucose metabolism disorders and outcome with cyclosporine versus tacrolimus. Am J Transplant 2007; 7: 1506-1514.

[38] Tamura K, Fujimura T, Tsutsumi T, *et al.* Transcriptional inhibition of insulin by FK506 and possible involvement of FK506 binding protein-12 in pancreatic beta-cell. Transplantation 1995; 59: 1016-1013.

[39] Oetjen E, Baun D, Beimesche S, *et al.* Inhibition of human insulin gene transcription by the immunosuppressive drugs cyclosporine A and tacrolimus in primary, mature islets of transgenic mice. Mol Pharmacol 2003; 63: 1289-1295.

[40] Ikeuchi M, Kida K, Goto Y, *et al. In vivo* and *in vitro* effects of cyclosporin A on glucose transport by soleus muscle of mice. Biochem Pharmacol 1992; 43: 1459-1463.

[41] Kutkuhn B, Hollenbeck M, Heering P, *et al.* Development of insulin resistance and elevated blood pressure during therapy with cyclosporin A. Blood Press 1997; 6: 13-20.

[42] Asberg A, Karsten M, Voitovich MH, *et al.* Calcineurin inhibitor effects on glucose metabolism and endothelial function following renal transplantation. Clin Transplant 2009; 23: 511-518.

[43] Asberg A, Berg KJ, Hartmann A. Each administration of cyclosporin A enhances skin microvascular reactivity in renal transplant recipients. Microvasc Res 2000; 60: 81-90.

[44] Burroughs TE, Lentine KL, Takemoto SK, *et al.* Influence of early post transplantation Prednisone and calcineurine inhibitor dosages on the incidence of new-onset diabetes. Clin J Am Soc Nephrol 2007; 2: 517-523.

[45] Kahan BD. Forty years of publications of Transplant Proceedings - the second decade: the cyclosporine revolution. Transplant Proc 2009; 41: 1423-1437. .

[46] Bloom RD, Reese PP. Chronic kidney disease after non-renal solid organ transplantation. J Am Soc Nephrol 2007; 18:3031-3041.

[47] Nankivell BJ, Borrows RJ, Fung CL, *et al.* Evolution and pathophysiology of renal-transplant glomerulosclerosis. Transplantation 2004; 78: 461-468.

[48] Weir MR, Ward MT, Blahut SA, *et al.* Long-term impact of discontinued or reduced calcineurin inhibitor in patients with chronic allograft nephropathy. Kidney Int 2001; 59: 1567-1573.

[49] Hestin D, Mertes PM, Hubert J, *et al.* Relationship between blood pressure and rennin, angiotensin II and atrial natriuretic factor after renal transplantation. Clin Nephrol 1997; 48: 98-103.

[50] Morales JM, Dominguez-Gill B. Impact of tacrolimus and mycophenolate mofetil combination on cardiovascular risk-profile after kidney transplantation. J Am Soc Nephrol 2006; S3: S296-S303.

[51] Ponticelli C, Campise MR. Neurological complications in kidney transplant recipients J Nephrol 2005; 18: 521-528.

[52] Bechstein WO. Neurotoxicity of calcineurin inhibitors: impact and clinical management. Transpl Int 2000; 13: 313-326.

[53] Gaston RS. Current and evolving immunosuppressive regimens in kidney transplantation. Am J Kid Dis 2006; 47(S2): S3-S21.

[54] Kaufman DB, Shapiro R, Lucey MR, *et al.* Immunosuppression: practice and trends. Am J Transplant 2004; 4: S28-53.

[55] Halloran PF. Immunosuppressive drug for kidney transplantation. N Engl J Med 2004; 35: 2715-2729.

[56] Golshayan D, Pascual M, Vogt B. Mycophenolic acid formulation in adult renal transplantation-update on efficacy and tolerability. Ther Clin Risk Manag 2009; 5: 341-351.

[57] Morris R, Hoyt E, Murphy MP, *et al.* Mycophenolic acid morpholinoethil ester (RS-61443) is a new immunosuppressant that prevents and halts heart allograft rejection by selective inhibition of T- and B-cell purine synthesis. Transplant Proc 1990; 22: 1659-1662.

[58] Allison AC, Kowalski WJ, Muller CJ, *et al.* Mycophenolic acid and Brequinar, inhibitors of purine and pyrimidine synthesis, block thw glycosylation of adhesion molecules. Transplant Proc 1993, 25: 67-70.

[59] Sollinger HW, Deierhoi MH, Belzer FO, *et al.* RS-61443-A phase one clinical trial and pilot rescue study. Transplantation 1992; 53: 428-432.

[60] Roche Pharmaceuticals: Cell Cept package insert. Nutley, NJ, Roche Pharmaceuticals 2004.

[61] Meier-Kriesche HU, Ojo AO, Leichtman AB, *et al.* Interaction of Mycophenolate Mofetil and HLA matching on renal allograft survival. Transplantation 2001; 71: 398-401.

[62] Zucker K, Rosen A, Tsaroucha A, *et al.* Augmentation of Mycophenolate Mofetil pharmacokinetics in renal transplant patients receiving Tacrolimus and Cell Cept combination therapy. Transplant Proc 1997; 29: 334-336.

[63] Flechner SM, Goldfarb D, Modlin C, *et al.* Kidney transplantation without calcineurin inhibitors drugs: a prospective randomized trial of Sirolimus versus cyclosporine. Transplantation 2002: 74: 1070-1076.

[64] Van Gelder T, Hilbrands LB, Vanrenterghem Y, *et al.* A randomized double blind multicenter plasma-concentration controlled study of the safety and efficacy of oral mycophenolate mofetil for the prevention of acute rejection after kidney transplantation. Transplantation 1999; 68: 261-266.

[65] Tsaroucha AK, Zucker K, Esquenazi V, *et al.* Levels of mycophenolic acid and its glucuronide derivative in the plasma of liver, small bowel and kidney transplant patients receiving Tacrolimus and Cell Cept combination therapy. Transplant Immunol 2000; 8: 143-146.

[66] Salvadori M, Holzer H, de Mattos A, *et al.* The ERL B301 study groups. Enteric coated Mycophenolate Sodium is therapeutically equivalent to mycophenolate in *de novo* renal transplant patients. Am J Transplant 2004; 4: 231-236.

[67] Sollinger H. Enteric coated Mycophenolate Sodium: therapeutic equivalence to mycophenolate mofetil in *de novo* renal transplant patients. Transplant Proc 2004; S2: S517-S520.

[68] Hay N, Sonenberg N "Upstream and downstream of mTOR". Genes Dev 2004, 18: 1926–1945.

[69] Beevers C, Li F, Liu L, *et al.* Curcumin inhibits the mammalian target of rapamycin-mediated signaling pathways in cancer cells". Int J Cancer 2006,119: 757–764.

[70] Tokunaga C, Yoshino K, Yonezawa K .mTOR integrates amino acid- and energy-sensing pathways. Biochem Biophys Res Commun 2004, 313: 443–446.

[71] Andrassy J, Graeb C, Rentsch M, *et al.* mTOR inhibition and its effect on cancer in transplantation. Transplantation 2005; 80: S171–S174.

[72] Sehgal SN. Sirolimus: its discovery, biological properties, and mechanism of action. Transplant Proc 2003; 35: 7S–14S.

[73] Sehgal SN. Rapamune (RAPA, rapamycin, sirolimus): mechanism of action immunosuppressive effect results from blockade of signal transduction and inhibition of cell cycle progression. Clin Biochem 2006; 39: 484–489.

[74] Mehrabi A, Fonouni H, Kashfi A, *et al.* The role and value of sirolimus administration in kidney and liver transplantation. Clin Transplant 2006; 20 Suppl 17: 30–43.

[75] Guba M, von Breitenbuch P, Steinbauer M, *et al.* Rapamycin inhibits primary and metastatic tumor growth by antiangiogenesis: involvement of vascular endothelial growth factor. Nat Med 2002; 8: 128–135.

[76] Andrassy J, Graeb C, Rentsch M, *et al.* mTOR inhibition and its effect on cancer in transplantation. Transplantation 2005; 80: S171-S174.

[77] Calne R, Collier D, Lim S, *et al.* Rapamycin for immunosuppression for organ allografting. Lancet 1989; 2: 227.

[78] Morris RE, Meiser BM. Identification of a new pharmacological action for an old compound. Med Sci Res 1989; 17: 609-610.

[79] Chen H, Wu J, Xu D, *et al.* Reversal of ongoing heart, kidney and pancreas rejection and suppression of accelerated heart allograft rejection in the rat by rapamycin. Transplantation 1993; 56: 661-666.

[80] Wang M, Stepkowski SM, Ferraresso M, *et al.* Evidence that rapamycin rescue therapy delays rejection of major and minor histocompatible heart allografts in rats. Transplantation 1992; 54: 704-709.

[81] Longoria JL, Roberts RF, Marboe CC, *et al.* Sirolimus potentiates cyclosporine in prevention of acute lung rejection. J Thorac Cardiovasc Surg 1999; 117: 715-718.

[82] Qi S, Xu D, Peng J, *et al.* Synergistic effect of rapamycin and cyclosporine in prevention of acute kidney allograft rejection in the mouse. Microsurgery 1999; 19: 344-347.

[83] Stepkowski SM, Tian L, Napoli KL, *et al.* Synergistic mechanisms by which sirolimus and cyclosporine inhibit rat heart and kidney allograft rejection. Clin Exp Immunol 1997; 108: 63-68.

[84] Vu MD, Qi S, Xu D, *et al.* Tacrolimus and sirolimus in combination are not antagonistic but produce extended graft survival in cardiac transplantation in the rat. Transplantation 1997; 64: 1853-1856.

[85] Kahan BD for The Rapamune US Study Group: Efficacy of sirolimus compared with azathioprine for reduction for acute renal allograft rejection: a randomized multicenter study. Lancet 2000; 356: 194-202.

[86] MacDonald A for The Rapamune Global Study Group: a worldwide phase III randomized, controlled safety and efficacy study of a sirolimus/cyclosporine regimen. Transplantation 2001; 71: 271-280.

[87] Oberbauer R, Kreis H, Johnson, *et al.* Long-term improvement in renal function with sirolimus after early cyclosporine withdrawal in renal transplant recipients: 2-years results of the Rapamune Mainteinance Regimen Study. Transplantation 2003; 76: 364-370.

[88] Stallone G, Di Paolo S, Schena A, *et al.* Early withdrawal of cyclosporine A improves 1-year graft structure and function in sirolimus treated patients. Transplantation 2003; 75:998-1003.

[89] Kreis H, Oberbauer R, Campistol JM, *et al.* for The Rapamune Mainteinance Regimen Trial. Long-term benefits with sirolimus-based therapy after early cyclosporine withdrawal. J Am Soc Nephrol 2004; 15: 809-817.

[90] Legendre G, Brault Y, Morales JM, *et al.* for The Rapamune Mainteinance Regimen Trial. Factors influencing glomerular filtration rate in renal transplantation after cyclosporine withdrawal using sirolimus-based therapy: a multivariate analysis of results at five years. Clin Transplant 2007; 21: 330-336.

[91] Pontrelli P, Rossini M, Infante B, *et al.* Rapamycin inhibits PAI-1 expression and reduces interstitial fibrosis and glomerulosclerosis in chronic allograft nephropathy. Transplantation 2008; 85: 125-134. .

[92] Stallone G, Infante B, Schena A. Rapamycin for treatment of chronic allograft nephropathy in renal transplant patients. J Am Soc Nephrol 2005; 16: 3755-3762.

[93] Schena F.P, Pascoe MD, Alberu J, *et al.* Conversion from calcineurin inhibitors to sirolimus manteinance therapy in renal allograft recipients: 24-months efficacy and safety results from the CONVERT trial. Transplantation 2009, 87: 233-242.

[94] Flechner SM, Goldfarb D, *et al.* Kidney transplantation with sirolimus and mycophenolate mofetil-based immunosuppression: five-years results of a randomized prospective trial compared to calcineurin inhibitor drugs. Transplantation 2007 ; 83: 883-892.

[95] Stallone G, Schena A, Infante B, *et al.* Sirolimus for Kaposi's sarcoma in renal transplant recipients. N Eng J Med 2005 ; 352 : 1317-1323.

[96] Campistol J.M, Eris J, Oberbauer R, *et al.* Sirolimus therapy after early cyclosporine withdrawal reduces the risk for cancer in adult renal transplantation. J Am Soc Nephrol 2006; 17: 581-589. .

[97] Kaplan BD. Current approaches to the use of sirolimus in renal transplantation. Transplant Proc 2009; 41: 3011-3015.

[98] Franz MG, Steed DL, Robson MC. Optimizing healing of the acute wound by minimizing complication. Curr Probl Surg 2007; 44: 691-763.

[99] Knight R, Villa M, Laskey R, *et al.* Risk factors for impaired wound healing in sirolimus-treated renal transplant recipients. Clin Transplant 2007; 21: 460-465.

[100] Schaffer M, Schier R, Napirei M, *et al.* Sirolimus impaires wound healing. Langenbeks Arch Surg 2007; 392: 297-303.

[101] Morris RE, Cao W, Huang X, *et al.* Rapamycin (sirolimus) inhibits vascular smooth muscle DNA synthesis *in vitro* and suppresses narrowing in arterial allografts and balloon- injured carotid arteries: Evidence that rapamycin antagonizes growth factor action on immune and nonimmune cells. Transplant Proc 1995; 27: 430-431.

[102] Zhu J, Wu J, Frizell E, *et al.* Rapamycin inhibits hepatic stellate cell proliferation *in vitro* and limits fibrogenesis in an *in vivo* model of liver fibrosis. Gastroenterology 1999; 117: 1198-1204.

[103] Langer RM, Kahan BD. Incidence, therapy and consequences of lymphocele after sirolimu/cyclosporine/prednisone immunosuppression in renal transplant recipients. Transplantation 2002; 74: 804-808.

[104] Huber S, Bruns CJ, Schmid G, *et al.* Inhibition of the mammalian target of rapamycin impedes lymphoangiogenesis. Kidney Int 2007; 71: 771-777.

[105] Hoogeveen RC, Ballantyne CM, Pownall HJ, *et al.* Effect of sirolimus of the metabolism of APO-B100 containing lipoproteins in renal transplant patients. Transplantation 2001; 72: 1244-1250. .

[106] Elloso MM, Azrolan N, Sehgal SN, *et al.* Protective effects of the immunosoppressant sirolimus against aortic atherosclerosis in APO-E deficient mice. Am J Transplant 2003; 3: 562-569.

[107] Varghese Z, Fernando R, Moorhead JF, *et al.* Effects of sirolimus on mesangial cells cholesterol homeostasis: a novel mechanism for its action against lipid-mediated injury in renal allograft. Am J Physiol Renal Physiol 2005; 289: F43-F48.

[108] Yang K, Li D, Luo M, *et al.* Generation of HSP60-specific regulatory Tcell and effect on atheroscelorisis. Cell Immunol 2006; 243: 90-95.

[109] Ma KL, Ruan XZ, Powis SH, *et al.* Antiatherosclerotic effects of sirolimus on human vascular smooth muscle cells. Am J Physiol Heart Circ Physiol 2007; 292: H2721-2728.

[110] Teutonico A, Schena FP, Di Paolo S. Glucose metabolism in renal transplant recipients: effect of calcineurin inhibitor withdrawal and conversion to sirolimus. J Am Soc Nephrol 2005; 16: 3128-3135.

[111] Pham PT, Pham PC, Danovitch GM, *et al.* Sirolimus associated pulmonary toxicity. Transplantation 2004; 77: 1215-1220.

[112] Champion L, Stern M, Israel-Biet D, *et al.* Sirolimus-associated pnemonitis: 24 cases in renal transplant recipients. Ann Int Med, 2006; 144: 505-509.

[113] Mahalati K, Murphy DM, West ML. Bronchiolitis obliterans and organizing pneumonia in renal transplant recipients. Transplantation 2000; 69: 1531-1535.

[114] Letavernier E, Legendre C. mToR inhibitors-induced proteinuria: mechanisms, significance, and management. Transplant Rev 2008; 22: 125-130.

[115] Letavernier E, Bruneval P, Mandet C, *et al.* High sirolimus levels may induce focal segmental glomerulosclerosis *de novo*. Clin J Am Soc Nephrol 2007; 2: 326-333.

[116] Diekmann F, Budde K, Oppenheimer F, *et al.* Predictors of success in conversion from calcineurin inhibitor to sirolimus in chronic allograft dysfunction. Am J Transplant 2004; 4: 1869-1875.

[117] Schuurman HJ, Cottens S, Fuchs S, *et al.* SDZ RAD, a new rapamycin derivative: synergism with cyclosporine. Transplantation 1997; 64: 32-35.

[118] Nashan B, Curtis J, Ponticelli C, *et al.* Everolimus and reduced-exposure cyclosporine in *de novo* renal-transplant recipients: a three-year phase II, randomized, multicenter, open-label study. Transplantation 2004; 78: 1332-1340.

[119] Lorber MI, Mulgaonkar S, Butt KM, *et al.* Everolimus versus mycophenolate mofetil in the prevention of rejection in *de novo* renal transplant recipients: a 3-year randomized, multicenter, phase III study. Transplantation 2005; 80: 244-252.

[120] Vítko S, Margreiter R, Weimar W, *et al.* Three-year efficacy and safety results from a study of everolimus versus mycophenolate mofetil in *de novo* renal transplant patients. Am J Transplant 2005; 5: 2521-2530.

[121] Pascual J. Everolimus in clinical practice--renal transplantation. Nephrol Dial Transplant 2006; 21 (Suppl 3): 18-23.

[122] Szczech L.A, Berlin JA, Aradhye S, *et al.* Effect on anti-lymphocite induction therapy on renal allograft survival: a meta-analysis. J Am Soc Nephrol 1997; 1771-1777.

[123] Annual report of the U.S. Organ Procurement and Transplantation Network and the Scientific Registry of Transplant Recipients: Transplant Data 1994-2003. Department of Health and Human Services, Health Resources and Services Administration, Healthcare System Bureau, Division of Transplantation, Rockville; MD; United Network for Organ Sharing, Richmond, VA; University Renal Research and Education Association, Ann Arbor, MI. Available at: http://www.optn.org/AR2004/default.htm.

[124] Annual report of the U.S. Organ Procurement and Transplantation Network and the Scientific Registry of Transplant Recipients: Transplant Data 1993-2002. Department of Health and Human Services, Health Resources and Services Administration, Healthcare System Bureau, Division of Transplantation, Rockville, MD; United Network for Organ

Sharing, Richmond, VA; University Renal Research and Education Association, Ann Arbor, MI. Available at: http://www.optn.org/AR2003/default.htm.

[125] Nashan B, Moore R, Amlot P, *et al.* Randomized trial of Basiliximab versus placebo for control of acute cellular rejection in renal allograft recipients. Lancet 1997; 350: 1193-1198.

[126] Vincenti F, Kirkman R, Light S, *et al.* Interleukin-2-receptor blockade with Daclizumab to porevent acute rejection in renal transplantation. N Engl J Med 1998; 338: 161-165.

[127] Bunnapradist S, Daswani A, Takemoto SK. Patterns of administration of antibody induction therapy and their associated outcomes. Clin Transpl 2002; 351-358.

[128] Mourad G, Garrigue V, Squifflet JP, *et al.* Induction versus noninduction in renal transplant recipients with tacrolimus-based immunosuppression. Transplantation 2001; 72: 1050-1055.

[129] Brennan DC, Flavin K, Lowell JA, *et al.* A randomized, double-blind comparison of Thymoglobulin versus Atgam for induction immunosuppressive therapy in adult renal transplant recipients. Transplantation 1999; 67: 1011-1018.

[130] Ciancio G, Burke GW, Gaynor JJ, *et al.* A randomized trial of thymoglobulin *vs.* alemtuzumab (with lower dose maintenance immunosuppression) *vs.* daclizumab in renal transplantation at 24 months of follow-up. Clin Transplant 2008; 22: 200-210.

[131] Cibrik D.M, Kaplan B, Meier-Kriesche HU. Role of anti-interleukin-2 receptor antibodies in kidney transplantation. Bio Drugs 2001; 15: 655-666.

[132] Vanrenterghem YF, Messiaen T. Nephrotoxicity of immunosuppressive agents. Adv Nephrol Necker Hosp 2001; 31: 285 293.

[133] Webster AC, Playford EG, Higgins G, *et al.* Interleukin 2 receptor antagonists for kidney transplant recipients. Cochrane Database Syst Rev 2004; 1:CD003897.

[134] Sageshima J, Ciancio G, Chen L, *et al.* Anti-interleukin-2 receptors antibodies-basiliximab and daclizumab-for the prevention of acute rejection in renal transplantation. Biol Targ Ther 2009; 3: 319-336.

[135] Morris PJ, Russel NK. Alemtuzumab (Campath-1H): a systematic review in organ trasplantation. Transplantation 2006, 81: 1361-1367.

[136] Watson CJ, Bradley JA, Friend PJ, *et al.* Alemtuzumab (Campath 1 H) induction therapy in cadaveric kidney transplantation-Efficacy and safety at five years. Am J Transplant 2005; 5: 1347-1353.

[137] Ciancio G, Burke GW, Gaynor JJ, *et al.* A randomized trial of three renal transplant induction antibodies: early comparison of tacrolimus, mycophenolate mofetil, and steroid: dosing, and newer immune-monitoring. Transplantation 2005; 80: 457-465.

[138] Knechtle SJ, Fernandez LA, Pirsch JD, *et al.* Campath-1H in renal transplantation: the University of Wisconsin experience. Surgery 2004; 136: 754-760.

[139] Friend PJ, Rebello P, Oliveira D, *et al.* Successful treatment of renal allograft rejection with a humanized antilymphocyte monoclonal antibody. Transplant Proc 1995; 27: 869-870.

[140] Basu A, Ramkumar M, Tan HP, *et al.* Reversal of acute cellular rejection after renal transplantation with Campath-1H. Transplant Proc 2005; 37: 923-926. .

[141] Ciancio G, Burke GW, Gaynor JJ, *et al.* The use of Campath-1H as induction therapy in renal transplantation: preliminary results. Transplantation 2004; 78: 426-433.

[142] Margreiter R, Klempnauer J, Neuhaus P, *et al.* Alemtuzumab (Campath-1H) and tacrolimus monotherapy after renal transplantation: results of a prospective randomized trial. Am J Transplant 2008; 8: 1480-1485.

[143] Alausa M, Almagro U, Siddiqi N, *et al.* Refractory acute kidney transplant rejection with CD20 graft infiltrates and successful therapy with rituximab. Clin Transplant 2005; 19: 137-140.

[144] Becker YT, Becker BN, Pirsch JD, *et al.* Rituximab as treatment for refractory kidney transplant rejection. Am J Transplant 2004; 4: 996-1001.

[145] Munoz AS, Rioveros AA, Cabanayan-Casaola CB, *et al.* Rituximab in highly sensitized kidney transplant recipients. Transplantation Proceedings 2008; 40: 2218-2221.

[146] Sawada T, Fuchinou S, Teraoka S. Successful A1-to-o AB0-incompatibile kidney transplantation after a preconditioning regimen consisting of anti-CD20 monoclonal antibody infusion, splenectomy, and double-filtration plasmapheresis. Transplantation 2002; 74: 1207-1210.

[147] Gloor JM, Lager DJ, Fidler ME, *et al.* A comparison of splenectomy versus intensive posttransplant antidonor blood group antibody monitoring without splenectomy in AB0-incompatibile kidney transplantation. Transplantation 2005; 80: 1572-1577.

[148] Gloor JM, DeGoey SR, Pineda AA, *et al.* Overcoming a positive crossmatch in living-donor kidney transplantation. Am J Transplant 2003, 3: 1017-1023.

[149] Vo AA, Lukovsky M, Toyoda M, *et al.* Rituximab and intravenous immune globulin for desensitization during renal transplantation. N Engl J Med 2008; 359: 242-251.

[150] Tyden G, Genberg H, Tollemar J, *et al.* A randomized double blind placebo-controlled study of single-dose rituximab as induction in renal transplantation. Transplantation 2009; 87: 1325-229.

[151] Vincenti F. Costimulation blockade in autoimmunity and transplantation. J Allergy Clin Immunol 2008, 121: 299-306.

[152] Biancone L, Segoloni G, Turello E, *et al.* Expression of inducible lymphocyte costimulatory molecules in human renal allograft. Nephrol Dial transplant 1998; 13. 716-722.

[153] Vincenti F, Larsen C, Durrbach A, *et al.* Costimulation blockade with Belatacept in renal transplantation. N Engl J Med 2005; 353: 770-781.

[154] Latek R, Fleener C, Lamian V, *et al.* Assessment of Belatacept-mediated costimulation blockade through evaluation of CD80/86-receptor saturation. Transplantation 2009; 87: 926-933.

[155] Billingham RE, Brent L, Medawar PB. Actively acquired tolerance of foreign cells. Nature 1953; 172: 603.

[156] Kuhr CS, Allen MD, Junghanss C, *et al.* Tolerance to vascularized kidney grafts in canine mixed hematopoietic chimeras. Transplantation 2002;73: 1487–1493.

CHAPTER 14

Minimization of Immunosuppression

Joshua J. Augustine and Donald E. Hricik*

Department of Medicine, University Hospitals Case Medical Center and Case Western Reserve University, Cleveland, Ohio, USA

Abstract: In an effort to reduce the long-term toxicities of immunosuppressant drugs, corticosteroid and calcineurin inhibitor-sparing immunosuppression protocols have become increasingly popular in managing kidney transplant recipients. The use of induction antibody therapy and potent residual immunosuppressants have increased the safety of steroid-free regimens, resulting in a paradigm shift towards earlier elimination of steroids after kidney transplantation. However, even in the modern era, results of randomized trials generally indicate that steroid elimination increases the risk of rejection compared to maintenance steroid therapy. Among calcineurin inhibitor-sparing strategies, withdrawal of these agents after their initial use in stable patients, or conversion to either mycophenolate mofetil or sirolimus in patients with renal dysfunction appears to yield the greatest benefit in preserving renal function. The outcomes of calcineurin inhibitor avoidance protocols have been mixed but have fallen into disfavor. The benefits of minimizing immunosuppression in kidney transplant recipients must be weighed against the risks of precipitating acute rejection or chronic allograft dysfunction. Additional research is needed to identify clinical and immune parameters that will enable selection of patients for whom the benefits outweigh the risks. In addition, the transplant community is in need of newer agents that can potently prevent rejection without the need for corticosteroids or calcineurin inhibitors.

Keywords: Immunosuppression, Corticosteroids, Calcineurin Inhibitors, Tacrolimus, Cyclosporine, Sirolimus, Everolimus, Calcineurin-Free Protocols, Tolerance, Mycophenolate Mofetil.

INTRODUCTION

The short-term outcomes of kidney transplantation have improved in recent years, and attention has shifted to the long-term outcomes of transplant recipients. Long-term survival of renal allografts has been influenced increasingly by co-morbidities that are related, in part, to immunosuppressive drugs. Death with a functioning graft is now a common cause of late allograft failure. Increasing enthusiasm has emerged for strategies that minimize the side effects of immunosuppressants with the hopes of prolonging patient survival by reducing the risks of associated infection, malignancy, chronic renal dysfunction, and cardiovascular disease. Efforts continue to focus on protocols that minimize exposure to either corticosteroids or calcineurin inhibitors (CNIs). Two general strategies have evolved: 1) *de novo* minimization, in which maintenance immunosuppression is often prescribed as monotherapy after treatment with lymphocyte depleting antibody therapy, and 2) *selective* minimization, in which one class of drug is either avoided, withdrawn or replaced within the context of traditional multi-drug immunosuppressive therapy.

DE NOVO MINIMIZATION STRATEGIES

Early attempts at *de novo* minimization of maintenance immunosuppression employed high doses of polyclonal antibodies for induction therapy. However, most recent experiences have encompassed the use of alemtuzumab, a humanized CD52-specific monoclonal antibody that induces profound and prolonged T cell depletion. Calne *et al.* first described the use of alemtuzumab and low doses cyclosporine (CsA) as monotherapy in 31 patients [1]. The incidence of acute rejection (AR) was 20% during the first posttransplant year. However, a report of the five year follow-up from this experience described an

***Address correspondence to Donald E. Hricik:** University Hospitals Case Medical Center, 11100 Euclid Avenue, Cleveland, Ohio 44106; Tel: 216-844-8060; Fax: 216-844-5204; E-mails: donald.hricik@uhhospitals.org or dhricik@aol.com.

Massimiliano Veroux and Pierfrancesco Veroux (Eds)

additional 14% incidence of AR after the first year [2], suggesting that alemtuzumab may simply delay the onset of immune injury to the graft.

Other trials exploring a potential tolerogenic effect of alemtuzumab have demonstrated relatively high rates of AR, sometimes with unusual histologic characteristics. Kirk *et al.* examined the effects of alemtuzumab alone, without maintenance immunosuppression, in seven patients, all of whom experienced early AR with a monocytic infiltrate [3]. Knechtle *et al.* used alemtuzumab with sirolimus monotherapy, and noted a 28% incidence of AR with 3 to 29 months of follow-up [4]. Many of AR episodes were humoral in nature, suggesting that this regimen may either fail to suppress or possibly augment the activity of B cells.

Shapiro *et al.* described outcomes of kidney transplant recipients with single pretransplant doses of alemtuzumab and methylprednisolone, followed by tacrolimus (TAC) monotherapy [5]. "Spaced weaning" of TAC to less than daily therapy was achieved in 42% of patients. The rate of AR was only 6.8% in the first year, although AR increased after spaced weaning of TAC. Recent follow-up data from the same experience revealed a 20% incidence of *de novo* donor specific antibody formation after spaced weaning [6].

SELECTIVE MINIMIZATION STRATEGIES

Currently, the most popular selective minimization strategies encompass either corticosteroid or calcineurin inhibitor sparing regimens.

Steroid Sparing Protocols

The history of steroid-free immunosuppression in kidney transplantation has been the subject of recent comprehensive reviews [7, 8]. In the past decade, there has been a paradigm shift towards earlier elimination or even avoidance of steroids, although a large portion of the published experience is based on uncontrolled experiences from single centers [9-12], large prospective but non-randomized multicenter trials [13], or registry analyses [14, 15]. Reports from some of these experiences [11, 13, 14] suggest that the use of steroid-free immunosuppression is associated with better graft and patient survival than observed in patients who receive steroids. However, each of these non-randomized studies is likely flawed by selection bias. The remainder of this section will focus on recent randomized studies of early steroid elimination using CNI therapy in combination with mycophenolate mofetil (MMF) (summarized in Table **1**).

The Astellas Steroid Withdrawal Study Group performed a doubled blinded, placebo-controlled study in 386 patients who were randomized to either maintenance therapy with prednisone or early withdrawal of steroids 7 days following transplantation [16]. Patients were treated with a combination of TAC and MMF after induction therapy with either rabbit anti-thymocyte globulin or an anti-IL2 receptor antibody. Importantly, patients randomized to maintenance steroid therapy received only 5 mg of prednisone daily by 6 months posttransplant.

Table 1: Randomized trials of early steroid elimination with CNI/MMF therapy

Study (Ref #)	n	CNI	Induction	Steroid 1-yr AR rate	Exposure
Vincenti *et al.* [27]	83	CsA	Basiliximab	5 days	20% in CSWD *vs.* 16% in CCS (NS)
FREEDOM [19]	338	CsA	Basiliximab	7 days	26% in CSWD *vs.* 15% in CCS (p<0.05)
CARMEN [24]	538	TAC	Daclizumab*	1 day	17% in both groups
ATLAS [21] in CCS (6 months)	451	TAC	None	1 day	31% in CSWD *vs.* 8%
Astellas [16] in CCS (p=0.04)	396	TAC	ATG	7 days	12% in CSWD *vs.* 6% (p=<0.001)

*Only steroid elimination group received daclizumab, CNI, calcineurin inhibitor, MMF, mycophenolate mofetil; CsA, cyclosporine; TAC, tacrolimus; ATG, anti-thymocyte globulin; CSWD, corticosteroid withdrawal group; CCS, chronic corticosteroid group; AR, acute rejection.

No differences were observed at five years in the proportion of patients experiencing the primary endpoint (a composite of death, graft loss, or moderate/severe acute rejection) with 15.7% of patients reaching the endpoint in the steroid withdrawal arm *versus* 14.4% in the control arm. After one year of follow-up, an interim analysis indicated that the incidence of biopsy-proven AR was more common in the steroid withdrawal group (12% *vs.* 6% , p=0.04) [17]. At five years, a trend persisted for more biopsy proven acute rejection in the steroid withdrawal group at 17.8% *vs.* 10.8% in the steroid-treated group (p=0.058). Protocol biopsies were not performed, but biopsy-proven chronic allograft nephropathy (CAN) was found in 9.9% of patients withdrawn from steroids *vs.* 4.1% of the group maintained on prednisone at 4 years (p=0.03). It is not clear whether CAN in these cases was related to immune injury or to CNI toxicity, but this finding is consistent with that of a small randomized trial that found an increase in allograft fibrosis in protocol biopsies in steroid-free patients despite rates of AR comparable to a control group maintained on steroids [18].

Another finding in the Astellas trial was that MMF dose reduction was more common in the steroid withdrawal group. MMF was reduced for leukopenia in 52% of steroid-free patients *vs.* 27% of patients maintained on prednisone, confirming the salutary effect of corticosteroids on leukopenia and raising the possibility that reduction of MMF doses may have contributed to the increase incidence of rejection. Renal function and graft survival remained similar in the two groups at five years, suggesting that the increase in acute rejection and CAN did not negatively affect allograft function or survival.

The FREEDOM study was a prospective trial in which kidney transplant recipients treated with basiliximab, CsA and enteric-coated mycophenolic sodium were randomly allocated to one of three arms: 1) steroid avoidance, 2) early steroid withdrawal at 7 days, or 3) maintenance prednisone. After one year of follow-up, the incidence of AR was 31.5%, 26.1% and 15%, respectively, (p=0.05 comparing steroid-free groups to the steroid treated group) [19]. Renal function, graft survival and patient survival were equivalent in the 3 groups after one year. Roughly half of patients in this trial did not achieve target C2 CsA levels and this may have contributed to the risk of AR.

One interesting observation from the FREEDOM study is that, among patients randomized to one of the two steroid-free arms of study, approximately 40% had returned to steroid therapy after one year of follow-up [19]. Recently, Schold *et al.* performed retrospective analysis of data from the Scientific Registry of Transplant Recipients (SRTR) to determine the frequency of and risk factors for renewal of steroid therapy in 24, 218 kidney transplant recipients initially discharged without steroids between 2002 and 2008 [20]. During that period, 22 percent of patients renewed steroid therapy. However, the frequency of steroid renewal decreased from 47 percent in 2002 to 16 percent in 2008. Among deceased donor transplant recipients, significant risk factors for renewal of steroids included African-American ethnicity, Medicaid as primary payer, interstitial nephritis as cause of kidney failure, PRA>30%, retransplantation, HLA mismatching, and donor age > 60 years. Among living donor transplant recipients, additional risk factors included duration of dialysis and use of an unrelated donor. Compared to patients who were never withdrawn from steroids (n=60, 429) or to those who remained off of steroids at 6 months (n=18, 591), 4-year graft survival was significantly worse in patients who returned to steroid therapy. Results of this analysis confirm that most of the risk factors associated with renewal of steroid therapy and poor long term graft survival are variables traditionally associated with “high risk”. Many previous studies, focusing on the excellent outcomes of patients who remain off of steroids for long periods of time, have been flawed by selection bias. Data from the current study confirm excellent outcomes in patients who remain off of steroid therapy, but suggest that a substantial minority of patients requiring renewal of steroids does poorly over the long term.

There is a growing consensus that induction antibody therapy is an important adjunct to successful early elimination of steroids. Moreover, polyclonal antibody therapy may convey an advantage over anti-IL2 receptor antibodies. In the Astellas trial, AR at three years occurred in 22.7% of steroid-free patients who received basiliximab *vs.* 12.8% of patients who received ATG (p=0.08), despite a greater percentage of deceased donors in the ATG group [16]. The European-based ATLAS study examined two different steroid-free regimens by randomizing 451 patients to one of three arms 1) basiliximab and TAC monotherapy, 2) TAC and MMF without induction antibody therapy, or 3) TAC, MMF, and steroids without induction antibodies. After 6 months, the incidence of biopsy-proven AR was 26.1%, 30.5%, and 8.2%, respectively ($p<0.001$) [21].

Reported metabolic benefits of steroid-free immunosuppression have been variable in recent reports. A large European trial demonstrated no difference in weight gain between an early steroid elimination group *vs.* a low-dose maintenance steroid group [22]. In the Astellas trial, after five years of follow-up, earlier differences in weight gain and in the incidence of new onset diabetes mellitus (NODAT) requiring treatment were no longer statistically significant, although insulin usage was lower in patients withdrawn from steroids (3.7% *vs.* 11.6%, $p=0.049$) [16]. Kumar *et al.* found low rates of NODAT in a steroid elimination cohort despite high TAC target levels and a high percentage of black recipients [23]. Other steroid elimination trials using TAC have also shown minimal NODAT, but no appreciable benefit of early steroid withdrawal on hyperlipidemia [24-26]. In the Astellas trial, lipid profiles were not significantly different after five years [16].

The wisdom of withdrawing steroids from high risk patients remains controversial. Highly sensitized patients have been excluded from recent trials [16, 21, 27]. African Americans appear to have a disproportionate risk for acute and subclinical rejection after steroid withdrawal [28, 29]. In the Astellas Study, the incidence of acute rejection after withdrawal of steroids was not influenced by ethnicity [16]. However, it could be argued that investigators may have been reluctant to enroll African Americans in a randomized trial of steroid withdrawal. Our own experience, in which steroids are withdrawn as a standard of practice for all patients, suggests that African Americans are at higher risk for AR. Among 133 primary transplant recipients subjected to this protocol, the cumulative incidence of AR was 23.6% in African Americans *versus* 7.7% in white patients after one year ($p=0.02$) [30]. The larger experience of Kumar *et al.* however, suggests that an aggressive approach to recognizing and treating subclinical AR *via* routine surveillance biopsies may result in long-term outcomes that are comparable to non-African Americans [29]. Based on our recent findings which suggest a correlation between hemodialysis exposure and T cell alloreactivity [31], longer dialysis vintage may pose a greater risk of AR than ethnicity and could be an additional risk factor for AR after steroid elimination.

Calcineurin Inhibitor Sparing Studies

CNI sparing regimens include conversion protocols in which these agents are substituted for another class of immunosuppressant, withdrawal protocols in which the CNIs are withdrawn at some arbitrary point posttransplant in stable patients, and avoidance protocols in which CNIs are avoided completely.

Calcineurin Inhibitor Conversion

Conversion from CNIs to other agents has been attempted most often in patients with chronic allograft dysfunction, based on the premise that elimination of the CNI will preserve renal function over time. In uncontrolled trials, MMF has been used to facilitate CNI minimization or withdrawal in a number of studies [32-34]. In one of the largest experiences, Weir *et al.* studied 118 patients with chronic allograft nephropathy in whom treatment with MMF was initiated to facilitate either elimination (n=18) or a 50% reduction in the dose of CsA or tacrolimus (n=100) [34]. Mean follow-up after conversion was 1.8 years. Approximately half of patients subjected to a 50% dose reduction exhibited stable or improved renal function.

A number of studies have reported outcomes after conversion from CNIs to sirolimus for kidney transplant recipients with renal dysfunction. Recently, Mulay *et al.* published a meta-analysis of five randomized trials including 1040 patients and 25 non-randomized studies including 977 patients [35]. Four trials [36-39] have reported estimates of glomerular filtration rate (GFR) at baseline and at end of follow-up in patients who had documented chronic allograft dysfunction and who were randomized either to remain on CNI therapy or to convert to sirolimus. In all four studies, the change from baseline creatinine clearance was positive in the sirolimus conversion group and negative in the control arm remaining on a CNI (Fig. **1**). Six non-randomized studies [40-45] measured creatinine clearance at baseline and at study end and collectively showed a mean increase of 5.7 ml/min ($p=0.003$) [35]. A number of uncontrolled studies [46-50] have used only serum creatinine concentration as an estimate of renal function at baseline and after conversion to sirolimus, but collectively indicate a mean decrease in serum creatinine concentration of 0.19 mg/dl (p=0.004) [35]. Since publication of the meta-analysis by Mulay *et al.* [35] another large but uncontrolled experience has been reported by Wali *et al.* who substituted sirolimus for CNIs in 136 patients with moderate to severe renal allograft dysfunction (mean serum creatinine concentration of 3.8 $\pm$ 0.2 mg/dl prior to conversion). This maneuver led to significant improvement in graft function in 74% of patients [51].

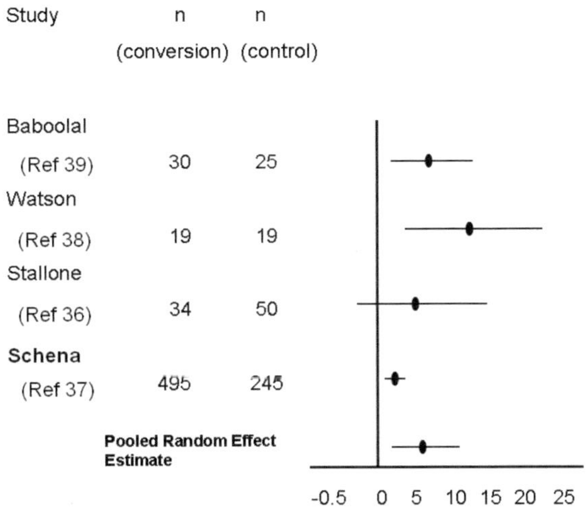

Figure 1: Change from baseline in creatinine clearance after conversion to sirolimus in randomized controlled trials: results of a meta-analysis. Adapted from reference [35].

Among randomized CNI conversion trials, the largest has been the CONVERT trial, in which 830 patients receiving either tacrolimus or cyclosporine and exhibiting renal allograft dysfunction were randomized to either conversion to sirolimus (n=555) or continued treatment with the CNI (n=275) [37]. Patients were stratified into 2 groups according to baseline estimated GFRs of either 20-40 ml/min or greater than 40 ml/min. Study of patients in the arm with baseline GFRs of 20-40 ml/minute was aborted prematurely by the study's data safety monitoring board because of a statistically higher incidence of the safety end-points.

For patients with baseline estimated GFRs > 40 ml/min at the time of enrollment, *on therapy* analysis revealed an overall improvement in filtration rate at 2 years in patients randomized to conversion (62.6 ml/min (n=370) *versus* 59.9 ml/min (n=201), p =0.009) after 2 years of follow-up. 19.8% of patients randomized to conversion discontinued sirolimus because of adverse events, the most common of which were hyperlipidemia, diarrhea, anemia, and edema. The incidence of AR following randomization was 7.8% in converters and 6.5% in non-converters (p=0.555). An important finding of the CONVERT trial has been the observation that improvement in GFR after conversion to sirolimus is inversely related to the degree of urine protein excretion prior to conversion. Results from the CONVERT trial also suggest an increase in urinary protein excretion following conversion in some patients. The tendency to develop worsening proteinuria was related to baseline histopathology. A higher Banff total sum score (p<0.001) and the percent of sclerotic glomeruli at baseline (p=0.007) were significantly correlated with increased protein excretion after conversion to sirolimus [37].

Calcineurin Inhibitor Withdrawal

A meta-analysis of 13 randomized studies of CsA withdrawal completed before 1999 found that elimination of CsA increased the risk of subsequent acute rejection by 11% without exerting a statistically significant impact on long-term graft survival [52]. More recent reports have described the benefits and risks of withdrawing CsA in stable patients previously treated with CsA and either MMF- or sirolimus-based immunosuppression and the outcomes are summarized in Table **2**. While some, but not all of these trials have shown that CNI withdrawal may improve long-term renal function compared to CNI maintenance, each of these large randomized trials has shown that CNI withdrawal is associated with an incremental risk of acute rejection [53-58]. For example, Abramowicz *et al.* reported the results of a multicenter trial in which kidney transplant recipients previously maintained on CsA, MMF, and steroids were randomly allocated to CsA withdrawal (n=85) or CsA continuation (n=85) [53]. Within 9 months of randomization, acute rejection occurred in 10.6% of patients in the withdrawal group and 2.4% of the continuation group. A trend toward improvement in creatinine clearance in the withdrawal group was statistically significant only if patients with AR were excluded. In the Cyclosporine Avoidance Eliminates Renal-toxicity (CAESAR) trial, 535 kidney transplant recipients initially treated with daclizumab, cyclosporine, mycophenolate and steroids were randomized either to cyclosporine withdrawal (weaned between 4 and 6 months), or to one of two cyclosporine maintenance groups. At 6 months, prior to elimination of cyclosporine in the experimental arm, the cumulative incidence of biopsy–proven acute rejection was similar in each arm (24.7% in the withdrawal arm and 26.2% in the standard cyclosporine dose arm). By 12 months, the cumulative incidence of acute rejection was 38% in the withdrawal group *versus* 27.5% in the group maintained standard doses of cyclosporine ($p<0.05$). The incremental incidence of acute rejection following cyclosporine elimination in the experimental arm was 13.3%. Despite successful withdrawal of cyclosporine in 88/151 patients (58%) originally randomized to the experimental arm, there was no significant improvement in measured GFR at 12 months in the entire group (50.8 *versus* 48.6 ml/min; p=NS), although the subgroup that successfully came off of CNI did enjoy better renal function.

Table 2: Acute rejection rates and changes in GFR after CNI withdrawal based on intention to treat

Ref (no)	Pts (n)	Timing of CNI Withdrawal (months)	Incidence of AR After Randomization (%)		Follow-up (months)	Residual Drugs After CNI Withdrawal	GFR (ml/min) at End of Study	
			W/D	Control			W/D	Control
[53]	187	6	10.6	2.4	12	MMF, CS	NR	
[54]	84	3	11.3	5.0	12	MMF, CS	73.2	61.9
[55]	212	6	22.0	1.4	24	MMF, CS	NR	
[56]	536	4	13.3	1.3	12	MMF, CS	50.9	48.6
[57]	246	2	14.0	6.2	12	Sir, CS	65.3	56.4
[59]	525	3	9.8	4.2	12	Sir, CS	63	57

Pts, patients; AR, acute rejection; W/D, withdrawal group; MMF, mycophenolate mofetil; CS, corticosteroids; Sir, sirolimus; NR, not reported.

Two randomized multicenter trials have assessed the benefits and risks of CsA withdrawal in kidney transplant recipients initially treated with CsA, sirolimus, and corticosteroids. In the study of Johnson *et al.* patients were randomized 3 months after transplantation to CsA withdrawal (n=215) or CsA continuation (n=215) [54]. Two years after randomization, the incidence of acute rejection was 9.8% in the withdrawal group and 5.1% in the continuation group. At 12 months, serum creatinine concentration was significantly better in the withdrawal group (142 *vs.* 158 umol/L, $p < 0.001$). Analysis of the outcomes of patients enrolled in this trial have been published with four years of follow-up and continue to suggest better renal function in the group of patients randomized to CsA withdrawal [58]. In a similar study, Gonwa *et al.* randomized primary cadaveric kidney transplant recipients at the time of transplantation to CsA withdrawal between 2 and 3 months posttransplant (n=100) or continued treatment with CsA, sirolimus and steroids (n=97) [59]. AR occurred in 22% of patients randomized to CsA withdrawal and in 18.6% of those randomized to CsA continuation. At 12 months, serum creatinine concentrations were lower in the withdrawal group, even when patients experiencing rejection were included in the analysis.

Calcineurin Inhibitor Avoidance

Two uncontrolled trials have reported CNI avoidance in patients treated with daclizumab induction therapy followed by maintenance treatment with MMF and corticosteroids. Tran *et al.* used such a regimen in 45 living or cadaveric kidney transplant recipients followed for 8 months at a single center [60]. The incidence of biopsy-proven AR was 31%. At the end of study, 48% of patients remained off of CNIs and graft survival was 95%. Vincenti *et al.* studied 98 patients in a similar study performed at multiple centers [61]. Biopsy-proven rejection occurred in 53% of patients within 12 months of follow-up. Graft survival was 96% but only 38% of the patients remained off of CIs by the end of the study.

Sirolimus also has been used with corticosteroids and either azathioprine or MMF to facilitate CNI avoidance. In a multicenter trial, Groth *et al.* randomized patients to receive either sirolimus, azathioprine, and steroids (n=41) or CsA, azathioprine, and steroids (n=42) [62]. The incidence of AR within 6 months of transplantation was 41% and 38%, respectively. Calculated GFRs were consistently lower in the sirolimus group, reaching statistical significance at 12 and 16 months posttransplant. Kreis *et al.* performed a similar, randomized study comparing maintenance therapy with sirolimus, MMF and steroids (n=40) to CsA, MMF, and steroids (n=38) [63]. The incidence of AR at 12 months was 27.5% and 18.4%, respectively. GFR was consistently better after 1 month in the sirolimus group. Induction antibody therapy was not used in either of these studies.

Flechner *et al.* reported the results of a single center trial in which primary kidney recipients were randomized to receive sirolimus, MMF and steroids (n=31) or CsA, MMF, and steroids (n=30) [64]. Patients in both arms received induction therapy with basiliximab. After follow-up of 18 months, the incidence of acute rejection was 6.4% in the sirolimus group and 16.6% in the CsA group. Serum creatinine concentration was significantly lower in sirolimus-treated patients beyond the third study month. In contrast, a larger randomized trial by Larsen *et al.* failed to demonstrate any differences in GFR measured by iothalamate clearance in kidney transplant patients treated with rabbit ATG and randomized to receive either TAC and MMF or sirolimus and MMF [65].

More recently, two larger multicenter trials have been performed to compare sirolimus-based immunosuppression to CNI-based immunosuppression. In the SPEISSER trial, 145 renal transplant recipients were randomized to receive either sirolimus or CsA. All patients received polyclonal antibodies, MMF, and steroids [66]. The primary endpoint, glomerular filtration rate estimated by the Nankivell formula, and was not significantly different between groups at 12 months. There were also no differences in graft or patient survival rates, nor in the incidence of acute rejection. Study drug discontinuation was higher in the sirolimus arm (28.2% *vs.* 14.9%).

Results from the SPEISSER study differ somewhat from those of the much larger Efficacy Limiting Toxicity Elimination (ELITE) - Symphony study trial that was ambitiously designed to test the benefit and risks of three CNI minimization regimens, including CNI avoidance. In the SYMPHONY trial [67], 1645 were randomized either to a control group treated with standard-dose cyclosporine (based on target trough blood levels), mycophenolate mofetil (MMF) and corticosteroids, or to one of three experimental groups who received induction antibody therapy with daclizumab, maintenance therapy with MMF and steroids and either 1) low-dose cyclosporine, 2) low-dose tacrolimus, or 3) low-dose sirolimus - the latter group essentially constituting a CNI avoidance arm. Estimated glomerular filtration rate, calculated by the Cockcroft-Gault formula, was the primary endpoint. After one year of follow-up, patients receiving low-dose tacrolimus had the highest GFR (65.4±27 ml/min), the lowest rate of biopsy-proven acute rejection (12.3%), and highest rate of graft survival (94.2%). In this group, estimated GFR and the incidence of acute rejection were statistically superior to the control group. The worst outcomes occurred in low-dose sirolimus, CNI avoidance group that exhibited the lowest GFR (56.7±27 ml/min), the lowest rate of graft survival (89.3%), and the highest rate of biopsy-proven acute rejection (37.2%).

CONCLUSIONS

De novo minimization protocols employing T cell depleting antibody induction therapy do not induce tolerance in all human kidney transplant recipients. However, the term "prope" tolerance has been used to describe the state of minimal maintenance immunosuppression achieved in many patients subjected to these protocols. Randomized trials are needed to further assess the benefits and risks of such protocols. Targeting select patient populations and monitoring patients aggressively for the development of humoral rejection may increase the safety of such protocols.

The majority of kidney transplant recipients can safely undergo early steroid elimination with CNI therapy in combination with MMF, although most randomized studies and meta-analyses of randomized studies continue to show a greater risk of AR in patients who stop steroids. Induction therapy appears to improve outcomes after early steroid elimination. The finding of increased graft fibrosis after steroid withdrawal in some recent trials is concerning, and illustrates the importance of long term follow-up in such studies.

Collectively, recent experiences with CNI conversion or withdrawal suggest that minimization of CNIs is generally associated with improved renal function over relatively short periods of time. When attempted in patients receiving MMF or sirolimus-based therapy, these strategies are associated with a relatively low risk of AR. Results of CNI avoidance studies have been mixed. Longer follow-up is need to determine whether the short-term benefits of minimizing CNIs will translate into prolonged patient or graft survival.

REFERENCES

[1] Calne R, Moffatt SD, Friend PJ, *et al.* Campath IH allows low-dose cyclosporine monotherapy in 31 cadaveric renal allograft recipients. Transplantation 1999; 68:1613-1616.

[2] Watson CJ, Bradley JA, Friend PJ, *et al.* Alemtuzumab (CAMPATH 1H) induction therapy in cadaveric kidney transplantation--efficacy and safety at five years. Am J Transplant 2005; 5:1347-1353.

[3] Kirk AD, Hale DA, Mannon RB, *et al.* Results from a human renal allograft tolerance trial evaluating the humanized CD52-specific monoclonal antibody alemtuzumab (CAMPATH-1H). Transplantation 2003; 76:120-129.

[4] Knechtle SJ, Pirsch JD, Fechner JH, *et al.* Campath-1H induction plus rapamycin monotherapy for renal transplantation: results of a pilot study. Am J Transplant 2003; 3:722-730.

[5] Tan HP, Kaczorowski DJ, Basu A, *et al.* Living donor renal transplantation using alemtuzumab induction and tacrolimus monotherapy. Am J Transplant 2006; 6:2409-241.

[6] Shapiro R, Zeevi A, Basu A, *et al.* Monitoring for donor-specific antibody (DSA) and outcomes after spaced weaning in adult renal transplant recipients [Abstract]. Am J Transplant 2007; 7[Suppl 2]:200-201.

[7] Bodziak KA, Hricik DE. Minimizing the side effects of immunosuppression in kidney transplant recipients. Current Opinion in Organ Transplantation 2003; 8:160-166.

[8] Augustine JJ, Hricik DE. Steroid sparing in kidney transplantation: Changing paradigms, improving outcomes, and remaining questions. Clin J Am Soc Nephrol 2006; 1:1080-1089.

[9] Cole E, Landsberg D, Russell D, *et al.* A pilot study of steroid-free immunosuppression in the prevention of acute rejection in renal allograft recipients. Transplantation 2001; 72:845-850.

[10] Birkeland SA. Steroid-free immunosuppression after kidney transplantation with antithymocyte globulin induction and cyclosporine and mycophenolate maintenance therapy. Transplantation 1998; 66:1207-1210.

[11] Matas AJ, Kandaswamy R, Gillingham KJ, *et al.* Prednisone-free maintenance immunosuppression: A 5-year experience. Am J Transplant 2005; 5:2473-2478.

[12] Kaufman DB, Leventhal JR, Axelrod D, *et al.* Alemtuzumab induction and prednisone-free maintenance immunotherapy in kidney transplantation: comparison with basiliximab induction--long-term results. Am J Transplant 2005; 5:2539-2548.

[13] Opelz G, Dohler B, Laux G. Long-term prospective study of steroid withdrawal in kidney and heart transplant recipients. Am J Transplant 2005; 5:720-728.

[14] Luan FL, Steffick DE, Gadegbeku C, *et al.* Graft and patient survival in kidney transplant recipients selected for *de novo* steroid-free maintenance immunosuppression. Am J Transplant 2009; 9: 160-168.

[15] Knight SR, Morris PJ. Steroid avoidance or withdrawal after renal transplantation increases the risk of acute rejection but decreases cardiovascular risk. A meta-analysis. Transplantation 2010; 89: 1-14.

[16] Woodle E, First M, Pirsch J, *et al.* Astellas Corticosteroid Withdrawal Study Group. A prospective, randomized, double-blind, placebo-controlled multicenter trial comparing early (7 day) corticosteroid cessation *versus* long-term, low-dose corticosteroid therapy. Ann Surg 2008: 248: 564-577.

[17] Woodle ES. Fujisawa Steroid Withdrawal Study Group: A randomized, double-blinded, placebo-controlled trial of early corticosteroid cessation *versus* chronic corticosteroid maintenance therapy [Abstract]. Am J Transplant 2005; 5[Suppl 11]:54.

[18] Laftavi MR, Stephan R, Stefancik B, *et al.* Randomized prospective trial of early steroid withdrawal compared with low-dose steroids in renal transplant recipients using serial protocol biopsies to assess efficacy and safety. Surgery 2005; 137:364-371.

[19] Vincenti F, Schena F, Paraskevas S, *et al.* FREEDOM Study Gropup. A randomized, multicenter study of steroid avoidance, early steroid withdrawal or standard steroid therapy in kidney transplant recipients. Am J Transplant 2008: 8: 307-316.

[20] Schold JD, Santos A, Rehman S, *et al.* The success of continued steroid avoidance after kidney transplantation in the US. Am J Transplant 2009; 9: 2768-2776.

[21] Vitko S, Klinger M, Salmela K, *et al.* Two corticosteroid-free regimens-tacrolimus monotherapy after basiliximab administration and tacrolimus/mycophenolate mofetil-in comparison with a standard triple regimen in renal transplantation: results of the ATLAS study. Transplantation 2005; 80:1734-1741.

[22] Van de Ham ECH, Kooman JP, Christiaans MHL, *et al.* Weight changes after renal transplantation: a comparison between patients on 5-mg maintenance steroid therapy and those on steroid-free immunosuppressive therapy. Transpl Int 2003; 16:82-87.

[23] Kumar MS, Heifets M, Moritz MJ, *et al.* Safety and efficacy of steroid withdrawal two days after kidney transplantation: analysis of results at three years. Transplantation 2006; 81:832-839.

[24] Rostaing L, Cantarovich D, Mourad G, *et al.* Corticosteroid-free immunosuppression with tacrolimus, mycophenolate mofetil, and daclizumab induction in renal transplantation. Transplantation 2005; 79:807-814.

[25] Gallon LG, Winoto J, Leventhal JR, *et al.* Effect of prednisone *versus* no prednisone as part of maintenance immunosuppression on long-term renal transplant function. Clin J Am Soc Nephrol 2006; 1:1029-1038.

[26] Pascual J, van Hooff JP, Salmela K, *et al.* Three-year observational follow-up of a multicenter, randomized trial on tacrolimus-based therapy with withdrawal of steroids or mycophenolate mofetil after renal transplant. Transplantation 2006; 82:55-61.

[27] Vincenti F, Monaco A, Grinyo J, *et al.* Multicenter randomized prospective trial of steroid withdrawal in renal transplant recipients receiving basiliximab, cyclosporine microemulsion and mycophenolate mofetil. Am J Transplant 2003; 3:306-311.

[28] Ahsan N, Hricik D, Matas A, *et al.* Prednisone withdrawal in kidney transplant recipients on cyclosporine and mycophenolate mofetil--a prospective randomized study. Steroid Withdrawal Study Group. Transplantation 1999; 68:1865-1874.

[29] Kumar MS, Moritz MJ, Saaed MI, *et al.* Avoidance of chronic steroid therapy in African American kidney transplant recipients monitored by surveillance biopsy: 1-year results. Am J Transplant 2005; 5:1976-1985.

[30] Padiyar A, Augustine JJ, Bodziak KA, *et al.* Influence of African American ethnicity on acute rejection after early steroid withdrawal in primary kidney transplant recipients. Transplant Proc 2010; 42:1643-1647.

[31] Augustine JJ, Poggio ED, Clemente M, *et al.* Hemodialysis vintage, black ethnicity, and pretransplantation antidonor cellular immunity in kidney transplant recipients. J Am Soc Nephrol 2007; 18:1602-1606.

[32] Hueso M, Boyer J, Seron D, *et al.* Low-dose cyclosporine and mycophenolate mofetil in renal allograft recipients with suboptimal renal function. Transplantation 1998; 66: 1727-1731.

[33] Houde I, Isenring P, Boucher D, *et al.* Mycophenolate mofetil, an alternative to cyclosporine A for long-term immunosuppression in kidney transplantation? Transplantation 2000; 70: 1251-1253.

[34] Weir MR, Ward MT, Blahut SA, *et al.* Long-term impact of discontinued or reduced calcineurin inhibitor in patients with chronic allograft nephropathy. Kidney Int 2001; 4: 1567-1573.

[35] Mulay AV, Cockfield S, Stryker R, *et al.* Conversion from calcineurin inhibitors to sirolimus for chronic renal allograft dysfunction: a systematic review of the evidence. Transplantation 2006; 82: 1153-1162.

[36] Stallone G, Infante B, Schena A, *et al.* Rapamycin for treatment of chronic allograft nephropathy in renal transplant patients. J Am Soc Nephrol 2005; 16: 3755-3762.

[37] Schena FP, Pascoe MD, Alberu J, *et al.* Conversion from calcineurin inhibitors to sirolimus maintenance therapy in renal allograft recipients: 24-month efficacy and safety results from the CONVERT trial. Transplantation 2009; 87: 233-242.

[38] Watson CJE, Firth JE, Williams PF, *et al.* A randomized controlled trial of late conversion from CNI-based to sirolimus-based immunosuppression following renal transplantation Am J Transplant 2005; 5: 2496-2503.

[39] Baboolal K. Six month interim analysis of a phase III prospective, randomized study to compare conversion from calcineurin inhibitors to rapamycin in established renal allograft recipients with mild to moderate renal insufficiency [abstract] Am J Transplant 2004: 4 (S8): 220.

[40] Paczek L, Dedocova J, Matl I, Ohanka E. An open non comparative pilot study of renal function after conversion from cyclosporine to sirolimus in stable renal allograft recipients with mild to moderate renal insufficiency [Abstract] 2003; 3: (S5): 217.

[41] Peddi VR, Jensik S, Pescovitz M, *et al.* An open-label pilot study evaluating the safety and efficacy of converting from calcineurin inhibitors to sirolimus in established renal allograft recipients with moderate renal insufficiency. Clin Transplant 2005; 19: 130-136.

[42] Wali RK, Richards A, Cunningham R, *et al.* Can we change the progressive decay in graft function after the onset of chronic allograft nephropathy in the recipients of kidney allografts? [Abstract]. Am J Transplant 2003; 3 (S5): 336.

[43] Moneim HA, Fletchner SM, George P, *et al.* Conversion to and from sirolimus in renal and hepatic transplant recipients treated with calcineurin inhibitors: effect on renal function [Abstract]. Am J Transplant 2005; 5 (S11): 376.

[44] Hoecker N, Feneberg R, Koepf S, *et al.* Switch of immunosuppression from calcineurin inhibitors to sirolimus in pediatric renal transplant recipients with CNI toxicity [Abstract] Am J Transplant 2005; 5 (S11): 497.

[45] Bumbea V, Kamar N, Ribes D, *et al.* Long term results in renal transplant patients with allograft dysfunction after switching from calcineurin inhibitors to sirolimus. Nephrol Dial Transplant 2005; 20: 2517-2523.

[46] Crowley KL, Hardinger KL, Koch M, *et al.* A single center experience with sirolimus conversion therapy in renal allograft recipients [Abstract]. Am J Transplant 2003; 3 (S5): 354.

[47] Diekmann F, Waiser J, Fritsche L, *et al.* Conversion to rapamycin in renal allograft recipients with biopsy-proven calcineurin inhibitor induced nephrotoxicity. Transplant Proc 2001; 33: 3234-3235.

[48] Egidi MF, Cowan PA, Naser A, Gaber AO. Conversion to sirolimus in solid organ transplantation: a single-center experience. Transplant Proc 2003; 35: 131S-137S.

[49] Hadaya K, Wissing M, Broeders N, Abramaowicz D. Nephrotic range proteinuria and other severe adverse events after conversion to sirolimus in renal transplantation: is high exposure to sirolimus responsible? [Abstract] Am J Transplant 2004; 4 (S8): 433.

[50] Lacha J, Bartosova K, Matl I, *et al.* Sirolimus associated proteinuria. Study in kidney and heart recipients after calcineurin inhibitor withdrawal and in kidney transplant recipients with sirolimus *de novo* immunosuppression. [Abstract] Am J Transplant 2005; 5: 414.

[51] Wali RK, Mohanlal V, Ramos E, *et al.* Early withdrawal of calcineurin inhibitors and rescue immunosuppression with sirolimus-based therapy in renal transplant recipients with moderate to severe renal dysfunction. Am J Transplant 2007; 7: 1572-1583.

[52] Kasiske BL, Chakkera HA, Louis TA, Ma JZ. A meta-analysis of immunosuppression withdrawal trials in renal transplantation. J Am Soc Nephrol 2000; 10:1910-1917.

[53] Abramowicz D, Manas D, Lao M, *et al.* Cyclosporine withdrawal from a mycophenolate mofetil-containing immunosuppressive regimen in stable kidney transplant recipients: a randomized, controlled study. Transplantation 2002; 74: 1725-1734.

[54] Schnuelle, P, van der Heide, JH, Tegzess, A, *et al.* Open randomized trial comparing early withdrawal of either cyclosporine or mycophenolate mofetil in stable renal transplant recipients initially treated with a triple drug regimen. J Am Soc Nephrol 2002; 13:536-543.

[55] Smak Gregoor, PJ, de Sevaux RG, Ligtenberg G, Hoitsma AJ, Hene RJ, Weimar W, Hilbrands LB, van Gelder T. Withdrawal of cyclosporine or prednisone six months after kidney transplantation in patients on triple drug therapy: a randomized, prospective, multicenter study. J Am Soc Nephrol 2002; 13:1365-1373.

[56] Ekberg H, Grinyo J, Nashan B, *et al.* Cyclosporine sparing with mycophenolate mofetil, daclizumab and corticosteroids in renal allograft recipients: the CAESAR Study. Am J Transplant 2007; 7:560-570.

[57] Johnson RWG, Kreis H, Oberbauer R, *et al.* Sirolimus allows early cyclosporine withdrawal in renal transplantation resulting in improved renal function and lower blood pressure. Transplantation 2001; 72: 777-786.

[58] Oberbauer R, Segoloni G, Campistol JM, *et al.* Early cyclosporine withdrawal from a sirolimus-based regimen results in better graft survival and renal function at 48 months after transplantation. Transplant Int 2005; 18: 22-28.

[59] Gonwa TA, Hricik DE, Brinker K, *et al.* Improved renal function in sirolimus-treated renal transplant patients after early cyclosporine elimination. Transplantation 2002; 74: 1560-1567.

[60] Tran HTB, Acharya MK, McKay DB, *et al.* Avoidance of cyclosporine in renal transplantation: effects of daclizumab, mycophenolate mofetil, and steroids. J Am Soc Nephrol 2000; 11: 1903-1909.

[61] Vincenti F, Ramos E, Brattstrom C, *et al.* Multicenter trial exploring calcineurin inhibitors avoidance in renal transplantation. Transplantation 2002; 71: 1282-1287.

[62] Groth CG, Backman L, Morales JM, *et al.* Sirolimus (rapamycin)-based therapy in human renal transplantation. Similar efficacy and different toxicity compared with cyclosporine. Transplantation 1999; 67: 1036-1042.

[63] Kreis H Cisterne JM, Land W, *et al.* Sirolimus in association with mycophenolate mofetil induction for the prevention of acute graft rejection in renal allograft recipients. Transplantation 2000; 69:1252-1260.

[64] Flechner SM, Goldfarb D, Modlin C, *et al.* Kidney transplantation without calcineurin inhibitor drugs: a prospective, randomized trial of sirolimus *versus* cyclosporine. Transplantation 2002; 74: 1070-1076.

[65] Larsen S, Dean PG, Stegall MD, *et al.* Complete avoidance of calcineurin inhibitors in renal transplantation: a randomized trial comparing sirolimus and tacrolimus. Am J Transplant 2006; 6: 514-522.

[66] Buchler M, Caillard S, Barbier S, *et al.* Sirolimus *versus* cyclosporine in kidney recipients receiving Thymoglobulin, mycophenolate mofetil and a 6-moth course of steroids. Am J Transplant 2007; 7: 2522-2531.

[67] Ekberg H, Tedesco-Silva H, Demirbas A, *et al.* Reduced exposure to calcineurin inhibitors in renal transplantation. N Engl J Med 2007;357: 2562-2575.

CHAPTER 15

Protocol Biopsies in Renal Transplantation

David Rush*

Transplant Manitoba Adult Kidney Program, University of Manitoba, Winnipeg, MB, Canada

Abstract: Protocol biopsies in renal transplant patients are those that are obtained at preimplantation and at predetermined times post-transplant, even in the absence of renal dysfunction. These biopsies have been invaluable for the study of the "natural history" of allograft histopathology, and have indeed revealed unexpected acute and chronic lesions in well-functioning grafts. Many centres, including ours, are attempting to develop non-invasive biomarkers of early graft injury. However, it is our view that until such tests have been developed and validated, the protocol biopsy will remain a useful tool for the management of renal transplant patients.

Keywords: Renal Transplantation, Protocol Biopsies, Subclinical Acute, Chronic Pathology.

INTRODUCTION

Protocol biopsies have disclosed the early "subclinical" phase of a number of lesions in renal transplant recipients with well functioning grafts, and have thus contributed significantly to the characterization of the natural history of several important entities. These include acute inflammatory states, such as subclinical acute rejection and subclinical peritubular capillaritis, and early chronic lesions, such as interstitial fibrosis and tubular atrophy (IF/TA) and transplant glomerulopathy (TG). An emerging literature suggests that subclinical acute rejection, peritubular capillaritis, IF/TA and TG are associated with subsequent graft dysfunction and loss. The early recognition of these histological changes may therefore provide the opportunity to modify the immunosuppressive regimen and potentially improve both long-term patient and graft survival. Indeed, until non-invasive biomarkers for these pathologies are developed and validated, protocol biopsies may be required for optimal patient care.

SUBCLINICAL ACUTE INFLAMMATION

Subclinical (Cellular) Rejection

Our group in Winnipeg was the first to report that acute rejection – as defined in the Banff schema [1] – was present in up to one-third of well-functioning renal allografts in the first three months in transplant patients receiving the earlier formulation of cyclosporine (CsA), azathioprine and prednisone, and the term "subclinical rejection" was coined [2]. It is however of historical interest that at the Necker Hospital in Paris, Dr. Jean Crosnier described what he called "latent crisis", referring to histological edema and lymphocytic infiltrates in eight patients with normal graft function in whom "systematic (*i.e.* protocol) biopsies" had been procured, and in whom the kidneys became less swollen after treatment with corticosteroids in five cases [3].

Our initial definition of "subclinical" rejection was quite stringent, as it required that the serum creatinine be within 10% of baseline, and that the Banff score was unequivocally "rejection" – *i.e.* "ai2at2" or greater - that is Type I A rejection at a minimum. Subsequent reports in both adults [4-11] and children [12, 13] have confirmed these findings. More recently, several authors have included "borderline" rejection (*e.g.*, ai1at1) in the subclinical rejection category [4, 6, 8-10]. This is most important in patients who in addition have IF/TA, as is discussed below.

In a series of 330 consecutive protocol biopsies in patients on a CsA-based therapeutic regimen and a

***Address correspondence to David Rush:** Transplant Manitoba Adult Kidney Program. 820 Sherbrook Street, Room GE441A, Winnipeg, MB, Canada R3A 1R9; Tel: 204-787-3437; Fax: 204-787-3326; E-mail: drush@hsc.mb.ca

Massimiliano Veroux and Pierfrancesco Veroux (Eds)

prevalence of subclinical rejection of 15%, we found that 75% of subclinical rejection was Banff Type I A and 24 % was Type I B; arteritis (Banff II A or greater) was found in a minority of cases [14]. More recently however, subclinical antibody-mediated rejection has been reported in ABO-incompatible transplants [14] and in transplant patients presensitized to donor HLA antigens [15, 16]. (See also the section on Subclinical peritubular capillaritis.)

Risk Factors for Subclinical Rejection

Histoincompatibility and Presensitization

Subclinical rejection is associated with histoincompatibility between the donor and recipient. In the Winnipeg studies, the prevalence of subclinical rejection in patients biopsied between months one to three was 0-25% with zero Class II mismatches; 30-32% with one class II mismatch; and 30-63% in patients with two Class II mismatches [17]. A correlation between HLA mismatches and the prevalence of subclinical rejection has been reported also by others [7, 11]. Moreover, subclinical rejection is more prevalent in patients presensitized to donor Class I or Class II HLA antigens [18]. Therefore, subclinical rejection appears to be an alloimmune response triggered by either mismatching of, or presensitization to the major histocompatibility antigens.

Immunosuppressive Regimen

The prevalence of subclinical rejection varies depending on whether antibody induction is used or not and on the maintenance immunosuppressive regimen. The first studies using protocol biopsies were in patients that did not receive antibody induction that were treated with CsA-based immunosuppressive regimens [3, 5, 6, 19-21] with [21] or without [3, 5, 6, 19, 20]. MMF. The prevalence of subclinical rejection between months one to three was approximately 25-30%. In some studies, the use of CsA microemulsion [22, 23] and MMF [11, 22, 23] reduced the prevalence of subclinical rejection; but this was not always the case [21]. The introduction of tacrolimus (TAC) with [7, 8, 10, 22, 23] or without [4] MMF reduced the prevalence of subclinical rejection, compared to that observed with CsA. For example Jurewicz reported a prevalence of subclinical rejection of 18% (that included "borderline" rejection) at three months in recipients of kidneys from deceased donors treated with TAC, azathioprine and prednisone [4], compared to our finding of 25-30% [2]. Nankivell *et al.* reported subclinical rejection (including borderline) in over 50% at one month that was virtually abolished at three, six and 12 months in patients on TAC and MMF [23]. Gloor *et al.* reported a similar prevalence of subclinical rejection of only 2.6% at three months in patients on TAC and MMF; however more than 60% of patients had received living donor grafts, and more than 50% had received antibody induction [8]. In very early biopsies (at a mean time eight days post-transplant) in patients receiving TAC and steroids, plus MMF in most, Shapiro *et al.* reported a 21% prevalence of borderline rejection and a prevalence of 25% of Type I or Type II rejection, despite stable or improving function [7]. We have recently reported a randomized, prospective, multicentre study that used TAC, MMF and prednisone as baseline immunosuppression in which the overall prevalence of subclinical rejection between months one to six was only about 4%, although it ranged from 0% at two months to 8.9% at six months [24] .

In contrast to the large amount of data on protocol biopsies in patients using calcineurin inhibitors (CNI), the reports on early protocol biopsies in patients receiving sirolimus (SRL) are very few. In one study [9], protocol biopsies were performed at three months in patients randomized to SRL and low dose TAC ("CNI-sparing"), or SRL and MMF ("CNI-free"). Subclinical rejection was found in 6% and IF/TA in 53% of patients in the CNI sparing regimen, whereas in the CsA-free regimen subclinical rejection and IF/TA were each seen in 15% of patients. In another study, 40 renal transplant patients with HIV infection were treated with basiliximab induction, SRL, CsA and prednisone. Protocol biopsies were obtained at one, six, 12 and 24 months post-transplant. The prevalence of subclinical rejection was 29% at the combined biopsy time points [25]. A more recent study has compared four different immunosuppressive regimens (without steroids) and monitored the patients with sequential protocol biopsies. In this study, 50 adult patients each were randomized to CsA/MMF, CsA/SRL, TAC/MMF and TAC/SRL. Protocol biopsies were done at one, two, six and 12 months and then yearly for five years. In the first year the prevalence of subclinical rejection was 22%, 8%, 16% and 6% respectively, in the order of immunosuppression regimen indicated above [26].

Time Post-Transplant

The prevalence of subclinical rejection decreases over time. In adults, after the first year, the overall prevalence of subclinical rejection was approximately 18% [23], and at two years it was 8.9% in patients on TAC and 9.2% in patients on CsA [27]. In a follow-up of our prospective study of TAC and MMF-based immunosuppression, the prevalence of subclinical rejection at 24 months was only 1% [28]. In children, the prevalence of subclinical rejection also decreased over time in one study, albeit less markedly. The prevalence of subclinical rejection in this study was 50%, 32%, 19% and 16% at one, two, three and five years post-transplant, respectively [12].

Pathogenicity of Subclinical Rejection

The treatment of subclinical rejection has been shown to reduce IF/TA [19] and improve graft function in two randomized studies in recipients of deceased [21] or living donor kidneys [29]. In both of the above studies, the immunosuppressive regimen was based on CsA. In the earlier study from our group, the standard formulation CsA was used in combination with azathioprine; whereas in the second study, CsA microemulsion or TAC, the latter in a small minority, were used in combination with MMF. The prevalence of subclinical rejection in the first three months post-transplantation was approximately 30% in the first study and approximately 15% in the second. In other studies, the pathogenicity of subclinical rejection is suggested by the fact that IF/TA develops in adult recipients of deceased donor kidneys in whom subclinical rejection is diagnosed but not treated [5, 6, 22]. In a cohort of adult recipients of living donor grafts followed for 10 years, the diagnosis of subclinical rejection at 14 days post-transplant was associated with a significantly worse graft survival even if treated, perhaps because there was an increased incidence of late clinical rejection in such patients [11]. In children, the finding of subclinical rejection in serial protocol biopsies (done at one, two, three and five years) was associated with progression of IF/TA and other changes of chronic injury as scored using the chronic allograft damage index (CADI) [30], as well as with decreased renal function and lower graft survival [12].

The pathogenicity of subclinical rejection is supported also by the immunohistochemical characterization of the graft-infiltrating cells and by the analysis of the genes present in the graft across the range of acute inflammation. In the most recent and complete of such studies, Hoffman *et al.* concluded that subclinical rejection and clinical rejection are probably different stages of the same process, as the differences in the phenotype of the infiltrating cells and the gene transcriptional findings observed between the two were quantitative more than qualitative. In clinical rejection however, one novel finding was the increased expression of T-bet, a maturation factor for cytotoxic T cells [31]. Our group in Winnipeg has also studied the phenotypic and activation marker profile of graft-infiltrating cells by immunochemical methods [32] as well as the transcripts for a more limited number of pro-inflammatory and cytotoxic genes [33]. Our conclusions from these studies were essentially the same as those of Hoffman *et al.* [31]. However, more recently, it has been suggested that patients with subclinical rejection in whom the infiltrate has a higher percentage of regulatory T-cells may have a better outcome than those in whom the infiltrate has fewer of these cells [34], and that in patients with borderline rejection that are untreated, those without regulatory T-cells progress to rejection, whereas those with regulatory T-cells don't [35]. It should be noted, however, that regulatory T-cells are found also in clinically rejecting allografts, where their function might be to limit the extent of inflammatory injury [31, 36].

Subclinical Peritubular Capillaritis

Although the Banff schema had always had a score for inflammation in the glomerular capillaries (glomerulitis), there had been no scoring of inflammation in the peritubular capillaries (PTC) until recently [37]. The association between PTC inflammation in early cellular or antibody-mediated rejection and the development of chronic rejection at later time points was first reported by Aita *et al.* [38]. Moreover, Lerut *et al.* demonstrated that PTC inflammation found in a protocol biopsy at three months post-transplant was associated with chronic rejection at one year [39]. In the most comprehensive study on the subject to date, Gibson *et al.* retrospectively analyzed 688 biopsies (46 pre-implantation, 461 protocol and 181 done for clinical indications) and scored these as previously proposed in the Banff Conferences of 2003 and 2005

[37]. Peritubular capillaritis was found in 26.3% of biopsies overall, with a greater prevalence in clinically indicated biopsies (45.5%) as compared to protocol biopsies (17.6%). Of interest, however, in the subgroup of patients with PTC inflammation in protocol biopsies, those with diffuse capillaritis in at least one protocol biopsy had a significant decrease in glomerular filtration rate, as assessed by the Cockroft-Gault equation, when compared to the group that never had PTC inflammation [37]. More recently, our group has found subclinical capillaritis in patients that were biopsied at various times post-transplant because of the *de novo* development of a donor-specific antibody. This work was presented at the American Transplant Congress held in San Diego, USA, in May 2010 (Nickerson *et al.* Am J Transplant 2010; 10 (S4): 124).

SUBCLINICAL INTERSTITIAL FIBROSIS AND TRANSPLANT GLOMERULOPATHY

Interstitial Fibrosis

The more frequent sampling of the tubulo-interstitial space in small biopsy cores makes the scoring of IF/TA more convenient as an outcome measure than the scoring of the less available glomerular and vascular lesions. Moreover, the precise quantitation of the volume of interstitial fibrosis that can be obtained by histomorphometry [40] and with the use of collagen-specific stains such as Sirius Red using image-analysis techniques [41, 42] has been proposed as a more reliable index of tubulointerstitial injury than that determined by the semiquantitative scoring of the Banff [1] and CADI systems [30].

Protocol biopsies obtained in the first year post-transplant have shown a rapid increase in the prevalence of IF/TA. Nankivell *et al.* showed that, compared to biopsies performed at implantation or at one or two weeks, IF/TA increased by a factor of 10 over the first post-transplant year, with less of an increase over the subsequent nine years [43]. In a similar study of shorter duration with biopsies done at one, two, three and six months, our group reported negligible IF/TA at one and two months with a five-fold increase at six months [20]. The prevalence of IF/TA, a designation that is now preferred over the equally non-specific term CAN, in protocol biopsies at three to four months is between 24 and 42% [5, 6, 44], at six months it is approximately 40% [10, 45], and at one year it is approximately 50% [12, 46]. The prevalence of IF/TA is approximately between 50% and 90% at two years [5, 22, 27]. All of the above studies were performed in patients under CsA-based immunosuppression, except for the latter in which the presence of IF/TA was compared between CsA and TAC-treated patients, in both of whom the prevalence of IF/TA was approximately 70% [27]. In our study using TAC and MMF, the prevalence of IF/TA (specifically ci + ct $\geq$2) increased from approximately 2.5% at implantation, to between 20 to 35% at six months, and to between 40 to 50% at 24 months [28].

Finally, recent studies have reported the prevalence of IF/TA in protocol biopsies in patients on sirolimus [26, 47-51]. In one study [47], approximately 32% of patients switched to SRL at three months had new onset IF/TA at one year, as compared to 65% of those maintained on cyclosporine. However this was not confirmed in a recent randomized study in which the extent of fibrosis was assessed morphometrically [48]. In another study, patients randomized to SRL had a 34% prevalence of IF/TA at two years as compared to almost 80% for those on cyclosporine. In a third study, at five years IF/TA was present in 54% of CsA/MMF, 11.6% of CsA/SRL, 38% of TAC/MMF and 14% of TAC/SRL-treated patients, respectively [28]. Finally, other studies have reported that patients randomized to SRL and maintained on that drug had a modest but significantly reduced IF/TA score as compared to patients randomized to and maintained on TAC [50] or CsA [51].

In most of the above studies the histopathological scoring was done according to the Banff schema [2], but in others the CADI system (that includes interstitial fibrosis among other variables) has been used [52, 53]. In one of these [51], protocol biopsies were obtained from patients in the USA and Tricontinental Roche studies at baseline, one and three years (n=739 for all biopsies). In these patients that were treated with CsA, MMF and prednisone, the mean CADI score more than doubled between baseline and 12 months and more than tripled by 36 months.

Risk Factors for Interstitial Fibrosis and Tubular Atrophy

The risk factors for the development of interstitial fibrosis can be arbitrarily defined as "early" –*i.e.* associated with fibrosis at or before one year, or late – *i.e.* associated with fibrosis after one year. By multivariate analysis, a number of risk factors have been correlated with the development of IF/TA that occurs in the first six to 12 months post-transplant. These include donor age, recipient gender (female), ischemia-reperfusion, subclinical and clinical rejections, delayed graft function, nephrocalcinosis related to hyperparathyroidism, and donor age [6, 19, 24, 45, 53]. Fibrosis beyond one year has been correlated with donor age, subclinical and clinical rejections, infection with cytomegalovirus, and episodes of presumed cyclosporine nephrotoxicity in some studies [12, 22, 27, 46, 47, 49] but not others [48]. Most of the data on SRL that were obtained in randomized studies [28, 46-49], with one exception [48] although preliminary, suggest that a maintenance drug regimen that includes a calcineurin inhibitor (CNI) may be a risk factor for late onset interstitial fibrosis. It should be pointed out that, in order to establish with certainty that fibrosis is of new onset (and therefore attributable to post-transplant events), either a pre-implantation biopsy should have been obtained, or that a very early biopsy – *e.g.,* at one month post-transplant – is available. This does not occur in all protocol biopsy studies reported. In our study using TAC and MMF, the only risk factor for IF/TA (ci + ct $\geq$2) at 24 months was having been the recipient of a kidney from a deceased donor; whereas there was significantly less IF/TA in those patients whose hypertension was treated with angiotensin-converting enzyme inhibitors or angiotensin II receptor blockers than in those in whom other types of antihypertensives were used [28].

Significance of IF/TA in Protocol Biopsies

The detection of IF/TA in protocol biopsies procured as early as three to six months post-transplant in well functioning transplants has been correlated with later allograft dysfunction and loss [6, 20, 41, 44]. Similarly, increased chronic scores reported with the CADI system [30] at one year [52] or two years [53], have been correlated with graft losses at three and six years, respectively. Furthermore, the more precise quantitation of interstitial fibrosis at six months using morphometry [40] or Sirius Red staining [41] has been correlated with graft survival and time to graft failure, respectively. However, it has now become apparent that patients with concomitant interstitial inflammation and fibrosis may have a greater risk of graft dysfunction and loss than those patients with fibrosis alone, as has been reported in adults [20, 41, 54, 55]and in children [12]. The degree of inflammation may be irrelevant – *i.e.* it may be below the Banff threshold for rejection [54, 55]. Indeed, a recent study using sequential protocol biopsies showed that persistent inflammation below the Banff threshold for rejection was associated with decreased renal function after one or two years [56].

Transplant Glomerulopathy

The early histological and clinical descriptions of TG in adults [57, 58] and children [59] refer to its usual presentation late post-transplantation, although earlier presentations were also recognized [58, 59], typically with graft dysfunction, proteinuria and a poor prognosis. With the use of protocol biopsies, the Mayo Clinic group at Rochester has contributed greatly to the clinical and pathological understanding of this entity [54, 60].

The cumulative incidence of TG increases from 4% at one year to approximately 20% at five years. In 50% of cases the diagnosis is subclinical – *i.e.* it is found on protocol biopsy; and most of these are found in the first 15 months post-transplant. The early diagnosis of TG may be made in patients that do not have significant proteinuria or impaired renal function, and TG may exist in the absence of other histological changes such as IF/TA [60]. The prognosis is the worst of all pathologies diagnosed on protocol biopsy [54]. Risk factors for TG detected on protocol biopsy are prior rejection and presensitization to class II HLA antigens [60].

SUMMARY

Immunological risk factors are undoubtedly important in determining graft survival, as demonstrated by the correlation between graft survival and HLA matching [61]. Moreover, a recent study has shown that most graft losses are due to alloreactivity, particularly alloantibody against donor HLA [62]. Protocol biopsies have shown that much of this alloreactivity, at least early on, is subclinical. The optimal use of immunosuppressive agents requires that anti-donor alloimmune response be detected by non-invasive tests that would allow for frequent determinations of that response. The urine may be the best medium to look for candidate tests and our group is examining the use of specific chemokines [63], as well as interrogating the urine proteome [64] and metabolome [65] in an attempt to develop such a test.

REFERENCES

[1] Racusen LC, Solez K, Colvin RB, *et al.* The Banff 97 working classification of renal allograft pathology. Kidney Int 1999; 55:713-723.

[2] Rush DN, Henry SF, Jeffery JR, *et al.* Histological findings in early routine biopsies of stable renal allograft recipients. Transplantation 1994; 57:208-211.

[3] J. Crosnier. Résultats de l'homotransplantation chez l'homme. In La transplantation rénale. J. Hamburger, J. Crosnier, J. Dormont, J.F. Bach, eds. Flammarion Médecine-Sciences, Paris, 1971, 203-267.

[4] Jurewicz WA. Immunological and nonimmunological risk factors with tacrolimus and Neoral in renal transplant recipients: an interim report. Transplant Proc 1993; 31(Supp 7A):64S-66S.

[5] Legendre C, Thervet E, Skhiri H, *et al.* Histologic features of chronic allograft nephropathy revealed by protocol biopsies in kidney transplant recipients. Transplantation 1998; 65:1506-1509.

[6] Nankivell BJ, Fenton-Lee CA, Kuypers DR, *et al.* Effect of histological damage on long-term kidney transplant outcome. Transplantation 2001; 71:515-523.

[7] Shapiro R, Randhawa P, Jordan ML, *et al.* An analysis of early renal transplant protocol biopsies – the high incidence of subclinical tubulitis. Am J Transplant 2001; 1:47-50.

[8] Gloor JM, Cohen AJ, Lager DJ, *et al.* Subclinical rejection in tacrolimus-treated renal transplant recipients. Transplantation 2002; 73:1965-1968.

[9] Lo A, Egidi MF, Gaber LW, *et al.* Comparison of sirolimus-based calcineurin inhibitor-sparing and calcineurin inhibitor-free regimens in cadaveric renal transplantation. Transplantation 2004; 77:1228-1235.

[10] Moreso F, Serón D, Carrera M, *et al.* Baseline immunosuppression is associated with histological findings in early protocol biopsies. Transplantation 2004; 78:1064-1068.

[11] Choi BS, Shin MJ, Shin SJ, *et al.* Clinical significance of an early protocol biopsy in living-donor renal transplantation; ten-year experience at a single center. Am J Transplant 2005; 5:1354-1360.

[12] Shishido S, Asanuma H, Nakai H, *et al.* The impact of repeated subclinical acute rejection on the progression of chronic allograft nephropathy. J Am Soc Nephrol 2003; 114:1046-1052.

[13] Birk PE, Stannard KM, Konrad HB, *et al.* Surveillance biopsies are superior to functional studies for the diagnosis of acute and chronic renal allograft pathology in children. Pediatr Transplant 2004; 8:29-38.

[14] Rush D. Controversies in Nephrology: Protocol biopsies should be part of the routine management of kidney transplant recipients. Am J Kid Dis 2002; 40:671-673.

[15] Gloor JM, Cosio FG, Rea DJ, *et al.* Histologic findings one year after positive crossmatch or ABO incompatible living donor kidney transplantation. Am J Transplant 2006; 6:1841-1847.

[16] Kraus ES, Parekh ES, Oberai P, *et al.* Subclinical rejection in stable positive crossmatch kidney transplant patients: incidence and correlations. Am J Transplant 2009; 9:1826-1834.

[17] Rush DN, Grimm P, Gough J, *et al.* Predicting rejection: Is early diagnosis achievable and important? Graft 1999; 2:S31-S35.

[18] Karpinski M, Rush D, Jeffery J, *et al.* Flow cytometric cross-matching in primary renal transplant recipients with a negative anti-human globulin enhanced cytotoxicity cross-match. J Am Soc Nephrol 2001; 12:2807-2814.

[19] Rush DN, Nickerson P, Gough J, *et al.* Beneficial effects of treatment of early subclinical rejection: a randomized study. J Am Soc Nephrol 1998; 9:2129-2134.

[20] Nickerson P, Jeffery JR, Gough J, *et al.* Identification of clinical and histopathologic risk factors for diminished renal function 2 years posttransplant. J Am Soc Nephrol 1998; 9:482-487.

[21] Nickerson P, Jeffery JR, Gough J, *et al.* Effect of increasing baseline immunosuppression on the prevalence of clinical and subclinical rejection: a pilot study. J Am Soc Nephrol 1999; 10:1801-1805.

[22] Nankivell BJ, Borrows RJ, Fung CLS, *et al.* The natural history of chronic allograft nephropathy. N Eng J Med 2003; 349:2326-2333.

[23] Nankivell BJ, Borrows RJ, Fung CLS, *et al.* Natural history, risk factors, and impact of subclinical rejection in renal transplantation. Transplantation 2004; 78:242-249.

[24] Rush D, Arlen D, Boucher A, *et al.* Lack of benefit of early protocol biopsies in renal transplant patients receiving TAC and MMF: a randomized study. Am J Transplant 2007; 7:2538-45.

[25] Kumar MSA, Sierka DR, Damask AM, *et al.* Safety and success of kidney transplantation and concomitant immunosuppression in HIV-positive patients. Kidney Int 2005; 67:1622-1629.

[26] Kumar MSA, Saeed MI, Ranganna K, *et al.* Comparison of four different immunosuppression protocols without long-term steroid therapy in kidney recipients monitored by surveillance biopsy: Five-year outcomes. Transplant Immunol 2008; 20:32-42.

[27] Solez K, Vincenti F, Filo RS. Histopathologic findings from 2-year protocol biopsies from a U.S. multicenter kidney transplant trial comparing tacrolimus versus cyclosporine: a report of the FK506 Kidney Transplant Study Group. Transplantation 1998; 66:1736-1740.

[28] Rush DN, Cockfield SM, Nickerson PW, *et al.* Factors associated with progression of interstitial fibrosis in renal transplant patients receiving tacrolimus and mycophenolate mofetil. Transplantation. 2009; 88:897-903.

[29] Kurtkoti J, Sakhuja V, Sud K, *et al.* The utility of 1- and 3-month protocol biopsies on renal allograft function: a randomized controlled study. Am J Transplant 2008; 8:317-323.

[30] Isoniemi HM, Krogerus L, von Willebrand E, *et al.* Histopathological findings in well-functioning, long-term allografts. Kidney Int 1992; 41:155-160.

[31] Hoffman FC, Hale DA, Kleiner DE, *et al.* Functionally significant renal allograft rejection is defined by transcriptional criteria. Am J Transplant 2005; 5:573-581.

[32] Grimm PC, McKenna R, Nickerson P, *et al.* Clinical rejection is distinguished from subclinical rejection by increased infiltration by a population of activated macrophages, J Am Soc Nephrol 1999; 10:1582-1589.

[33] Lipman ML, Shen Y, Jeffery JR, *et al.* Immune-activation gene expression in clinically stable renal allograft biopsies: molecular evidence for subclinical rejection. Transplantation 1998; 66:1673-1681.

[34] Bestard O, Cruzado JM, Rama I, *et al.* Presence of FoxP3+regulatory T cells predicts outcome of subclinical rejection of renal allografts. J Am Soc Nephrol 2008; 19:2020-2026.

[35] Mansour H, Homs S, Desvaux D, *et al.* Intragraft levels of Foxp3 mRNA predict progression in renal transplants with borderline change, J Am Soc Nephrol 2008; 10:2277-2281.

[36] Veronese F, Rotman S, Smith RN, *et al.* Pathological and clinical correlates of FOXP3+ cells in renal allografts during acute rejection. Am J Transplant 2007; 7:914-922.

[37] Gibson IW, Gwinner W, Bröcker V, *et al.* Peritubular capillaritis in renal allografts: prevalence, scoring system, reproducibility and clinicopathological correlates. Am J Transplant 2008; 8:819-825.

[38] Aita K, Yamaguchi Y, Horita S, *et al.* Peritubular capillaritis in early renal allograft is associated with the development of chronic rejection and chronic allograft nephropathy. Clin Transplant 2005; 19:20-26.

[39] Lerut E, Naesens M, Kuypers DR, *et al.* Subclinical peritubular capillaritis at 3 months is associated with chronic rejection at 1 year. Transplantation 2007; 83:1416-1422.

[40] Nicholson ML, McCulloch TA, Harper SJ, *et al.* Early measurement of interstitial fibrosis predicts long-term renal function and graft survival in renal transplantation. Br J Surgery 1996; 83:1082-1085.

[41] Grimm PC, Nickerson P, Gough J, *et al.* Computerized image analysis of Sirius Red-stained renal allograft biopsies as a surrogate marker to predict long-term allograft function. J Am Soc Nephrol 2003; 14:1662-1668.

[42] Encarnación MM, Griffin MD, Slezak JM, *et al.* Correlation of quantitative digital image with the glomerular filtration rate in chronic allograft nephropathy. Am J Transplant 2003; 4:248-256.

[43] Nankivell BJ, Borrows RJ, Fung CL, *et al.* Delta analysis of posttransplantation tubulointerstitial damage. Transplantation. 2004; 78:434-441.

[44] Serón D, Moreso F, Bover J, *et al.* Early protocol renal allograft biopsies and graft outcome. Kidney Int 1997; 51:310-316.

[45] Schwarz A, Mengel M, Gwinner W, *et al.* Risk factors for chronic allograft nephropathy after renal transplantation: a protocol biopsy study. Kidney Int 2005; 67:341-348.

[46] Serón D, Moreso F, Fulladosa X, *et al.* Reliability of chronic allograft nephropathy diagnosis in sequential protocol biopsies. Kidney Int 2002; 61:727-733.

[47] Ruiz JC, Campistol JM, Grinyó JM, *et al.* Early Cyclosporine A withdrawal in kidney-transplant recipients receiving Sirolimus prevents progression of chronic pathologic allograft lesions. Transplantation 2004; 78:1312-1318.

[48] Servais A, Meas-Yedid V, Toupance O, *et al.* Interstitial fibrosis quantification in renal transplant recipients randomized to continue cyclosporine or convert to sirolimus. Am J Transplant. 2009; 9:2552-2560.

[49] Flechner SM, Kurian SM, Solez K, *et al.* *De novo* kidney transplantation without use of calcineurin inhibitors preserves renal structure and function at two years. Am J Transplant 2004; 4:1776-1785.

[50] Dean PG, Grande JP, Sethi S, *et al.* Kidney transplant histology after one year of continuous therapy with sirolimus compared with tacrolimus. Transplantation 2008; 85:1212-1215.

[51] Mota A, Arias M, Taskinen EI, *et al.* Sirolimus-based therapy following early cyclosporine withdrawal provides significantly improved renal histology and function at 3 years. Am J Transplant 2004; 4:953-961.

[52] Isoniemi H, Taskinen E, Hayry P. Histological chronic allograft damage index accurately predicts chronic renal allograft rejection. Transplantation 1994; 58:1195-1198.

[53] Yilmaz S, Tomlanovich S, Mathew T, *et al.* Protocol core needle biopsy and histologic chronic allograft damage index (CADI) as surrogate end point for long-term graft survival in multicenter studies. J Am Soc Nephrol 2003; 14:773-779.

[54] Cosio FG, Grande JP, Wadei H, *et al.* Predicting subsequent decline in kidney allograft function from early surveillance biopsies. Am J Transplant 2005; 5:2464-2472.

[55] Moreso F, Ibernón M, Goma M, *et al.* Subclinical rejection associated with chronic allograft nephropathy in protocol biopsies as a risk factor for late graft loss. Am J Transplant 2006; 6:747-752.

[56] Mengel M, Gwinner W, Schwarz A, *et al.* Infiltrates in protocol biopsies from renal allografts. Am J Transplant 2007; 7:356-365.

[57] Zollinger HU, Moppert J, Thiel G, *et al.* Morphology and pathogenesis of glomerulopathy in cadaver kidney allografts treated with antilymphocyte globulin. Curr Top Pathol 1973; 57:1-48.

[58] Maryniak M, First MR, Weiss MA. Transplant Glomerulopathy: evolution of morphologically distinct changes. Kidney Int 1985; 27:799-806.

[59] Habib R, Broyer M. Clinical significance of allograft glomerulopathy. Kidney Int 1993; 44 (Suppl 43):S95-98.

[60] Gloor JM, Sethi S, Stegall MD, *et al.* Transplant glomerulopathy: subclinical incidence and association with alloantibody. Am J Transplant 2007; 7:2124-32.

[61] Opelz G, Wujciak T, Dohler B, *et al.* HLA compatibility and organ transplant survival. Collaborative transplant study. Rev Immunogenet 1999; 1:334-342.

[62] El-Zoghby ZM, Stegall MD, Lager DJ, *et al.* Identifying specific causes of kidney allograft loss. Am J Transplant 2009; 9:527-535.

[63] Schaub S, Nickerson P, Rush D, *et al.* Urinary CXCL9 and CXCL10 levels correlate with the extent of subclinical tubulitis. Am J Transplant 2009; 9:1347-1353.

[64] Schaub S, Rush D, Wilkins J, *et al.* Proteomic-based detection of urine proteins associated with acute renal allograft rejection. J Am Soc Nephrol 2004; 15:219-227.

[65] Rush D, Somorjai R, Deslauriers R, *et al.* Subclinical rejection – a potential surrogate marker for chronic rejection – may be diagnosed by protocol biopsy or urine spectroscopy. Ann Transplant 2000; 5:44-49.

CHAPTER 16

Quality of Life After Kidney Transplantation

Kris Denhaerynck[1], Fabienne Dobbels[2], Jürg Steiger[3] and Sabina De Geest[1,2,*]

[1]*Institute of Nursing Science, University of Basel, Basel, Switzerland;* [2]*Center for Health Services and Nursing Research, Katholieke Universiteit Leuven, Leuven, Belgium and* [3]*Department of Transplant Immunology and Nephrology, University Hospital Basel, Basel, Switzerland*

Abstract: This literature review summarizes the research on quality of life (QoL) in kidney transplant recipients. After clarification and discussion of conceptual issues in view of QoL, the following topics are reviewed: comparisons of QoL pre- to post-transplant, post-transplant QoL of kidney transplant recipients to that of other chronically ill patients and of healthy subjects, correlates of QoL, and interventions designed to enhance QoL in kidney transplantation. Gaps in the state-of-the-art evidence, from conceptual, content, and methodological perspectives, are highlighted, and directions for future research are discussed.

Keywords: Quality of Life, Kidney Failure, Chronic/Psychology/Surgery, Kidney Transplantation, Marginal Donor, SF-36, Adherence to Therapy.

INTRODUCTION

Two treatment options are currently available for patients who suffer from end-stage renal disease. Either they receive a kidney transplant or dialysis treatment. The latter solution is time-consuming and uncomfortable for the patient, and offers less favorable survival prospects than transplantation. Transplantation outperforms dialysis in terms of disability-adjusted life years [1, 2]. However, though transplantation is cost-effective and longer-lasting, the threat of declining graft function over time remains a major concern [3]. Maintaining transplant functionality requires a meticulous life-long intake of immunosuppressive medication. Non-adherence to it may result in long-term damage to the transplanted kidney [4, 5]. Additionally, long-term outcomes may be jeopardized by side-effects of the immunosuppression, which include the development of new co-morbidities such as malignancies [6], infections [7], or cardiovascular complications [8]. Thus, though transplantation offers a life of reduced disability, it remains a chronic condition: patients remain dependent on a life-long therapeutic regimen.

Long-term transplantation success has traditionally been measured by objective measures such as rejection and survival rates. Increasingly, however, this evaluation includes the patient's perceived quality of life (QoL). Although it is often used as an umbrella term [9] to covering such concepts as functionality, health status, life conditions, behavior, happiness, lifestyle, symptoms, *etc.* [10], the transplant literature generally refers to QoL as the perceived multidimensional impact of a disease on physical, mental and social functionality, a conceptualization derived from the World Health Organization's holistic definition of health as "a state of complete physical, mental and social well-being and not merely absence of disease or infirmity" [11]. A number of authors have criticized this definition, arguing that the selection of factors that make life valuable should be left to a patient's own discretion, and may include non-health-related aspects [12, 13]. Moreover, it is common practice in transplant research to gauge QoL based on 'perceived health status' data, despite the fact that both theoretical and empirical evidence indicates that patients' perceived health status is not equivalent to a quality judgment of this status [12]. A life that seems undesirable from an external perspective may entirely fulfill expected quality standards in the eye of the person living it (*i.e.* the 'disability paradox') [14]. While health status is an important determinant of QoL, denoting the concept 'quality of life'/'health-related quality of life' is misleading.

***Address correspondence to Sabina De Geest:** Institute of Nursing Science, University of Basel, Bernoullistrasse 28, 4056 Basel, Switzerland; Tel: +41612673040; Fax: +41612670955; E-mail:sabina.degeest@unibas.ch

Massimiliano Veroux and Pierfrancesco Veroux (Eds)

This article reviews and summarizes the literature on quality of life in adult kidney transplant patients. In line with current practice, we have included all studies listing their primary outcome variable as 'QoL', regardless of its conceptualization. More specifically, we have built on the review of Dew *et al.*, who published a comprehensive review on this topic in 1997 [15]. Focusing on the large body of literature that has since been published, we excluded the literature Dew *et al.* had already reviewed, leaving a review period spanning from 1996 to the first half of 2009.

Our search strategy included the databases of Medline, Cinahl, and Psycinfo and was aimed at identifying original empirical research on quality of life in adult kidney transplant patients, using the following (combination of) search terms: (kidney OR renal) AND transplant* AND (quality of life OR QOL OR HRQOL OR health status OR life satisfaction OR well-being). A total of 175 abstracts were found. For this review, 65 articles were returned (see Table **1**), which could be categorized under the following themes: comparisons of pre- and post-transplant QoL, long-term trends in post-transplant QoL, QoL comparisons with other transplant and other chronically ill populations, correlates or determinants of QoL, and QoL enhancing interventions. Each of these themes will be addressed in this review

OVERVIEW OF THE LITERATURE

Of the 65 studies included (Table **1**), the majority were cross-sectional (n=36), followed by prospective cohort studies (n=16) and randomized controlled trials (n=6). Studies were conducted mainly in Europe (n=28) or North-America (n=20), but other regions (n=17) were also represented. As instruments to measure QoL, the Medical outcomes study-Short Form (SF-36) [16] and Sickness Impact Profile (n=6) [17] were used most often.

Comparisons of Post-Transplant and Pre-Transplant Quality of Life

The majority of studies comparing pre- and post-transplant QoL use a cross-sectional design involving one sample of transplant recipients and one of patients awaiting transplants. The remainder prospectively monitors pre-transplant patients through the post-transplantation period. Regardless of their design, however, all show that QoL improves with transplantation [15, 18-30]. Pre- to post-transplant gains are most consistently noted for physical functionality and global QoL [15, 31-33]. However, evidence of improvement in psychological and social functionality is either moderate [15, 34] or too weak to detect [31, 35]. In accordance with the disability paradox described earlier, patients rate their overall QoL as much higher than that in various functional domains, which may reflect a redefinition of life and what it signifies, despite problems in specific aspects of post-transplant functionality [36].

It has been observed that patients who undergo dialysis expect higher QoL gains post-transplant than actually occur [37, 38]. Reasons may be that the patients are not appropriately informed about the treatment after transplantation or do not fully understand the information provided to them. Many of their expectations may not materialize (such as not performing planned traveling after their transplant) [38]. Or they may expect a complete cure from transplantation and freedom from kidney disease treatment, whereas transplantation remains a chronic condition, demanding lifelong treatment alongside active engagement in health care to battle pre-existing and emerging co-morbidities, all of which confronts them with a more nuanced reality [37].

The evidence reported above is derived from quantitative studies indicating that patients show improved QoL after transplantation. Nevertheless, the qualitative study of Orr *et al.* [26] indicates a subgroup of patients who do not follow this general trend. During focus group discussions among 26 patients divided into four groups, one older woman frankly stated that her quality of life had declined since transplantation (although her focus group colleagues attributed this to the effects of advanced age). Another patient showed

Table 1: Quality of life after kidney transplantation: review of literature

Study	Design	Setting	Sample Size and In/Exclusion Criteria	Operationalization of QoL
Aasebo 2005 [61]	RCT	Norway	124 adult RTx, 3w post-Tx, ≥ 95mmHg Excluded: hypersensitivity to calcium-channel blockers or ACE inhibitors, myocardial infarction in previous 6 months and/or stenosis of graft artery	SF-36
Akman 2007 [88]	Cross-sectional	Turkey	68 cadaveric renal Tx waiting list patients	SF-36
Bakewell 2001 [20]	Cross sectional	UK	60 Asian patients > 3m on renal replacement therapy (RTx/haemo-/peritoneal dialysis), matched with 60 European counterparts	Kidney disease and quality o life – short form
Balaska 2003 [35]	Prospective cohort	Greece	85 RTx patients on cyclosporine, steroid & MMF. With creatinine clearance <200 mmol; creatinine =<1.5mg/dl; no rejection, no depression treated with antidepressives	SF-36
Basok 2009 [25]	Cross-sectional	Turkey	106 RTx women	SF-36
Blake 2000 [58]	Cross-sectional	Ireland (multi-center)	60 RTx, 49 haemo- & 35 peritoneal dialysis patients between 18-65y and at least 3 months on the therapy	SF-36
Capocasale 2007 [27]	Cross-sectional	Italy	17 diabetic I patients with renal failure	QoL: anedoctic evidence
Cetingok 2005 [69]	Cross-sectional	USA	219 adult RTx, liver & pancreas Tx	1) Sickness Impact Profile, 2) Quality of Life Index 3) a general quality of life ite 4) Adult self image scales
Chan 2006 [82]	Prospective multi-center cohort	International	278 adult RTx, ≥ 1m post-tx; ≥ 2w on MMF Excluded: not-MMF-related GI symptoms, AR <1m before study start, hospitalized, acute medical intervention	Gastro-intestinal quality of li index
Chang 2004 [90]	Quasi-experimental study	USA	180 adult RTx, no pre-tx diabetes, literate English	1) Sickness impact profile 2) Ferran's and Power's Qua of Life Index 3) Adult Self-Image Scale
Chisholm 2007 [60]	Cross-sectional	US	130 adult RTx patients with functioning graft	SF-12v2
Christensen 2002 [63]	Prospective cohort	US	95 adult, English speaking RTx	Sickness Impact profile
Cofan 2007 [89]	Prospective cohort	Spain	18 stable cadaveric RTx patients ≥ 6 m; between 35-70y, on calcineurin inhibitors, MMF & steroids; and with mild gastrointestinal disorders. Excluded: severe renal failure; acute rejection in past 6m; cardiovascular disease in past 12m; uncontrolled hypertension; hyperthyroidism; severe liver disease; or kidney-pancreas Tx	Gastrointestinal Quality of L Index, measured at baseline 8w
Cornella 2008 [52]	Cross-sectional	US	52 older (> 60y) RTx patients, who were at least 1y in follow up	SF-36
Cure 2008 [44]	Prospective cohort	US	7 diabetic Islet after RTx	1) Health status questionnair 2) Diabetes quality of life questionnaire

Table 1: cont….

Dobbels [55]	Cross-sectional	Belgium	143 RTx patients, 29 heart, 75 liver, 67 lung Tx	EuroQoL	Better
Ekberg 2007 [49]	Cross-sectional	Scandinavian countries	4232 RTx patients	SF-36v2	QoL l Correl sympt
Fallon 1997 [43]	Cross-sectional	UK	30 RTX with > 200mmol/l creatinine clearance. Excluded: significant or co-morbid event which might have affected QoL perception	One item asking for QoL before and after Tx (5-point scale)	Increa betwe
Franke 2006 [77]	Pre-post intervention	Germany	64 RTx pts who switched from cyclosporine to tacrolimus because of side effects. Inclusion criteria: >6m cya based, and one of the following criteria: hypertension (blood pressure ≥18.7 kPa systolic or ≥12 kPa diastolic despite antihypertensive treatment), total cholesterol ≥4.65 mmol/L despite lipid lowering treatment, and disabling gum hyperplasia and/or hypertrichosis requiring intervention	1) SF-36 2) End-Stage Renal Disease Symptom Checklist measured at baseline & 7w	Increa switch
Fujisawa 2000 [21]	Cross-sectional	Japan (2 centers)	117 RTx & 114 haemodialysis patients Excluded if answering < 50% of questions on at least 1 scale	SF-36	Higher pain, g functic hemod
Griva 2002 [40]	Cross-sectional	UK	347 RTx, 1 16y, ≥ 3m post-Tx, not concurrently hospitalized, not treated for rejection or infection, fluent English	SF-36	Worry comor physic
Gross 2004 [91]	Pre-post intervention study	USA	20 adult solid organ Tx patients (85% Rtx), English literate, mentally intact, Minneapolis St-Paul area, have telephone, on standard Tx follow up care	SF-36 measured pre-intervention, post-intervention and 3m	QoL d
Hathaway 1998 [24]	Prospective cohort study	USA	68 adult RTx patients, non-diabetic	1) Sickness Impact profile 2) Ferran's & Powel's QoL index 3) Adult self image scales measured at baseline, 6 & 12m	QoL ir at sam Higher employ less ho
Jofré 1998 [23]	Prospective cohort study	Spain	88 haemo- and peritoneal dialysis patients who received RTx in the upcoming two years	1) Karnofsky Scale 2) Sickness Impact Profile	Qol im
Kachuee 2007 [73]	Cross-sectional	Iran	125 adult stable RTx patients. Excluded: elevated serum creatinine level or any concomitant acute disease	SF-36	Higher functio health
Khedmat 2007 [67]	Cross-sectional	Iran	136 stable 1st RTx patients > 6m post-Tx	SF-36	Lower single/ as reas
Kontodimopoulos 2009 [48]	Cross-sectional	Greece, multi-center	874 adult RTx, >1y post-Tx, without cognitive problems, able to understand Greek	SF-36	Tx pati genera except
Liu 2008 [51]	Cross-sectional	US	138 adult RTx patients with functioning graft	SF-36	Lower older. I genera womer
Lumsdaine 2005 [29]	Prospective cohort study	UK (2 centers)	49 adult RTx patients	WHOQOL-Bref	Both p increas scores QoL hi
Manu 2001 [53]	Descriptive	Romania	92 RTX; 66 hemodialysis; 21 urolithasis & renal failure (Romania)	SF-36	QoL hi > tx >

Table 1: cont….

Matas 2002 [64]	Prospective cohort study	US	4247 recipients of a solid organ transplant taking Sandimmune or Neoral and who had been transplanted for at least 90 d	Life Satisfaction Index
Mitsui 2009 [97]	Cross-sectional	Japan	43 RTx patients >6m post-Tx	QoL score
Molnar 2007 [74]	Cross sectional	Canada	785 cadaveric RTx patients	Kidney Disease QoL-SF
Moloney 2005 [57]	Cross-sectional	Ireland	173 RTx, > 16y, attending dermatology clinic	Dermatology Life Quality In
Moons 2003 [47]	Cross-sectional	Belgium (3 centers)	350 adult RTx patients, ≥ 6m post-tx and/or ≥ 6m on tacrolimus, 1st tx. Excluded: multi-transplants	1) Euroqol-5 dimensions 2) Euroqol-VAS 3) SF-36
Neipp 2006 [41]	Cross-sectional	Germany	139 adult RTx patients, > 15y after Tx. Excluded: multi-organ recipients at time of study	1) SF-36 2) the Disease-specific kidne transplant questionnaire
Noohi 2007[62]	Cross-sectional	Iran	162 RTx patients	SF-36
Noohi 2007[75]	Cross-sectional	Iran	88 RTx patients, of stable clinical condition, no acute concomitant disease, >6m post-tx	SF-36
Nourbala 2007 [72]	Case-control matched for age, sex, total family income, & educational level	Iran	205 RTx patients, 69 hemodialysis patients, 100 healthy controls. Inclusion: stable clinical conditions, absence of acute concomitant diseases/infections, > 6m on hemodialysis if RTx and an overall elapsed time of at least 6 months postTx and satisfactory state of kidney function if dialysis	SF-36
Oberbauer 2003 [78]	RCT	International multi-center study	361 (118 sirolimus + steroids ; 126 sirolimus + steroids + cyclosporine). Excluded: Banff grade 3 acute/vascular rejection in month preceding random assignment, dialysis dependency, serum creatinine level > 400 μM, inadequate renal function to support CsA elimination	1) SF-36 2) the Disease-specific kidne transplant questionnaire
Oppenheimer 2008 [80]	RCT (phase III/IV substudy)	Spain	156 RTx patients on 1) standard CsA, 2) low CsA, 3) low tacrolimus and 4) low sirolimus	SF-36, measured at 1, 3, 6, a 12 months post-transplant
Orr 2007 [26]	Qualitative	UK	26 patients in 4 focus groups	
Ortega 2000 [34]	Cross-sectional	Spain (multi-center)	210 RTx ≥ 3m. Excluded: significant Mini-Mental State Examination score ≤ 17 points, 2) Graft loss during data collection 170 haemodialysis	1) Karnofsky performance s 2) Sickness impact profile 3) SF-36
Özçürümez 2004 [39]	Descriptive	Turkey	49 RTx	a question about the level of satisfaction with quality of l after transplantation
Painter 2002 [98]	RCT	US	167 RTx within 2m after Tx. Excluded if rejection/psychiatric/neurological disorder precluding participation; orthopedic limitations precluding exercise testing/training; unavailable for regular follow-up; contra-indications to exercise testing as established be the American Heart Association/American College of Sports Medicine, medical complications preventing regular participation.	SF-36

Table 1: cont….

Painter 2003 [50]	RCT	US	adult RTx, N= 14 standard maintenance immunosuppression, including prednisone; N=9 rapid withdrawal of steroids using Simulect® Excluded if positive T-cell cross match or ABO incompatibility against the donor; multiple organ transplants; evidence of transplant rejection; increased risk for graft rejection; panel reactive antibody level >30% at the time of T; HIV positivity; active hepatitis; history of malignancy; history of myocardial infarction within six months prior to the study; or cardiac arrhythmias or other severe or unstable medical conditions, orthopedic or musculoskeletal disorders preventing completion of the exercise testing or any absolute contraindications to exercise testing as established by the American Heart Association or American College of Sports Medicine	SF-36	Larger compo withdra prednis
Panagopoulou 2009 [99]	Cross-sectional	Greece	48 RTx patients, 40 haemo-, 36 peritoneal dialysis	1) Rating QoL & Health status on a scale from 0 (very bad) to 10 (excellent), 2) Functional status Karnovsky scale (0-100)	Karnov Tx (no
Pérez-San-Gregorio 2006 [100]	Prospective cohort study	Spain	166 Liver Tx, RTx (42.8%), Heart Tx patients	A Questionnaire of Quality of Life focusing on physical, role, social, emotional, and cognitive issues, measured immediately after Tx, and after 1y	Negati and lon
Pinson 2000 [54]	Prospective cohort study	US	24 RTx, 53 liver, 33 heart, 27 lung Tx patients,	1) Karnovsky Performance Status 2) SF-36 3) Psychosocial Adjustment to Illness Scale	QoL hi Rtx pat lung T RTx pa similar
Reimer 2005 [76]	Prospectice cohort study	Germany	RTx patients (63 taking tacrolimus and 63 in a matched cyclosporin micro-emulsion group)	1) SF-36 2) the ESRD Symptom Checklist - Transplantation Module measured at baseline and 1y	QoL hi instrum
Rosenberger 2005 [59]	Cross-sectional	Slovakia (2 centers)	128 adult RTx, >3m and <7y post-transplant	SF-36	Older a educati hospita predict
Rosenberger 2006 [65]	Cross-sectional	Slovakia (2 centers)	138 adult RTx, >3m and <7y post-transplant. Excluded: dementia or severe mental retardation	SF-36	Predict <40y: s stress f 40–59y housek from ac >60y: l hospita from ac
Russ 2007 [79]	RCT	US	361 RTx patients, >13y Group 1) siro+CsA+ST (n=178); group 2) siro+ST (n=183) with gradual elimination of CsA Exclusion: Banff grade 3 AR or vascular rejection within 4w before randomization, post-tx dialysis dependency, serum creatinine >400 µm, or inadequate renal function that precluded elimination of CsA	1) SF-36 2) Kidney Transplant Questionnaire measured at 3, 12, 24 & 36 months	SF-36: health, favouri KTQ: scores
Sayin 2008 [33]	Cross-sectional	Turkey	75 haemo-, 41 peritoneal dialysis, 20 RTx	SF-36	Tx pati than di lower t

Table 1: cont….

Shah 2006 [66]	Cross-sectional	US	50 RTx patients free of acute medical problems	Quality of Life Scale
Smith 2008 [38]	Cross-sectional	US	307 pts on waiting list for Tx	1) QoL on a scale of 0-100, SF-12
	Prospective cohort		33 (post-Tx op 6 & 12m)	
Suresh-kumar 2006 [32]	Cross-sectional	US	120 type 1 diabetes pts (cadaver kidney RTx; living donor RTx; pancreas-kidney tx; wait-listed pts)	1) Diabetes QoL questionna 2) SF-36, 3) Quality of well-being questionnaire
	Prospective cohort		29 type 1 diabetes pts (pancreas-kidney Tx, cadaver kidney Tx)	idem ditto measured over 3 years
Suzuki 2008 [28]	Prospective cohort	Japan	8 Type I diabetics with living pancreas and RTx	SF-36 v2, measured at pre-t 12 & 24 months
Tanriverdi 2004 [46]	Cross-sectional	Turkey	49 RTx patients; 45 healthy controls	SF-36
Tomasz 2003 [19]	Cross-sectional	Poland	83 RTx & 61 haemodialysis patients	WHOQOL-100
Tsuji-Hayashi 1999 [42]	Cross-sectional	Japan	472 RTx patients, ≥ 16y, ≥ 1y post-tx	SF-36
Virzi 2007 [30]	Prospective cohort	Italy	48 adult living RTx patients	SF-36, measured at 1m pre- 6 m post-Tx
Yildrim 2006 [18]	Cross-sectional	Turkey	104 haemo-, 186 peritoneal dialysis, 356 RTx patients	1) the Patient Satisfaction Questionnaire III (PSQ-18), the '15D'

Abbreviations: QoL: quality of life; RCT: randomized controlled trial; (R)Tx : (renal) transplantation; w=week, m=month, y=year; SF-36: medical outc signs of disappointment with the QoL increase, complaining, for example, about the medications' side effects. A small sub-sample of recipients reporting dissatisfaction with their post-transplant QoL also occurs in the descriptive study of Özçürümez [39]. Though the overall trend in both studies was toward improved QoL, it would be very interesting to focus on the deviating subgroups because they may provide deeper insight into what determines suboptimal QoL [40].

Long-Term Post-Transplant Quality of Life

Most studies investigating quality of life over time have a prospective design and focus on the early post-transplant period. A minority have follow-up periods beyond 5 years post-transplant. The project spanning the longest period is actually a cross-sectional study, comparing different groups of patients with functioning grafts between transplantation and up to 32 years post-transplant. This study found that long-term QoL scores are mainly comparable to those of recipients within the first year post-transplant – the exception being physical functionality, where scores declined [41]. Similar results can also be found in other reports [31, 42], although it should be noted that focusing on patients with functioning grafts may introduce survival bias. Alternative views on the trajectory of QoL over time suggest that QoL follows a rather U-shaped pattern. After the first year post-transplant, for example, Fallon *et al.* found that QoL dipped, recovering after approximately five years [43]. A similar observation is reported in a 3-year follow up study by Cure *et al.* [44], in which QoL declined after the first year post-transplant. One possible explanation is that the observed U-form actually reflects two simultaneous processes – the downturn process resulting from the summed effect of QoL-lowering factors (*i.e.* comorbidities, age and the long-term immunosuppressive therapy) – the upward trend from a survival bias of healthier counterparts staying in the study.

Comparison with other Populations

Notwithstanding the obvious improvements that result from transplantation, transplant patients do not typically regain a QoL equivalent to the general population regarding physical functionality, social activity or general perceived health [15, 31, 42, 45-52]. Not all studies, however, confirmed these results [25, 34, 40, 53], although this was likely due to a lack of statistical power.

Compared to other chronically ill populations (*e.g.*, other transplant groups, urolithiasis patients), kidney transplant patients show similar or higher QoL, at least with respect to physical function and overall QoL perceptions [15, 53]. In two studies, kidney transplant recipients appeared to have higher QoL in the immediate post-transplant period than heart, liver and lung transplant recipients [54, 55], even approaching the level of the general population [55]. However, unlike heart, liver and lung transplant recipients, their scores tended not to increase during the first two post-transplant years [54]. Another study showed that more than 10 years post-transplant, the QoL of kidney transplant patients was comparable to that of heart transplant recipients, but lower than that of long term liver transplant recipients regarding psychological functionality and general health perception [56].

Correlates or Determinants of Quality of Life

To organize the presentation of the found correlates of QoL in the following section of this article, we subdivided them according to whether they were socio-demographic, condition-, treatment-, or healthcare team/worker-related.

Socio-Demographic Correlates

Compared to men, women show lower levels of QoL regarding both physical and mental functionality [18, 34, 50, 51, 57, 58]. Increased age is also associated with lower QoL [23, 51, 59, 60], particularly for the physical component [34, 58, 61, 62]. In contrast, mental health functions show improvement in some studies [40, 61, 62]. This may be because older patients accumulate more coping or adaptation skills, or have stronger social networks, which are clearly beneficial for QoL [63]. Patients who live in close relationships have a higher social and psychological QoL than those who do not [18, 24, 41, 64-67].

QoL is higher among individuals who have received higher education [18, 34, 59, 67] or are employed [18, 24, 41, 58, 68]. These two factors may, in fact, be related: education may ensure employment, and consequently a higher income [40], leading to better healthcare access/insurance [64, 69], a stronger social support network and greater levels of personal satisfaction [70]. Note that post-transplant employment rates are comparable to pre-transplant levels, ranging between 30 and 60% [31, 70]. It is not entirely clear why more patients do not re-enter the workforce after transplantation. Fear of rejection, physical impairment, the depressed situation of the labor market, and lack of willingness to give up disability benefits have all been put forward to explain high post-transplant unemployment rates [31]. The fact that a considerable proportion of kidney transplant patients have passed or are approaching retirement age [71] may also be an explanation.

Another demographic variable that has been linked to QoL is ethnicity. This is often a proxy for social class, as it is linked with education and employment. White persons show the highest QoL, followed by African Americans, followed in turn by other ethnicities [60]. Despite their excellent graft outcomes, people from Asian descent demonstrate low physical and psychological QoL compared to people of European decent, which may be explained by the conditions of social deprivation they often live in (*i.e.* suboptimal living circumstances in terms of job opportunities and housing) [20].

Condition- Related Correlates

Poorer QoL is associated with factors such as co-morbidity (*e.g.*, presence of diabetes, ischemic heart disease), postoperative complications [20, 23, 31, 40, 42, 58, 61, 64, 67, 68], pain [72, 73] and restless legs [74]. Longer periods spent on dialysis [40, 60] and longer cold ischemic time [61] are linked negatively with the physical component of a patient's functioning. Higher numbers of histocompatibility antigen mismatches are associated with decreased mental functionality [61]. The latter analysis was not controlled for age, but not for type of donation. However, no differences in QoL were observed between living and deceased donor recipients [40, 61].

The following psychological factors correlate with higher overall QoL: fewer depressive symptoms [47, 63, 65, 68], less transplant-related worrying [40] and less perceived effect of the illness on the recipients' functionality [66]. Patients with psychiatric disorders, or who hold the opinion that preoperative information is inadequate, are more dissatisfied post-transplant [39]. Quality of sleep correlates positively with mental and physical health [73] and negatively with anxiety/depressed mood [75].

Treatment-Related Factors

One of the most widely investigated treatment related factors is the immunosuppressive regimen. Patients who have been prescribed steroid-free regimens show higher social functionality, general mental health [47], vitality and physical component scores than patients receiving steroids [50]. Likewise, patients on tacrolimus-based regimens show higher scores than on tacrolimus-free regimens [45, 76, 77]. Higher scores regarding vitality and psychosocial functions are also observed in patients receiving sirolimus/steroid-based therapy as compared to those receiving sirolimus/steroid plus cyclosporine therapy [78, 79]. One four-group randomized controlled study in which a regimen of mycophenolate and corticosteroids was supplemented with low doses or tacrolimus, cyclosporine, and sirolimus, respectively, did not yield QoL data significantly different from the standard high-dose cyclosporine treatment [80].

It can be argued that the differences in QoL between the drugs reflect their side effect profiles as experienced by the patient. Examples of side effects associated with lower QoL [68, 78] are sexual dysfunction [64, 81], skin related symptoms (*e.g.*, dry, itchy skin, acne, genital warts, gland hyperplasia) [57], headache [64] and gastrointestinal complaints [77, 82]. Though none of these are serious in terms of mortality risk, all are important from a patient's viewpoint. The patient viewpoint on side-effects is increasingly recognized as relevant, as the symptoms experienced are an important determinant both of QoL and of non-adherence [65, 83-87], two inter-related variables [88]. One rather small study (n=18) supporting the association between side-effects and QoL shows that improved gastro-intestinal QoL can be detected in deceased-donor recipients given an enteric-coated mycophenolate formula as compared to those receiving the standard mycophenolate mofetil medication [89].

Healthcare Team- and Healthcare System-Related Factors

Few studies have been published on the relationship between healthcare team/system-related factors and QoL. We found one report, that reported a lower QoL among patients who were insured under the American Medicare program [60]. More research is needed on this important category of factors.

Quality of Life Enhancing Interventions

A small number of studies examine interventions designed to enhance quality of life. One tested an interdisciplinary treatment approach, consisting of: 1) proactive, patient-initiated care to prevent transplant-related morbidities; 2) employment/vocational counseling; and 3) enhanced social support, finding QoL improvements in a cost-effective way [90]. Using a pre-post design, another intervention study evaluated the effect of mindfulness therapy, showing promising results in reducing depression, anxiety, and symptom distress. However, no effect on QoL was demonstrated [91].

DISCUSSION

One of the most important outcomes of this review was our confirmation of previous research in this domain that QoL is higher post-transplant than pre-transplant. Though it may not be restored to the level of a healthy person, the overall level of QoL after kidney transplantation is comparable to that of other chronically ill populations, and may be considered good to excellent in the majority of cases. Dissatisfaction with post-transplant QoL was expressed by a small minority of recipients. Because the vast majority of published research is quantitative, there is ample room for in-depth exploration of topics using qualitative methods (*e.g.,* why certain patients report declining QoL). One shortcoming of the reviewed studies is that most of them were from the immediate post-transplant period, when QoL improvements tend to be most apparent. Knowledge of long-term QoL trends is scant. Where available, it is collected in part by cross-sectional studies, which are of limited value in answering longitudinal questions, as they compare patients at different post-transplant times to each other rather than following up individuals over time.

As a second important group of findings, we found evidence linking QoL with several socio-demographic (*e.g.,* social support), condition-related (*e.g.,* comorbidities), treatment-related (*e.g.,* immunosuppressive regimens), and healthcare team/system-related (*i.e.* insurance) factors. Despite the fact that the latter category may contain a number of powerful QoL determinants, it was underrepresented as a source of correlates. Future research for determinants of QoL should therefore attach a high priority to healthcare system factors. Appropriate research models to investigate data structures involving system-level data have already been successfully implemented in other disciplines, such as in education (*e.g.,* effects of school-level variables on pupil achievement) or other medical area's (*e.g.,* variables related to general practices explaining patients' treatment success) [92-94]. Analogous study design and analysis strategies as the ones used in these fields could be used to focus on factors influencing QoL in kidney transplantation. More specifically, a multi-level framework representing patient-related factors, nested within a hierarchical set of healthcare system variables, should be conceived as a guide for the design of system-oriented multi-center studies [94, 95].

However, before such large-scale research is initiated, conceptual problems surrounding the term 'quality of life' should be resolved. Despite the lack of consensus on such a definition, little effort is currently being made to clarify the conceptual and theoretical underpinnings of QoL [96]. Such groundwork represents the most urgent research priority in QoL research: it is fundamental to the sound construction of a relevant body of knowledge upon which to base QoL enhancing interventions.

CONCLUSIONS

In summary, this literature review on quality of life in kidney transplant recipients confirms that transplantation restores QoL to a level satisfactory to the majority of patients, although a small number express disappointment in the degree of improvement, and QoL may decline over time. The knowledge to fully understand the processes that determine QoL is not yet available; however, given the increased importance of QoL in the evaluation of kidney transplantation outcomes, researchers should proceed by studying predictors of QoL. First, though, they should pursue a sound conceptualization of quality of life.

REFERENCES

[1] Kaminota M. Cost-effectiveness analysis of dialysis and kidney transplants in Japan. Keio J Med 2001;50:100-108.

[2] de Wit GA, Ramsteijn PG, de Charro FT. Economic evaluation of end stage renal disease treatment. Health policy (Amsterdam, Netherlands). 1998;44:215-232.

[3] Ponticelli C. Renal transplantation 2004: where do we stand today? Nephrol Dial Transplant 2004;19:2937-2947.

[4] Denhaerynck K, Dobbels F, Cleemput I, *et al.* Prevalence, consequences, and determinants of nonadherence in adult renal transplant patients: a literature review. Transpl Int. 2005;18:1121-1133.

[5] Lerut E, Kuypers DR, Verbeken E, *et al.* Acute rejection in non-compliant renal allograft recipients: a distinct morphology. Clin Transplant 2007;21:344-351.

[6] Kauffman HM, Cherikh WS, McBride MA, *et al.*Post-transplant *de novo* malignancies in renal transplant recipients: the past and present. Transpl Int. 2006;19:607-620.

[7] Parasuraman R, Yee J, Karthikeyan V, del Busto R. Infectious complications in renal transplant recipients. Adv Chronic Kid Dis. 2006;13:280-294.

[8] Ojo AO. Cardiovascular complications after renal transplantation and their prevention. Transplantation. 2006;82:603-611.

[9] Feinstein AR. Clinimetric perspectives. J Chronic Dis. 1987;40:635-640.

[10] Simko LC. Adults with congenital heart disease: utilizing quality of life and Husted's nursing theory as a conceptual framework. Critical care nursing quarterly. 1999;22:1-11.

[11] WHO. Constitution of the WHO: Basic documents. Geneva: World Health Organisation 1948.

[12] Moons P. Why call it health-related quality of life when you mean perceived health status? Eur J Cardiovasc Nurs. 2004;3:275-277.

[13] Gill TM, Feinstein AR. A critical appraisal of the quality of quality-of-life measurements. JAMA. 1994;272:619-626.

[14] Albrecht GL, Devlieger PJ. The disability paradox: high quality of life against all odds. Social science & medicine (1982). 1999 Apr;48(8):977-988.

[15] Dew MA, Switzer GE, Goycoolea JM, *et al.* Does transplantation produce quality of life benefits? A quantitative analysis of the literature. Transplantation. 1997;64:1261-1273.

[16] Ware JE, Jr., Sherbourne CD. The MOS 36-item short-form health survey (SF-36). I. Conceptual framework and item selection. Medical care. 1992;30:473-483.

[17] Bergner M, Bobbitt RA, Kressel S, *et al.* The sickness impact profile: conceptual formulation and methodology for the development of a health status measure. Int J Health Serv. 1976;6:393-415.

[18] Yildirim A. The importance of patient satisfaction and health-related quality of life after renal transplantation. Transplant Proc. 2006;38:2831-2834.

[19] Tomasz W, Piotr S. A trial of objective comparison of quality of life between chronic renal failure patients treated with hemodialysis and renal transplantation. Ann Transplant. 2003;8:47-53.

[20] Bakewell AB, Higgins RM, Edmunds ME. Does ethnicity influence perceived quality of life of patients on dialysis and following renal transplant? Nephrol Dial Transplant. 2001;16:1395-1401.

[21] Fujisawa M, Ichikawa Y, Yoshiya K, *et al.* Assessment of health-related quality of life in renal transplant and hemodialysis patients using the SF-36 health survey. Urology. 2000;56:201-206.

[22] Cameron JI, Whiteside C, Katz J, Devins GM. Differences in quality of life across renal replacement therapies: a meta-analytic comparison. Am J Kidney Dis. 2000;35:629-637.

[23] Jofre R, Lopez-Gomez JM, Moreno F, *et al.* Changes in quality of life after renal transplantation. Am J Kidney Dis. 1998;32:93-100.

[24] Hathaway DK, Winsett RP, Johnson C, *et al.* Post kidney transplant quality of life prediction models. Clin Transplant 1998;12:168-174.

[25] Basok EK, Atsu N, Rifaioglu MM, *et al.* Assessment of female sexual function and quality of life in predialysis, peritoneal dialysis, hemodialysis, and renal transplant patients. Int Urol Nephrol 2009;41:473.

[26] Orr A, Willis S, Holmes M, *et al.* Living with a kidney transplant: a qualitative investigation of quality of life. J Health Psych 2007;12:653-662.

[27] Capocasale E, Busi N, Mazzoni MP, *et al.* Simultaneous kidney-pancreas transplantation: the Parma Center experience. Acta Biomed. 2007;78:123-127.

[28] Suzuki A, Kenmochi T, Maruyama M, *et al.* Evaluation of quality of life after simultaneous pancreas and kidney transplantation from living donors using short form 36. Transplant Proc 2008;40:2565-2567.

[29] Lumsdaine JA, Wray A, Power MJ, *et al.* Higher quality of life in living donor kidney transplantation: prospective cohort study. Transpl Int. 2005;18:975-980.

[30] Virzi A, Signorelli MS, Veroux M, *et al.* Depression and quality of life in living related renal transplantation. Transplant Proc 2007;39:1791-1793.

[31] Overbeck I, Bartels M, Decker O, *et al.* Changes in quality of life after renal transplantation. Transplant Proc 2005;37:1618-1621.

[32] Sureshkumar KK, Patel BM, Markatos A, *et al.* Quality of life after organ transplantation in type 1 diabetics with end-stage renal disease. Clin Transplant 2006;20:19-25.

[33] Sayin A, Mutluay R, Sindel S. Quality of life in hemodialysis, peritoneal dialysis, and transplantation patients. Transplant Proc 2007;39:3047-3053.

[34] Rebollo P, Ortega F, Baltar JM, *et al.* Health related quality of life (HRQOL) of kidney transplanted patients: variables that influence it. Clin Transplant 2000;14:199-207.

[35] Balaska A, Moustafellos P, Gourgiotis S, *et al.* Changes in health-related quality of life in Greek adult patients 1 year after successful renal transplantation. Exp Clin Transplant. 2006;4:521-524.

[36] Simmons RG, Klein S, Simmons RL. Gift of life. NY: John Wiley & Sons 1977.

[37] Cleemput I, Kesteloot K, De Geest S, *et al.* Health professionals' perceptions of health status after renal transplantation: a comparison with transplantation candidates' expectations. Transplantation 2003;76:176-182.

[38] Smith D, Loewenstein G, Jepson C, *et al.* Mispredicting and misremembering: patients with renal failure overestimate improvements in quality of life after a kidney transplant. Health Psychol. 2008;27:653-658.

[39] Ozcurumez G, Tanriverdi N, Colak T, *et al.* The psychosocial impact of renal transplantation on living related donors and recipients: preliminary report. Transplant Proc 2004;36:114-116.

[40] Griva K, Ziegelmann JP, Thompson D, *et al.* Quality of life and emotional responses in cadaver and living related renal transplant recipients. Nephrol Dial Transplant 2002;17:2204-11.

[41] Neipp M, Karavul B, Jackobs S, *et al.* Quality of life in adult transplant recipients more than 15 years after kidney transplantation. Transplantation. 2006;81:1640-1644.

[42] Tsuji-Hayashi Y, Fukuhara S, Green J, *et al.* Health-related quality of life among renal-transplant recipients in Japan. Transplantation. 1999;68:1331-1335.

[43] Fallon M, Gould D, Wainwright SP. Stress and quality of life in the renal transplant patient: a preliminary investigation. J Adv Nurs 1997;25:562-270.

[44] Cure P, Pileggi A, Froud T, *et al.* Improved metabolic control and quality of life in seven patients with type 1 diabetes following islet after kidney transplantation. Transplantation 2008;85:801-812.

[45] Bohlke M, Rocha M, Gomes RH, *et al.* Tacrolimus and quality of life after kidney transplantation--a multicenter study. Clin Transplant 2006;20:504-508.

[46] Tanriverdi N, Ozcurumez G, Colak T, *et al.* Quality of life and mood in renal transplantation recipients, donors, and controls: preliminary report. Transplant Proc 2004;36:117-119.

[47] Moons P, Vanrenterghem Y, Van Hooff JP, *et al.* Health-related quality of life and symptom experience in tacrolimus-based regimens after renal transplantation: a multicentre study. Transpl Int. 2003;16:653-664.

[48] Kontodimopoulos N, Pappa E, Niakas D. Gender- and age-related benefit of renal replacement therapy on health-related quality of life. Scand J Car Sci 2009:24.

[49] Ekberg H, Kyllonen L, Madsen S, *et al.* Increased prevalence of gastrointestinal symptoms associated with impaired quality of life in renal transplant recipients. Transplantation. 2007;83:282-289.

[50] Painter PL, Topp KS, Krasnoff JB, *et al.* Health-related fitness and quality of life following steroid withdrawal in renal transplant recipients. Kidney Int 2003;63:2309-2316.

[51] Liu H, Feurer ID, Dwyer K, *et al.* The effects of gender and age on health-related quality of life following kidney transplantation. Journal of clinical nursing. 2008;17:82-89.

[52] Cornella C, Brustia M, Lazzarich E, *et al.* Quality of life in renal transplant patients over 60 years of age. Transplant Proc 2008;40:1865-1866.

[53] Manu MA, Radulescu S, Harza M, *et al* Quality of life assessed by SF-36 health survey in renal transplant patients. Transplant Proc 2001;33:1927-1928.

[54] Pinson CW, Feurer ID, Payne JL, *et al.*Health-related quality of life after different types of solid organ transplantation. Ann Surg. 2000;232:597-607.

[55] Dobbels F, Wernli-Fluri C, Denhaerynck K, *et al.* Comparison of perceived health status among solid organ transplant candidates. Clin Transplant 2009; epub ahead of print

[56] Karam VH, Gasquet I, Delvart V, *et al.* Quality of life in adult survivors beyond 10 years after liver, kidney, and heart transplantation. Transplantation. 2003;76:1699-1704.

[57] Moloney FJ, Keane S, O'Kelly P, *et al.* The impact of skin disease following renal transplantation on quality of life. Brit J Dermatol 2005;153:574-578.

[58] Blake C, Codd MB, Cassidy A, O'Meara YM. Physical function, employment and quality of life in end-stage renal disease. J Nephrol 2000;13:142-149.

[59] Rosenberger J, van Dijk JP, Nagyova I, *et al.* Do dialysis- and transplantation-related medical factors affect perceived health status? Nephrol Dial Transplant. 2005;20:2153-2158.

[60] Chisholm MA, Spivey CA, Nus AV. Influence of economic and demographic factors on quality of life in renal transplant recipients. Clin Transplant 2007;21:285-293.

[61] Aasebo W, Midtvedt K, Hartmann A, Stavem K. Predictors of health-related quality of life in hypertensive recipients following renal transplantation. Clin Transplant 2005;19:756-762.

[62] Noohi S, Karami GR, Lorgard-Dezfuli-Nejad M, *et al.* Are all domains of quality of life poor among elderly kidney recipients? Transplant Proc. 2007;39:1079-1081.

[63] Christensen AJ, Raichle K, Ehlers SL, Bertolatus AJ. Effect of family environment and donor source on patient quality of life following renal transplantation. Health Psychol. 2002;21:468-476.

[64] Matas AJ, Halbert RJ, Barr ML, *et al.* Life satisfaction and adverse effects in renal transplant recipients: a longitudinal analysis. Clin Transplant 2002;16:113-121.

[65] Rosenberger J, van Dijk JP, Nagyova I, *et al.* Predictors of perceived health status in patients after kidney transplantation. Transplantation. 2006;81:1306-1310.

[66] Shah VS, Ananth A, Sohal GK, *et al.* Quality of life and psychosocial factors in renal transplant recipients. Transplant Proc. 2006;38:1283-1285.

[67] Khedmat H, Karami GR, Pourfarziani V, *et al.* A logistic regression model for predicting health-related quality of life in kidney transplant recipients. Transplant Proc 2007;39:917-922.

[68] Muehrer RJ, Becker BN. Life after transplantation: new transitions in quality of life and psychological distress. Semin Dial 2005;18:124-131.

[69] Cetingok M, Hathaway DK, Winsett RR. Differences in quality of life before transplantation among transplant recipients with respect to selected socioeconomic variables. Progress in transplantation (Aliso Viejo, Calif. 2005;15:338-344.

[70] Keown PA. Composite outcomes in renal transplantation using cyclosporine. Transplant Proc 2004;36:35S-9S.

[71] Administration HRaS. Annual Report of the U.S. Organ Procurement and Transplantation Network and the Scientific Registry of Transplant Recipients: Transplant Data 1997-2006. Rockville, MD: Healthcare Systems Bureau, Division of Transplantation; 2007.

[72] Nourbala MH, Hollisaaz MT, Nasiri M, *et al.* Pain affects health-related quality of life in kidney transplant recipients. Transplant Proc 2007;39:1126-1129.

[73] Kachuee H, Ameli J, Taheri S, *et al.* Sleep quality and its correlates in renal transplant patients. Transplant Proc 2007;39:1095-1097.

[74] Molnar MZ, Novak M, Szeifert L, *et al.* Restless legs syndrome, insomnia, and quality of life after renal transplantation. J Psychosomat Res 2007;63:591-597.

[75] Noohi S, Khaghani-Zadeh M, Javadipour M, *et al.* Anxiety and depression are correlated with higher morbidity after kidney transplantation. Transplant Proc; 2007;39:1074-1078.

[76] Reimer J, Franke GH, Philipp T, Heemann U. Quality of life in kidney recipients: comparison of tacrolimus and cyclosporine-microemulsion. Clin Transplant 2002;16:48-54.

[77] Franke GH, Trampenau C, Reimer J. Switching from cyclosporine to tacrolimus leads to improved disease-specific quality of life in patients after kidney transplantation. Transplant Proc 2006;38:1293-1294.

[78] Oberbauer R, Hutchison B, Eris J, *et al.* Health-related quality-of-life outcomes of sirolimus-treated kidney transplant patients after elimination of cyclosporine A: results of a 2-year randomized clinical trial. Transplantation. 2003;75:1277-1285.

[79] Russ G, Jamieson N, Oberbauer R, *et al.* Three-year health-related quality-of-life outcomes for sirolimus-treated kidney transplant patients after elimination of cyclosporine. Transpl Int. 2007;20:875-883.

[80] Oppenheimer F, Rebollo P, Grinyo JM, *et al.* Health-related quality of life of patients receiving low-toxicity immunosuppressive regimens: a substudy of the Symphony Study. Transplantation. 2009;87:1210-1213.
[81] Raiz L, Davies EA, Ferguson RM. Sexual functioning following renal transplantation. Health & social work. 2003;28:264-272.
[82] Chan L, Mulgaonkar S, Walker R, *et al.* Patient-reported gastrointestinal symptom burden and health-related quality of life following conversion from mycophenolate mofetil to enteric-coated mycophenolate sodium. Transplantation. 2006;81:1290-1297.
[83] Teixeira de Barros C, Cabrita J. Noncompliance with immunosuppressive therapy: prevalence and determinants. Transplant Proc 2000;32:2633.
[84] Moons P, De Geest S, Abraham I, *et al.* Symptom experience associated with maintenance immunosuppression after heart transplantation: patients' appraisal of side effects. Heart Lung 1998;27:315-325.
[85] Moons P, Vanrenterghem Y, van Hooff JP, *et al.* Steroids may compromise quality of life of renal transplant recipients on a tacrolimus-based regimen. Transplant Proc 2002;34:1691-1692.
[86] Artz MA, Boots JM, Ligtenberg G, *et al.* Conversion from cyclosporine to tacrolimus improves quality-of-life indices, renal graft function and cardiovascular risk profile. Am J Transplant. 2004;4:937-945.
[87] De Geest S, Abraham I, Moons P, *et al.* Late acute rejection and subclinical noncompliance with cyclosporine therapy in heart transplant recipients. J Heart Lung Transplant. 1998;17:854-863.
[88] Akman B, Uyar M, Afsar B. Adherence, depression and quality of life in patients on a renal transplantation waiting list. Transpl Int. 2007;20:682-687.
[89] Cofan F, Rosich E, Arias M, *et al* Quality of life in renal transplant recipients following conversion from mycophenolate mofetil to enteric-coated mycophenolate sodium. Transplant Proc 200;39:2179-2181.
[90] Chang CF, Winsett RP, Gaber AO, Hathaway DK. Cost-effectiveness of post-transplantation quality of life intervention among kidney recipients. Clin Transplant 2004;18:407-414.
[91] Gross CR, Kreitzer MJ, Russas V, *et al.* Mindfulness meditation to reduce symptoms after organ transplant: a pilot study. Advances in mind-body medicine. 2004;20:20-29.
[92] McLaughlin D, Drori G, Ross M. School-level Correlates of Academic Achievement: Student Assessment Scores in SASS Public Schools. In: Statistics NCfE, ed.: U.S. Department of Education 2000.
[93] Van der Niepen P, Woestenburg A, Brie H, *et al.* Effectiveness of valsartan for treatment of hypertension: patient profiling and hierarchical modeling of determinants and outcomes (the PREVIEW study). Ann Pharmacother 2009;43:849-861.
[94] Denhaerynck K, Desmyttere A, Dobbels F, *et al.* Nonadherence with immunosuppressive drugs: U.S. compared with European kidney transplant recipients. Progress in transplantation (Aliso Viejo, Calif. 2006;16:206-214.
[95] McLeroy KR, Bibeau D, Steckler A, Glanz K. An ecological perspective on health promotion programs. Health Educ Q. 1988;15:351-377.
[96] Moons P, Budts W, De Geest S. Critique on the conceptualisation of quality of life: a review and evaluation of different conceptual approaches. Int J Nurs Stud 2006;43:891-901.
[97] Mitsui T, Shimoda N, Morita K, *et al.* Lower urinary tract symptoms and their impact on quality of life after successful renal transplantation. Int J Urol. 2009;16:388-392.
[98] Painter PL, Hector L, Ray K, *et al.* A randomized trial of exercise training after renal transplantation. Transplantation. 2002;74:42-48.
[99] Panagopoulou A, Hardalias A, Berati S, Fourtounas C. Psychosocial issues and quality of life in patients on renal replacement therapy. Saudi J Kidney Dis Transpl. 2009;20:212-218.
[100] Perez-San-Gregorio MA, Martin-Rodriguez A, Diaz-Dominguez R, Perez-Bernal J. The influence of posttransplant anxiety on the long-term health of patients. Transplant Proc 2006;38:2406-2408.

CHAPTER 17

Graft-Transmitted Infection in Kidney Transplantation

Laetitia Albano[1], Marie-France Mamzer[2], Fanny Lanternier[3], Christophe Legendre[2] and Olivier Lortholary[3,4,*]

[1]Université de Nice Sophia-Antipolis, Unité médico-chirurgicale de Transplantation Rénale CHU de Nice; [2]Université Paris Descartes, Hôpital Necker Enfants malades, Service de Transplantation Rénale; [3]Université Paris Descartes, Hôpital Necker Enfants malades, Service de Maladies Infectieuses et Tropicales, Centre d'Infectiologie Necker Pasteur and [4]Institut Pasteur, Centre National de Référence Mycologie et Antifongiques, Unité de Mycologie Moléculaire, CNRS URA3012, Paris, France

Abstract: Transplanted organs can transmit infectious diseases to recipients with varying consequences depending on the pathogen, the infection status of the recipient and the effectiveness of treatment (curative and/or preventive). In this non-exhaustive review, we detailed the classical diseases transmitted by the transplanted kidney which can be easily detected in the deceased donor with the last recommendations of treatment, but also emerging infectious diseases due to the increasing mobility of populations (conventional tourism , transplant tourism, immigration .). New challenge in this field, is the earliest possible detection of infectious agents from the donor to guide the decision of organ harvesting and direct matching D/R . Pending the use of Nucleic Acid Testing in routine, it remains essential, in addition to conventional serological tests, to achieve a very specific examination, paying particular attention to record the countries visited by the donor, as well as performing systematic bacteriological and mycological analysis of preservation solution.

Keywords: Kidney Transplantation, Tissue Donor, Tissue and Organ Procurement, Bacterial Infection Transmission, Virus Disease Transmission, Parasitic Disease Transmission, Mycoses Transmission, Emigration and Immigration, Travel.

INTRODUCTION

Donor-derived infection complicates less than 1% of all transplant procedures [1]. Although it is a rare event, the transmission of an infection through a donor organ can result not only in the loss of the allograft, but also in death of the recipient. All infectious agents are transmissible through the graft: bacteria, viruses, fungi, parasites, and potentially prion (Table **1**). However, due to the limited supply of kidney donors, careful consideration should be made so as not to discard them without balancing potential risks and benefits for the patient. Infection transmission pathways after kidney transplantation are multiple. First, transplanted kidneys facilitate the transmission of infections from organ donors (most often preexisting latent infections in transplanted tissues, but also active donor infections at the time of organ recovery, and donor transfusion-acquired infection prior to organ recovery). Secondly organs may become infected with nosocomial organisms during recovery process, or through the contamination of the organ preservation solution (PS). Pretransplant infectious disease screening of potential organ donors and recipients is essential in order to identify infectious conditions which may contraindicate the allograft (Table **2**), to identify and treat pretransplant active infection, to define the risk of infection and guide preventative strategies. Even though there is a global consensus on the major infections for which screening has to be performed, there are some variations between regions and centers, due to epidemiology or to center practices in the types of screening used and actions taken as a result. Detection strategies depend on the frequency of microbial agents in donors, screening sensitivity, transmission rate, recipient injury and preventive/therapeutic alternatives. Therefore, most infectious diseases transmissions are expected and manageable. Still, some of the risks of transmission are known only after grafting (*e.g.,* PS contamination) or occur unexpectedly

***Address correspondence to Olivier Lortholary:** Université Paris Descartes, Hôpital Necker Enfants malades, Service de Maladies Infectieuses et Tropicales, Centre d'Infectiologie Necker Pasteur, Paris, France; Tel: 33 1 42 19 26 63; Fax: 33 1 44 49 54 40; E-mail: olivier.lortholary@nck.aphp.fr

Massimiliano Veroux and Pierfrancesco Veroux (Eds)

because the infection is unknown to the donor and therefore not screened before transplantation. Cluster of infections derived from deceased donors have nevertheless been described in this context. Knowing that many common pathogens (mainly viruses) that may be transmitted by grafts are ubiquitous, the recipient screening for viral infections as the serologic status is potentially crucial in determining the risk of infection. Pre-existing immunity against pathogens such as cytomegalovirus (CMV), Epstein-Barr Virus (EBV), herpes simplex (HSV), varicella-zoster virus (VZV), hepatitis B virus and *Toxoplasma gondii* protect the recipient from severe primo-infection due to these agents.

Table 1: Microorganisms transmitted through kidney graft. In bold, pathogens addressed in this chapter

Virus	Bacteria	Parasites
Human immunodeficiency virus	***Staphylococcus aureus***	***Toxoplasma gondii***
Cytomegalovirus	*Klebsiella* species	*Strongyloïdes stercoralis*
Epstein-Barr virus	Bacteroides fragilis	***Plasmodium* species**
Herpes simplex virus	***Pseudomonas aeruginosa***	***Trypanosma cruzi***
Varicella-zoster virus	***Escherichia coli***	*Echinococcus granulosus*
Human T-lymphotropic virus 1/2	*Salmonella* species	*Filariae*
Human herpesvirus-6	*Yersinia enterocolitica*	*Clonorchis* species
Human herpesvirus-7	***Treponema pallidum***	*Schistosoma* species
Human herpesvirus-8	*Brucella* species	
Hepatitis B	*Bartonella* species	**Fungi**
Hepatitis C	*Enterobacter* species	***Aspergillus* species**
Rabies	*Acinetobacter* species	***Candida* species**
Lymphocytic choriomeningitis virus		***Coccidioides immitis***
West Nile virus	**Mycobacteria**	***Histoplasma capsulatum***
BK virus	***Mycobacterium tuberculosis***	*Cryptococcus neoformans*
Parvovirus B19	Nontuberculous mycobacteria	

Table 2: Absolute infectious contraindication to organ donation

HIV
Active hepatitis B, West Nile Virus
Encephalitis of unknown origin
HSV encephalitis
Lymphocytic Choriomeningitis Virus
Rabies
Chikungunya virus if NAT positive
Malaria if cause of death
Disseminated tuberculosis
Disseminated fungal infection
Multiresistant bacteria if resistance unknown and/or adequate treatment not given
Chagas disease if cause of death
Leishmania if cause of death

DONOR SCREENING

Donor screening includes a comprehensive medical history evaluation concentrating on infections, vaccinations, and unusual exposures (residence in endemic area, even several years earlier, travel, drug use, risky sexual behavior, incarceration). Microbiological analysis results documents with drug-susceptibility testing are mandatory. Geographically restricted diseases require special attention (Table **3**) [2].

Table 3: Agents to screen according to donor travel geographical area

Infectious Agents	Geographical Areas
HTLV ½	Japan, Caraib, South America, Africa
HHV8	Mediterranean country, Africa
West Nile Virus	United-States, Middle-East, South-East Asia
Chagas disease	South United States, South America
Histoplasmosis	Africa, Caraib, Middle west United States, Central and South America, South East Asia
Coccioidomycosis	South West United States, Central and South America,

Viruses

HIV

It is one of the most prejudicial infections transmitted by the donor. The rate of transmission is high. Simonds [3] reports that among 34 kidney recipients of HIV+ donors, only one remained seronegative 6 months after transplantation. Screening of donors with a highly sensitive assay for the presence of HIV antibodies is routine in all centers [4]. Several cases of HIV transmission by donors who had not yet seroconverted and were antibody-negative at the time of harvest have been reported [3]. Thus, screening for HIV p24 antigen is also utilized in all potential organs donors. This is recommended in order to better define the risk of HIV infection than relying only on past history (risky sexual behavior, hemophilia, incarceration). American guidelines define high-risk donors and recommend to inform the potential recipient of the possibility of an increased risk of HIV transmission [4].

CMV

CMV primo-infection transmitted by the transplant occurs in more than 80% of couples D+/R- in the first months following transplantation. It can lead to CMV disease impacting graft and patient survival. CMV-seropositive recipients are also at risk for superinfection by CMV from a CMV-seropositive donor, especially in the setting of intense immunosuppression. The best approach for CMV disease in kidney recipients is prevention, but which strategy—prophylaxis or preemptive therapy—is optimal remains debatable. Ganciclovir and valganciclovir remain the best options for prevention of CMV disease in kidney recipients. In high-risk patients D+/R-, the American Society of Transplantation [5] recommends a universal prophylaxis based on 12–14 weeks with IV and/or oral ganciclovir, oral valganciclovir, or oral valacyclovir. Regarding the optimal duration of prophylaxis, a recent study suggests that extending the period of preventive treatment after kidney transplantation from classically 3 months to 6 months can better reduce the risk of CMV disease [6]. For intermediate risk D+/R+, preemptive therapy with oral valganciclovir or IV ganciclovir during 100 days is an acceptable option.

Epstein-Barr Virus (EBV)

Most of Post-Transplant Lymphoprolifertaive Disorders (PTLD) are associated with the Epstein Barr Virus (EBV). Although approximately 90% of adults are seropositive for this virus, less than 2% of transplant recipients will develop a PTLD, and despite this risk, kidney transplantation from EBV-D+ to EBV-R- is not contraindicated. Nevertheless, pretransplant EBV serologies are useful to target the highest PTLD risk group of seronegative recipients of a seropositive graft. These patients, mainly children, will develop a primary-infection which increases the risk of developing a PTLD. A close monitoring of this higher risk group by EBV-PCR is useful in order to guide preemptive interventions such as decreasing immunosuppression, which clinical presentation varies from isolated lymphadenopathy to systemic disease. Because of a possible allograft rejection, calcineurin inhibitor (CNI) minimization or conversion from a CNI to proliferation signal inhibitors might be useful for preventing development of PTLD and allograft rejection [7].

HBV

Organs procured from HBV-infected donors can transmit infection to the recipient. HBV transmission depends on stage of donor HBV infection, presence or absence of HBs antigen, and anti-HBs recipient immune status. Organ donors' serologic evaluation of HBV infection markers includes testing for hepatitis

B surface antigen (HBsAg), anti-hepatitis B surface antigen antibody (HBsAb), and antibody to hepatitis B core antigen (anti-HBc). HBsAg-positive donors are at high risk of transmitting HBV infection to the recipients and most of the organizations for organ procurement prohibit the use of kidneys from these donors. Kidneys from donors presenting either isolated HBsAb or IgG anti-HBc-positive/HBsAg-negative or both HBcAb and anti-HBc negative are unlikely to transmit HBV infection to their recipients. Indeed, an Italian study from De Feo *et al.* shows no clinical or biochemical manifestation of hepatitis B in 344 recipients AgHBs- grafted with 210 donors anti-HBc+/HbsAg- donors, five years after kidney transplantation [8]. Kidneys from HBsAg-positive donors who are negative for HBeAg carry little to no risk of transmitting HBV if their recipients are immune to HBV or HBsAg-positive [9]. Consequently, if HBsAg+ kidney is exclude from donation (or used in life-threatening situations with intensive prophylaxis), kidney from donor HBcAb+ can be considered if documented vaccination in vaccinated recipients and negative nuclear antigen testing (NAT) if donor vaccination is unknown [10].

Hepatitis C Virus (HCV)

HCV is transmitted by 50% to 100% of kidneys from HCV-D+ to HCV-R- [11]. American Society of Transplantation 2009 guidelines recommend the use of kidneys of HCV-D+ to HCV-RNA+-R+ [8], but such practice remains controversial due to data from large cohorts suggesting that kidney transplant with HCV-D+ is an independent risk of mortality [12, 13]. Kidney transplantation from HCV-D+ to HCV-R+ should only occur in recipients with chronic kidney disease stage 5 because studies indicate that transplanting HCV-D+ kidneys results in improved survival compared to wait-listed and dialyzed patients [14]. Future donors and recipients rapid nucleic acid testing (NAT) will allow kidney transplant from HCV-D+ to HCV-R+ with positive viremia [15].

Human T Cell Lymphotropic Virus Type I/II (HTLV-1/2)

HTLV-1/2 virus infection is endemic in Japan, Australia and parts of Africa with a seroprevalence below 15%. It causes adult T-cell leukemia-lymphoma, tropical spastic paraparesis-HTLV type I, vasculitis and myositis. Although the risk of transmission by solid organ transplantation is not yet defined, Gonzalez-Perez *et al.* described HTLV-I infection in several transplant recipients sharing the same donor 2 years after transplantation [16]. Since it is not clearly established if HTLV seropositivity in kidney recipient affects the development of T cell leukemia [17], a positive HTLV-1 screening in a potential donor must be considered according to the emergency status of the recipient.

Human Herpes Virus 8 (HHV-8)

Human herpes virus 8 (HHV-8) is a member of the Herpesviridae family. HHV-8 seroprevalence ranges from <5% in North America, northern Europe and Southeastern Asia, to 10–20% in certain Mediterranean countries, to more than 50% in sub-Saharan regions [18]. A strong association between HHV-8 and Kaposi Sarcoma (KS) has been assessed particularly in kidney recipients *via* two possible mechanisms: reactivation in patients infected before transplantation, and contamination through the infected organ donor. Some studies, using molecular, cytogenetic, immunohistochemical and immunofluorescent methods following the viral infection, have shown that organ-related transmission of HHV-8 could be more frequent than previously considered [19]. A recent study from the skin and organ transplantation group of the French Society of Dermatology has shown that among 64 kidney HHV -8-R- grafted with a HHV8-D+, 25% (n=16) seroconverted and 3/16 presented clinical manifestation of KS [20]. These results should not discourage grafting potentially HHV-8 infected donor kidneys, all the more so the incidence of KS in the D+/R- group (13%) was lower than in the R+ group (4.6%), but promote screening of HHV-8, prior to grafting, and to monitor recipients at risk for HHV-8-related disease development even if the results of the detection of HHV-8 antibodies were transmitted to the physicians retrospectively.

Emerging Viruses

Several emerging viral pathogens such as rabies [21], West Nile virus [22], and lymphocytic choriomeningitis [23] have been recently reported in kidney transplant recipients transmitted by the donors, underlining the importance to adjust screening on a regional basis for endemic or epidemic infections that can be transmitted with unusually severe presentation in recipients.

Rabies

Rabies is an acute fatal encephalitis caused by neurotropic viruses in the genus Lyssavirus, family Rhabdoviridae. The majority of rabies cases are caused by the bite of rabid mammals. After an incubation period of several weeks to months, the virus passes *via* the peripheral nervous system and replicates in the central nervous system. The few cases published in recipients of solid organ transplants are from donors with unclear neurological symptoms. This suggests a re-evaluation of strategies for screening organ donors presenting with neurological symptoms. Because there are no 100% sensitive *in vivo* tests that exclude rabies in a donor, an effort should be accomplished to obtain an exhaustive recent history before harvesting.

West Nile Virus (WNV)

Transmission of West Nile virus by organ transplantation is well documented [22]. It is a mosquito-borne flavivirus, native to Africa, Europe, and Western Asia which has become increasingly prevalent in North America since it was first recognized in New York in 1999. Eighty percent of infections are asymptomatic, 20% manifest a flu-like illness. Rarely, symptomatic patients develop meningitis or encephalitis. The morbidity and mortality associated with West Nile virus infection in transplant recipients is high. Potential treatment is restricted due to limited experience with this virus in the field of transplantation. Before the emergence of WNV in the USA, only few methods of diagnosis were available. Recently, there have been many developments in the field of WNV diagnosis and prevention. Diagnosis of WNV may be carried out serologically or by RT-PCR. The commercial IgM antibody capture assay tests positive in cerebral spinal fluid 3 to 5 days after onset of symptoms, even before serum antibody develops. Nucleic acid testing in plasma or cerebro-spinal fluid is the most useful diagnostic test [24].

Lymphocytic Choriomeningitis Virus (LCMV)

LCMV is a rodent-borne viral infectious disease that presents as aseptic meningitis. Its causative agent is a member of the family Arenaviridae. Although LCMV is most commonly recognized by causing neurological disease, infection without symptoms or mild febrile illnesses are common clinical manifestations. Humans are more likely to contract LCMV from house mice. In addition to pregnancy-related infection, inter-human transmission has also been documented in 3 clusters of donor-transmitted infection in 2003, 2005 and 2006 in the United States and Australia [23-25] leading to death in all but one kidney recipient who was treated by ribavirin and radical decrease in immunosuppressive therapy. Potential donors with aseptic meningitis should be screened for LCMV through PCR analysis of cerebral-spinal fluid.

Bacteria

Bacteremia

Organs transplanted from bacteremic donors rarely transmit bacterial infection, and the data show that these recipients outcome are not significantly worse than those of uninfected donors [26]. It is suggested that the use of such infected organs should proceed cautiously during the following circumstances [27]: bacteremia with a non virulent or immediately remedied organism, or *S. aureus* or *P. aeruginosa* caused bacteremia which subsides upon bactericidal therapy for at least 2 weeks, showing negative subsequent blood cultures one week after stopping antibiotics. In the case of meningitis, infection with organisms associated with a high risk of relapse and/or infectious metastasis (*e.g.*, *Listeria monocytogenes*) [28], endothelial tropism, or highly virulent (*e.g.*, *Staphylococcus* spp., *P. aeruginosa*, *Salmonella* spp.) should be considered a contra-indication to organ donation. A potential donor with bacterial meningitis should not be discarded if treated 24 to 48 hours by effective antimicrobial therapy following by 1 week to 10 days in recipients [29].

Syphilis

Transmission of syphilis by means other than sexual transmission is infrequent. Only one documented case has been reported [30]. Serologic testing of organ donors for syphilis is recommended, but evidence of donor syphilis infection (past or present) is not considered a contraindication to transplantation if prophylactic antibiotics are administered to the recipient.

Mycobacterium Tuberculosis

Although reactivation of latent tuberculosis (TB) is the usual mode of acquisition, donor transmission is possible [31]. Incidence of TB in Europe and America is respectively of 49 and 32 per 100 000 population (WHO, 2007). In case of transplant tourism, the principal place to buy an organ is South East Asia where TB incidence is higher (181 per 100000 populations, WHO, 2007). So, the risk of contracting TB through the graft is increased if the donor is originated from these countries. Tuberculosis in solid organ transplant recipients is associated with relatively high morbidity and mortality and is often extra-pulmonary. The screening in the potential donor is not efficient. When transmission is suspected, investigation of potential donor-transmitted tuberculosis requires rapid communication among physicians, transplant centers, and organ procurement organizations.

Parasites

Toxoplasma Gondii

T. gondii can be transmitted to the recipient *via* solid organ transplants leading to potentially fatal primo-infection in the seronegative recipients. Toxoplasma persists as encystments in heart muscle and recipients of heart transplants are particularly subject to Toxoplasmosis graft transmission. Fatal cases have also been observed following renal transplantation [32]. Without prophylaxis, less than 1% of kidney recipients acquire toxoplasmosis through the organ of a seropositive donor. The prevalence of *T. gondii* varies in the general population from 10% to 75% depending on the geographic area, therefore a mismatch of donor and recipient is common. Trimethoprim/sulfamethoxazole treatment currently prescribed for Pneumocystis prophylaxis is also efficient as Toxoplasma prophylaxis. However, some recipients cannot receive such treatment. Therefore, all donors should be screened for the presence of anti-*Toxoplasma* antibody. In case of D+/R-, Rogers *et al.* suggest treating with trimethoprim/sulfamethoxazole for the first 6 months after renal transplantation [32].

Malaria

Malaria is a rare infection in transplant patients and is mostly caused by transfusion of infected blood. However, in a few cases, transmission *via* a transplanted allograft has been described. Clear evidence of donor-to-host transmission *via* the graft has been described in five cases, including one heart (*P. falciparum*), one liver (*P. falciparum*) and three kidney graft recipients (all *P. vivax*) [33]. Fischer has reported donor-transmitted disease in 1 liver, 1 heart and 2 kidney recipients. Kidneys and heart recipients responded well to an anti-malaria treatment. Despite typical criterion, it seems logical to exclude donors deceased from malaria, however, not to exclude donors with a malaria history if the condition has been effectively treated. Recipient should receive the appropriate therapeutic regimen.

Chagas Disease

Transmission of Chagas disease (Tripanosoma cruzi) remains an important problem in endemic areas from the south of the United States to Argentina and Chile. Approximately 30% of infected patients have clinical manifestations of myocarditis and meningoencephalitis. Recipient's contamination through the kidney graft has already been described [34]. The rate of transmission in kidney transplant is estimated around 20%, and if transmission occurs, patients do not tend to have severe complications as demonstrated in several publications [35]. Two serologic-based tests including PCR techniques are required in all potential donors from endemic areas. If it is contraindicated to use donors with acute infection and heart from donor with chronic infection, there is no consensus on use of other organs from donor with chronic infection. However, strict follow up is mandatory if organs are transplanted [2].

Fungi

Graft-transmitted fungal infections are rare in comparison to bacterial and viral infection.

Invasive Fungal Infection

Invasive fungal infection is a contraindication to organ recovery [36]. Not only cases of candidemia, but also *Aspergillus* spp. infection, cryptoccocosis, and mucormycosis are of great concern to potential transplant recipients. Keating *et al.* [37] report the case of a donor with tracheal secretions positive for *Aspergillu fumigatus*. Three weeks after transplantation, the 2 kidney recipients studied developed multiple Aspergillus abscesses leading to transplantectomy. A recent review of the literature by Rammaert *et al.* [38] has retrieved 7 cases of renal graft mucormycosis presented as acute rejection in 4/7 recipients and graft arteritis in 3/7. Living unrelated donation in third world countries has been identified as a possible risk factor.

Quiescent Infection

Relevant to many endemic areas are the so-called quiescent infections, where some fungal mycoses remain silent in the donor and become reactivated in the recipient. Histoplasmosis transmission through donor organs has already been reported [39, 40]. It is endemic in certain areas of the United States, particularly in states bordering the Ohio River valley and the lower Mississippi River. It also common in caves in southern and East Africa. Limaye *et al.* describe the cases of two kidney recipients from the same deceased donor originated from the state of Kansas, United States, developed a disseminated histoplasmosis during the first year of transplantation [40]. The isolates were found to be identical in the 2 recipients and serological analysis of the donor indicated a high titer of antibodies against *Histoplasma capsulatum*. An appropriate treatment by amphotericin B resulted in recovery in both kidney recipients.

Coccidioides spp, also involved in fungi transmission by the graft, is a fungus endemic to the southwestern United States. Infection is caused by inhaling the spores of *Coccidioides immitis,* often found in desert regions. Donor-derived coccidioidomycosis has been documented, but its risk of transmission is not known. Wright *et al.* [41] described the American cases of a kidney and a liver recipients from the same donor with unrecognized active coccidoidomycosis at the time of death. Donor and recipients had never visited endemic areas. The 2 recipients died from rapidly disseminated infection. The recipient of the other kidney received prophylaxis by itraconazole during 3 months after other recipients' death and was still asymptomatic after 2 years. More recently, Coccidioidomycosis has been diagnosed in a lung transplant recipient acquired from the donor graft in France [42]. Serological screening for coccidioidomycosis in transplant donors or recipients coming from or residing in areas of endemicity is recommended. If a positive result is known subsequently to the transplantation, active illness must be excluded. Fluconazole or itraconazole prophylaxis should continue for 6 months. After transplantation, all patients should be monitored serologically every 3 to 4 months during the first year and yearly thereafter [2].

PRESERVATION SOLUTION SCREENING

In addition of donor and recipient infectious screenings, microbiological analysis of PS is essential to detect a graft contamination not related to the donor's active infection. Microbiological results are only available 2 -3 days after transplantation, therefore confirming PS graft contamination cannot prevent transplantation of infectious organs to the recipient. The most important focus in such instances is deciding the most appropriate management/therapy for these patients after transplantation.

Bacteria

The overall positivity rate of preservation solution cultures ranged from 5 to 23%. Many studies [43] have concluded that contamination of renal allografts by *Staphylococcus aureus*, *Escherichia coli* and *Pseudomonas aeruginosa*, because of vasculo-tropism could lead to renal graft arteritis, need to be treated preemptively before the onset of clinical manifestations. By contrast, contamination with skin contaminants does not pose a risk to the graft.

Fungi

Fungi represent 2 to 10% of all positive cultures. Routine culturing of PS at 30°C for five or more days established a 3.6% incidence of preservation solutions positive for *Candida* spp without subsequent consequence for the recipients who were treated with antifungals [44]. Fungal contamination of PS runs a low risk of renal graft arteritis and although it's fairly uncommon, such fungal arteritis carries high morbidity and mortality. A recent publication from the French Mycosis Study Group [45] suggests that organ contamination is the consequence of donor peritoneal contamination during recovery, with subsequent contamination of the preservation solution. Several recommendations have been proposed and are currently used in all renal transplant centres in France. Any digestive tract breach at the time of multiorgan recovery should be mentioned to the transplant teams. In addition, cultures of all individual organ preservation solutions should be completed, with any positive results notified to the transplant teams and the coordination centre. Moreover, when preservation solution cultures are positive for yeasts, efficient antifungal treatment is mandatory: $\geq$ 200 mg/dl of fluconazole is suggested as first line treatment for azole-susceptible *Candida* species; liposomal amphotericin B or an echinocandin should be administered for azole-resistant *Candida* species. The treatment can be pursued until all recipient cultures are negative. Any *Candida* species isolated from preservation solution from any organ should prompt repeated Doppler ultrasound. *Candida* isolates should be stored for further analysis by a reference laboratory whenever possible. Finally, when graft site candidiasis is documented, surgery should be discussed rapidly.

CONCLUSIONS

Almost all microorganisms have been transmitted *via* organs and tissue allograft, and while traditional screening strategies are effective in most cases, they are not sufficient to reduce the infection transmission risk to zero. Given the limited pool of donors, and the changing pattern of human life it has become necessary to consider new candidates, including those with infection at the time of donation, higher risk serologic profiles or social history indicating a particular risk. Moreover, immigration, and travel (international and domestic), a so called "transplantation tourism, " poses risks such as 'exotic' infectious diseases on recipients, which are often unknown to the donor, and unpreventable in some instances. Even if the disease is clinically detectable, the time to perform microbiological analysis and to obtain results is too long to decide to harvest the organ or not. In a near future, the use of nucleic acid testing could allow rapid detection of many pathogens at the same time, in order to discard an organ donor, or not, but also to guide a right match D/R (*e.g.,* in case of hepatitis). At the very least, we must improve the way to inform the recipient on the infectious risk.

REFERENCES

[1] Ison MG. The epidemiology and prevention of donor-derived infections. Adv Chronic Kidney Dis 2009 16:234-241.

[2] Martín-Dávila P, Fortún J, López-Vélez R, *et al.* Transmission of tropical and geographically restricted infections during solid-organ transplantation. Clin Microbiol Rev 2008 21:60-96.

[3] Simonds RJ. HIV transmission by organ and tissue transplantation. AIDS 1993 7 Suppl 2:S35-38.

[4] Guidelines for preventing transmission of human immunodeficiency virus through transplantation of human tissue and organs. Centers for disease control and prevention. MMWR Recomm Rep 1994 43(RR-8):1-17.

[5] Cytomegalovirus. Am J Transplant 2004, Nov;4 Suppl 10:51-58.

[6] Luan FL, Stuckey LJ, Park JM, *et al.* Six-Month prophylaxis is cost effective in transplant patients at high risk for cytomegalovirus infection. J Am Soc Nephrol 2009 20:2449-2458.

[7] Ohta H, Fukushima N, Ozono K. Pediatric post-transplant lymphoproliferative disorder after cardiac transplantation. Int J Hematol 2009 90:127-136.

[8] De Feo TM, Grossi P, Poli F, *et al.* Kidney transplantation from anti-hbc+ donors: Results from a retrospective italian study. Transplantation 2006;81:76-80.

[9] Natov SN, Pereira BJ. Transmission of viral hepatitis by kidney transplantation: Donor evaluation and transplant policies (part 1: Hepatitis B virus). Transpl Infect Dis 2002 4:117-123.

[10] Grossi PA, Fishman JA, AST Infectious Disease Community of Practice. Donor-Derived infections in solid organ transplant recipients. Am J Transplant 2009; 9 Suppl 4:S19-26.

[11] Pereira BJ, Wright TL, Schmid CH, Levey AS. A controlled study of hepatitis C transmission by organ transplantation. The New England organ bank hepatitis C study group. Lancet 1995; 345:484-487.

[12] Bucci JR, Matsumoto CS, Swanson SJ, *et al.* Donor hepatitis C seropositivity: Clinical correlates and effect on early graft and patient survival in adult cadaveric kidney transplantation. J Am Soc Nephrol 2002; 13:2974-2982.

[13] Fabrizi F, Bunnapradist S, Lunghi G, Martin P. Transplantation of kidneys from hcv-positive donors: A safe strategy? J Nephrol 2003;16:617-625.

[14] Fabrizi F, Messa P, Martin P. Current status of renal transplantation from hcv-positive donors. Int J Artif Organs 2009; 32:251-261.

[15] Covic A, Abramowicz D, Bruchfeld A, *et al.* Endorsement of the kidney disease improving global outcomes (KDIGO) hepatitis C guidelines: An European renal best practice (ERBP) position statement. Nephrol Dial Transplant 2009;24:719-727.

[16] González-Pérez MP, Muñoz-Juárez L, Cárdenas FC, *et al.* Human t-cell leukemia virus type I infection in various recipients of transplants from the same donor. Transplantation 2003;75:1006-1011.

[17] Tanabe K, Kitani R, Takahashi K, *et al.* Long-Term results in human t-cell leukemia virus type 1-positive renal transplant recipients. Transplant Proc 1998;30:3168-3170.

[18] Plancoulaine S, Gessain A. Epidemiological aspects of human herpesvirus 8 infection and of kaposi's sarcoma. Med Mal Infect 2005;35:314-321.

[19] Barozzi P, Luppi M, Facchetti F, *et al.*Post-Transplant Kaposi sarcoma originates from the seeding of donor-derived progenitors. Nat Med 2003; 9:554-561.

[20] Francès C, Marcelin AG, Legendre Ch, Chevret S, *et al.* The impact of preexisting or acquired kaposi sarcoma herpesvirus infection in kidney transplant recipients on morbidity and survival. Am J Transplant 2009;9:2580-2586.

[21] Srinivasan A, Burton EC, Kuehnert MJ, *et al.* Transmission of rabies virus from an organ donor to four transplant recipients. N Engl J Med 2005;352:1103-1111.

[22] Iwamoto M, Jernigan DB, Guasch A, *et al.* Transmission of West nile virus from an organ donor to four transplant recipients. N Engl J Med 2003;348:2196-2203.

[23] Fischer SA, Graham MB, Kuehnert MJ, *et al.* Transmission of lymphocytic choriomeningitis virus by organ transplantation. N Engl J Med 2006; 354:2235-2249.

[24] Zhang W, Wu J, Li Y, Li F, *et al.* Rapid and accurate *in vitro* assays for detection of west nile virus in blood and tissues. Transfus Med Rev 2009;23:146-154.

[25] Palacios G, Druce J, Du L, *et al.* A new arenavirus in a cluster of fatal transplant-associated diseases. N Engl J Med 2008;358:991-998.

[26] Freeman RB, Giatras I, Falagas ME, *et al.* Outcome of transplantation of organs procured from bacteremic donors. Transplantation 1999;68:1107-1111.

[27] Rubin RH, Fishman JA. A consideration of potential donors with active infection--is this a way to expand the donor pool? Transpl Int 1998;11:333-335.

[28] Skogberg K, Ruutu P, Tukiainen P, Valtonen VV. Nontuberculous mycobacterial infection in hiv-negative patients receiving immunosuppressive therapy. Eur J Clin Microbiol Infect Dis 1995;14:755-763.

[29] López-Navidad A, Domingo P, Caballero F, *et al.* Successful transplantation of organs retrieved from donors with bacterial meningitis. Transplantation 1997;64:365-368.

[30] Cortes NJ, Afzali B, MacLean D, *et al.* Transmission of syphilis by solid organ transplantation. Am J Transplant 2006;6:2497-2499.

[31] Singh N, Paterson DL. Mycobacterium tuberculosis infection in solid-organ transplant recipients: Impact and implications for management. Clin Infect Dis 1998;27:1266-1277.

[32] Rogers NM, Peh CA, Faull R, *et al.* Transmission of toxoplasmosis in two renal allograft recipients receiving an organ from the same donor. Transpl Infect Dis 2008;10:71-74.

[33] Fischer L, Sterneck M, Claus M, *et al.* Transmission of malaria tertiana by multi-organ donation. Clin Transplant 1999; 13:491-495.

[34] Figueiredo JF, Martinez R, da Costa JC, *et al.* Transmission of Chagas disease through renal transplantation: Report of a case. Trans R Soc Trop Med Hyg 1990;84:61-62.

[35] Riarte A, Luna C, Sabatiello R, *et al.* Chagas' disease in patients with kidney transplants: 7 years of experience 1989-1996. Clin Infect Dis 1999;29:561-567.

[36] Delmonico FL. Cadaver donor screening for infectious agents in solid organ transplantation. Clin Infect Dis 2000;31:781-786.

[37] Keating MR, Guerrero MA, Daly RC, *et al.* Transmission of invasive aspergillosis from a subclinically infected donor to three different organ transplant recipients. Chest 1996;109:1119-1124.

[38] Rammaert B, Lanternier F, Zahar J R, *et al.* Healthcare-Associated zygomycosis. Clin Infect Dis. 2012 Feb;54 Suppl 1:S44-54.

[39] Botterel F, Romand S, Saliba F, *et al.* A case of disseminated histoplasmosis likely due to infection from a liver allograft. Eur J Clin Microbiol Infect Dis 1999;18:662-664.

[40] Limaye AP, Connolly PA, Sagar M, *et al.* Transmission of histoplasma capsulatum by organ transplantation. N Engl J Med 2000;343:1163-1166.

[41] Wright PW, Pappagianis D, Wilson M, *et al.* Donor-Related coccidioidomycosis in organ transplant recipients. Clin Infect Dis 2003;37:1265-1269.

[42] Brugière O, Forget E, Biondi G, *et al.* Coccidioidomycosis in a lung transplant recipient acquired from the donor graft in France. Transplantation 2009;88:1319-1320.

[43] Sharma AK, Smith G, Smith D, *et al.* Clinical outcome of cadaveric renal allografts contaminated before transplantation. Transpl Int 2005;18:824-827.

[44] Matignon M, Botterel F, Audard V, *et al.* Outcome of renal transplantation in eight patients with candida sp. Contamination of preservation fluid. Am J Transplant 2008;8:697-700.

[45] Albano L, Bretagne S, Mamzer-Bruneel MF, *et al.* Evidence that graft-site candidiasis after kidney transplantation is acquired during organ recovery: A multicenter study in France. Clin Infect Dis 2009; 48:194-202.

CHAPTER 18

Infectious Complications of Kidney Transplantation

Paolo Antonio Grossi* **and Daniela Dalla Gasperina**

Department of Clinical Medicine, Section of Infectious Diseases, University of Insubria, Varese, Italy

Abstract: Improved immunosuppressive therapies for organ transplantation have reduced the incidence of allograft rejection while increasing susceptibility to opportunistic infections and virally mediated malignancies. Renal transplant recipients are susceptible to a broad range of infectious pathogens and infections often progress rapidly. Improved microbiologic diagnostic tools are used in the routine management of common infections and have allowed the definition of new clinical syndromes and of donor-derived infections. However, invasive diagnostic procedures are often required for accurate and timely diagnosis and are justified by the high morbidity and mortality of infection in this population. Early and specific microbiologic diagnosis is essential for guiding treatment and minimizing non-essential drug therapy.

Keywords: Kidney Transplantation, Infection, CMV, Donor-Derived Infection, EBV, Prophylaxis, Bacterial Infection, Viral Infection, Immunosuppression, Screening.

INTRODUCTION

Infectious complications after solid organ transplantation remains a field in evolution. Improved immunosuppressive therapies for organ transplantation have reduced the incidence of allograft rejection while increasing susceptibility to opportunistic infections and virally mediated malignancies [1]. Renal transplant recipients are susceptible to a broad range of infectious pathogens and infections often progress rapidly. Patients often will have nonspecific symptoms, making distinction of infection from non-infectious processes (eg, graft rejection, drug toxicity) difficult [2]. Traditional patterns of opportunistic infection after transplantation have also been altered by antifungal (including *Pneumocystis*) and antiviral prophylaxis (*i.e.* for *Cytomegalovirus* (CMV) and other *Herpesviruses*) and by the emergence of organisms with antimicrobial resistance [3]. Improved microbiologic diagnostic tools (*e.g.,* nucleic acid testing) are used in the routine management of common infections (*e.g.,* CMV, *Epstein-Barr virus* (EBV)) and have allowed the definition of new clinical syndromes (*e.g.,* BK polyomavirus (BKV) nephropathy) and of donor-derived infections [1]. However, invasive diagnostic procedures are often required for accurate and timely diagnosis and are justified by the high morbidity and mortality of infection in this population. Early and specific microbiologic diagnosis is essential for guiding treatment and minimizing non-essential drug therapy. Antimicrobial therapy frequently has in fact toxic effects that may involve interactions with immunosuppressive agents (*e.g.,* azole antifungal agents with calcineurin inhibitors). Detailed knowledge of pharmacokinetic and pharmacodynamic interactions between immunosuppressive and antimicrobial agents is required to prevent deleterious drug interactions and to appropriately recommend drug dose adjustments [4, 5].

RISK OF INFECTION

The risk of infection in the renal transplant recipient changes over time and is determined by the interaction of 2 factors: (1) the *epidemiologic exposures* of the patient including the timing, intensity, and virulence of the organisms to which the individual is exposed; and (2) the patient's *net state of immunosuppression*, a measure of all host factors potentially contributing to the risk for infection. Prophylactic strategies are based on the patient's known or likely exposures to infection according to the results of serologic testing and epidemiologic history.

***Address correspondence to Paolo Antonio Grossi:** Professor of Infectious Diseases, Department of Clinical Medicine, Section of Infectious Diseases, University of Insubria Ospedale di Circolo e Fondazione Macchi, Viale Borri, 57, 21100 Varese, Italy; Tel: +39-0332-393075; +39-0332-278234; Fax: +39-0332-393080; E-mail: paolo.grossi@uninsubria.it

Massimiliano Veroux and Pierfrancesco Veroux (Eds)

Epidemiologic Exposures

Epidemiologic exposures can be divided into four overlapping categories: donor- and recipient-derived infections, and community or nosocomial exposures.

Donor-Derived Infections

Viral, bacterial, parasitic, prion and fungal infections have been transmitted *via* organ and tissue allografts [3, 6]. Despite screening programs utilizing serologic testing and on a review of the potential donor's medical records and behavioral history, clusters of donor-derived infections in recipients persist although these are uncommon. Recent improvements in the microbiologic screening of donors have reduced this risk. The accuracy of exposure history and the availability of viral nucleic acid testing (NAT) have in fact the capacity to reduce the risk of disease transmission by detecting early stages of many infections including those due to human immunodeficiency virus (HIV), hepatitis B virus (HBV) and hepatitis C virus (HCV) in the 'window' period before antibody seroconversion develops. However, it should be recognized that the screening of organ donors for potential pathogens can never completely exclude the risk of disease transmission. The process of donor screening must continue to evolve with our knowledge about the ever-changing field of infectious diseases. The donor derived infections are more extensively discussed in the specific chapter of this eBook.

Recipient-Derived Infections

Infections in this category reflect colonization or latent infections that reactivate in the setting of immunesuppression [7, 8]. Active infection in transplant recipients should be eradicated before transplantation, since immunosuppression will exacerbate the infectious process. Furthermore, individualized epidemiologic histories can guide preventive strategies [9]. Common recipient-derived pathogens include *Mycobacterium tuberculosis*, certain parasites (*e.g.*, *Strongyloides stercoralis* and *T. cruzi*), viruses (*e.g.*, CMV, EBV, herpes simplex virus (HSV), varicella–zoster virus (VZV), HBV, HCV, and HIV), and endemic fungi (*e.g.*, *Histoplasma capsulatum and Coccidioides immitis* [3]. Infections that can be treated or controlled do not preclude transplantation.

Nosocomial Infections

Transplant recipients are uniquely vulnerable to colonization and infection resulting from nosocomial pathogens. Within the same institution, transplant recipients have been shown to have a significantly higher incidence of nosocomial infections than non-transplant patients [10]. Paralleling the trends in nosocomially acquired infections, antimicrobial resistance is increasingly recognized as a problem in all critically-ill patients, including dialysed patients and kidney transplant recipients [11]. Patients on the waiting list for renal transplantation may become colonized with antimicrobial-resistant organisms, including methicillin-resistant *Staphylococcus aureus (*MRSA) and *Staphylococcus epidermidis* (MRSE), vancomycin-resistant *Enterococcus* (VRE), and antimicrobial-resistant gram-negative bacteria, particularly extended-spectrum beta-lactamase (ESBL) producing *Escherichia coli* and *Klebsiella* spp. More recently carbapenem-resistant *P. aeruginosa,* multidrug resistant *Acinetobacter baumannii* and carbapenemase producing *Klebsiella pneumonia* (KPC) have emerged as major threat in the hospital settings [12, 13]. After transplantation, these pathogens may cause urinary tract infections (UTI), bacteremia or may infect hematomas, ascitic fluid, wounds, and catheters. Urinary tract and postoperative surgical infections are the most frequent and serious nosocomial infection in renal transplant recipients.

Community Acquired Infections

Exposures that are relatively benign in a normal host may lead to major infection after transplantation. Common microorganisms include those noted above, pathogens in soil such as aspergillus or nocardia species, *C. neoformans* in birds, and respiratory viruses with subsequent bacterial or fungal superinfection.

Net state of Immunosuppression

The net state of immunosuppression refers to all factors that contribute to the patient's risk of infection. The main determinants of risk are the dose, duration, and sequence of immunosuppressive therapies. When acute rejection is treated using high dose steroids or antilymphocyte therapies, such as thymoglobulins or monoclonal antibodies, the risk of infections increases for the next several months; this is particularly true for CMV, BKV, and EBV infection; however, bacterial, fungal, and parasitic infections also may occur [14].

STRATEGIES FOR PREVENTION OF INFECTIONS

The study of infectious diseases associated with transplantation focuses on the strategies for prevention of infection in transplant recipients.

A correct preventative approach, as well as detailed knowledge of the immunosoppressive therapy of the patient, can greatly improve the outcome of transplant recipients.

The main strategies for prevention of infections are the following:

1. Screening of recipient prior to solid organ transplantation.
2. Perioperative and post-transplant antimicrobial prophylaxis.
3. Post-transplant monitoring and preemptive strategies.
4. Pre-transplant counseling and strategies for post-transplant safe living.

Screening of Recipient Prior to Solid Organ Transplantation

All candidates to renal transplantation must undergo an accurate screening for infectious diseases, which should include: medical history and physical examination, serologic tests, procedures to indentify colonitation and latent or active infections, vaccination status and behavioral recommendation.

The first step in screening candidates is a thorough ***medical history***, including activities such as travel, hobbies, animal and environmental exposure history, that may increase the risk of infection in the post-transplant period. The close contacts with pigeons is associated with *Cryptococcus neoformans* infection, transplant candidates who are gardeners, landscapers, farmers, construction workers, or marijuana smokers have a higher risk of fungal colonization of the sinuses and airways than the general population and may have a higher risk of invasive fungal infection after transplant [14-16]. Table **1** outlines the recipient screening serologic tests and the actions required at the time of evaluation.

Although certain **screening tests** recommended by the American Society of Transplantation (AST) guidelines, such as serological testing for viruses (HIV, CMV, HSV, VZV, EBV, HBV and HCV), latent syphilis and *Toxoplasma gondii*, are obtained by virtually all kidney transplant centers, there is considerable center-to-center variation in the screening policy [16-18]. Other serologic tests may in fact be added depending on regionally important infections or clinical evaluation.

Table 1: Kidney transplantation cadaveric and living related: tests to be drawn on the recipient and the donor

For all Kidney Transplant Candidates		
HIV 1-2 Ab	If negative	to be checked every 6 months
	If recipient positive	ID consult for possible inclusion in specific protocol
HBsAg, HBsAb, HBcAb,	If HBsAg positive	HBV DNA; if positive ID/GI consult for staging and treatment. Combined liver and kidney transplantation should consedered if liver cirrhosis
	If HBsAb negative	HBV vaccine on the recipient
	If vaccinated	HBsAb titer (potential booster if necessary), to be repeated every 6 months

Table 1: cont…..

HCV Ab HCV-RNA qualitative	If positive	HCV-RNA quantitative and genotype; ID/GI consult for staging and treatment before transplant. Combined liver and kidney transplantation should consedered if liver cirrhosis
HAV Ab	If negative	HAV vaccine on recipients from endemic areas
CMV Ab (IgG)	If negative	to be checked every 6 months on the recipient
HSV 1-2 Ab (IgG)	If negative	to be checked every 6 months on the recipient
VZV Ab (IgG)	If negative	to be checked every 6 months on the recipient
EBV Ab (EBNA Ab, VCA IgG, IgM)	If VCA-IgG negative	to be checked every 6 months on the recipient
HHV8 Ab (lytic and latent Ab)	If positive	HHV8-DNA on whole blood with qualitative PCR; if positive quantitative PCR and careful clinical evaluation; if the living donor is HHV8-DNA positive on peripheral blood cancel donation or consider the use of the organs only for HHV8 Ab positive recipients
HHV6 Ab (IgG)	If negative	to be checked every 6 months on the recipient, particulary in pediatric recipients
Toxoplasma Ab (IgG)	If negative	to be checked every 6 months on the recipient
RPR/VDRL; TPPA/TPHA	If positive	if positive → ID consult for evaluation and treatment
Stool examination for ova and parasites	If positive	ID consult for evaluation and treatment
Tubercolin skin test (PPD) and/or IGRA	If positive	Ziehl Neelsen + cultures for mycobacteria (urine, sputum or gastric secretions and blood). PCR on urine, sputum or gastric secretions. ID consult for prophylaxis or treatment
Urine examination and urine culture	If positive	ID consult
Nose swab for MRSA	If positive	Mupirocin treatment and repeat q3 months
Skin swabs (axilla and groin) for MRSA/MRSE	If positive	Clorexidin for 5 days for skin decontamination and repeat q 3 months
Rectal swab for VRE	If positive	Contact isolation
Other tests on clinical indication		
For all Kidney Transplant Candidates from endemic areas		
Serologic test for: Strongyloides, Coccidioides, Trypanosoma, Histoplasma HTLV 1-2	If positive	ID consult

Ab = Antibody; ID = Infection Diseases; GI = Gastroenterology.

Initial screening for **viral hepatitis** (HBV and HCV) should be done at the time transplant assessment and all candidates with chronic hepatitis infection should be evaluated for staging of liver diseases and eligibility for therapy prior to transplant (see Hepatitis B and Hepatitis C section in this chapter) [19]. Abdominal ultrasound must be performed for identification of complications of HBV/HCV-related liver disease such as ascites, portal hypertension and hepatocarcinoma. In chronic hepatitis, the liver biopsy remains the *"gold standard"* for assessing the degree of hepatic inflammation and fibrosis as well as the prognosis of the disease. Biopsy is recommended in the assessment of kidney transplant candidates with chronic hepatitis to guide antiviral treatment decisions, identify those who are ineligible for kidney transplantation due to advanced liver disease and those who may be considered for combined (with liver) transplant [19, 20].

Potential kidney transplant recipients should be screened for **latent syphilis** with a nontreponemal test (rapid plasma reagin (RPR) or venereal disease research laboratory (VDRL)), as recommended by AST and

Centers for Disease Control and Prevention (CDC) guidelines [16-18, 21]. If the results are positive, the patient should undergo a specific treponemal test (*Treponema pallidum* particle agglutination assay (TPPA)). Recently, the availability of automatable treponemal enzyme and chemiluminescence immunoassays (EIA/CIA) has led some laboratories to adopt a reverse sequence of screening in which a treponemal EIA/CIA is performed first. However, CDC recommends that a specimen with reactive EIA/CIA results be tested reflexively with a quantitative nontreponemal test (*e.g.*, RPR or VDRL). If test results are discordant, the specimen should be tested reflexively using the TPPA test as a confirmatory treponemal test. Patients with discordant serologic results by EIA/CIA and RPR/VDRL testing whose sera are reactive by TPPA testing are considered to have past or present syphilis; if sera is TPPA nonreactive, syphilis is unlikely [21]. Traditionally, the fluorescent treponemal antibody absorption (FTA-ABS) test has been considered the *gold standard* treponemal test and still is used by some laboratories. However, the FTA-ABS test has lower specificity than other treponemal tests and probably lower sensitivity [22]. In addition to inherent subjectivity, the FTA-ABS test also requires trained personnel and a dedicated fluorescence microscope. For these reasons, CDC recommends that the FTA-ABS test not be used to confirm discordant treponemal screening results. Based on published sensitivity and specificity data, the TPPA test currently is considered to be the most suitable confirmatory treponemal test [23].

All positive test results should be reported promptly and concurrently to the Infections Diseases (ID) consultant. An assessment is needed of the patient's sexual risk factors and medical history, especially history of previous treatment for syphilis. A physical examination also should be performed to assess for evidence of syphilis, especially primary disease (*e.g.*, ulcerative genital or anal lesions). Patients with suspected primary syphilis should be treated and then retested with a nontreponemal test in several weeks. Previously untreated patients with discordant sera and a reactive TPPA should be treated pre-transplant according to CDC's 2010 Sexually Transmitted Diseases Treatment Guidelines [24].

Screening ***procedures to indentify colonitation and latent or active infections*** should include tuberculin skin test (TST) and/or interferon gamma release assay (IGRA) to screen for latent tuberculosis (TB) infection, stool examination for ova and parasite, stool culture, skin (axilla and groin) and nasal swab cultures for MRSA. A review of recent microbiological data and past infections is recommended. Patients awaiting renal transplants may have infected hemodialysis or peritoneal dialysis access sites or catheters, or complicated upper and/or lower-tract urinary infections. These infections should be fully treated before transplant. Patients with polycystic kidney disease who present with recurrent fevers should be assessed for occult infection in their native kidneys.

All transplant candidates should be evaluated for **latent tuberculosis** before transplantation with either TST or IGRA [25-27]. Because patients with end stage renal disease may have an increased incidence of anergy, historical information related to potential exposure or past untreated infection as well as chest radiographs should be included in the risk assessment. In transplant candidates with a TST and/or IGRA positive or clinical history suggesting infection with TB, a thorough evaluation for active disease should be performed, which may include chest computed tomography (CT) scan, sputum smear or bronchoalveolar lavage, blood and urine for *Mycobacterium tuberculosis* (microscopic, polymerase chain reaction assay using primers for *M. tuberculosis* and cultures). Public health authorities and guidelines recommend treatment of latent TB in persons who are actively immunosuppressed [26, 28]. The standard recommended treatment dose is isoniazid 5 mg/kg (maximum of 300 mg) daily (if hemodialysis dose after dialysis) for 6-9 months for adults, supplemented with vitamin B6 [29-32]. Prophylaxis with isoniazid has been proven to prevent TB in randomized studies involving kidney recipients [27, 30, 32, 33]. All patients should have baseline hepatic measurements of serum aspartate aminotransferase (AST), alanine aminotransferase (ALT), and bilirubin levels. They should receive follow-up evaluations at least monthly. Treatment of latent TB infection must be suspended if AST or ALT values increase 3-fold in patients with symptoms or 5-fold in patients with no accompanying symptoms. Although practice varies among centers, it is desirable to complete treatment with isoniazid before transplant, although the course can be completed post-transplant if a graft becomes available before treatment completion.

Parasites that are largely asymptomatic before transplantation may flourish and become clinically evident under immunosuppressive treatment [34]. Stool examinations for ova and parasites should be performed in all candidates. Strongyloides stercoralis hyperinfection has in fact been reported in immunosuppressed solid organ transplant recipients [35].

It is recommended that **vaccination** status be reviewed at the time of the first transplant clinic visit, that a vaccine strategy be developed at that time and that the vaccination status be reviewed once again at the time the patient is listed for transplantation. Every effort should be made to ensure that renal transplant candidates and their household members have completed the full course of recommended vaccinations prior to transplantation. Since the response to many vaccines is diminished in organ failure, transplant candidates should be immunized early in the course of their disease [36]. Live vaccines should not be administered after transplant. Pediatric candidates should complete standard vaccine series to the extent possible before transplant, including anti *Meningococcus* and *Heamophilus influenzae* b vaccine. Adult candidates should receive the following nonlive vaccines: yearly injected influenza vaccine (both seasonal and H1N1 influenza), pneumococcal polysaccharide vaccine (PPV-23) if not given within 5 years, hepatitis A and HBV vaccine series if seronegative, Td (tetanus-diphtheria vaccine) or Tdap (tetanus-diphtheria-acellular pertussis vaccine) if no tetanus vaccine given within the last 10 years [14].

Kidney transplant candidates who are nonimmune should be vaccinated for HBV as early in the course of their disease as possible [19, 37]. In those with end-stage renal disease, the proportion who develop a protective antibody response (anti-HBs $\geq$ 10 mIU/mL), however, is suboptimal even with double-dose regimens (55-67%) [38]. Seroconversion rates decrease with declining renal function [39]. Current recommended enhanced-potency (dialysis formulation) dose of recombinant hepatitis B vaccine in patients with end-stage renal disease is 40μg in at least three repeated doses [37, 40]. Revaccination is recommended in non-responders patients (antibody titer < 10mIU/mL). Annual measurements of HBsAb levels to identify those patients with antibodies levels lower than 10 mIU/ml who are not protected against the infection and to inform them on the use of a booster dose of hepatitis B vaccine has been recommended for dialysis patients by the US Advisory Committee on Immunization Practices [37, 41]. In addition, the European Consensus Group on Hepatitis B immunity has expanded this recommendation to include patients with impaired immune function [42].

Primary varicella acquired after transplant can be extremely severe and varicella vaccine (Oka vaccine) should be given to the candidate before transplant if seronegative for VZV (and if transplant is not anticipated within the next 3-4 weeks, because VZV vaccine is live), provided no contraindications are present [14, 43]. Multiple nonrandomized studies in subjects with end-stage renal disease have demonstrated that the Oka vaccine is safe and effective prior to transplant [44-47]. Data from a large French pediatric study support the use of pretransplant VZV vaccination in decreasing the risk of primary varicella and also zoster reactivation post-transplant [47]. Patients with end-stage organ disease have reduced seroconversion rates to varicella vaccination (~60%) [45, 46], so the standard two doses should be given prior to transplantation if practical with a minimal interval of 4-6 weeks [43, 48, 49].

The newly licensed Herpes Zoster vaccine contains approximately 15 times more plaque forming units of live virus then does current Oka varicella vaccines and so poses a risk of disseminated disease in immunosuppressed patients. This vaccine has not been studied in patients with end-organ disease and is currently not recommended for pretransplant patients [43].

Transplant recipients with anogenital *Human papillomavirus* (HPV) infection are at 20-100-fold increased risk of cervical intraepithelial neoplasia and other anogenital malignancies [50]. In addition, transplant recipients are at high risk for HPV-related warts and skin cancers. Although there have not been any specific studies of HPV vaccine involving transplant recipients and candidates to date, preliminary studies in HIV-positive patients suggest that HPV vaccines would be safe and immunogenic even in immunosuppressed patients [51]. Therefore, HPV vaccine should be administered to nonpregnant female transplant candidates aged 9-26 years if they have not yet been vaccinated; the series is three doses at 0, 2 and 6 months, as per current guidelines [52, 53]. However, transplant recipients may still receive the HPV vaccine safely as it is not a live vaccine [50].

Perioperative and Post-Transplant Antimicrobial Prophylaxis

Perioperative Prophylaxis

A number of studies have clearly demonstrated that antimicrobial prophylaxis significantly decreases postoperative infection rates in renal transplant recipients [54-60]. Based on the available literature, the routine use of systemic antimicrobial prophylaxis is justified in patients undergoing kidney transplantation and in patients undergoing donor nephrectomy (draft document of AST guidelines) [61]. The data do not indicate a significant difference between single-drug or multiple-drug antimicrobial regimens [54, 55, 58]. Also, there appear to be no significant differences in SSI rates between single-agent regimens employing anti-staphylococcal penicillins or cephalosporins and between single-dose or 24 hours and multidose regimens [54, 55, 57, 59, 60, 62-65]. Cefazolin for 24 hours was equivalent to seven days surgical prophylaxis in living-related kidney transplant donors [61]. The international recommendations for SSI prevention include limiting the use of vancomycin only when there is a MRSA or MRSE cluster or as alternative for penicillin allergic patients [66-68].

On the basis of the available literature and international guidelines, the possible surgical antibiotic prophylaxis strategies for patients undergoing kidney transplantation are summarized in Table **2**.

Table 2: Surgical antibiotic prophylaxis strategies for patients in kidney transplantation

Patient Features	Drug	Adult Dosages	Pediatric Dosages
Standard	Ampicillin/sulbactam	3 g IV at induction of anesthesia, and 1.5 g every 12 hours for 24-48 hours postoperatively	100 mg/kg IV divided every 6 hours
	Cycled every 3 months		
	Cefazolin	2 g IV at induction of anesthesia, repeat 1 g every 4 hours intraoperatively, followed by 1 g every 8 hours for 24-48 hours postoperatively	20 mg/kg IV at induction of anesthesia, repeated every 4 hours intraoperatively, and every 8 hours for 24-48 hours postoperatively
Allergic to penicillins	Vancomycin	1 g IV once at induction of anesthesia	10-15 mg/kg IV every 8 hours
MRSA positive	Vancomycin	1 g IV once at induction of anesthesia	10-15 mg/kg IV every 8 hours
Diverticulitis	Piperacillin/tazobactam	4.5 g IV at induction of anesthesia, and 2.25 g every 8 hours for 24-48 hours postoperatively	100 mg/kg IV at induction of anesthesia and 50 mg/kg every 8 hours for 24-48 hours postoperatively (Piperacillin/tazobactam safety and efficacy in pediatric patients have not been established)
Past UTI due to a specific pathogen (in recipient or donor)	Antibiotic therapy targeted according to the previous results		
Donor with bacteremia/meningitis	Early antibiotic therapy targeted according to the "second opinion" ID consult		
Others	ID consult		

ID = Infection Diseases.

Post-Transplant Prophylaxis

Most kidney transplant centers use trimethoprim-sulfamethoxazole prophylaxis (one single-strength tablet containing 80 mg of trimethoprim and 400 mg of sulfamethoxazole 3 times a week) for 3-6 months or for lifetime to prevent *Pneumocystis jirovecii* pneumonia as well as infections with *Toxoplasma gondii* and common urinary pathogens [34, 69, 70]. Low-dose trimethoprim sulfamethoxazole is well tolerated and should be used unless there is evidence that the patient has an allergy or interstitial nephritis. Alternative agents for prophylaxis against pneumocystis include dapsone, atovaquone, and pentamidine, but they are less effective than trimethoprim-sulfamethoxazole and lack the breadth of protection [3, 71]. The routine use of sulfamethoxazole/trimethoprim for prophylaxis of *Pneumocystis carinii* pneumonia and urinary tract infections resulted in an increase of resistance against this agent [13]. Therefore, it is preferable to limit antibiotic prophylaxis for the first 6 months to prevent pneumocystis pneumonia and donor-derived *Toxoplasma* infection.

Oral candidiasis is common and local prophylaxis with nystatin usually is given. Currently, there are insufficient data to recommend universal systemic antifungal prophylaxis in solid organ transplant (SOT) patients, particulary in kidney transplant recipients [72, 73]. A more rational approach is the targeted antifungal prophylaxis: the use of an antifungal agent in a subgroup of kidney transplant recipients with predisposing conditions that place them at higher risk of developing invasive fungal infections. This strategy may be adapted to the specific risk factors and continued for a variable period depending upon the persistence of risk factors. Targeted antifungal prophylaxis in SOT recipients is based on both risk factors and epidemiological exposure, since there is no clinically validated indirect test or molecular method for detecting fungi in clinical specimens. Identifying patients at the highest risk of infection is crucial to the development of an effective antifungal prophylaxis. The ideal antifungal agent to be used for prophylaxis is one that is proven to be efficacious, safe to the allograft and other organs, with predictable or no drug interactions, ease of administration, with minimal/manageable side effects, and affordable. It is also important to determine if the patient is at risk for *Candida* infection or at risk for mould infections, particularly due to *Aspergillus*, as this would require the choice of an agent with good anti-mould activity (Table **3**).

Table 3: Possible risk factors for invasive fungal infections in kidney transplant recipients

Risk Factors for Invasive Fungal Infections in Kidney Transplant Recipients		
Candida	***Aspergillus***	**Other Mould**
Retransplantation or reoperation	Retransplantation or reoperation	*Zygomicosis*
Candida colonization	Renal failure and renal replacement therapy	Renal failure
Broad spectrum antibiotics and durationof antibiotic use		Rejection and augmented immunosuppression
	Use of monoclonal antibodies	
High transfusion requirement	Pre or post-transplant *Aspergillus* colonization	Corticosteroid usage
Central venous catheters		
Renal replacement therapy	CMV infection	Exposure to antifungals not active against zygomycetes (*i.e.* voriconazole)
Graft rejection/dysfunction	Rejection and augmented immunosuppression	
Multivisceral transplantation		Poorly controlled diabetes mellitus
		Prolonged neutropenia
	Acquired hypogammaglobulinemia (IgG < 400mg/dL)	Iron chelation with deferoxamine
		Fusariosis
		Prolonged neutropenia
		Impaired macrophage function

Universal antiviral prophylaxis was commonly used for prevention of CMV infection in solid organ transplant patients and has resulted in significant reductions in CMV disease and CMV-related mortality. Antivirals are usually begun in the immediate or very early posttransplant period and continued for a finite period of time, often in the range of 3 to 6 months. Several antivirals have been evaluated for universal prophylaxis, including acyclovir, valacyclovir, IV ganciclovir, oral ganciclovir, and valganciclovir. In early studies, acyclovir was determined to be inferior to ganciclovir for prevention of CMV [74]. Late onset

CMV disease has been the most significant finding in all studies evaluating universal prophylaxis, defined as disease occurring after the discontinuation of prophylaxis. The determinants of late-onset CMV disease in patients receiving prophylaxis have not been fully elucidated, but are likely related to ongoing significant immunosuppression, accompanied by a lack of development of significant CMV specific cell-mediated immunity. Risk factors for late onset disease include Donor (D)+/Recipient (R) - (D+/R-) serostatus, higher levels of immunosuppression, and allograft rejection [75]. In the recently published International Consensus Guidelines, the majority of consensus conference participants favored the use of prophylaxis over preemptive therapy in the highest risk recipients (*e.g.*, D+/R-), based on the available data suggesting better graft survival and clinical outcomes [76]. The consensus recommendations were: both universal prophylaxis and preemptive strategies are viable approaches for prevention of CMVdisease (grade I of evidence); for the highest risk patients (D+/R-), prophylaxis may have some advantages over preemptive therapy (grade II/III of evidence); in kidney transplant recipients valganciclovir, IV or oral ganciclovir, or valacyclovir are recommended for prophylaxis (grade I of evidence); the duration of prophylaxis in D+/R- patients should be generally between 3 months (grade I of evidence) and 6 months (grade I of evidence); in R+ patients (with either D+ or D-), the majority of the experts felt that 3 months of antiviral medication should be used for kidney transplant recipients (grade I/II of evidence) [76].

However, based on their experience, the Authors believe that preemptive therapy is more effective as CMV preventive strategy [77-82]. However, diagnosis, prevention and treatment of CMV infection will be discussed in another chapter of this book.

HSV-specific prophylaxis should be considered for only HSV-1 and HSV-2 seronegative kidney recipients receiving a graft from a donor positive (R-/D+). In the unusual circumstance of a patient who is HSV seronegative, the risk of early posttransplant HSV infection is not well defined, though probable cases of HSV transmission from organs have been described [83]. In this setting, some clinicians may choose to give antiviral prophylaxis while others may consider close clinical monitoring [84]. Patients with a history of frequent clinical HSV-2 reactivations prior to transplant should receive antiviral prophylaxis with valacyclovir (500 mg bid) or famciclovir (500 mg bid) [84, 85]. Dosage adjustment for renal insufficiency is necessary if GFR is <50. Immunosuppression intensification for organ rejection has been associated with HSV-1 recurrence, though usually it is not a life-threatening situation.

Post-Transplant Monitoring and Preemptive Therapy

All kidney transplant recipients must undergo a post-transplant monitoring to detect early infections and/or reactivations (Table **4**).

Table 4: Post-transplant monitoring in kidney transplant recipients

Post-transplant Monitoring																					
Tests	**Time Checked**																				
	1 w	**2 w**	**3 w**	**4 w**	**5 w**	**6 w**	**7 w**	**8 w**	**9 w**	**10 w**	**11 w**	**12 w**	**4 m**	**5 m**	**6 m**	**7 m**	**8 m**	**9 m**	**10 m**	**11 m**	**12 m**
CMV-DNA quantitative *	x	x	x	x	x	x	x	x	x	x	x	x	x	x	x	x	x	x	x	x	x
HHV8-DNA	x			x				x				x	x	x	x						
EBV-DNA quantitative				x				x				x			x			x			x
HIV-Ab				x				x				x			x			x			x
HHV6-DNA				x								x			x						x
Decoy cells on urine and BKV-DNA on peripheral blood												x			x			x			x
Urine examination	x	x	x	x	x	x	X	x	x	x	x	x	x	x	x	x	x	x	x	x	X

and Urine colture																					
Lymphocyte immunophen otyping				x								x			x						X
Any negative serology (HCV, toxoplasma)												x			x			x			X

*If positive, twice a week.

In kidney transplantation, a recommended CMV prevention strategy requires CMV-DNA post-transplant monitoring and the pre-emptive therapy, especially when the logistics (short distance from the lab) will allow close patient monitoring. In preemptive therapy, laboratory monitoring is performed at regular intervals to detect early, asymptomatic viral replication. Once viral replication reaches a certain assay threshold, and hopefully before the development of symptoms, antiviral therapy is initiated to prevent the progression to clinical disease. The advantages of preemptive therapy include more selective drug targeting, decreased drug cost, and associated toxicities. Theoretically, a preemptive strategy may promote the development and maintenance of CMV-specific cell-mediated immunity by allowing low-level viral replication. Reactivation and primary infection must be monitored by quantitative CMV DNA. CMV DNA must be checked weekly for the first 3 months post-transplant, thereafter monthly and every time there is clinical suspicious of CMV infection. CMV DNA cutoff considered prognostic of progression from infection to disease is settled at **100, 000 cp/ml** (Amplicor®). Management is independent from the pre-transplant serostatus of the recipient and the match D/R: 1) If the DNAemia level is positive but below the cutoff (**100, 000 copies/ml**), check again twice a week until DNAemia clearance or start pre-emptive therapy if the DNAemia reaches the threshold of ≥100, 000 copies/ml; 2) If DNAemia level is positive above the cutoff, therapy should be started immediately and ID consult is required; 3) if DNAemia gets positive below the cutoff but patient suffers of a clinical picture suggestive of CMV disease, ID consult is required and other potential causes must be ruled out; 4) if DNAemia is positive, irrespectively from the level, in patients planned for having anti-rejection therapy, pre-emptive therapy needs to be started and to be continued until 2 consecutive negative DNAemia samples are obtained.

The preemtive strategy can be successfully applied to the prevention of other viral infections or reactivations, which can be monitored by molecular tests.

EBV may reactivate in EBV+ recipients, particularly if receiving intensified immunosuppression, eg, antilymphocyte therapy for steroid-refractory rejection. Quantitative EBV-DNA monitoring together with determination of EBV specific T cytotoxic activity measured by enzyme/linked immunospot (elispot®) must be checked at 1, 2, 3, 6, 9, 12 months post-transplant, thereafter every three months and for every patient with signs or symptoms suggestive of EBV symptomatic infection. EBV D+/R- status, more frequent in the pediatric patient, leads to high risk of developing primary EBV infection. If documented primary infection, EBV-DNA must be checked every 15 days.

HHV-6 is the viruses that cause roseola in infants and can reactivate rarely after transplant, often earlier than CMV, and cause cytopenia, fever, pneumonitis, hepatitis, and/or meningoencephalitis. The test of choice is PCR because 90% of adults are seropositive. HHV6-DNA must be checked weekly for the first 3 months post-transplant, thereafter monthly and every time there is clinical suspicious of HHV6 infection

HHV8-DNA detection on peripheral blood will be performed at day 30, 60, 90, 120, 150, 180 post-transplant, regardless of donor/recipient HHV8 serology. ID consult for further clinical evaluation if the HHV8-DNA detection is positive. HHV8-DNA will be detected, at any time after transplantation, on peripheral blood and on tissue samples in case of signs or symptoms suggestive for HHV8-related disease.

All patients undergoing kidney transplantation should be monitored for detection of decoy cells on urine and BKV-DNA on peripheral blood every 3 months during the first 2 years post-transplant, in case of graft dysfunction or renal biopsy.

All patients undergoing solid organ transplantation have to be screened for anti-HIV antibodies according to the following schedule: day 0 (just before transplant), day 30, 60, 180 after transplant, one year after transplant, every year or whenever clinically indicated.

The role of immunologic fungal tests, such as detection of galactomannan and ß-D-glucan in serum, in SOT recipients remains somewhat controvesial. The utility of the galactomannan test for the early diagnosis of invasive aspergillosis has been assessed in a limited number of studies in SOT recipients. According to recent meta-analysis, this assay may have greater utility in hematopoietic stem cell transplant recipients than in SOT recipients in whom the sensitivity and specificity of the test was 22% and 84%, respectively [86]. Because of the low frequency of invasive fungal infections in patients undergoing kidney transplantation and the lack of reliable surrogate markers that could allow prompt diagnosis, post-transplant monitoring with currently available immunologic fungal tests is not recommended.

Each kidney transplant recipients should be monitored for bacterial and fungal infections, expecially in the early post-transplantation period and if receiving intensified immunosuppression.

Urine specimens must be collected for culture twice during the first week, weekly for the first 3 months post-transplant, once every month for the next 3 months and whenever indicated by the presence of fever or symptoms suggestive of UTI.

The risk of bacterial and fungal infections after intensified immunosuppression is better managed by careful observation, minimization of environmental exposures, and early evaluation and treatment if symptoms occur.

Pre-Transplant Counseling and Strategies for Post-Transplant Safe Living

Prevention strategies for infection should not be limited to medications and vaccinations. A thorough education of the transplant recipient and his or her family is a very important preventive tool. Pretransplant classes and printed materials are helpful and should include information on handwashing/hand hygiene, environmental exposures, activities to avoid, food safety and handling, foodborne pathogens, pets and travel. It is also helpful for patients to have a general idea of the infections to which transplant patients are susceptible and the preventive strategies in use at their particular center [17, 18, 87].

In the face of organ shortages, each transplant center will need to weigh the risk-benefit ratio of using organs from donors with active or suspected infection (*i.e.* bacteremia, meningitis, HCV, ...) or organs from increased risk donors. Decisions regarding the use of organs from these donors reflect the urgency of transplantation for the recipient, the availability of alternative organs, and recipient informed consent [6]. It is recommended that the possible use of donors with potential risk of infections transmission be discussed with the patient at the time of transplant evaluation rather than when confronted with the availability of an organ from these donor and informed consent be signed at the time of listing and signed again at the time of availability of such an organ.

A major goal of transplantation is to be able to lead the patient to a healthy and normal life despite the risk of exposure to infectious agents will always be present. Various measures can be taken to reduce the risk of epidemiologic exposures in the hospital and in the community, and transplant recipients should be counseled in order to minimize the risk of infection [87]. The recommendations for a safe living after kidney transplantation are based on the general recognition that solid organ transplant recipients are at greatest risk of infection during the first 6 months after transplantation or when their immunosuppression is augmented for episodes of rejection. These recommendations should be tailored to the individual recipient by their health care providers with special consideration of the patient's degree of immunosuppression and personal circumstances (*i.e.* work, hobbies, travels, *etc.*) [87].

The AST infectious disease guidelines 2009 include a section with strategies for safer living, which covers food and water precautions, pets and animal contact, occupational and recreational hazards, precautions for West Nile virus and other vector-borne infections, ill contacts, and travel issues [87].

Transplant recipients with negative *Toxoplasma* serology should follow the guidelines to reduce the risk of acquiring toxoplasmosis [88]. A printed summary with the recommendation should be given to the patient before discharge after transplantation. The information should be discussed with the patient and family mebers to avoid misunderstanding (Table **5**).

Table 5: Recommendations for prevention of toxoplasmosis

RECOMMENDATIONS FOR PREVENTION OF TOXOPLASMOSIS
• Food should be cooked to safe temperatures. A food thermometer should be used to measure the internal temperature of cooked meat to ensure that meat is cooked all the way through. Beef, lamb, and veal roasts and steaks should be cooked to at least 145 F (63 C°), and pork, ground meat, and wild game should be cooked to 160 F (71 °C) before eating. Whole poultry should be cooked to 180 F (82 °C) in the thigh to ensure doneness.
• Fruits and vegetables should be peeled or thoroughly washed before eating
• Cutting boards, dishes, counters, utensils, and hands should always be washed with hot soapy water after they have contacted raw meat, poultry, seafood, or unwashed fruits or vegetables.
• Transplant patient should wear gloves when gardening and during any contact with soil or sand because cat waste might be in soil or sand. After gardening or contact with soil or sand, wash hands thoroughly.
• Transplant patients should avoid changing cat litter if possible. If no one else is available to change the cat litter, use gloves, then wash hands thoroughly. Change the litter box daily because *Toxoplasma* oocysts require several days to become infectious. Transplant patient should be encouraged to keep their cats inside and not adopt or handle stray cats. Cats should be fed only canned or dried commercial food or well-cooked table food, not raw or undercooked meats.
• The government and the meat industry should continue efforts to reduce *Toxoplasma* in meat.

GENERAL APPROACH TO DIAGNOSIS AND TREATMENT

The spectrum of infection in the immunocompromised host is quite broad. Given the toxicity of antimicrobial agents and the need for rapid interruption of infection, early specific diagnosis is essential in this population. Advances in diagnostic modalities (CT scan or magnetic resonance imaging scanning and molecular microbiologic techniques) may greatly assist in this process. However, given the diminished immune responses of the host and the frequency of multiple simultaneous processes, invasive procedures are often the preferred method for optimal care [4].

All transplant patients with a suspected severe infection require appropriate antimicrobial agents immediately; appropriate cultures must be obtained beforehand. Antimicrobial susceptibilities should be obtained for all bacterial isolates because antimicrobial resistance is increasingly common. Appropriate empiric antibiotic treatment, administered to the patient before identification of the pathogen or its antibiotic susceptibilities, decreases the fatality rate by one-half [89]. Initial antimicrobial therapy should include one or more drugs active against the likely pathogens (bacterial or fungal) involved at the presumed site of infection.

With the aim of achieving the highest efficacy, the choice of drugs takes into account complex issues related to the nature and source (nosocomial *vs.* community acquired) of the infection, the clinical syndrome, the patient's history (including drug intolerance), underlying risk factors (*i.e.* length of hospitalization, intensive care unit (ICU) admissions, previous antimicrobial chemotherapy exposure, concomitant medical problems), the local resistance patterns of the microorganisms and the pharmacokinetic (PK) and pharmacodynamic (PD) parameters of the selected drugs [90, 91].

At 48-72 h, antibiotic treatment should be reviewed on the basis of the results of initial cultures and the clinical response. Whenever possible, the spectrum should be narrowed, with the aim of containing costs, reducing the risk of emergence of resistant organisms, and minimizing the potential for drug toxicity or interactions. At the same time, it must be recognized and taken into account that some infections are polymicrobial (*e.g.*, intra-abdominal infections, most cases of necrotizing soft tissue infection), even if only a single pathogen is identified. If the presenting clinical syndrome is determined to be attributable to a non-infective cause, antibiotic therapy should be stopped promptly to minimize the risk of emergence of resistant pathogens.

Drug levels should be measured when these are available (vancomycin, aminoglycosides, voriconazole, *etc.*) and doses should be adjusted appropriately.

In a transplant recipient who is neutropenic and has fever or other signs or symptoms of infection, human granulocyte colony-stimulating factor (G-CSF) should be administered to increase the neutrophil count; several studies have shown no increased risk of rejection from G-CSF in kidney transplantation [92-94].

In a leukopenic transplant recipient with signs or symptoms of infection, consideration should be given to decreasing or temporarily discontinuing other medications that can cause leukopenia (eg, azathioprine, mycophenolate mofetil or cotrimoxazole).

In presence of an acute infection it may be reasonable to reduce the intensity of immune suppression. This should be done with caution to avoid the risk of inducing a graft rejection, that would result in an increase in immunosuppressive therapy. This may be useful mostly for patients with reactivation of latent viral infections (CMV, EBV, or BKV), fungal infections, or tuberculosis, in whom infection should be seen as evidence of excessive immune suppression. Particularly important in these cases is the reduction or withdrawal of the steroids.

An important aspect in managing post-transplant infections is the awareness of potential drug interactions between immunosuppressive medications and the antimicrobial agents [91]. The optimal outcome of management of any infection depends not only on the knowledge of the infecting organism and the antimicrobial sensitivity, but also on the prevention of adverse events from severe drug interactions and allograft dysfunction that results from drug interaction [5].

Generally, drug interactions can be grouped into 2 major types: pharmacokinetic and pharmacodynamic [95]. Knowledge of the interactions is very helpful to avoid some antimicrobial agent whenever possible, find an alternative, or modify the dose of immunosuppressive agent appropriately during coadministration. Monitoring drug levels in a controlled situation such as in hospital or in a transplant clinic is important when initiating or discontinuing the interacting antimicrobial agents. Occasionally, multiple drugs can augment the severity of interactions as can be seen with statins, macrolide antibiotics, and calcineurin inhibitors agents.

The degree of interactions between anti-infective agents and immunosuppressant is shown in Table **6**.

Table 6: Adverse effects and interactions between anti-infective agents and immunosuppressant

Anti-infective Agent (A)	**Adverse Effects**	**Interactions and Effects Immunosuppressants (B) (Import)**			**Comments**
		TAC	**CSA**	**Sirolimus**	
Macrolides	Prolonged QTc, tinnitus or deafness	↑ levels of B (++)	↑ levels of B (+)	No	Avoid concomitant drugs with potential to prolong QTc
Fluoriquinolones	Photosensivity, tendinopathy,	No	↑ levels of B (±) only cipro and ofloxa	No	Avoid concomitant drugs with potential to prolong QTc
Rifampicin	Hepatotoxicity	↓ levels of B (++)	↓ effect of B (++)	No	Discolors urine, tears, sweat, contact lens an orange-brownish color
Aminoglycosides	Nephro/ototoxicity	↑ nephrotoxicity (+)	↑ nephrotoxicity (+)	No	
Fluconazole	Hepatotoxicity	↑ levels of B (++) with toxicity	↑ levels of B (+) with toxicity	No	
Deoxycholate Ampho B	Nephrotoxicity, ↓ K and Mg serum levels	No	↑ nephrotoxicity of A (++)	No	
Liposomal Ampho B	Nephrotoxicity, Hepatotoxicity, ↓ K and Mg serum levels	No	↑ nephrotoxicity of A (++)	No	

Table 6: cont….

Voriconazole	Hepatotoxicity, transiet visual disturbance in 1/3 of patients	↑ levels of B (++) with toxicity (↓ *TAC doses of 67%)*	↑ levels of B (+) with toxicity (↓ *CSA doses of 50%)*	↑ levels of B (++)	Not IV if CrCl < 50 mL/min. Not in urine in active form
Posaconazole	Hepatotoxicity, nausea, vomiting	↑ levels of B (++) with toxicity (↓ *TAC doses of 1/3)*	↑ levels of B (+) with toxicity CSA clearance ↓ 16-33% (↓ *CSA doses of ¾)*	↑ levels of B (++)	High fat meal ↑ absorption
Caspofungin	Hepatotoxicity (mild), pruritus at infusion	↓ levels of B (++) AUC of TAC ↓ 25%	↑ levels of B (++) AUC of caspofungin ↑ 35%	No	↓doses in moderate to severe hepatic failure. No drug in CSF or urine
Micafungin	Hepatotoxicity (mild)	ND	No	↑ levels of B (+) AUC of sirolimus ↑21%	No drug in CSF or urine
Anidulafungin	Headache	No	↑ levels of B (+) AUC of anidulafungin ↑ 22%	ND	No dose adjustments for renal or hepatic insuff. No drug in CSF or urine
Protease inhibitors	Multiple effects	↑ levels of B (+++)	↑ levels of B (+++)	↑ levels of B (+++)	ID expert needed

COMMON INFECTIONS AFTER RENAL TRANSPLANTATION

Urinary Tract Infections

UTI is the most common infection in renal transplant recipients, ranging from 6% to 86% and accounting for approximately 40-50% of all infectious complications [96-103]. These infections are detected frequently within one month post-transplant and can be seen in high rates within the first year [13, 64, 104].

Many risk factors for UTI in renal allograft recipients are similar to those in the general population, such as advanced age, female gender and diabetes [13, 105, 106]. Similarly anatomical factors predisposing to UTI like urinary stasis, reflux and stones are more prominent in renal transplant recipients [107]. Specific potential risk factors include pre-transplant UTI, prolonged period of haemodialysis before transplantation, polycystic kidney disease and retransplantation [13, 105]. Operative risk factors include organism transmission with the graft, allograft trauma, cadaveric graft with prolonged ischemic time and technical complications associated with ureteral anastomosis [64, 105, 108]. Postoperative factors include the use of ureteral stents, duration of urinary bladder catheterization, length of hospital stay, impaired graft function and acute rejection episodes (Table 7) [13, 64, 105, 108].

The causative organisms are similar to those causing UTI in the general population: gram-negative bacterial infections account for more than 70% and *Escherichia coli* is the most common clinical isolate [104, 105, 109]. Howerer, resistant pathogens such as ESBL-producing *Klebsiella*, vancomycin-resistant *Enterococcus* spp, *Pseudomonas aeruginosa*, and *Candida* spp have all emerged as significant pathogens [5, 13, 110].

Renal transplant recipients with UTIs are more likely to be clinically asymptomatic compared to non-immunocompromised patients. On the other hand, UTI is often associated with acute pyelonephritis and rapidly developing bacteraemia, particularly during the early post-transplant period. Therefore, careful surveillance is necessary to identify and eliminate these infections. Importantly, UTIs have been shown to be the most common source of bacteraemia in renal transplant recipients [111, 112]. Patients are at especially high risk for UTI in the first month post-transplant, when the bacteraemia-associated mortality is around 11%.

Interestingly, UTIs did not increase the risk for renal graft loss but were significantly associated with increased mortality. In contrast, post-transplant acute pyelonephritis was associated with an impairment of long term allograft function but not with the mortality of the patients [113].

Table 7: Potential risk factors involved in the development of UTIs after kidney transplantation

Female gender
Advanced age
Pre-transplant UTIs
Prolonged period of haemodialysis before transplantation
Intensive immunosuppression
Acute rejection episodes
Impaired graft function
Bladder catheter postoperatively
Technical complications associated with ureteral anastomosis
Intraoperative ureteral stents
Surgical manipulation of the graft (allograft trauma)
Contaminated graft perfusion solution
Diabetes mellitus
History of vesicoureteral reflux
History of polycystic kidney disease
Deceased donor
Schistosomiasis

Surgical site Infections (SSI)

The incidence of SSI in kidney transplant recipients ranged from 0% to 11% with antimicrobial prophylaxis to 2% to 7.5% without systemic prophylaxis [13, 64, 104, 110, 114-116]. The majority of these infections were superficial in nature and were detected within 30 days post-transplantation [13, 104, 114, 115]. Surgical site infections were found in 2% to 4% of living-related kidney transplant donors who received antimicrobial prophylaxis [61]. Risk factors for SSI after kidney transplantation include contamination of organ perfusate, patient factors pre-transplant of diabetes, chronic glomerulonephritis and obesity, factors related to the procedure, such as ureteral leakage and hematoma formation, type of immunosuppressive therapy, in particular sirolimus-containing regimens, and postoperative complications of acute graft rejections, reoperation and delayed graft function [64, 110, 114, 117, 118]. These infections are usually caused by gram-positive organisms, particularly *Staphylococcus* species (including *S. aureus* and *S. epidermidis*) and *Enterococcus* species, gram-negative organisms (*E.coli*, *Enterobacter* species, *Klebsiella* species and *Pseudomonas aeruginosa*), and rarely by yeast with *Candida* species [13, 56, 59, 64, 65, 104, 110, 119, 120].

Hepatitis B

The prevalence of overt carriers of HBsAg among dialysed patients is 0-7% in developed countries and 10-20% in developing ones [121]. Acquisition of HBV on dialysis is now uncommon in the majority of dialysis centers. For the most part HBsAg positivity can be attributed to standard risk factors (birth in endemic country, vertical transmission, injection drug use, sexual transmission), although dialysis-associated outbreaks continue to be reported [122].

In these subjects, the frequent normality of the liver function tests makes clinical judgment difficult, confirming the fundamental role of the virological markers (quantitative HBV-DNA) and of the liver biopsy to distinguish between active and inactive carriers [123]. In kidney transplant, the rate of HBsAg carrier can be estimated in 10-20% of cases and it is associated with a significantly higher risk of death (OR 2.49, 95% CI), independently by the viremic condition (active or inactive carrier), and the presence of chronic hepatitis shows an accelerated course towards cirrhosis (5.3-12% year), decompensation and hepatocarcinoma [124, 125]. No controlled trials for the treatment of HBV with either interferon (IFN) or nucleos(t)ides analogues (NAs) in dialysed patients or in kidney transplants are currently available.

Interferon can be used to treat dialysed patients with chronic hepatitis B, but it is contraindicated in transplanted patients. Short-term administration of lamivudine monotherapy is effective but when the drug is withdrawn, viremia rebounds and hepatitis relapses in most cases. Continuous administration of lamivudine monotherapy for 3-4 years is able to obtain long-term suppression of HBV replication and may prevent the development of liver related complications and mortality [126]. Secondary treatment failure is caused by the emergence of YMDD which in some patients herald hepatitic flares and progression of the liver disease.

In *active carriers* candidates for kidney transplant, the indication to therapy is confirmed, both in pre-transplant (with NAs or IFN, when tolerated) and post-transplant phase (only NAs in view of the high risk of IFN-induced rejection) [123].

For the *inactive carrier* patients, pre-transplant and during dialysis there is no indication for prophylaxis, however biochemical and virological monitoring is advised. Instead, therapy should be used in the re-activated forms (HBV DNA ≥20, 000 IU/mL), especially if associated with significant liver damage (HAI score > 4 and/or signs of fibrotic disease by noninvasive methods). Post-transplant, instead, there is an indication to prophylaxis, in relation to the available data on mortality in HBV carriers, independently from their virological condition [124].

In HBsAg negative and HBcAb positive recipients of kidney transplant the presence of subclinical manifestations (low levels of circulating HBV DNA detectable with amplified techniques post-transplant) without seroreversion has been reported in over 95% of the cases [124, 125, 127, 128]. In this condition, HBsAg monitoring is the only requirement and prophylaxis or therapy should be started only if seroreversion and/or hepatitis, occurs [123].

Hepatitis C

Historically, the prevalence of HCV in patients with end-stage renal disease has been up to 10-fold that of the general population; however with strict adherence to routine infection control practices and screening of blood products, the prevalence has declined over the past decade, averaging 7.8% in U.S. hemodialysis units [129]. Initial screening for antibody to HCV should be done at the time of transplant assessment using a third- or fourth generation enzyme immunoassay (EIA). The third-generation assay has improved sensitivity compared to older assays and false negative EIAs are rare even in the setting of immunosuppressed patients [130, 131]. However, in transplant candidates or recipients with negative HCV serology and persistent unexplained liver enzyme abnormalities, qualitative HCV RNA testing to rule out false negative testing should be considered [19]. In those with positive HCV serology, quantitative HCV RNA and HCV genotype should be determined to confirm current infection. All candidates with chronic HCV infection should undergo staging of liver disease with abdominal ultrasound and liver biopsy [19, 37, 132]. Those without advanced fibrosis (METAVIR stage F0-F2) should be listed for transplant [133-135]; however IFN-based therapy should be considered prior to transplant [19, 136]. Those with bridging fibrosis or compensated cirrhosis should undergo IFN-based therapy and may be listed for transplant if a sustained virological response (SVR) is achieved. Those with decompensated cirrhosis are generally not considered candidates for isolated renal transplant but may be considered for combined liver-kidney transplant [19, 132, 137]. Treatment of HCV infection prior to kidney transplant has been shown to have a benefit on posttransplant outcomes [138]. Pretransplant HCV therapy in renal transplant candidates, however, is associated with suboptimal SVR rates and a higher rate of adverse events and discontinuation due to intolerability than in the general population. With standard IFN monotherapy, the overall SVR rate is 37% and ranges from 13% to 75% with PEG-IFN monotherapy [132]. Most of the studies are small and many have not reported the response rate by genotype.

The kidneys play a major role in the catabolism and filtration of both IFN and ribavirin; thus, their clearances may be affected in subjects with chronic kidney-disease (CKD) [139, 140]. The clearance of pegylated interferon is affected in those with CKD, although hemodialysis does not affect its clearance [141]. Hence, the AASLD (American Association for the Study of Liver Diseases) guidelines recommend subcutaneous weekly doses of 1 μg/kg of peginterferon alpha-2b or 135 μg of peginterferon alpha-2a [142] to patients with stage 3-5 CKD. Because ribavirin is eliminated by the kidney and if overdosed might result in dramatic anemia, ribavirin therapy is contraindicated when creatinine clearance is <50 mL/min [143]. However, several case series have examined the use of ribavirin in combination with IFN-based therapy in patients with chronic HCV and poor renal function [144-149]. The largest series published so far on the combined use of peginterferon alpha-2a plus ribavirin in hemodialysis patients obtained a SVR rate of 97% (34/35) in the treated patients (peginterferon alpha-2a plus ribavirin) *versus* 0% (0/35) in untreated controls [150]. These findings have not been confirmed in further reports where the SVR rate ranges between 7% and 71% [151].

With regard to this combined therapy, the AASLD guidelines state that ribavirin can be used in combination with interferon with a markedly reduced daily dose with careful monitoring for anemia and other adverse effects [142].

REFERENCES

[1] Fishman JA and the ATS Infectious Diseases Community of Practice. Introduction: Infection in solid-organ transplant recipients. Am J Transplant 2009; 9: S3-S6.

[2] Fishman JA, Rubin RH. Infection in organ-transplant recipients. N Engl J Med 1998; 338: 1741-1751.

[3] Fishman JA. Infection in solid-organ transplant recipients. N Engl J Med 2007; 357: 2601-2614.

[4] Fishman JA. Infection in Renal Transplant Recipients. Semin Nephrol 2007; 27: 445-461.

[5] Parasuraman R, Yee J, Karthikeyan V, del Busto R. Infectious Complications in Renal Transplant Recipients. Adv Chronic Kidney Dis 2006; 13: 280-294.

[6] Grossi P, Fishman JA and the ATS Infectious Diseases Community of Practice. Donor-Derived infections in solid organ transplant recipients. Am J Transplant 2009; 9: S19-S26.

[7] Avery RK. Infections and immunizations in organ transplant recipients: a preventive approach. Cleve Clin J Med 1994; 61: 386-392.

[8] Avery RK. Prophylactic strategies before solid-organ transplantation. Curr Opin Infect Dis 2004; 17: 353-356.

[9] Preiksaitis JK, Green M, Avery RK. Guidelines for the prevention and management of infectious complications of solid organ transplantation. Am J Transplant 2004; 4 (Suppl. 10): 5-166.

[10] Singh N. Nosocomial infections in solid organ transplant recipients. In: C. Glen Mayall, Ed. *Hospital Epidemiology and Infection Control*. 3rd edition. Philadelphia, Lippincott Williams & Wilkins, 2004; pp. 985-1009.

[11] Singh N, Gayowski T, Rihs JD, *et al.* Evolving Trends in Multiple-Antibiotic-Resistant Bacteria in Liver Transplant Recipients: A Longitudinal Study of Antimicrobial Susceptibility Patterns. Liver Transpl 2001; 7: 22-26.

[12] Menezes FG, Wey SB, Peres CA, *et al.* Risk factors for surgical site infection in kidney transplant recipients. Infect Control Hosp Epidemiol 2008; 29: 771-773.

[13] Alangaden GJ, Thyagarajan R, Gruber SA, *et al.* Infectious complications after kidney transplantation: current epidemiology and associated risk factors. Clin Transplant. 2006; 20: 401-409.

[14] Avery RK. Infectious Disease Following Kidney Transplant: Core Curriculum 2010. Am J Kidney Dis 2010; 55: 755-771.

[15] Coffman KL. The debate about marijuana usage in transplant candidates: recent medical evidence on marijuana health effects. Curr Opin Organ Transplant 13: 189-195.

[16] Avery RK. Recipient Screening Prior to Solid-Organ Transplantation. Clin Infect Dis 2002; 35: 1513-1519.

[17] Screening of Donor and Recipient Prior to Solid Organ Transplantation. Am J Transplant 2004; 4(Suppl 10): 10-20.

[18] Fischer SA, Avery RK and the AST Infectious Disease Community of Practice. Screening of Donor and Recipient Prior to Solid Organ Transplantation. Am J Transplant 2009; S7-S18.

[19] Levitsky J, Doucetteb K and the AST. Infectious Diseases Community of PracticeViral Hepatitis in Solid Organ Transplant Recipients. Am J Transplant 2009; 9 (Suppl 4): S116–S130.

[20] Morales JM, Campistol JM. Transplantation in the patient with hepatitis C. J Am Soc Nephrol 2000; 11: 1343-1353.

[21] Centers for Disease Control and Prevention. Discordant Results from Reverse Sequence Syphilis Screening- Five Laboratories, United States, 2006–2010. Morb Mortal Wkly Rep 2011; 60: 134-137.

[22] Marangoni A, Sambri V, Storni E, *et al.* *Treponema pallidum* surface immunofluorescence assay for serologic diagnosis of syphilis. Clin Diagn Lab Immunol 2000;7: 417-421.

[23] Cole MJ. Comparative evaluation of 15 serological assays for the detection of syphilis infection. Eur J Clin Microbiol Infect Dis 2007; 26: 705-713.

[24] Centers for Disease Control and Prevention. Sexually Transmitted Diseases Treatment Guidelines, 2010. Morb Mortal Wkly Rep 2010; 59: 1-110.

[25] *Mycobacterium tuberculosis*, in Guidelines for the Prevention and Management of Infectious Complications of Solid Organ Transplantation. Am J Transplant 2004; 4(Suppl 10): 37-41.

[26] Subramanian A, Dorman S and the AST Infectious Diseases Community of Practice: *Mycobacterium tuberculosis* in Solid Organ Transplant Recipients. Am J Transplant 2009; 9 (Suppl 4): S57-S62.

[27] Currie AC, Knight SR, Morris PJ. Tuberculosis in Renal Transplant Recipients: The Evidence for Prophylaxis. Transplantation 2010; 90: 695-704.

[28] Controlling Tuberculosis in the United States. This Official Joint Statement of the American Thoracic Society, the Centers for Disease Control and Prevention, and the Infectious Diseases Society of America was approved by the ATS Board of Directors, June 2004, the Centers for Disease Control and Prevention, November 2004, and the IDSA Board of Directors, March 2005. Am J Respir Crit Care Med 2005; 172: 1169-1227.

[29] Singh N, Paterson DL. *Mycobacterium tuberculosis* infection in solidorgan transplant recipients: impact and implications for management. Clin Infect Dis 1998; 27: 1266-1277.

[30] John GT, Thomas PP, Thomas M, *et al.* A double-blind randomized controlled trial of primary isoniazid prophylaxis in dialysis and transplant patients. Transplantation 1994; 57: 1683-1684.

[31] EBPG Expert Group in Renal Transplantation. European best practice guidelines for renal transplantation. Section IV: Long-term management of the transplant recipient. IV.7.2. Late infections. Tuberculosis. Nephrol Dial Transplant 2002; 17(Suppl 4): 39-43.

[32] Vikrant S, Agarwal SK, Gupta S, *et al.* Prospective randomized control trial of isoniazid chemoprophylaxis during renal replacement therapy. Transpl Infect Dis 2005; 7: 99-108.

[33] Agarwal SK, Gupta S, Dash SC, *et al.* Prospective randomised trial of isoniazid prophylaxis in renal transplant recipient. Int Urol Nephrol 2004; 36: 425-431.

[34] Kotton CN, Lattes R and the AST Infectious Disease Community of Practice. Parasitic Infections in Solid Organ Transplant Recipients. Am J Transplant 2009; 9; S234-S251.

[35] Marty FM. Strongyloides hyperinfection syndrome and transplantation: a preventable, frequently fatal infection. Transpl Infect Dis 2009; 11: 97-99.

[36] Danzinger-Isakov L, Kumar D and the AST Infectious Disease Community of Practice. Guidelines for Vaccination of Solid Organ Transplant Candidates and Recipients. Am J Transplant 2009; 9; S258-S262.

[37] Kidney Disease: Improving Global Outcomes (KDIGO) Transplant Work Group. KDIGO clinical practice guideline for the care of kidney transplant recipients. Am J Transplant 2009; 9(Suppl 3): S1–S157.

[38] Keating GM, Noble S. Recombinant hepatitis B vaccine (Engerix- B): A reviewof its immunogenicity and protective efficacy against hepatitis B. Drugs 2003; 63: 1021-1051.

[39] DaRoza G, Loewen A, Djurdjev O, *et al.* Stage of chronic kidney disease predicts seroconversion after hepatitis B immunization: Earlier is better. Am J Kidney Dis 2003; 42: 1184-1192.

[40] Duchini A, Goss JA, Karpen S, Pockros PJ. Vaccinations for Adult Solid-Organ Transplant Recipients: Current Recommendations and Protocols. Clin Microbiol Rev 2003; 16:357-364.

[41] Recommendations for preventing transmission of infections among chronic hemodialysis patients. MMWR Recomm Rep 2001; 50: 1-43.

[42] Are booster immunisations needed for lifelong hepatitis B immunity? European Consensus Group on Hepatitis B Immunity. Lancet 2000; 355: 561–565.

[43] Pergam SA, Limaye AP and the AST Infectious Diseases Community of Practic Varicella Zoster Virus (VZV) in Solid Organ Transplant Recipients. Am J Transplant 2009; 9 (Suppl 4): S108–S115.

[44] Geel A, Zuidema W, van Gelder T, *et al.* Successful vaccination against varicella zoster virus prior to kidney transplantation. Transplant Proc 2005; 37: 952–953.

[45] Furth SL, Hogg RJ, Tarver J, *et al.* Varicella vaccination in children with chronic renal failure. A report of the Southwest Pediatric Nephrology Study Group. Pediatr Nephrol 2003; 18: 33–38.

[46] Webb NJ, Fitzpatrick MM, Hughes DA, *et al.* Immunisation against varicella in end stage and pre-end stage renal failure. Trans-Pennine Paediatric Nephrology Study Group. Arch Dis Child 2000; 82: 141-143.

[47] Broyer M, Tete MJ, Guest G, *et al.* Varicella and zoster in children after kidney transplantation: Long-term results of vaccination. Pediatrics 1997; 99: 35-39.

[48] Burroughs M, Moscona A. Immunization of pediatric solid organ transplant candidates and recipients. Clin Infect Dis 2000; 30: 857-869.

[49] Levin MJ. Varicella vaccination of immunocompromised children. J Infect Dis 2008; 197(Suppl 2): S200–S206.

[50] Kwak EJ, Julian K and the AST Infectious Diseases Community of Practice Human Papillomavirus Infection in Solid Organ Transplant Recipients. Am J Transplant 2009; 9 (Suppl 4): S151-S160.

[51] Anderson JS, Hoy J, Hillman R, *et al.* A randomized, placebocontrolled, dose-escalation study to determine the safety, tolerability, and immunogenicity of an HPV-16 therapeutic vaccine in HIV-positive participants with oncogenic HPV infection of the anus. J Acquir Immune Defic Syndr. 2009; 52 : 371-381.

[52] Markowitz LE, Dunne EF, Saraiya M, *et al.* Quadrivalent Human Papillomavirus Vaccine: Recommendations of the Advisory Committee on Immunization Practices (ACIP). MMWR Recomm Rep 2007; 56(RR-2): 1–24.

[53] Avery RK, Michaels M. Update on Immunizations in Solid Organ Transplant Recipients: What Clinicians Need to Know. Am J Transplant 2008; 8: 9-14.

[54] Tilney NL, Strom TB, Vineyard GC, *et al.* Factors contributing to the declining mortality rate in renal transplantation. N Engl J Med 1978; 299: 1321-1325.

[55] Cohen J, Rees AJ, Williams G. A prospective randomized controlled trial of perioperative antibiotic prophylaxis in renal transplantation. J Hosp Infect 1988; 11: 357-363.

[56] Hoy WE, May AG, Freeman RB. Primary renal transplant wound infections. N Y State J Med 1981; 81: 1469-1473.

[57] Muakkassa WF, Goldman MH, Mendez-Picon G, *et al.* Wound infections in renal transplant patients. J Urol 1983; 130: 17-19.

[58] Novick AC. The value of intraoperative antibiotics in preventing renal transplant wound infections. J Urol 1981; 125: 151-152.

[59] Judson RT. Wound infection following renal transplantation. Aust N Z J Surg 1984; 54: 223-224.

[60] Del Rio G, Dalet F, Chechile G. Antimicrobial prophylaxis in urologic surgery: does it give some benefit? Eur Urol 1993; 24: 305-312.

[61] Zomorrodi A, Buhluli A. Is antibiotic usage necessary after donor nephrectomy? A single center experience. Saudi J Kidney Dis Transpl 2008; 19: 200-205.

[62] Kohlberg WI, Tellis VA, Bhat DJ, *et al.* Wound infections after transplant nephrectomy. Arch Surg 1980; 115: 645-646.

[63] Capocasale E, Mazzoni MP, Tondo S, *et al.* Antimicrobial prophylaxis with ceftriaxone in renal transplantation. Prospective study of 170 patients. Chemotherapy 1994; 40: 435-440.

[64] Dantas SPRE, Kuboyama RH, Mazzali M, Moretti ML. Nosocomial infections in renal transplant patients: risk factors and treatment implications associated with urinary tract and surgical site infections. J Hosp Infect 2006; 63: 117-123.

[65] Pfundstein J, Roghmann M-C, Schwalbe RS, *et al.* A randomized trial of surgical antimicrobial prophylaxis with and without vancomycin in organ transplant patients. Clin Transplant 1999; 13: 245-252.

[66] Mangram AJ, Horan TC, Pearson ML, *et al.* Guideline for prevention of surgical site infection. Infect Control Hosp Epidemiol 1999; 20: 250-269.

[67] Gemmell CG, Edwards DI, Fraise AP, *et al.* Guidelines for the prophylaxis and treatment of methicillin-resistant Staphylococcus aureus (MRSA) infections in the UK. J Antimicrob Chemother 2006; 57: 589-608.

[68] Bolon MK, Morlote M, Weber SG, *et al.* Glycopeptides are no more effective than beta-lactam agents for prevention of surgical site infection after cardiac surgery: A meta-analysis. Clin Infect Dis 2004; 38: 1357-1363.

[69] Soave R. Prophylaxis strategies for solid-organ transplantation. Clin Infect Dis 2001; 33(suppl 1): s26-s31.

[70] Martin SI, Fishman JA and the AST Infectious Diseases Community of Practice. Pneumocystis Pneumonia in Solid Organ Transplant Recipients. Am J Transplantation 2009; 9 (Suppl 4): S227–S233.

[71] Rodriguez M, Fishman JA. Prevention of infection due to Pneumocystis spp. in human immunodeficiency virus-negative immunocompromised patients. Clin Microbiol Rev 2004; 17: 770-782.

[72] Cruciani M, Mengoli C, Malena M, *et al.* Antifungal prophylaxis in liver transplant patients: a systematic review and meta-analysis. Liver Transpl 2006; 12 : 850-858.

[73] Playford EG, Webster AC, Sorell TC, Craig JC. Antifungal agents for preventing fungal infections in solid organ transplant recipients. Cochrane Database Syst Rev 2004; (3): CD004291.

[74] Rubin RH, Kemmerly SA, Conti D, *et al.* Prevention of primary cytomegalovirus disease in organ transplant recipients with oral ganciclovir or oral acyclovir prophylaxis. Transpl Infect Dis 2000; 23: 112-117.

[75] Razonable RR, Rivero A, Rodriguez A, *et al.* Allograft rejection predicts the occurrence of late-onset cytomegalovirus (CMV) disease among CMV-mismatched solid organ transplant patients receiving prophylaxis with oral ganciclovir. J Infect Dis 2001; 184: 1461-1464.

[76] Kotton CN, Kumar D, Caliendo AM, *et al;* on behalf of The Transplantation Society International CMV Consensus Group International Consensus Guidelines on the Management of Cytomegalovirus in Solid Organ Transplantation. Transplantation 2010; 89: 779-795.

[77] Grossi P, Minoli L, Percivalle E, *et al.* Clinical and virological monitoring of human cytomegalovirus infection in 294 heart transplant recipients. Transplantation 1995; 27; 59: 847-851.

[78] Grossi P, Kusne S, Rinaldo C, *et al.* Guidance of ganciclovir therapy with PP65 antigenemia in cytomegalovirus-free recipients of livers from seropositive donors. Transplantation 1996; 61: 1659-1660.

[79] Kusne S, Grossi P, Irish W, *et al.* Cytomegalovirus PP65 antigenemia monitoring as a guide for preemptive therapy: a cost effective strategy for prevention of cytomegalovirus disease in adult liver transplant recipients. Transplantation 1999; 68: 1125-1131.

[80] Lilleri D, Baldanti F, Gatti M, *et al.* Clinically-Based Determination of Safe DNAemia Cutoff Levels for Preemptive Therapy or Human Cytomegalovirus Infections in Solid Organ and Hematopoietic Stem Cell Transplant Recipients. J Med Virol 2004; 73: 412-419.

[81] Gerna G, Baldanti F, Torsellini M, *et al.* Evaluation of cytomegalovirus DNAaemia versus pp65-antigenaemia cutoff for guiding preemptive therapy in transplant recipients: a randomized study. Antiviral Therapy 2007; 12: 63-72.

[82] Baldanti F, Lilleri D, Gerna G. Monitoring human cytomegalovirus infection in transplant recipients. J Clinical Virology 2008; 41: 237-241.

[83] Basse G, Mengelle C, Kamar N, *et al.* Disseminated herpes simplex type 2 (HSV-2) infection after solid-organ transplantation. Infection 2008; 36: 62-64.

[84] Zuckerman R, Wald A and the AST Infectious Diseases Community of Practice Herpes Simplex Virus Infections in Solid Organ Transplant Recipients. Am J Transplant 2009; 9 (Suppl 4): S104-S107.

[85] Conant MA, Schacker TW, Murphy RL, *et al.* Valaciclovir versus aciclovir for herpes simplex virus infection in HIV-infected individuals: Two randomized trials. Int J STD AIDS 2002; 13: 12-21.

[86] Pfeiffer CD, Fine JP, Safdar N. Diagnosis of invasive aspergillosis using a galactomannan assay: A meta-analysis. Clin Infect Dis 2006; 42: 1417-1427.

[87] Avery RK, Michaels MG and the AST Infectious Diseases Community of Practice. Strategies for Safe Living Following Solid Organ Transplantation. Am J Transplant 2009; 9 (Suppl 4): S252–S257.

[88] CDC Preventing Congenital Toxoplasmosis. MMWR 2000 March 31, 2000 / 49(RR02); 57-75.

[89] Ibrahim EH, Sherman G, Ward S, *et al.* The influence of inadequate antimicrobial treatment of bloodstream infections on patient outcomes in the ICU setting. Chest 2000; 118: 146-155.

[90] Grossi P, Dalla Gasperina D. Antimicrobial treatment of sepsis. Surg Infect 2006; 7: S87-91.

[91] Thomas LD, Miller GG and the AST Infectious Diseases Community of Practice. Interactions between Antiinfective Agents and Immunosuppressants. Am J Transplantation 2009; 9 (Suppl 4): S263–S266.

[92] Schmaldienst S, Bekesi G, Deicher R, *et al.* Recombinant human granulocyte colony-stimulating factor after kidney transplantation: a retrospective analysis to evaluate the benefit or risk of immunostimulation. Transplantation 2000; 69: 527-531.

[93] Turgeon N, Hovingh GK, Fishman JA, *et al.* Safety and efficacy of granulocyte colony-stimulating factor in kidney and liver transplant recipients. Tranplant Infect Dis 2000: 2: 15-21.

[94] Hartmann EL, Gatesman M, Roskopf-Somerville J, *et al.* Management of leukopenia in kidney and pancreas transplant recipients. Clin Transplant 2008: 22: 822-828.

[95] Srinivas TR, Meier-Kriesche HU, Kaplan B. Pharmacokinetic principles of immunosuppressive drugs. Am J Transplant 2005; 5: 207-217.

[96] Säemann M, Hörl WH. Urinary tract infection in renal transplant recipients. Eur J Clin Invest 2008; 38: 58-65.

[97] Schmaldienst S, Hörl WH. Bacterial infections after renal transplantation. Contrib Nephrol 1998; 124: 18–24.

[98] Schmaldienst S, Dittrich E, Hörl WH. Urinary tract infections after renal transplantation. Curr Opin Urol 2002; 12: 125-130.

[99] Takai K, Tollemar J, Wilczek HE, Groth CG. Urinary tract infections following renal transplantation. Clin Transplant 1998; 12: 19-23.

[100] Rubin RH. Infectious disease complications of renal transplantation. Kidney Int 1993; 44: 221-236.

[101] Karakayali H, Emiroglu R, Arslan G, Bilgin N, Haberal M. Major infectious complications after kidney transplantation. Transplant Proc 2001; 33: 1816-1817.

[102] Giral M, Pascuariello G, Karam G, *et al.* Acute graft pyelonephritis and long-term kidney allograft outcome. Kidney Int 2002; 61: 1880-1886.

[103] Chuang P, Parikh CR, Langone A. Urinary tract infections after renal transplantation: a retrospective review at two US transplant centers. Clin Transplant 2005; 19: 230-235.

[104] Maraha B, Bonten H, van Hooff H, *et al.* Infectious complications and antibiotic use in renal transplant recipients during a 1-year follow-up. Clin Microbiol Infect 2001; 7: 619-625.

[105] Muñoz P. Management of urinary tract infections and lymphocele in renal transplant recipients. Clin Infect Dis 2001; 33(suppl 1): S53-57.

[106] Argani H, Rahnama AMA, Amjadi M, *et al.* The role of stent and cotrimoxazole in prevention of UTI after kidney transplantation. Transplant Proc 2001; 33: 2667.

[107] de Souza RM, Olsburgh J. Urinary tract infection in the renal transplant patient. Nat Clin Pract Nephrol 2008; 4 : 252-264.

[108] Fisher SA. Infections in the transplant recipient. Med Health R I. 2002; 85(4): 125-127.

[109] Rice JC, Peng T, Kuo YF, *et al.* Renal allograft injury is associated with urinary tract infection caused by Escherichia coli bearing adherence factors. Am J Transplant 2006; 6: 2375-2783.

[110] Menezes FG, Wey SB, Peres CA, *et al.* Risk factors for surgical site infection in kidney transplant recipients. Infect Control Hosp Epidemiol. 2008; 29: 771-773.

[111] Martinez-Marcos F, Cisneros J, Gentil M, *et al.* Prospective study of renal transplant infections in 50 consecutive patients. Eur J Clin Microbiol Infect Dis 1994; 13: 1023–1028.

[112] Audard V, Amor M, Desvaux D, *et al.* Acute graft pyelonephritis: a potential cause of acute rejection in renal transplant. Transplantation 2005; 80: 1128-1130.

[113] Pellé G, Vimont S, Levy PP, *et al.* Acute pyelonephritis represents a risk factor impairing long-term kidney graft function. Am J Transplant 2007; 7: 899-907.

[114] Ramos A, Asensio A, Muñoz E, *et al.* Incisional surgical site infection in kidney transplantation. Urology 2008; 72: 119-23.

[115] Celik A, Sifil A, Cavdar C, *et al.* Outcome of renal transplantation: 7-year experience. Transplant Proc 2001; 33: 2657-2659.

[116] Stephan RN, Munschauer CE, Kumar MSA. Surgical wound infection in renal transplantation. Outcome data in 102 consecutive patients without perioperative systemic antibiotic coverage. Arch Surg 1997; 132: 1315-1319.

[117] Schmaldienst S, Hoerl WH. Bacterial infections after renal transplantation. Nephron 1997; 75: 140-153.

[118] Sawyer RG, Pelletier SJ, Pruett TL. Increased early morbidity and mortality with acceptable long-term function in severely obese patients undergoing liver transplantation. Clin Transplantation 1999; 13: 126-130.

[119] Lai M-K, Huang C-C, Chu S-H, *et al.* Surgical complications in renal transplantation. Transplant Proc 1994; 26: 2165-2166.

[120] Rubin RH, Wolfson JS, Cosimi AB, *et al.* Infection in the renal transplant recipient. Am J Med 1981; 70: 405-411.

[121] Burdick RA, Bragg-Gresham JL, Woods JD, *et al.* Patterns of hepatitis B prevalence and seroconversion in hemodialysis units from three continents: The DOPPS. Kidney Int 2003; 63: 2222-2229.

[122] Kondili LA, Genovese D, Argentini C, *et al.* Nosocomial transmission in simultaneous outbreaks of hepatitis C and B virus infections in a hemodialysis center. Eur J Clin Microbiol Infect Dis 2006; 25: 527-531.

[123] Marzano A, Angelucci E, Andreone P, *et al.* Prophylaxis and treatment of hepatitis B in immunocompromised patients. Dig Liver Dis 2007; 39: 397-408.

[124] Fabrizi F, Martin P, Dixit V, *et al.* HBsAg sieropositive status and survival after renal transplantation: meta-analysis of observational studies. Am J Transplant 2005; 5: 2913-2921.

[125] Berger A, Preiser W, Kachel HG, *et al.* HBV reactivation after kidney transplantation. J Clin Virol 2005; 32: 162-165.

[126] Fabrizi F, Dulai G, Dixit V, *et al.* Lamivudine for the treatment of hepatitis B virus-related liver disease after renal transplantation: meta-analysis of clinical trials. Transplantation 2004; 77: 859-864.

[127] Knoll A, Pietrzyk M, Loss M,*et al.* Solid organ transplantation in HBsAg-negative patients with antibodies to HBV core antigen: low risk of HBV reactivation. Transplantation 2005; 79: 1631-1633.

[128] De Feo TM, Grossi P, Poli F, *et al.* Kidney transplantation from anti-HBc positive donors: results from a retrospective Italian study. Transplantation 2006; 81: 76-80.

[129] Finelli L, Miller JT, Tokars JI, *et al.* National surveillance of dialysis associated diseases in the United States, 2002. Semin Analysis 2005; 18: 52-61.

[130] Gretch DR. Use and interpretation of HCV diagnostic tests in the clinical setting. Clin Liver Dis 1997; 1: 543-557.

[131] Sandhu J, Preiksaitis JK, Campbell PM, *et al.* Hepatitis C prevalence and risk factors in the northern Alberta dialysis population. Am J Epidemiol 1999; 150: 58–66.

[132] Berenguer M. Treatment of chronic hepatitis C in hemodialysis patients. Hepatology 2008; 48: 1690-1699.

[133] Mathurin P, Mouquet C, Poynard T, *et al.* Impact of hepatitis B and C virus on kidney transplantation outcome. Hepatology 1999; 29: 257-263.

[134] Kamar N, Rostaing L, Selves J, *et al.* Natural history of hepatitis C virus-related liver fibrosis after renal transplantation. Am J Transplant 2005; 5: 1704-1712.

[135] Alric L, Di-Martino V, Selves J, *et al.* Long-term impact of renal transplantation on liver fibrosis during hepatitis C virus infection. Gastroenterology 2002; 123: 1494-1499.

[136] Weclawiak H, Kamar N, Ould-Mohamed A, *et al.* Treatment of Chronic Hepatitis C Virus Infection in Dialysis Patients: An Update. Hepat Res Treat 2010; 2010:267412.

[137] [No authors listed]. KDIGO. Clinical practice guidelines for the prevention, diagnosis, evaluation, and treatment of hepatitis C in chronic kidney disease. Kidney Int 2008; 73: S1-2.

[138] Gonzalez-Roncero F, Gentil MA, Valdivia MA, *et al.* Outcome of kidney transplant in chronic hepatitis C virus patients: Effect of pretransplantation interferon-alpha2b monotherapy. Transplant Proc 2003; 35: 1745-1747.

[139] Bocci V, Pacini A, Muscettola M. Renal filtration, absorption and catabolism of human alpha interferon. J Interferon Res 1981; 1: 347-352

[140] Glue P. The clinical pharmacology of ribavirin. Semin Liver Dis 1999; 19 Suppl 1: 17-24.

[141] Gupta SK, Pittenger AL, Swan SK, *et al.* Single-dose pharmacokinetics and safety of pegylated interferon-α2b in patients with chronic renal dysfunction. J Clin Pharmacol 2002; 42: 1109-1115.

[142] Ghany MG, Strader DB, Thomas DL, Seeff LB. Diagnosis, management, and treatment of hepatitis C: an update. Hepatology 2009; 49: 1335-1374.

[143] Brochot E, Castelain J, Duverlie G, *et al.* Ribavirin monitoring in chronic hepatitis C therapy: anaemia versus efficacy. Antiviral Therapy 2010; 15: 687-695.

[144] Bruchfeld A, Lindahl K, Reichard O, *et al.* Pegylated interferon and ribavirin treatment for hepatitis C in haemodialysis patients. J Viral Hep 2006; 13: 316-21.

[145] Bruchfeld A, Stahle L, Andersson J, *et al.* Ribavirin treatment in dialysis patients with chronic hepatitis C virus infection–a pilot study. J Viral Hep 2001; 8: 287-292.

[146] Carriero D, Fabrizi F, Uriel AJ, *et al.* Treatment of dialysis patients with chronic hepatitis C using pegylated interferon and low-dose ribavirin. Int J Artif Organs 2008; 31: 295-302.

[147] Mousa DH, Abdalla AH, Al-Shoail G, *et al.* Alpha-interferon with ribavirin in the treatment of hemodialysis patients with hepatitis C. Transplantation Proc 2004; 36: 1831-1834.

[148] Tan AC, Brouwer JT, Glue P, *et al.* Safety of interferon and ribavirin therapy in haemodialysis patients with chronic hepatitis C: Results of a pilot study. Nephrol Dial Transplant 2001; 16: 193-195.

[149] van Leusen R, Adang RP, de Vries RA, *et al.* Pegylated interferon alfa-2a (40 kD) and ribavirin in haemodialysis patientswith chronic hepatitis C. Nephrol Dial Transplant 2008; 23: 721-725.

[150] Rendina M, Schena A, Castellaneta NM, *et al.* The treatment of chronic hepatitis C with peginterferon alfa-2a (40 kDa) plus ribavirin in haemodialysed patients awaiting renal transplant. J Hepatology 2007; 46: 768-374.

[151] Fabrizi F, Messa P, Basile C, Martin P. Hepatic disorders in chronic kidney disease. Nat Rev Nephrol 2010; 6: 395-403.

CHAPTER 19

Impact of Polyomavirus BK and Cytomegalovirus on the Kidney Allograft

Ilkka Helanterä[1,*,†], Adrian Egli[2,3,†], Petri Koskinen[1], Hans H. Hirsch[2,4] and Irmeli Lautenschlager[5]

[1]*Department of Medicine, Division of Nephrology; Helsinki University Hospital, and University of Helsinki, PL 263, FI-00029 HUS, Helsinki, Finland;* [2]*Transplantation Virology, Institute for Medical Microbiology, Department of Biomedicine, University of Basel, Petersplatz 10, CH-4003 Basel, Switzerland;* [3]*Department of Medicine, University Hospital Basel, Petersgraben 4, CH-4031 Basel, Switzerland;* [4]*Infectious diseases & Hospital Epidemiology, Department of Internal Medicine, University Hospital Basel, Petersgraben 4, CH-4031 Basel, Switzerland and* [5] *Department of Virology, Helsinki University Hospital, and University of Helsinki, PL 400, FI-00029 HUS, Helsinki, Finland*

Abstract: After polyomavirus BK was recognized as a pathogen causing severe nephropathy in transplant recipients, infections in renal transplant patients receiving more potent immunosuppressive medication have raised increasing concern. As no effective treatment of BK-virus nephropathy is available, the prevention of this condition, which often leads to graft loss, is of outmost importance. Recently, new data of the pathogenesis of replication and immune responses to BK virus have been reported. In addition to the well-characterized direct effects caused by clinical CMV infections, also multiple indirect immunomodulatory effects of CMV have been postulated. Experimental data of the indirect effect of CMV have associated CMV with acute and chronic injury of the kidney graft, but in the recent years, also some clinical evidence has associated persistent CMV infection of the transplant with detrimental long-term effects.

The aim of this chapter is to review the pathophysiology of the effect of viruses to the kidney allograft, with special emphasis on the two probably most important viruses challenging the survival of the graft, namely polyomavirus BK and cytomegalovirus.

Keywords: Chronic Allograft Nephropathy, Cytomegalovirus, Polyomavirus BK, Polyomavirus JC, Polyomavirus Associated Nephropathy, Graft Function, Prophylaxis, Ganciclovir, Valganciclovir.

INTRODUCTION

The survival of transplanted kidneys has improved significantly in the past decades with the introduction of more potent immunosuppressive drugs, which effectively prevent acute rejection. However, the long-term survival has not improved accordingly [1]. Chronic allograft injury leads to slow decline in kidney graft function and eventually to graft loss. This injury is thought to be caused by non-immunological damage to the graft caused by cold ischemia and increased donor and recipient age, immunological damage, and chronic calcineurin inhibitor toxicity. In the recent years, data has been accumulating about viral infections causing damage to kidney allograft and impairing long-term graft function and survival.

The incidence of infections is increased in transplant recipients as a result of unspecific suppression of cellular immune functions of the host by immunosuppressive drugs, and the burden of viral causes has been increasing in the recent years due to more potent immunosuppressive compounds [2]. Polyomavirus BK only emerged in the last decade as the leading cause of functional renal decline and kidney transplant loss [3]. Modern potent immunosuppressive medication has increased the risk of infections caused by polyomaviruses and increasing interest by both clinicians and researchers has been directed to polyomaviruses. As no effective treatment exists, the prevention of polyomavirus BK-associated nephropathy (PyVAN) by reducing immunosuppression at an early time point of detection BKV replication is currently regarded as the most successful strategy.

***Addresss correspondence to Ilkka Helanterä:** Helsinki University Hospital, Nephrology Clinic, Kasarmikatu 11-13, Po Box 263, FI-00029 HUS, Helsinki, Finland; Tel: +358-9-471 88203; Fax: +358-9-471 88400; Emails: ilkka.helantera@helsinki.fi

†Ikka Helanterä and Adrian Egli gave equal contribution to the chapter.

Massimiliano Veroux and Pierfrancesco Veroux (Eds)

Virus replication causes direct injury to the host cell and organ by cell lysis, *e.g.*, tissue-invasive CMV infections in the intestines (CMV colitis), the liver (CMV hepatitis), the lung (CMV pneumonitis) and other target tissues. When virus replication occurs in a transplanted organ, immune control is not only impaired due to the necessary immunosuppression to avoid rejection, but also due to an impaired response of the presented viral epitopes in an allo-MHC-I context. In addition, the injury caused by inflammatory reaction to viral replication, experimental models and clinical observations associate CMV with so-called indirect effects including acute rejection and chronic histopathological changes in the kidney allograft [4-6].

In this chapter, we review the pathogenesis and mechanisms of virus-associated injury in the kidney, focusing on polyomaviruses and CMV.

POLYOMAVIRUSES BK (BKV) AND JC (JCV)

Currently, 8 human polyomaviruses (PyV) have been identified. Polyomaviruses BK (BKV) and JC (JCV) have significant impact in transplant patients, but the role of WU, KI, and Merkel-cell carcinoma associated polyomavirus in immunosuppressed hosts is still undetermined. Moreover, human PyV-6 and PyV-7 have been identified in skin swabs of otherwise healthy individuals suggesting that the range of PyV as skin colonizers may be significantly larger than previously thought. In addition, the recently discovered Tichodyplasia spinnulosa virus is the eighth human PyV, which may cause skin proliferations and alopecia in immunosuppressed patients. Human polyomaviruses are non-enveloped DNA-viruses, with the genome consisting of a circular double-stranded DNA of about 5.2kB. The viral genome encodes early proteins (small T and large T antigen), and late proteins (viral capsid protein (VP) 1 to 3 and agno protein). Gangliosides GD1b and GT1b serve as cellular entry receptors for BKV and serotonergic 5HT2AR for JCV [7, 8]. In addition to renal proximal tubular epithelial cells and urinary tract epithelium, polyomavirus BK is able to infect brain cells and lymphocytes [9-11]. The receptor and host characteristics of the other human PyV are currently undefined.

BKV and JCV infect up to 80% of the population [12, 13]. Primary infection occurs usually in early childhood and is asymptomatic, but may present as fever, malaise, and flu-like symptoms; also anecdotal cases of cystitis have been reported [14]. After primary infection, polyomaviruses BK and JC remain latent in the kidney and genitourinary tract epithelium [9, 15]. Low-level replication and secretion of polyomaviruses in the urine is found in healthy immunocompetent individuals, with a predominance of JC virus [16]. In healthy donors, BKV was found in the urine in 10% of samples in median 3.5 log copies/ml, and JCV in about 20% samples in median 5 log copies/ml [13, 17-19]. Viremia is rarely observed in immunocompetent individuals [10].

Polyomavirus-Associated Nephropathy (PyVAN)

The incidence of PyVAN after kidney transplantation is between 1-10% in different transplant populations receiving different immunosuppression [20-23]. Premature functional decline is found in 60-90% cases, and PyVAN may lead to graft loss in as much as 50% cases [24].

Table 1: Histological patterns of polyomavirus-associated nephropathy (PVAN) [24]. Interstitial fibrosis, tubular atrophy, and interstitial inflammation scored according to the Banff scheme [25, 26]

	PyVAN A	PyVAN B	PyVAN C
Viral cytopathic changes	Minimal to mild (infected tubules in 0-25% of biopsy core)	Mild to severe (infected tubules in ≥10% of biopsy core)	Variable
Interstitial Inflammation	Insignificant	Moderate to severe	Variable
Tubular atrophy and interstitial fibrosis	Insignificant	Mild	Moderate to severe

Three morphological patterns of PyVAN are identified histologically, based on the extent of inflammatory infiltrates and fibrosis in the biopsy: Pattern A (viral cytopathic changes in architecturally normal renal parenchyma), pattern B (combination of viral cytopathic changes and focal areas of tubular atrophy, interstitial fibrosis and interstitial inflammation), and pattern C (variable viral cytopathic changes in diffusely scarred renal parenchyma) (Table **1**, Figs. **1** and **2**) [24].

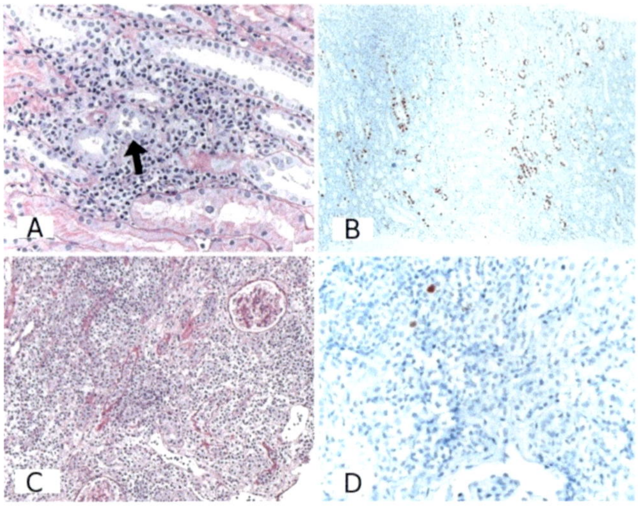

Figure 1: (A) A kidney biopsy 3 months after transplantation showing polyoma-virus associated nephropathy: dense focal lymphohistiocytic infiltrates in the cortical and medullary interstitial space with mild tubulitis. (B) Numerous infected tubular epithelial cells in the cortex and medulla positively stained for SV40 antigen. (C) A second biopsy 6 months post-transplant showing massive diffuse lymphohistiocytic infiltrates affecting the whole cortical and medullary space with severe tubulitis. (D) Only few SV40 antigen- positive tubular epithelial cells. From: Schaub S, Mayr M, Egli A, Binggeli S, Descoeudres B, Steiger J, Mihatsch MJ, Hirsch HH. Transient allograft dysfunction from immune reconstitution in a patient with polyoma BK-virus- associated nephropathy. Nephrol Dial Transplant. 2007 Aug; 22(8): 2386-90. Reproduced with permission from the authors and publisher (Oxford University Press).

In addition to the characteristic nuclear viral inclusion in tubular epithelial cells, confirmation of the diagnosis of PyVAN requires detection of the virus in the biopsy, usually by immunohistochemical detection of SV40 large T-antigen, which identifies both BK and JC viruses (Fig. **1**) [24]. Because of the focal nature of PyVAN, sampling error can be minimized by obtaining more than 2 biopsy cores, but a negative biopsy cannot rule out PyVAN.

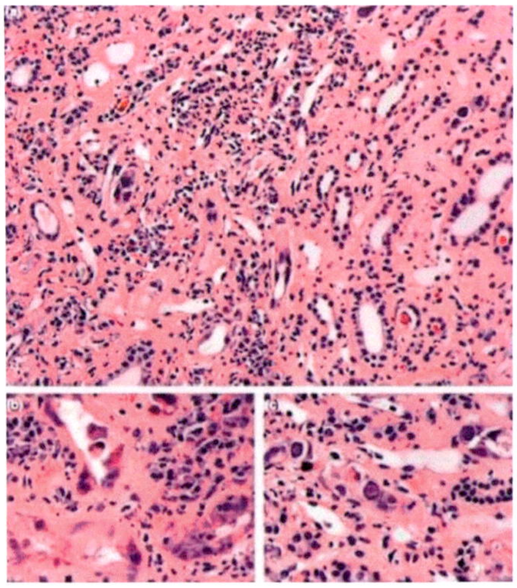

Figure 2: Plasma cell-rich polyomavirus nephropathy. (A) Abundant plasma cells present around the virus infected tubules in the medulla. H–E, Magnification 130x. (B,C) Typical viral inclusions in the tubular epithelial cells. H–E, Magnification 200x. From: Kemény E, Hirsch HH, Eller J, Dürmüller U, Hopfer H, Mihatsch MJ. Plasma cell infiltrates in polyomavirus nephropathy. Transplant Int 2010; 23: 397-406. Reproduced with permission from the authors and the copyright holder (Blackwell Publishing).

Several risk factors for PVAN have been suggested, but probably the most important factor is the higher intensity of immunosuppression, especially immunosuppressive regimens using tacrolimus and MMF [3, 21, 24]. Also acute rejection and anti-rejection treatments increases the risk of PyVAN [22, 27]. In accordance of these findings, the incidence of PyVAN may be very low in low-risk populations with conservative immunosuppression and low frequency of acute rejections [28]. Other risk factors for PyVAN include HLA mismatch [27], HLA C7 negative donor or recipient [29], male gender and older donor age [24]. Also viral factors, such as capsid serotype, replicative fitness, and non-coding control region (NCCR) rearrangements, contribute to the risk of PVAN [19, 30, 31]. Donor seropositivity, recipient seronegativity, and lack of BKV-specific cellular immune memory compartment have also been associated with increased risk of BKV infections and PyVAN [29, 32, 33].

Possible Mechanisms of BKV Related Allograft Injury

The pathogenesis of PyVAN is not yet fully elucidated. However, *in vitro* BKV replication has been shown to induce several genes involved in cell division and DNA replication and to down-regulate immune and defense response genes [34]. Increased expression of markers of cytotoxic T-cell function IFN-γ and perforin has been observed in the kidney during PVAN [35], and increased proinflammatory cytokine response was observed in samples with BK viruria, including upregulation of cytokines IL-3 and IL-6 [36]. In addition to direct cytopathic injury in the kidney caused by BKV, it may also contribute to the graft damage indirectly by upregulating inflammation in the kidney, leading to repair responses. Fibrosis and loss of functional kidney substance is a key event in kidney injury, also in association with PyVAN, and transforming growth factor-beta (TGF-β) is a key molecule in the development of renal fibrosis. BKV is shown to directly upregulate TGF-β and several components of the TGF-β-signalling pathway, and increased transcription of profibrotic molecules TGF-β, CTGF, and matrix metalloproteinases MMP-2 and -9 has been observed during PyVAN [35, 37]. Upregulation of TGF-β- signalling by BKV may be a central mechanism by which BKV triggers graft fibrosis. On the other hand, TGF-β induces BKV gene expression, and may be involved in reactivation of BKV, further stimulating BKV replication and associated kidney injury [38]. TGF-β is also an important inducer of epithelial-mesenchymal transition (EMT), a process mediating kidney fibrosis and late graft deterioration after transplantation. Induction of molecules associated with EMT has also been observed during PyVAN [35].

Prolonged BKV replication leads to accumulation of rearrangements in the virus non-coding control region (NCCR) harbouring major transcription sites. Deletions and insertions into the NCCR have been associated with increased early gene expression, replication capacity, and cytopathology of BKV *in vitro* [19]. In clinical settings, NCCR rearrangements appeared first in urine, followed by plasma. Patients with NCCR rearrangements showed 20-fold higher plasma viral loads and a more rapid progression to PVAN [19, 39].

Polyomavirus Specific Immune Responses

Neutralizing antibodies targeting BKV major capsid protein VP1 inhibit host cell infection [40], although evidence suggests that the amount of antibody activity correlates more to recent BKV antigen exposure rather than protection from polyomavirus replication [13, 32, 41]. Also JCV specific antibodies have been linked to more antigen exposure in healthy individuals [13]. Highest risk for BKV infection after kidney transplantation was found in seropositive recipients receiving a kidney from a seropositive donor. Also the risk of viruria was associated with donor serostatus and increased with increasing donor antibody titers [29]. In this context, the infiltration of the renal allograft with plasma cells has been noted (Fig. **2**), which may indicate a response to prolonged BKV replication [42]. Interestingly, IgM plasma cell infiltrates in biopsies correlated positively with titers of circulating anti-BK virus IgM antibodies.

The control of BKV replication is achieved mainly through BKV-specific T-cells. After kidney transplantation, low BKV-specific T-cell control is associated with higher plasma and intragraft BKV loads and increased risk for PyVAN [33, 43]. Specific immune responses to BKV large T-antigen have been found important in clearing BKV replication, but also studies with other stimulants to BKV- specific T-cells support the importance of cellular immune responses in the control of BKV infection after kidney transplantation [43-46]. Furthermore, immunosuppressive drugs are shown to reduce the function and quantity of BKV-specific T-cells [47], and evidence shows inhibition of BKV-specific T-cell function with more intense immunosuppression [48]. Although BKV-specific immune effectors are crucial to contain and eventually clear infected cells with active replication, it has been observed that the desired immune reconstitution may be associated with detrimental effects called immune reconstitution (inflammatory) syndrome (IRS or IRIS) [49]. These responses may be worse in patients with better HLA-matching [50] and high persisting BKV replication [45], thereby appearing reminiscent to responses to JCV in the CNS of HIV-AIDS patients with progressive multifocal leukoencephalopathy [51]. The inflammatory infiltrates are difficult to distinguish from concurrent rejection and may require similar treatment with steroid pulses.

Diagnosis, Screening, and Prevention of BKV Infections

After kidney transplantation, BKV shedding in the urine can be found in up to 30% of samples, with approximately 1000-fold higher viral loads compared to healthy individuals. JCV shedding in the urine is detected in 20-50% of samples, with a similar fold increase in viral loads compared to healthy individuals [20, 22, 52]. BK viremia is seen in about 30% patients with viruria, and BK viruria precedes viremia by median of four weeks [22, 53]. BK viremia serves as a surrogate marker for PyVAN; the negative predictive value for the development of PyVAN with no BK viremia is 100%, and positive predictive value with BK viremia is approximately 50% [14]. In addition, in patients with PyVAN, BKV loads are markedly higher compared to patients with no PyVAN [22], and BKV plasma loads of more then 4 logs copies/ml are associated with a high sensitivity and specificity of >95% to PyVAN [54]. Also JCV has been rarely associated with nephropathy in up to 5% cases with PyVAN, with lower viral loads compared to BKV [20]. Screening of polyomavirus is recommended from urine with either decoy cells or by quantification of BKV-DNA or RNA by PCR, and quantitative plasma PCR should be performed in positive cases. In cases of urine DNA load $>10^7$ copies/ml or plasma DNA load $>10^4$ copies/ml, a biopsy should be performed to confirm the diagnosis of PyVAN. After intervention viral load should be monitored with 2-4 weeks interval [24].

As no specific treatment for BKV exists, the most effective intervention is to prevent the development of PyVAN by reducing immunosuppression when viremia or high-level viruria is observed. No consensus of the optimal intervention exists, and various strategies of reducing immunosuppression can be applied, including a switch from tacrolimus to cyclosporine, reduction of calcineurin inhibitor doses and trough level targets, or reduction or discontinuation of MMF [24, 55]. As reconstitution of immune control of the infection and clearance of viremia takes from 4-12 weeks [52], early intervention is recommended. Recent data from Basel indicate that this intervention may not only be successful in the preemptive situation (described by Brennan 2005 and Ginevri 2007), but may also be successful when cases of histologically confirmed definitive PyVAN are diagnosed subsequent to the initial intervention [56]. Guidelines about the monitoring and treatment of PyVAN have been recently published [55, 57]. Antiviral activity against BKV has been shown *in vitro* by leflunomide, cidofovir, and fluoroquinolones. No randomized controlled trials have been performed with any of these drugs, and only empirical use of these agents is described. Evidence suggests that concentrations required for effective antiviral activity may not be achievable in clinical settings [58, 59], although some evidence exists of using cidofovir in treating hemorrhagic cystitis after hematopoietic stem cell transplantation [60]. In addition, the use of cidofovir after kidney transplantation is limited by nephrotoxicity. Further randomized controlled studies are required to define the role of antiviral medications in the treatment of polyomavirus BK infections. A new antiviral compound, CMX001, a cidofovir-derivate with high lipophilicity and reduced toxicity might possibly be a future option for the treatment of polyomavirus infections [61].

CYTOMEGALOVIRUS (CMV)

Cytomegalovirus (CMV) is a member of the betaherpesvirus subfamily, belonging to the family of herpesviruses. Human cytomegalovirus is a large DNA- virus of 150-200 nm in diameter, consisting of a linear double-stranded DNA of approximately 230 kbp. Monocytes, macrophages, lymphocytes, and hematopoietic precursor cells are the main cell types of CMV infection and replication. In addition, CMV is able to infect several tissues, including most of the parenchymal organs, salivary glands, eye, gastrointestinal and genitourinary tract, and is also able to replicate in several cell types, including epithelial cells, endothelial cells, fibroblasts, smooth muscle cells and macrophages. The cellular entry of CMV remains yet to be fully elucidated, but due to the wide range of cells CMV is able to infect, the receptor is thought to be widely distributed, and may be a complex of several molecules. One suggested candidate molecule has been epidermal growth factor receptor [62]; others include cellular integrins [63] and PDGFR-α [64].

Primary infection of CMV occurs commonly during the first two decades of life and is usually asymptomatic, but may present as a mononucleosis-like syndrome, or rarely as hepatitis or pneumonia. The seroprevalence of CMV varies between 40 and 100% in different countries. Primary CMV infection leads to a life-long latency. During latency, the main reservoir of CMV is thought to be blood leucocytes, mainly mononuclear cells, but also hematopoietic progenitor cells have been documented to carry latent viral DNA [65]. During latency, CMV can be transmitted *via* blood products and transplanted organs.

CMV Infections in Kidney Transplant Recipients

After kidney transplantation, approximately 5-20% of recipients suffer from symptomatic CMV infection [66]. CMV seronegative recipients of a kidney from a seropositive donor are at highest risk of symptomatic CMV infection; without prophylaxis activation of the virus can be detected in more than 60% and symptomatic infection in approximately 50% of recipients. In CMV seropositive recipients asymptomatic viral reactivation can be detected in up to 60-70% with a significantly lower frequency of symptomatic infections, ranging between 16-20% [66]. CMV has been associated with increased cardiovascular complications [67], increased gastrointestinal complications [68, 69], and with the development of post-transplant diabetes mellitus after kidney transplantation [70].

CMV and Allograft Histopathology

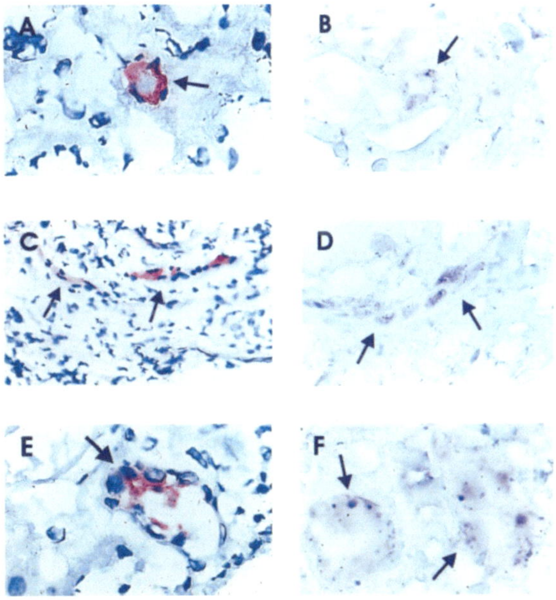

Figure 3: The demonstration of CMV pp65- antigen by immunoperoxidase staining and CMV-DNA *in situ* hybridization from frozen sections of 6 months protocol biopsies. (A) A strong positive staining of CMV antigen in the endothelium of a small blood vessel (arrow); (B) A blood vessel expressing endothelial CMV-DNA (arrow); (C) A moderate expression of CMV antigen in the capillary wall (arrows); (D) Capillaries with a moderate expression of CMV-DNA (arrows); (E) A tubule showing a strong positive staining of CMV antigen (arrow); (F) A strong expression of CMV-DNA in tubular wall epithelium (arrows). (Original magnification 400 x). From: Helanterä I, Koskinen P, Törnroth T, Loginov R, Grönhagen-Riska C, Lautenschlager I. The Impact of Cytomegalovirus Infections and Acute Rejection Episodes on the Development of Vascular Changes in 6 Months Protocol Biopsies of Cadaveric Kidney Allograft Recipients. Transplantation 2003; 75 (11): 1858-1864. Reproduced with permission from the authors and publisher (Lippincott, Williams and Wilkins).

CMV infections have been associated with the rejection process of kidney allografts already since the 1970s, and since then several studies have suggested an association between CMV and acute rejection [6, 71, 72]. Some studies have showed an association of only symptomatic CMV infection (CMV disease) with acute rejections [73], and some studies have failed to show any association [74].

Similarly, CMV infection has been associated with inferior graft survival already since the 1980s [75], and findings of impaired graft function and survival in patients with previous CMV infections have been confirmed also in the modern era of immunosuppressive drugs and diagnostic tests for CMV [76-79], although also controversial evidence exists [74, 80]. A recent randomized study comparing oral ganciclovir prophylaxis and preemptive therapy in kidney transplant recipients showed increased graft survival in the prophylaxis group with fewer CMV infections detected [81].

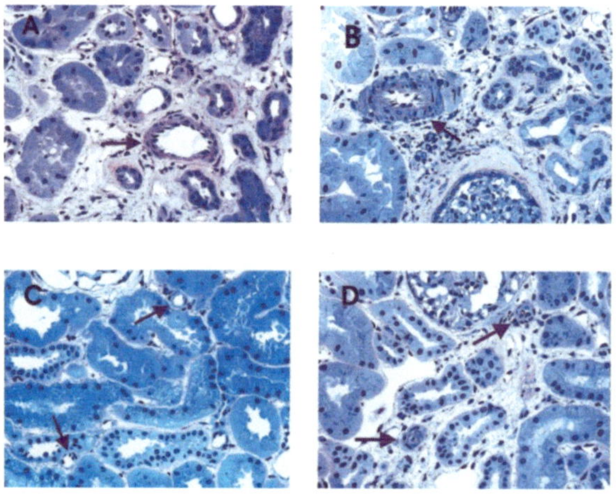

Figure 4: Six months protocol biopsies of kidney allografts. (A) Small artery (*arrow*) in a biopsy of a recipient without previous history of CMV infection or acute rejection episodes. (B) Small artery with intimal thickening in a biopsy of a recipient with intragraft CMV and a history of acute rejection episodes (*arrow*). (C) Small arterioles in a biopsy of a control recipient (*arrows*). (D) Biopsy specimen from the same recipient as in B, showing two small occluded arterioles, (May-Grunwald- Giemsa stain, magnification 400 x). From: Helanterä I, Koskinen P, Törnroth T, Loginov R, Grönhagen-Riska C, Lautenschlager I. The Impact of Cytomegalovirus Infections and Acute Rejection Episodes on the Development of Vascular Changes in 6 Months Protocol Biopsies of Cadaveric Kidney Allograft Recipients. Transplantation 2003; 75 (11): 1858-1864. Reproduced with permission from the authors and publisher (Lippincott, Williams and Wilkins).

Although the association of CMV and chronic dysfunction of kidney allograft has been discussed for decades, the evidence on histological level of the impact of CMV infection on the development of chronic rejection in kidney allografts, previously referred as chronic allograft nephropathy, has still been lacking. CMV has been associated with glomerulopathic changes in the allograft [82, 83], but only a few studies in the modern era have addressed the association of CMV with histopathologic changes in renal allograft. The association of CMV infection with biopsy-proven chronic rejection has been reported in the presence of previous acute rejection episodes [84], and in a recent analysis of three months protocol biopsies in patients with CMV infections closely monitored after transplantation, increased interstitial fibrosis and tubular atrophy was seen only in patients with high CMV viral loads, but not in all patients with CMV infection [85]. In our own study of a material of 6 months protocol biopsies, previous history of CMV infection was not associated with any histopathological changes, but increased vascular changes were recorded in patients with histological evidence of either CMV pp65 antigen or DNA detected in the kidney biopsy together with previous history of acute rejection (Figs. **3** and **4**) [5].

Persistent CMV in the Kidney Allograft

In vitro, CMV is able to infect most cell types of the kidney, including glomerular, tubular and endothelial cells [86]. *In vivo*, the virus has been detected in transplanted kidneys in several studies [87, 88], and CMV may also to persist in the allograft for months after viremia and active infection [89]. Similar findings of persistent CMV-DNA in the allograft, together with increased histopathological changes, have been described after liver transplantation [90, 91]. Persistent CMV DNA or protein expression has also been found in various tubular, glomerular, and vascular structures in kidney transplant biopsies taken more than 30 days after the last positive CMV finding in blood or urine. This persistent replication of CMV in the graft, detected several weeks or even months after systemic infection, was associated with reduced graft function at one and two years after transplantation and reduced graft survival compared to patients with no intragraft CMV (Fig. **3**) [89].

Possible Mechanisms of CMV Related Injury

CMV infection may cause direct injury to the graft due to viral replication and cell injury, and also the inflammatory reaction to the injury and increased production of proinflammatory cytokines by T-cells, including TNF-α, IFN-γ, IL-1 and IL-2, may stimulate the rejection cascade. However, there are also several indirect immunomodulatory mechanisms by which CMV may stimulate the alloresponse and also contribute to the stereotypical histopathological reaction of kidney injury, characterized eventually as tubular atrophy, interstitial fibrosis, glomerulosclerosis and arteriosclerosis.

CMV directly or indirectly induces the production of several proinflammatory cytokines involved in T-cell activation, such as IL-1, IL-2, TNF-α [92-94], and adhesion molecules ICAM-1 and VCAM-1 [95, 96], which are key molecules in the initiation of the alloresponse. Chemokines are also important mediators of inflammation in transplant rejection, and CMV genome is known to encode chemokine analogues (UL146 and UL147) and chemokine receptor analogues (UL33, UL78, US27, US28), through which the virus is able to modify immune response and to stimulate cellular responses [97, 98].

TNF-α is thought to be a central molecule in the inflammatory process leading to activation of adhesion molecules and stimulation of synthesis and release of growth factors TGF-β and PDGF, which induce smooth muscle proliferation in the vascular wall and collagen synthesis by fibroblasts. CTGF, upregulated by TGF- β, is especially important in the generation of fibrosis [99, 100]. As CMV induces the production of TNF-α, and TNF-α may also be a key molecule in the activation of CMV from latency during alloresponse, TNF-α is thought to be a central molecule in the continuous allograft injury and inflammation associated with persistent CMV [101, 102]. In addition to TNF-α also other molecular pathways are probably involved in reactivation of CMV from latency [103]. Chronic kidney injury is characterized by tubular atrophy, and TNF-α – TNF-R1 pathway may also be involved in the CMV associated increased tubular apoptosis [104]. *Via* cytokine induction, but also directly CMV may induce the expression of TGF-β, PDGF, CTGF and VEGF [105-108], all thought to be key molecules in the profibrotic and vasculopathic response in the kidney.

All these molecular mechanisms are further supported by findings in experimental rat models of chronic kidney allograft rejection, in which CMV increased inflammation, enhanced the development of vascular changes, and increased the generation of fibrosis [4, 109, 110]. In addition, increased expression of adhesion molecules (ICAM-1, VCAM-1) and growth factors (TGF-β, PDGF, CTGF) was associated with CMV infection [110-112]. Experimental data also indicate that CMV upregulates several genes involved in the processes of wound repair and angiogenesis, contributing to the development of chronic allograft injury [113].

Our recent clinical findings suggest persistent cytomegalovirus replication in the allograft as a new possible risk factor for poorer early kidney allograft function and survival [89, 114]. Previous studies have only analyzed the association of CMV infection or disease with rejections or graft function and survival, and the presence of intragraft CMV has not been recorded. Our results suggest that it could be particularly the persistence of CMV in the graft that is associated with long-term damage of the allograft and inferior outcome after transplantation, possibly explaining the controversial findings in previous studies. Indirectly *via* inflammatory response to infection, but also directly, persistent CMV could induce the expression of adhesion molecules and production of cytokines, which result in growth factor response and contribute to the early development of chronic changes in the graft and finally, to the deterioration of graft function. Our findings of increased expression of the profibrotic and vasculopathic growth factors TGF-β and PDGF, and adhesion molecule ICAM-1 in biopsies with persistent intragraft CMV support this hypothesis (Fig. **5**) [114].

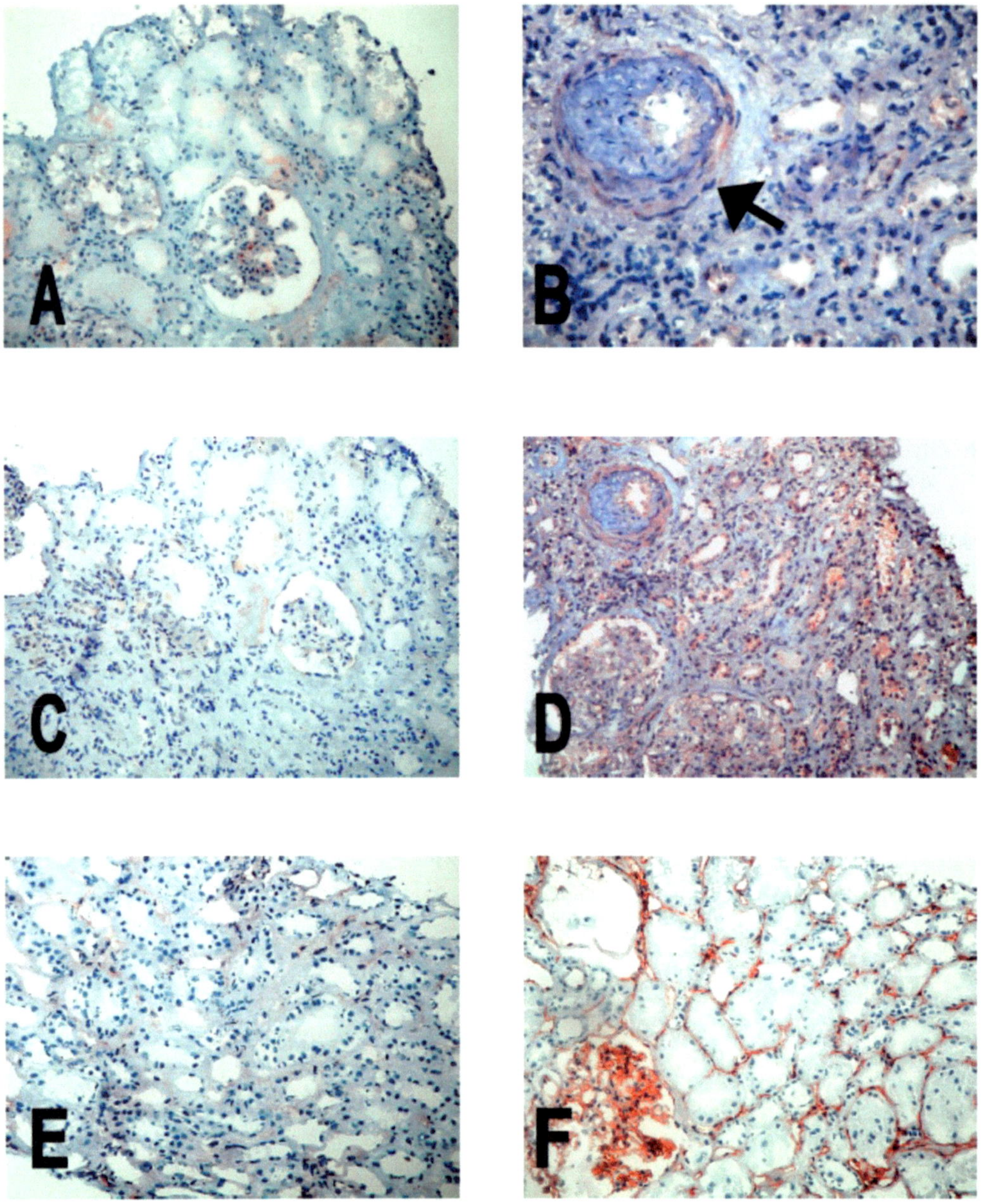

Figure 5: The expression of TGF- β, PDGF-AA and ICAM-1 in frozen sections of kidney biopsies. (A) The expression of TGF- β in a biopsy from a control patient, and (B) positive staining in medial smooth muscle cells and endothelial cells in an artery (arrow), and in tubular epithelial cells in a biopsy from a patient with persistent CMV infection in the graft. (C) The expression of PDGF-AA in a biopsy from a control patient, and (D) strong positive staining in vascular endothelial and medial smooth muscle cells, tubular epithelial cells, and glomerular cells in a biopsy from a patient with persistent CMV infection in the graft. (E) The expression of ICAM-1 in a biopsy from a control patient, and (F) strong positive staining in peritubular capillary structures and in glomerular structures in a biopsy from a patient with persistent CMV infection in the kidney allograft. (Magnification 200 x). From: Helanterä I, Loginov R, Koskinen P, Törnroth T, Grönhagen- Riska C, Lautenschlager I. Persistent cytomegalovirus infection is associated with increased expression of TGF-beta1, PDGF-AA and ICAM-1 and arterial intimal thickening in kidney allografts. Nephrol Dial Transplant. 2005 Apr;20(4): 790-796. Reproduced with permission from the authors and publisher (Oxford University Press).

These novel findings highlight the importance of adequately screening and preventing CMV infections after transplantation.

Diagnosis, Prevention and Treatment of CMV

The diagnosis of CMV infections is in most centers nowadays based on quantitative PCR to detect CMV DNA in preferably whole blood, but also from plasma samples [115-119]. The semiquantitative assay for the detection of CMV pp65 antigen in blood leukocytes, developed in the late 1980s, is also sensitive and accurate for the diagnosis of CMV infections [120, 121], but PCR methods, which are less laborious and can be easily standardized and automated, have mostly replaced it. CMV proteins or genome can be demonstrated also in tissue sections of biopsy material. Serology has an important role prior to transplantation in evaluating the donor and recipient, but after transplantation serology has only a limited diagnostic value.

CMV infection can be treated with a specific antiviral agent, the nucleoside analogue ganciclovir, which prevents viral replication but does not completely eliminate the virus. Other antiviral agents include foscarnet and cidofovir, the use of which is severely limited by their nephrotoxicity. Because of the high morbidity, costs, and even mortality associated with CMV, prophylaxis is recommended for high-risk groups for at least 3 months after transplantation [55]. Prolonging the prophylaxis in seronegative recipients of a kidney from a seropositive donor to 6 months probably reduces the incidence of late-onset CMV infection [119, 122]. Nowadays the most common agent used for CMV prophylaxis is valganciclovir, an oral valine ester of ganciclovir. However, late-onset CMV infection occurring after prophylaxis is a common problem in high-risk patients [123]. Viral load screening or seroconversion are shown to be poor predictors of late-onset CMV disease in these patients [124, 125]. As the control of CMV replication and infection after transplantation is achieved mainly by CD8+ and CD4+ T-cell mediated immune responses [126, 127], a novel strategy to predict CMV infection could be to measure CMV-specific T-cell responses [128-130]. Another strategy of prevention of CMV disease is preemptive treatment, in which patients are frequently monitored and antiviral therapy is administered when evidence of CMV viremia is detected, before clinical symptoms develop. This strategy can be used especially in seropositive recipients with lower risk for infection to prevent unnecessary exposure to antiviral medications [119].

Table 2: Effects of polyomavirus BK and CMV in the transplanted kidney

	BK Virus	**CMV**
Acute and direct effects in the kidney	• Cytopathic effect in tubular cells • Interstitial inflammation • Graft dysfunction	• Cytopathic effects (inclusions) • Interstitial inflammation • Glomerulitis • Graft dysfunction
Indirect and long-term effects in the kidney	• Inflammatory cytokine response (IFN-γ, IL-3, IL-6) • Profibrotic response (TGF-β, CTGF, matrix collagens, epithelial-mesenchymal transition)	• Stimulation of inflammation and alloresponse (TNF-α, IFN-γ, IL-1, IL-2, ICAM-1, VCAM-1) • Profibrotic and vasculopathic response (TGF-β, CTGF, PDGF)
Common effects of BK virus and CMV in the graft	• Persisting replication in the graft • Inflammatory response in the graft • Irreversible damage and loss of substance; intersitial fibrosis and tubular atrophy • Graft dysfunction and failure	

CONCLUSIONS

Viral infections commonly complicate the clinical course of a kidney transplant recipient.

Although rarely life threatening, several viral infections, mainly polyomavirus BK and cytomegalovirus, are associated with morbidity and damage in the allograft and poorer graft survival. Much is already known about the association of these viruses with injury in the kidney, but the underlying mechanisms of indirect injury in clinical transplantation still need to be clarified. The suggested mechanisms are summarized in Table **2** and Fig. **6**. Prevention and effective treatment of these infections is of great importance in reducing the long-term harmful effects of BKV and CMV.

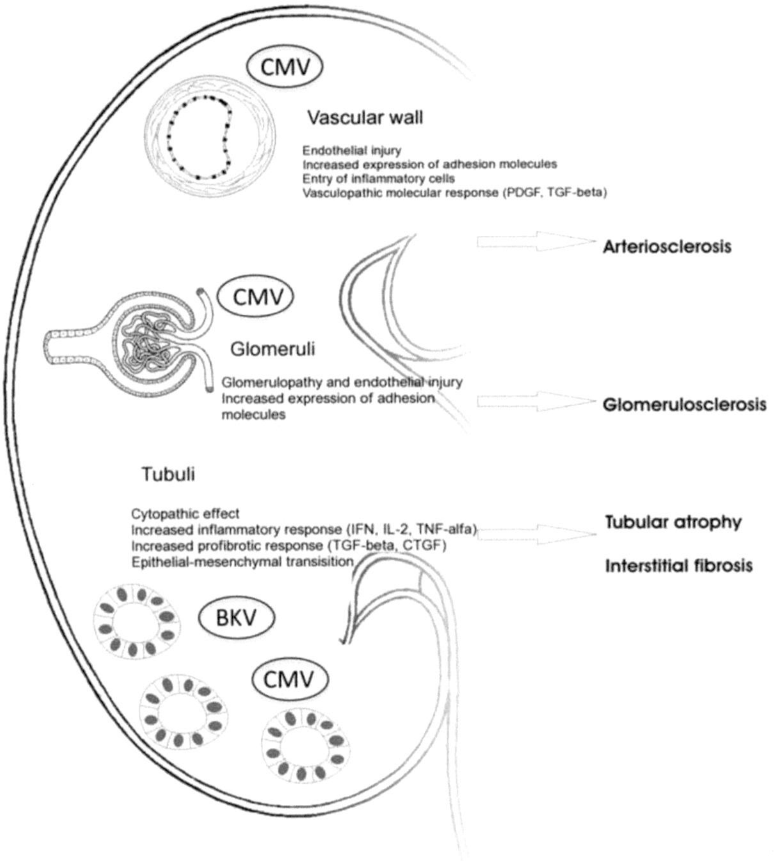

Figure 6: Possible mechanisms of the allograft injury caused by BKV and CMV.

REFERENCES

[1] Meier-Kriesche HU, Schold JD, Kaplan B. Long-term renal allograft survival: have we made significant progress or is it time to rethink our analytic and therapeutic strategies? Am J Transplant 2004; 4: 1289-1295.

[2] Dharnidharka VR, Caillard S, Agodoa LY, Abbott KC. Infection frequency and profile in different age groups of kidney transplant recipients. Transplantation 2006; 81: 1662-1667.

[3] Binet I, Nickeleit V, Hirsch HH, *et al.* Polyomavirus disease under new immunosuppressive drugs: a cause of renal graft dysfunction and graft loss. Transplantation 1999; 67: 918-922.

[4] Lautenschlager I, Soots A, Krogerus L, *et al.* Effect of cytomegalovirus on an experimental model of chronic renal allograft rejection under triple-drug treatment in the rat. Transplantation 1997; 64: 391-398.

[5] Helanterä I, Koskinen P, Törnroth T,*et al.* The impact of cytomegalovirus infections and acute rejection episodes on the development of vascular changes in 6-month protocol biopsy specimens of cadaveric kidney allograft recipients. Transplantation 2003; 75: 1858-1864.

[6] Sagedal S, Nordal KP, Hartmann A, *et al.* The impact of cytomegalovirus infection and disease on rejection episodes in renal allograft recipients. Am J Transplant 2002; 2: 850-856.

[7] Low JA, Magnuson B, Tsai B, Imperiale MJ. Identification of gangliosides GD1b and GT1b as receptors for BK virus. J Virol 2006; 80: 1361-1366.

[8] Elphick GF, Querbes W, Jordan JA, *et al.* The human polyomavirus, JCV, uses serotonin receptors to infect cells. Science 2004; 306: 1380-1383.

[9] Chesters PM, Heritage J, McCance DJ. Persistence of DNA sequences of BK virus and JC virus in normal human tissues and in diseased tissues. J Infect Dis 1983; 147: 676-684.

[10] Dolei A, Pietropaolo V, Gomes E, *et al.* Polyomavirus persistence in lymphocytes: prevalence in lymphocytes from blood donors and healthy personnel of a blood transfusion centre. J Gen Virol 2000; 81: 1967-1973.

[11] Behzad-Behbahani A, Klapper PE, Vallely PJ, Cleator GM. BK virus DNA in CSF of immunocompetent and immunocompromised patients. Arch Dis Child 2003; 88: 174-175.

[12] Knowles WA, Pipkin P, Andrews N, *et al.* Population-based study of antibody to the human polyomaviruses BKV and JCV and the simian polyomavirus SV40. J Med Virol 2003; 71: 115-123.

[13] Egli A, Infanti L, Dumoulin A, *et al.* Prevalence of polyomavirus BK and JC infection and replication in 400 healthy blood donors. J Infect Dis 2009; 199: 837-846.

[14] Hirsch HH, Steiger J. Polyomavirus BK. Lancet Infect Dis 2003; 3: 611-623.

[15] Boldorini R, Veggiani C, Barco D, Monga G. Kidney and urinary tract polyomavirus infection and distribution: molecular biology investigation of 10 consecutive autopsies. Arch Pathol Lab Med 2005; 129: 69-73.

[16] Polo C, Perez JL, Mielnichuck A, *et al.* Prevalence and patterns of polyomavirus urinary excretion in immunocompetent adults and children. Clin Microbiol Infect 2004; 10: 640-644.

[17] Kitamura T, Aso Y, Kuniyoshi N, *et al.* High incidence of urinary JC virus excretion in nonimmunosuppressed older patients. J Infect Dis 1990; 161: 1128-1133.

[18] Rossi A, Delbue S, Mazziotti R, *et al.* Presence, quantitation and characterization of JC virus in the urine of Italian immunocompetent subjects. J Med Virol 2007; 79: 408-412.

[19] Gosert R, Rinaldo CH, Funk GA, *et al.* Polyomavirus BK with rearranged noncoding control region emerge *in vivo* in renal transplant patients and increase viral replication and cytopathology. J Exp Med 2008; 205: 841-852.

[20] Drachenberg CB, Hirsch HH, Papadimitriou JC, *et al.* Polyomavirus BK versus JC replication and nephropathy in renal transplant recipients: a prospective evaluation. Transplantation 2007; 84: 323-330.

[21] Mengel M, Marwedel M, Radermacher J, *et al.* Incidence of polyomavirus-nephropathy in renal allografts: influence of modern immunosuppressive drugs. Nephrol Dial Transplant 2003; 18: 1190-1196.

[22] Hirsch HH, Knowles W, Dickenmann M, *et al.* Prospective study of polyomavirus type BK replication and nephropathy in renal-transplant recipients. N Engl J Med 2002; 347: 488-496.

[23] Sachdeva MS, Nada R, Jha V, *et al.* The high incidence of BK polyoma virus infection among renal transplant recipients in India. Transplantation 2004; 77: 429-431.

[24] Hirsch HH, Brennan DC, Drachenberg CB, *et al.* Polyomavirus-associated nephropathy in renal transplantation: interdisciplinary analyses and recommendations. Transplantation 2005; 79: 1277-1286.

[25] Racusen LC, Solez K, Colvin RB, *et al.* The Banff 97 working classification of renal allograft pathology. Kidney Int 1999; 55: 713-723.

[26] Racusen LC, Colvin RB, Solez K, *et al.* Antibody-mediated rejection criteria - an addition to the Banff 97 classification of renal allograft rejection. Am J Transplant 2003; 3: 708-714.

[27] Awadalla Y, Randhawa P, Ruppert K, *et al.* HLA mismatching increases the risk of BK virus nephropathy in renal transplant recipients. Am J Transplant 2004; 4: 1691-1696.

[28] Helanterä I, Ortiz F, Auvinen E, *et al.* Polyomavirus BK and JC infections in well matched Finnish kidney transplant recipients. Transpl Int 2009; 22: 688-693.

[29] Bohl DL, Storch GA, Ryschkewitsch C, *et al.* Donor origin of BK virus in renal transplantation and role of HLA C7 in susceptibility to sustained BK viremia. Am J Transplant 2005; 5: 2213-2221.

[30] Randhawa PS, Khaleel-Ur-Rehman K, Swalsky PA, *et al.* DNA sequencing of viral capsid protein VP-1 region in patients with BK virus interstitial nephritis. Transplantation 2002; 73: 1090-1094.

[31] Randhawa P, Zygmunt D, Shapiro R, *et al.* Viral regulatory region sequence variations in kidney tissue obtained from patients with BK virus nephropathy. Kidney Int 2003; 64: 743-747.

[32] Ginevri F, De Santis R, Comoli P, *et al.* Polyomavirus BK infection in pediatric kidney-allograft recipients: a single-center analysis of incidence, risk factors, and novel therapeutic approaches. Transplantation 2003; 75: 1266-1270.

[33] Comoli P, Azzi A, Maccario R, *et al.* Polyomavirus BK-specific immunity after kidney transplantation. Transplantation 2004; 78: 1229-1232.

[34] Grinde B, Gayorfar M, Rinaldo CH. Impact of a polyomavirus (BKV) infection on mRNA expression in human endothelial cells. Virus Res 2007; 123: 86-94.

[35] Mannon RB, Hoffmann SC, Kampen RL, *et al.* Molecular evaluation of BK polyomavirus nephropathy. Am J Transplant 2005; 5: 2883-2893.

[36] Sadeghi M, Daniel V, Schnitzler P, *et al.* Urinary proinflammatory cytokine response in renal transplant recipients with polyomavirus BK viruria. Transplantation 2009; 88: 1109-1116.

[37] Gupta G, Ishwad C, Gasper G, *et al.* BK Virus upregulates TGF-beta as well as specific components of the TGF-beta signaling pathway. Am J Transplant 2006; 6: 119-120.

[38] Abend JR, Imperiale MJ. Transforming growth factor-beta-mediated regulation of BK virus gene expression. Virology 2008; 378: 6-12.

[39] Olsen GH, Hirsch HH, Rinaldo CH. Functional analysis of polyomavirus BK non-coding control region quasispecies from kidney transplant recipients. J Med Virol 2009; 81: 1959-1967.

[40] Knowles WA. Propagation and assay of BK virus. Methods Mol Biol 2001; 165: 19-31.

[41] Leuenberger D, Andresen PA, Gosert R, *et al.* Human polyomavirus type 1 (BK virus) agnoprotein is abundantly expressed but immunologically ignored. Clin Vaccine Immunol 2007; 14: 959-968.

[42] Kemeny E, Hirsch HH, Eller J, *et al.* Plasma cell infiltrates in polyomavirus nephropathy. Transpl.Int. 2010; 23: 397-406.

[43] Binggeli S, Egli A, Schaub S, *et al.* Polyomavirus BK-specific cellular immune response to VP1 and large T-antigen in kidney transplant recipients. Am J Transplant 2007; 7: 1131-1139.

[44] Chen Y, Trofe J, Gordon J, *et al.* Interplay of cellular and humoral immune responses against BK virus in kidney transplant recipients with polyomavirus nephropathy. J Virol 2006; 80: 3495-3505.

[45] Hammer MH, Brestrich G, Andree H, *et al.* HLA type-independent method to monitor polyoma BK virus-specific CD4 and CD8 T-cell immunity. Am J Transplant 2006; 6: 625-631.

[46] Li J, Melenhorst J, Hensel N, *et al.* T-cell responses to peptide fragments of the BK virus T antigen: implications for cross-reactivity of immune response to JC virus. J Gen Virol 2006; 87: 2951-2960.

[47] Egli A, Kohli S, Dickenmann M, Hirsch HH. Inhibition of polyomavirus BK-specific T-Cell responses by immunosuppressive drugs. Transplantation 2009; 88: 1161-1168.

[48] Ginevri F, Azzi A, Hirsch HH, *et al.* Prospective monitoring of polyomavirus BK replication and impact of pre-emptive intervention in pediatric kidney recipients. Am J Transplant 2007; 7: 2727-2735.

[49] Schaub S, Mayr M, Egli A, *et al.* Transient allograft dysfunction from immune reconstitution in a patient with polyoma BK-virus-associated nephropathy. Nephrol Dial Transplant 2007; 22: 2386-2390.

[50] Drachenberg CB, Papadimitriou JC, Mann D, *et al.* Negative impact of human leukocyte antigen matching in the outcome of polyomavirus nephropathy. Transplantation 2005; 80: 276-278.

[51] Hirsch HH, Kaufmann G, Sendi P, Battegay M. Immune reconstitution in HIV-infected patients. Clin Infect Dis. 2004; 38: 1159-1166.

[52] Funk GA, Gosert R, Hirsch HH. Viral dynamics in transplant patients: implications for disease. Lancet Infect Dis 2007; 7: 460-472.

[53] Nickeleit V, Klimkait T, Binet IF, *et al.* Testing for polyomavirus type BK DNA in plasma to identify renal-allograft recipients with viral nephropathy. N Engl J Med 2000; 342: 1309-1315.

[54] Drachenberg CB, Hirsch HH, Ramos E, Papadimitriou JC. Polyomavirus disease in renal transplantation: review of pathological findings and diagnostic methods. Hum Pathol 2005; 36: 1245-1255.

[55] Kidney Disease: Improving Global Outcomes (KDIGO) Transplant Work Group. KDIGO clinical practice guideline for the care of kidney transplant recipients. Am J Transplant 2009; 9 Suppl 3: S1-155.

[56] Schaub S, Hirsch HH, Dickenmann M, *et al.* Reducing immunosuppression preserves allograft function in presumptive and definitive polyomavirus-associated nephropathy. Am J Transplant 2010; 10: 2615-2623.

[57] Hirsch HH, Randhawa P, AST Infectious Diseases Community of Practice. BK virus in solid organ transplant recipients. Am J Transplant 2009; 9 Suppl 4: S136-46.

[58] Bernhoff E, Gutteberg TJ, Sandvik K, *et al.* Cidofovir inhibits polyomavirus BK replication in human renal tubular cells downstream of viral early gene expression. Am J Transplant 2008; 8: 1413-1422.

[59] Farasati NA, Shapiro R, Vats A, Randhawa P. Effect of leflunomide and cidofovir on replication of BK virus in an *in vitro* culture system. Transplantation 2005; 79: 116-118.

[60] Cesaro S, Hirsch HH, Faraci M, *et al.* Cidofovir for BK virus-associated hemorrhagic cystitis: a retrospective study. Clin Infect Dis 2009; 49: 233-240.

[61] Rinaldo CH, Gosert R, Bernhoff E, *et al.* 1-O-hexadecyloxypropyl cidofovir (CMX001) effectively inhibits polyomavirus BK replication in primary human renal tubular epithelial cells. Antimicrob Agents Chemother 2010; 54: 4714-4722.

[62] Wang X, Huong SM, Chiu ML, *et al.* Epidermal growth factor receptor is a cellular receptor for human cytomegalovirus. Nature 2003; 424: 456-461.

[63] Feire AL, Koss H, Compton T. Cellular integrins function as entry receptors for human cytomegalovirus *via* a highly conserved disintegrin-like domain. Proc Natl Acad Sci U.S.A. 2004; 101: 15470-15475.
[64] Soroceanu L, Akhavan A, Cobbs CS. Platelet-derived growth factor-alpha receptor activation is required for human cytomegalovirus infection. Nature 2008; 455: 391-395.
[65] Sinclair J, Sissons P. Latency and reactivation of human cytomegalovirus. J Gen Virol 2006; 87: 1763-1779.
[66] Sagedal S, Nordal KP, Hartmann A, *et al.* A prospective study of the natural course of cytomegalovirus infection and disease in renal allograft recipients. Transplantation 2000; 70: 1166-1174.
[67] Humar A, Gillingham K, Payne WD, *et al.* Increased incidence of cardiac complications in kidney transplant recipients with cytomegalovirus disease. Transplantation 2000; 70: 310-313.
[68] Kaplan B, Meier-Kriesche HU, Jacobs MG, *et al.* Prevalence of cytomegalovirus in the gastrointestinal tract of renal transplant recipients with persistent abdominal pain. Am J Kidney Dis 1999; 34: 65-68.
[69] Lempinen M, Halme L, Sarkio S, *et al.* CMV findings in the gastrointestinal tract in kidney transplantation patients, patients with end-stage kidney disease and immunocompetent patients. Nephrol Dial Transplant 2009; 24: 3533-3539.
[70] Hjelmesaeth J, Sagedal S, Hartmann A, *et al.* Asymptomatic cytomegalovirus infection is associated with increased risk of new-onset diabetes mellitus and impaired insulin release after renal transplantation. Diabetologia 2004; 47: 1550-1556.
[71] Pouteil-Noble C, Ecochard R, Landrivon G, *et al.* Cytomegalovirus infection--an etiological factor for rejection? A prospective study in 242 renal transplant patients. Transplantation 1993; 55: 851-857.
[72] Reinke P, Fietze E, Ode-Hakim S, *et al.* Late-acute renal allograft rejection and symptomless cytomegalovirus infection. Lancet 1994; 344: 1737-1738.
[73] Reischig T, Jindra P, Svecova M, *et al.* The impact of cytomegalovirus disease and asymptomatic infection on acute renal allograft rejection. J Clin Virol 2006; 36: 146-151.
[74] Dickenmann MJ, Cathomas G, Steiger J,*et al.* Cytomegalovirus infection and graft rejection in renal transplantation. Transplantation 2001; 71: 764-767.
[75] Rubin RH, Tolkoff-Rubin NE, Oliver D, *et al.* Multicenter seroepidemiologic study of the impact of cytomegalovirus infection on renal transplantation. Transplantation 1985; 40: 243-249.
[76] Tong CY, Bakran A, Peiris JS, *et al.* The association of viral infection and chronic allograft nephropathy with graft dysfunction after renal transplantation. Transplantation 2002; 74: 576-578.
[77] Giral M, Nguyen JM, Daguin P, *et al.* Mycophenolate mofetil does not modify the incidence of cytomegalovirus (CMV) disease after kidney transplantation but prevents CMV-induced chronic graft dysfunction. J Am Soc Nephrol 2001; 12: 1758-1763.
[78] Nett PC, Heisey DM, Fernandez LA, *et al.* Association of cytomegalovirus disease and acute rejection with graft loss in kidney transplantation. Transplantation 2004; 78: 1036-1041.
[79] Sagedal S, Hartmann A, Nordal KP, *et al.* Impact of early cytomegalovirus infection and disease on long-term recipient and kidney graft survival. Kidney Int 2004; 66: 329-337.
[80] Akposso K, Rondeau E, Haymann JP, *et al.* Long-term prognosis of renal transplantation after preemptive treatment of cytomegalovirus infection. Transplantation 1997; 63: 974-976.
[81] Kliem V, Fricke L, Wollbrink T, *et al.* Improvement in long-term renal graft survival due to CMV prophylaxis with oral ganciclovir: results of a randomized clinical trial. Am J Transplant 2008; 8: 975-983.
[82] Richardson WP, Colvin RB, Cheeseman SH, *et al.* Glomerulopathy associated with cytomegalovirus viremia in renal allografts. N Engl J Med 1981; 305: 57-63.
[83] Rao KV, Hafner GP, Crary GS, *et al.* *De novo* immunotactoid glomerulopathy of the renal allograft: possible association with cytomegalovirus infection. Am J Kidney Dis 1994; 24: 97-103.
[84] Humar A, Gillingham KJ, Payne WD, *et al.* Association between cytomegalovirus disease and chronic rejection in kidney transplant recipients. Transplantation 1999; 68: 1879-1883.
[85] Reischig T, Jindra P, Hes O, *et al.* Effect of cytomegalovirus viremia on subclinical rejection or interstitial fibrosis and tubular atrophy in protocol biopsy at 3 months in renal allograft recipients managed by preemptive therapy or antiviral prophylaxis. Transplantation 2009; 87: 436-444.
[86] Ustinov JA, Loginov RJ, Mattila PM, *et al.* Cytomegalovirus infection of human kidney cells *in vitro*. Kidney Int 1991; 40: 954-960.
[87] Andersen CB, Ladefoged SD, Lauritsen HK, *et al.* Detection of CMV DNA and CMV antigen in renal allograft biopsies by *in situ* hybridisation and immunohistochemistry. Nephrol Dial Transplant 1990; 5: 1045-1050.

[88] Liapis H, Storch GA, Hill DA, *et al.* CMV infection of the renal allograft is much more common than the pathology indicates: a retrospective analysis of qualitative and quantitative buffy coat CMV-PCR, renal biopsy pathology and tissue CMV-PCR. Nephrol Dial Transplant 2003; 18: 397-402.

[89] Helanterä I, Koskinen P, Finne P, *et al.* Persistent cytomegalovirus infection in kidney allografts is associated with inferior graft function and survival. Transpl Int 2006; 19: 893-900.

[90] Arnold JC, Portmann BC, O'Grady JG, *et al.* Cytomegalovirus infection persists in the liver graft in the vanishing bile duct syndrome. Hepatology 1992; 16: 285-292.

[91] Lautenschlager I, Höckerstedt K, Jalanko H, *et al.* Persistent cytomegalovirus in liver allografts with chronic rejection. Hepatology 1997; 25: 190-194.

[92] Iwamoto GK, Monick MM, Clark BD, *et al.* Modulation of interleukin 1 beta gene expression by the immediate early genes of human cytomegalovirus. J Clin Invest 1990; 85: 1853-1857.

[93] Geist LJ, Monick MM, Stinski MF, Hunninghake GW. The immediate early genes of human cytomegalovirus upregulate expression of the interleukin-2 and interleukin-2 receptor genes. Am J Respir Cell Mol Biol 1991; 5: 292-296.

[94] Smith PD, Saini SS, Raffeld M,*et al.* Cytomegalovirus induction of tumor necrosis factor-alpha by human monocytes and mucosal macrophages. J Clin Invest 1992; 90: 1642-1648.

[95] Sedmak DD, Knight DA, Vook NC, Waldman JW. Divergent patterns of ELAM-1, ICAM-1, and VCAM-1 expression on cytomegalovirus-infected endothelial cells. Transplantation 1994; 58: 1379-1385.

[96] Craigen JL, Grundy JE. Cytomegalovirus induced up-regulation of LFA-3 (CD58) and ICAM-1 (CD54) is a direct viral effect that is not prevented by ganciclovir or foscarnet treatment. Transplantation 1996; 62: 1102-1108.

[97] Streblow DN, Soderberg-Naucler C, Vieira J, *et al.* The human cytomegalovirus chemokine receptor US28 mediates vascular smooth muscle cell migration. Cell 1999; 99: 511-520.

[98] van Cleef KW, Smit MJ, Bruggeman CA, Vink C. Cytomegalovirus-encoded homologs of G protein-coupled receptors and chemokines. J Clin Virol 2006; 35: 343-348.

[99] Grotendorst GR. Connective tissue growth factor: a mediator of TGF-beta action on fibroblasts. Cytokine Growth Factor Rev. 1997; 8: 171-179.

[100] Phanish MK, Winn SK, Dockrell ME. Connective tissue growth factor-(CTGF, CCN2)--a marker, mediator and therapeutic target for renal fibrosis. Nephron Exp Nephrol 2010; 114: 83-92.

[101] Fietze E, Prosch S, Reinke P, *et al.* Cytomegalovirus infection in transplant recipients. The role of tumor necrosis factor. Transplantation 1994; 58: 675-680.

[102] Reinke P, Prosch S, Kern F, Volk HD. Mechanisms of human cytomegalovirus (HCMV) (re)activation and its impact on organ transplant patients. Transpl Infect Dis 1999; 1: 157-164.

[103] Zhang Z, Kim SJ, Varghese T, *et al.* TNF receptor independent activation of the cytomegalovirus major immediate early enhancer in response to transplantation. Transplantation 2008; 85: 1039-1045.

[104] Krogerus L, Soots A, Loginov R, *et al.* CMV increases tubular apoptosis through the TNF-alpha-TNF-R1 pathway in a rat model of chronic renal allograft rejection. Transpl Immunol 2008; 18: 232-236.

[105] Michelson S, Alcami J, Kim SJ, *et al.* Human cytomegalovirus infection induces transcription and secretion of transforming growth factor beta 1. J Virol 1994; 68: 5730-5377.

[106] Zhou YF, Yu ZX, Wanishsawad C, *et al.* The immediate early gene products of human cytomegalovirus increase vascular smooth muscle cell migration, proliferation, and expression of PDGF beta-receptor. Biochem Biophys Res Commun 1999; 256: 608-613.

[107] Markiewicz M, Smith EA, Rubinchik S, *et al.* The 72-kilodalton IE-1 protein of human cytomegalovirus (HCMV) is a potent inducer of connective tissue growth factor (CTGF) in human dermal fibroblasts. Clin Exp Rheumatol 2004; 22: 31-34.

[108] Reinhardt B, Schaarschmidt P, Bossert A, *et al.* Upregulation of functionally active vascular endothelial growth factor by human cytomegalovirus. J Gen Virol 2005; 86: 23-30.

[109] Inkinen K, Soots A, Krogerus L, *et al.* Cytomegalovirus increases collagen synthesis in chronic rejection in the rat. Nephrol Dial Transplant 2002; 17: 772-779.

[110] Yilmaz S, Koskinen PK, Kallio E, *et al.* Cytomegalovirus infection-enhanced chronic kidney allograft rejection is linked with intercellular adhesion molecule-1 expression. Kidney Int 1996; 50: 526-527.

[111] Kloover JS, Soots AP, Krogerus LA, *et al.* Rat cytomegalovirus infection in kidney allograft recipients is associated with increased expression of intracellular adhesion molecule-1 vascular adhesion molecule-1, and their ligands leukocyte function antigen-1 and very late antigen-4 in the graft. Transplantation 2000; 69: 2641-2647.

[112] Inkinen K, Soots A, Krogerus L, *et al.* Cytomegalovirus enhance expression of growth factors during the development of chronic allograft nephropathy in rats. Transpl Int 2005; 18: 743-749.

[113] Dumortier J, Streblow DN, Moses AV, *et al.* Human cytomegalovirus secretome contains factors that induce angiogenesis and wound healing. J Virol 2008; 82: 6524-6535.

[114] Helanterä I, Loginov R, Koskinen P, *et al.* Persistent cytomegalovirus infection is associated with increased expression of TGF-beta1, PDGF-AA and ICAM-1 and arterial intimal thickening in kidney allografts. Nephrol Dial Transplant 2005; 20: 790-796.

[115] Pang XL, Chui L, Fenton J, *et al.* Comparison of LightCycler-based PCR, COBAS amplicor CMV monitor, and pp65 antigenemia assays for quantitative measurement of cytomegalovirus viral load in peripheral blood specimens from patients after solid organ transplantation. J Clin Microbiol 2003; 41: 3167-3174.

[116] Piiparinen H, Höckerstedt K, Groönhagen-Riska C, Lautenschlager I. Comparison of two quantitative CMV PCR tests, Cobas Amplicor CMV Monitor and TaqMan assay, and pp65-antigenemia assay in the determination of viral loads from peripheral blood of organ transplant patients. J Clin Virol 2004; 30: 258-266.

[117] Razonable RR, Brown RA, Wilson J, *et al.* The clinical use of various blood compartments for cytomegalovirus (CMV) DNA quantitation in transplant recipients with CMV disease. Transplantation 2002; 73: 968-973.

[118] Caliendo AM, St George K, Allega J, *et al.*Distinguishing cytomegalovirus (CMV) infection and disease with CMV nucleic acid assays. J Clin Microbiol 2002; 40: 1581-1586.

[119] Kotton CN, Kumar D, Caliendo AM, *et al.* International consensus guidelines on the management of cytomegalovirus in solid organ transplantation. Transplantation 2010; 89: 779-795.

[120] Gerna G, Lilleri D. Monitoring transplant patients for human cytomegalovirus: Diagnostic update. Herpes 2006; 13: 4-11.

[121] The TH, van den Berg AP, Harmsen MC, *et al.* The cytomegalovirus antigenemia assay: a plea for standardization. Scand J Infect Dis Suppl 1995; 99: 25-29.

[122] Humar A, Lebranchu Y, Vincenti F, *et al.* The efficacy and safety of 200 days valganciclovir cytomegalovirus prophylaxis in high-risk kidney transplant recipients. Am J Transplant 2010; 10: 1228-1237.

[123] Helanterä I, Kyllönen L, Lautenschlager I, *et al.* Primary CMV infections are common in kidney transplant recipients after 6 months valganciclovir prophylaxis. Am J Transplant 2010; 10: 2026-2032.

[124] Humar A, Mazzulli T, Moussa G, *et al.* Clinical utility of cytomegalovirus (CMV) serology testing in high-risk CMV D+/R- transplant recipients. Am J Transplant 2005; 5: 1065-7100.

[125] Humar A, Paya C, Pescovitz MD, *et al.* Clinical utility of cytomegalovirus viral load testing for predicting CMV disease in D+/R- solid organ transplant recipients. Am J Transplant 2004; 4: 644-649.

[126] Sester M, Sester U, Gartner B, *et al.* Levels of virus-specific CD4 T cells correlate with cytomegalovirus control and predict virus-induced disease after renal transplantation. Transplantation 2001; 71: 1287-1294.

[127] Bunde T, Kirchner A, Hoffmeister B, *et al.* Protection from cytomegalovirus after transplantation is correlated with immediate early 1-specific CD8 T cells. J Exp Med 2005; 201: 1031-1036.

[128] Kumar D, Chernenko S, Moussa G, *et al.* Cell-mediated immunity to predict cytomegalovirus disease in high-risk solid organ transplant recipients. Am J Transplant 2009; 9: 1214-1222.

[129] Egli A, Binet I, Binggeli S, *et al.* Cytomegalovirus-specific T-cell responses and viral replication in kidney transplant recipients. J Transl Med 2008; 6: 29.

[130] Mattes FM, Vargas A, Kopycinski J, *et al.* Functional impairment of cytomegalovirus specific CD8 T cells predicts high-level replication after renal transplantation. Am J Transplant 2008; 8: 990-999.

CHAPTER 20

Epidemiology of Cancers After Kidney Transplantation and Role of Viral Infections

Pierluca Piselli[1,*], Enrico Girardi[1], Diego Serraino[2], Vincenzo Puro[1], Claudia Cimaglia[1] and Giuseppe Ippolito[1]

[1]*Department of Epidemiology, National Institute for Infectious Diseases "L. Spallanzani", Rome, Italy and* [2]*Unità di Epidemiologia e Biostatistica, IRCCS Centro di Riferimento Oncologico, Aviano, Italy*

Abstract: Kidney transplantation (KT) is an increasingly used medical procedure for treating otherwise fatal end stage renal diseases (ESRD); this success was obtained with the use of potent immunosuppressive agents able to reduce the risk of rejection of transplanted organs, but exposing patients to an increased risk of opportunistic diseases such infections or cancers, this latter representing nowadays the second major cause of morbidity and mortality after KT. KT recipients (KTR) experience a 2- to 4-fold increase of *de novo* post-transplant malignancies (PTM) when compared to the general population, particularly skin cancers, urological malignancies and virus-related cancers such as non-Hodgkin lymphoma (NHL) or Kaposi's sarcoma (KS) with up to 100-fold augmented risk when compared to the general population. Given the improved graft and patient survival that have lengthened the observation period for the natural history of immunosuppressed recipients and their increasing age, we can expect that over the next decades mortality from malignancy may represents the leading cause of death in transplanted patients. As the immunosuppression *per se* and various potentially oncogenic viruses play a major role in cancer development after transplant, a better definition of this phenomenon can lead to the adoption of preventive measure to reduce the risk of PTM or the implementation of better screening protocols to earlier detect malignancies. This chapter examines, from an epidemiological point of view, the incidence, etiology and prognosis of malignancies after kidney transplantation with a focus on those associated with viral infections.

Keywords: Post-Transplant Malignancies, Viruses and Cancer, Kaposi's Sarcoma, Epstein-Barr Virus, Post-Transplant Lymphoproliferative Disorders, Skin Cancer, Renal Cell Carcinoma, Everolimus, Sirolimus.

INTRODUCTION

Kidney transplantation (KT) is an increasingly used medical procedure for treating otherwise fatal end-stage renal diseases (ESRD), with numbers of transplant recipients doubling in last decades. In 2008, more than 16000 individuals received a kidney transplant in USA, and 1600 in Italy. The main reason of this success is to be attributed to the use of potent agents able to reduce the risk of rejection of the transplanted organs acting as immunosuppressant of the natural immune response against a *non-self* tissue/organ; nowadays, 5-year survival rate after KT is more than 90% in most centers and with an acute rejection rate resulting in graft loss less than 5% [1]. However, the chronic use of immunosuppression to prevent unwanted rejection of the grafted organ, conversely expose the recipient to an increased risk of opportunistic diseases such infections or cancers [2].

The relationship between malignancies development and the immune response was firstly described in the early 1900s by Ehrlich, who established the so-called theory of "immunological surveillance". This theory is based on the principles that the neoplastic cells are antigenic and for this reason can be destroyed by the immune response of the organism and that immune depression is associated with a higher incidence of cancer [3].

Since the beginning of the transplantation era in the late 1960s, an increased frequency of certain cancers in people treated with anti-rejection drugs after organ transplantation was described.

***Address correspondence to Pierluca Piselli:** INMI "L. Spallanzani" IRCCS, Dipartimento di Epidemiologia, *Via* Portuense 292 – 00149 Rome, Italy; Tel: +39 0655170900; E-mail: pierluca.piselli@inmi.it

The Fourth Report of the Human Kidney Transplant Registry (HKTR) in 1965, describing the results of the 672 kidney transplants performed in the world so far, detailed the first two tumors (both fatal and donor derived) [4]. First description of *de novo* malignancies after KTR dated 1969, when 13 post-transplant primary malignancies (all fatal, of which 7 lymphomas) were reported from HKTR data, with a calculated cancer incidence 5- to 8-fold increased than general population [5]. In the same year, Israel Penn and transplant pioneer Thomas Starzl described five lymphomas in living donor KTR [6], and Dr. Penn later founded the Cincinnati Transplant Tumor Registry or CTTR (named after his death in 1999, Israel Penn International Transplant Tumor Registry), the first international registry in the World who is still able to report data on more than 15,000 transplant related malignancies collected on a voluntary base by transplantation centers' members, founding all the present knowledge in this field [7].

The same malignancies, namely, non-Hodgkin lymphoma (NHL), Kaposi's sarcoma (KS), non-melanoma skin cancers, are the commonest neoplastic manifestations in the course of HIV infection or AIDS, another type of acquired immunodeficiency [8].

Initially, malignancy was a sideline in the management of transplant recipients, since cancer specific morbidity and mortality comprised only a small proportion of the total, in a group of patients where leading mortality risks was associated with immunological or non immunological graft failure. As the risk of acute rejection and subsequent graft loss diminished due to the introduction of better immunosuppressive regimens, frequency of malignancies dramatically increased. Given the improved graft and patient survival that have lengthened the observation period for the natural history of immunosuppressed recipients and their increasing age, we can expect that over the next decades mortality from malignancy may represent the leading cause of death in transplanted patients.

Actually, the overall incidence of any kind of malignancy has been estimated at 20% after 10 years of chronic immunosuppression [9]. Several studies have shown that kidney transplanted patients experience a 3- to 5-fold increase of *de novo* post-transplant malignancies (PTM) when compared to the general population, particularly skin cancers, urological malignancies and virus-related cancers such as non-Hodgkin lymphoma (NHL) or Kaposi's sarcoma (KS) with up to 100-fold augmented risk [10].

Other neoplastic complications in the transplanted patients could arise not only from *de novo* PTM, but with the recurrence of pre-existing cancers or cancer transmitted from donor organs, addressing the need of a careful pre-transplant screening procedure.

In any case, survival among renal transplanted recipients with advanced cancer is often poor and treatment options are limited, due to presence of important co-morbidities such as cardiovascular disease or infection; finally, treatment of malignancies with potent chemotherapeutic drugs can cause graft rejection or strong adverse effects that can heavily affect graft functionality [2].

ROLE OF VIRAL INFECTIONS

Certain viral infections predispose transplant recipients to specific type of malignancies (see Table **1**). The impairment of immune-control due to the immunosuppressive treatment, could lead to the reduction or elimination of virus-specific cytolytic responses, facilitating the expansion of virus-infected cells either through primary viral infection or reactivation of latent infection [2, 11].

The implicit capacity of several viruses to immortalize infected cells disrupting the cell-cycle control, in a setting of induced lowered immunesurveillance could lead to tumorigenesis and this ability is thought to closely correlate with overall or cumulative exposure to immunosuppression [12].

A paradigmatic example of this capability is given by Epstein-Barr Virus (EBV). EBV primary infection occurs normally in the first few years of life (up to 90% of adolescents are found to be EBV-seropositives), predominantly without any evident disease, but delayed primary infection could lead to mononuclear cells proliferation resulting in lymphoprolifearitive disorders ranging from benignant (mononucleosis) to malignant (*i.e.* Burkitt's lymphoma) forms [13]. More frequently, primary infection results in the establishment of a dormant latent phase in which EBV-genome is maintained in an episomal form in the infected cell and its progeny, through the action of EBV-nuclear antigens 1 and 2 (EBNA-1 and EBNA-2) [14]. The viral genome encodes also for trans-membrane molecule LMP-1 (Latent Membrane Protein 1) that during the latent phase activates, *via* second messengers, NF-κB protein, leading to the production of important transcription factors and anti-apoptotic proteins, ensuring the immortalization of infected cells [13]. In the immunocompetent host the immunesurveillance can control, without efficiently eliminating, overgrowth of EBV-infected cells, but a transient or permanent immunosuppression unbalances this equilibrium leading eventually to uncontrolled tumour growth [15].

Table 1: Virus related to post-transplant malignancies

Virus	Malignancy
EBV	Lymphoma and lymphoproliferative disorders
HPV	Cervical cancer Penis cancer Anal cancer Vulvar carcinoma Tonsillar cancer Non-melanoma skin cancer
HHV-8	Kaposi's Sarcoma Primary effusion lymphoma (PEL)
HBV	Hepatocellular carcinoma
HCV	Hepatocellular carcinoma Lymphoma and lymphoproliferative disorders
SV40	B-cell lymphoma
HTLV-1	Lymphoma and lymphoproliferative disorders

EBV: Epstein-Barr Virus; HPV: Human papillomoviruses; HHV-8: Human Herpesvirus 8; HBV: Hepatitis B Virus; HCV: Hepatitis C Virus; SV40: Simian Virus 40; HTLV-1: Human T-lymphotrophic virus 1.

In the transplanted patients there are two different possibilities of EBV-driven tumour growth, or in re-activation of latent persistent EBV-infection (especially in the first months after transplant when immunosuppression is higher) or as the effect of an uncontrolled EBV-primary infection in an EBV-negative recipient [16].

A similar situation is represented by the re-activation of HHV-8 infection in the development of Kaposi's Sarcoma after transplantation or HTLV-1 infection and lymphomagenesis geographically relevant respectively in Mediterranean/Middle East and Asian countries where prevalence of infection in the general population and prior transplantation is higher [17, 18].

Given this link between immunosuppression and viral-oncogenesis, is not surprising that in transplanted patients virus-related tumours such as lymphomas, ano-genital cancer, Kaposi's sarcoma or hepatocellular cancer are at a markedly increased risk while non-viral-related solid malignancies such as breast and prostatic cancers are not increased. Consequently the overall increased risk of malignancy in transplanted can be ascribed principally to those form of cancers, pointing the relevance of tailored programs to prevent, early diagnose and manage these kind of malignancies [10].

DE NOVO POST-TRANSPLANT MALIGNANCIES

Cancer of the Skin

Non-melanocytic skin cancers are the most common PTM found in renal recipients, affecting up to 82% of renal recipients within 20 years after transplantation [19].

Skin cancers in transplanted patients have several peculiarities compared to those found in the general population. In the general population usually non-melanoma skin cancers predominantly occur after 60 or

70 years of age, while in transplanted patients is diagnosed at a younger age; multiple skin lesions (even up to 100) are frequently found, requiring several surgical procedures [20]. Frequently, the same patient that experiences a skin cancer may have another primary cancer either before or after the skin lesion [10, 21].

While in the general population basal cell carcinomas (BCC) outnumber squamous cell carcinomas (SCC) with a ratio of 5 to 1, the proportion is inverted 1:4 to 5 in several series of studied performed in renal recipients [22]. SCC occurs at least 25 times more frequently in renal recipients than in the general population. This kind of tumour that in the general population not so frequently metastatizes, shows a more aggressive behaviour and accounts for the majority of lymph node metastases and deaths from skin cancers [23].

Among skin cancers that frequently occur after KT, is Merckel's cell tumours a cancer of neuroendocrine origin, that present especially in the transplant a high tendency to spread and is associated with a high mortality [24].

Another important cancer of epithelial origin after KT is lip cancer, which in several international series was found up to 30-times more frequently in KTR than in the general population [25]. Lip cancer like all other skin cancers is associated with the duration and level of immunosuppression and UV exposure [26].

Skin cancers occur, as in the general population, on sun exposed areas like head, neck or upper extremities; risk rises with the degree of sunshine and cumulative UV exposure and is higher in light-skinned individuals. For this reason skin cancers are more frequently found in kidney recipients from Nordic countries like Norway or Sweden with pale skin [27, 28] and even more in countries with a elevated sun exposure like Australia, where moreover most of the population is of Anglo-Saxon origin (Australia is the country with the higher incidence of skin cancer even in the general population) [19]. Even if the choice of a specific immunosuppression protocol does not clearly appear to play a role in risk of skin cancer, some studies demonstrated that *in vitro* azathioprine sensitizes DNA to ultraviolet A (UVA) radiation, enhancing the effect of sun exposure [19].

As previously mentioned, viral infection plays an etiologic role in the development of many post-transplant malignancies. Moreover, immunosuppression can play a permissive role in the pathogenesis of viral infections such as human papilloma virus (HPV), and this is in accordance with great incidence of skin warts after transplant and with recent findings that HPV nucleotide sequences are frequently found in SCC of transplant recipients [29, 30].

Although transplant recipients have a lower risk for melanoma than for other skin cancers, the risk has been reported to be increased by a factor of 2 to 4 in Europe, Australia and North America as compared with the risk in the general population, occurring mainly in patients with fair skin, light hair and eyes [20]. Transmission of a melanoma from a donor with undiagnosed metastatic tumor can give rise to the development of metastatic melanoma in the recipient with poor outcome.

Management of skin cancers in KTR depends on the type of lesion and its extension; superficial tumors can be managed with cryotherapy or curettage, while thicker lesions need surgical excision with histologic examination to assess their aggressive behavior. Adjuvant radiotherapy or combination chemotherapy is recommended for more aggressive lesions, but in the case of metastatic forms response to treatment is often poor [20, 31]

In general skin cancers are associated with increased level of immunosuppression, thus explaining why patients with higher degree of allograft mismatch are at increased risk of skin cancers, especially SCC, mostly because of the heavier immunosuppression received [32]. In the same direction are some reports that cessation of immunosuppression appears to slow or even reverse skin tumor growth [33].

The newer class of immunosuppressive drug, the proliferation signal inhibitors drugs (PSI, Everolimus or Sirolimus, inhibitors of the mToR signalling pathway), are now used in combination with calcineurin inhibitors (CNI) drugs (Cyclosporin CsA, or Tacrolimus, TAC) [34]. Moreover PSI have shown to have also anti-proliferative and anti-angiogenesis actions, leading to the speculation of their preferred use in diminishing PTM incidence at least in patients at higher risk, as switch therapy after cancer diagnosis [35]. The use of PSI in combination with other CI or alone reduce the total immunosuppression, so the promising effects of cancer reduction and lower recurrence rate reported in the treatment of Kaposi's Sarcoma (see below) or in the treatment of skin cancer must be better studied to identify if these effects are linked to the diminished immunosuppression or to the direct anti-proliferation effect of the drugs [36].

Post-Transplant Lymphoproliferative Disorders (PTLD)

Post-transplant lymphoproliferative disorders (PTLD), are the second form of malignancies that occurs in KTR (1 to 5% cumulative incidence), but represent the most serious neoplastic complications occurring after transplantation [37].

PTLD are a complex group of conditions in which B cells (or less frequently, <10%, T cells) proliferate, ranging from a benign self-limited form of lymphoproliferation such as infectious mononucleosis-like illness or polyclonal lymphoid hyperplasia, to monoclonal malignancies such as lymphomas characterize to be aggressive, widely disseminated disease which may take a fulminant course [38]. Patients with PTLD appear to have different histological findings, a more aggressive clinical course, less likelihood of responding to conventional treatments for lymphoma and poorer outcomes when compared to immunocompetent hosts who develop malignant lymphomas [38].

More than 90% of PTLD are associated with latent Epstein-Barr virus (EBV) infection, and infection with EBV is the essential event underlying almost all PTLD [38].

There is no universally accepted PTLD definition and several classification systems have been proposed based on morphology, clonality and disruption of nodal architecture [39]. Neoplastic forms should be defined by two of the following three characteristics: a) Destruction of the lymph node structure; b) Monoclonality (regardless of morphology) and c) Evidence of EBV infection in the neoplastic cells.

The World Health Organization (WHO) classification of PTLD (2001), one of the most used, divides PTLD in three major groups [40]:

1. Hyperplastic PTLD Early lesions: including infectious mononucleosis and plasma cell hyperplasia.

2. Polymorphic PTLD Polyclonal B-cell proliferation with cytogenetic abnormalities and immunoglobulin (Ig) rearrangements suggestive of early malignant transformation.

3. Monomorphic PTLD Including B- and T-cell lymphomas, plasmacytoma-like lesions and myeloma, Hodgkin's and Hodgkin's-like lymphoma – characterized by monoclonality representing a single EBV infection event and cytogenetic abnormalities and Ig gene rearrangements.

The relevance of early lesions is often underestimated, because often they resemble more generic and unspecific malaise with fever and asthenia; still, without any treatment benign lesions can evolve to frankly malignant forms, hardly to treat and manage.

Primary infection with EBV is the main risk factor for PTLD development, as shown by the fact that PTLD incidence in EBV-seronegative recipients who receive a seropositive organ is several times greater than in EBV-seropositive patients. Risk is even higher if the patient is also seronegative for CytomegaloVirus (CMV) infection and the donor is seropositive, given the capacity of CMV infection to act as a negative immunomodulant agent, but also a direct effect of CMV in lymphocyte transformation has been speculated [41].

The higher incidence found in pediatric KTR respect to adults counterparts, can be almost entirely explained by the higher proportion of EBV-seronegative (*naïve*) patients in the pediatric as opposed to the adult population where the prevalence of EBV-seropositivity reaches >90% [42].

The progression from early lesions to malignant forms of PTLD can happen in the absence of T lymphocyte control of EBV infection [38, 43]. There is a strong evidence linking EBV with non-Hodgkin's Lymphoma (NHL) not only in transplanted patients but also in patients with primary immunodeficiency diseases or AIDS, pointing the relevance of the role of immune system in controlling abnormal lymphoproliferation [44].

PTLD can be divided in two forms according to time after transplantation at onset and EBV-positivity. A first group, consisting up to 60% of all PTLD forms, is diagnosed earlier after transplantation (in the first 12 months after KTR) and they are almost all EBV-positive [45].

A second minor group is diagnosed later (median time 4 years after KTR) and is mostly EBV-negative. Alternate viruses agents were proposed to explain those EBV-negative PTLD, such as CMV, polyomaviruses and Hepatitis C Virus (HCV), but also a secondary loss of EBV viral genome after EBV-driven initiation has been suggested [45, 46]. Independently from EBV-positivity or not, the two groups of PTLD show a similar prognosis [38].

Immunosuppression plays a relevant role in PTLD development. Transplants of organs requiring heavier immunosuppression (intestine, lung or heart) have a higher incidence of PTLD than liver or even more than kidney transplants; in the same group of transplants heavier protocols of immunosuppression (high dose, multidrug immunosuppression) are associated with a higher risk in all kind of transplants [38, 47].

Induction therapy with monoclonal (OKT3) or polyclonal anti-lymphocyte (ATG or thymoglobulin) antibodies has been associated with a 2-fold increased risk of PTLD (especially when used as anti-rejection therapy) [48, 49], but more recently lower dosage of ATG or thymoglobulin seems to be associated, conversely, to a decreased risk of PTLD [50].

Antibody inductions against the IL-2 receptor do not seem to imply a higher risk [48]. Comparing other common immunosuppressive drugs, mycophenolate mofetil (MMF) seems associated to a lower risk when compared to azathioprine (AZA) containing protocols [51], while among calcineurin inhibitors, TAC is associated with a higher risk of PTLD than CsA [48, 52].

Successful treatment of early lesions can be achieved with diminishing (or stopping) immunosuppression [53], which has to be considered as the first line approach for PTLD management. Virtually all other therapies have been combined with high-dose antiviral therapy, usually acyclovir, even if there is still little evidence of their significance in improving the outcome, so it is difficult to assess the true utility of antivirals as adjuncts to other treatments in PTLD treatment [37]. Even malignant forms of PTLD can be treated lowering immunosuppression, but the other side of this approach is the elevated risk of graft rejection, especially in non-renal allograft recipients; in KTR immunosuppression withdrawal can be considered as an option with the almost unavoidable graft loss and return to dialysis treatment [10]. However, PTLD that fails to respond adequately to reduced immunosuppression has a very high mortality (50–90%) [54].

The use of systemic chemotherapy (cyclophosphamide, doxorubricin, vincristine and prednisone, CHOP) to treat PTLD as it happens with lymphomas in immunocompetent patients is the common practice, even if it is not without adverse, even fatal, effects [10].

Since most of malignant PTLD, of the B-lineage, express CD20 antigen, use of anti-CD20 antibody rituximab, that have shown encouraging benefits in the treatment of lymphomas in the immunocompetent patient, is still now under extensive investigation. First reports have already shown good results in decreasing recurrence and improving survival rate in KTR but with a higher number of doses given than in the general population cases of lymphoma [55].

Promising results came from pre-clinical data suggesting that Everolimus has *in vitro* anti-growth effect on PTLD-derived cell lines. There is currently limited clinical data on the use of PSI in the management of PTLD, but data from nine European Transplant centres on conversion to PSI and subsequent minimization or withdrawal of CNIs was analysed in 19 renal transplant recipients with PTLD and remission was observed in 15 patients, suggesting that those drugs may assist with the management of PTLD following renal transplantation [56].

Prognosis of malignant PTLD depends on the type of diseases; in the US Renal Data System (USRDS) data 10-year survival rates varied from 26% for patients with myeloma, 39% with leukemia to 42% with NHL and 55% for those patients affected with Hodgkin's disease [57].

Factors associated with prolonged survival are younger age at diagnosis, solitary site of disease (especially if limited at the allograft), resectable lesions and manageability of the disease with immunosuppression reduction, while the presence of disease in the central Nervous System (CNS) represents the worst prognostic indicators because the inability of appropriate therapy to penetrate the CNS [58].

Kaposi's Sarcoma

In 1872, Moritz Kaposi, a Hungarian dermatologist, described five men with aggressive "idiopathic multiple pigmented sarcomas of the skin", describing a new malignancy, that later was name after him, that can manifest as either a cutaneous or a visceral involvement [59].

Kaposi's Sarcoma (KS) is a tumor originating from either endothelial or spindle cells that occurs in 4 forms [60]. The first form denominated "Classic form" is diagnosed in older persons (male to female ratio is 15:1) of Mediterranean, Eastern Europe or Jewish descent. A second form, the "Endemic form", is seen in sub-Saharan Africa and affects primarily young adults and young children. A third form, "Epidemic" or "AIDS-associated form", is the most common cancer seen in HIV–infected persons (prevalently homosexual men) [8].

The last form of KS is the "iatrogenic form" and is a relatively common malignancy of solid-organ transplant recipients (with a lower male to female ratio 3:1), occurring 100- to 1000-fold (depending on the reference population) more often than in aged-matched control subjects, with an incidence ranging from <0.5% to 5% [61].

Considering the peculiar geographic distribution of Kaposi's sarcoma prompted the speculation about an infective agent as well as its possibility of sexual transmission. In 1994 Chang and colleagues identified DNA fragments of a previously unrecognized herpesvirus, from KS lesions. The new virus named HHV-8 or KS-associated herpesvirus (KSHV) is a member, together with EBV, of the gammaherpesvirus subfamily sharing the possibility, once internalized in the host cell to cause immortalization [11].

HHV-8 can be found in all KS forms, and is considered a necessary, but not sufficient, cause for KS development, but is also associated with other two forms of rare malignancies principally in immunosuppressed subjects: Primary Effusion Lymphoma (PEL) and Castelmann's disease [62, 63].

In the United States, Northern or Western Europe, or Eastern countries (Japan, Taiwan), KS occurs in less than 0.5% of all transplant recipients [10, 18, 28, 61, 64], but is more common among KTR from those areas associated with classic and endemic forms like Mediterranean Countries (including Italy) [65-67] or of the Middle East reaching 5%, often representing the major group reaching up to 70% of all PTM cases observed [68-71].

This higher frequency of KS in some areas reflects the higher prevalence of infection with HHV-8 that is lower than 5% in North America, Northern Europe and Asia, but reaches 10-30% in most Mediterranean countries (including Italy and particularly Southern regions) and Middle East, and more than 50% in Central and Southern Africa [17].

In a series of 2099 organ-transplant recipients studied at the Toronto Hospital, Kaposi's sarcoma developed in 12 (0.6 percent), 9 of whom were of Italian origin [72]. Analyzing data from US Organ Procurement and Tissue Network (OPTN) on more than 234, 000 KTs, 65 KS cases were identified (0.06%), but among them risk was 2-fold increased in Hispanics and 4-times higher in non US citizens where 7 KS were diagnosed, 5 of which in recipient form Middle East and 1 from Italy [73].

The mean age at diagnosis of post-transplant KS is around 40s, so at least 20-years younger than mean age at diagnosis of Classic KS cases [61], but very few cases are diagnosed in pediatric transplanted patients [74].

KS after transplant usually appears early (a mean interval is 12 months in most series). The evidence that more than 80% of transplant recipients with KS are seropositive for HHV-8 before transplantation and the short time after transplantation at KS onset indicate that most cases of post-transplantation KS apparently develop as a result of viral reactivation [75-78].

The risk of developing a KS in pre-transplant HHV-8 seropositive renal recipients is by far greater than in seronegative subjects [79, 80]. For this reason pre-KT antibody screening appears to be useful for indentifying high-risk patients, at least in areas with high HHV-8 prevalence [81].

However, several epidemiologic data suggest that HHV-8 can be also transmitted from the donor, giving rise to acute infection and eventually to malignant transformation [82]. Some studies have reported that cells form KS lesions display phenotypic and genotypic features of donor origin [83], but these events have to be considered more rare than expected and however of minor importance on the total number of KS [84, 85].

Aggressive immunosuppression (particularly with CNI drugs), is an important risk factor as for HHV-8 re-activation as for post-transplant KS development. Even the course of KS depends on the level of immunosuppression, since lesions can regress on discontinuation or minimization of immunosuppressive therapy, but frequently the condition can recurs after re-transplantation or fully reintroduction of immunosuppressive therapy [20].

If KS is not diagnosed or treated soon enough, mortality is substantial, especially in patients with visceral disease affecting up to 40% of all KS cases developed after KT, in which mortality may reach 50% [86]. Excision or cryotherapy is often used to resolve cutaneous lesions but recurrence is quite frequent. Chemotherapeutic treatment (among others with blomycin, vincristine, vinblastine and doxorubricin, cisplatin) can be effective as well as radiotherapy or treatment with interferon, but these treatment have to considered with caution because of graft rejection and subsequent loss [60].

As described earlier, introduction of PSI represent a promising option to decrease PTM incidence or at least their recurrence [34]. Use of Rapamycin derivative have been shown to block vascular endothelial growth factor (VEGF) production *in vitro,* and *in vivo* in animal models this effect has shown to block new angiogenesis [87]. Recent studies have shown that an important phase in HHV-8 tumorigenesis is the production of the viral G-protein-coupled receptor (vGPCR), an oncoprotein that increases the secretion of VEGF and up-regulation of its receptor [88].

For all these reason KS represents an important target for PSI, and several studies have shown, in KTR affected by KS, that after reduction of immunosuppression the conversion to PSI in combination with CI or alone with low therapeutic doses of MMF, may lead to regression of KS either of skin or visceral lesions [34]. The potentiality of PSI to reduce KS recurrence seems to be due to the reduction of the total immunosuppression more than their intrinsic anti-tumoral effect, since using a higher dosage of PSIs can lead to tumor recurrence [89]. With the increasing experience with PSIs, the true potential of this drug will be realized to be a critical element to reduce the impact of KS on the long-term outcomes of kidney transplantation.

Renal Cell Carcinoma

Primary *de novo* renal cell carcinoma (RCC) can develop after KT (either in the native kidney or, but more rarely, in the donated organ), with a 10-fold increased incidence when compared to the general population [90].

Acquired cystic kidney disease (ACKD), that is the consequences of the persistence of uremic state in patients with ESRD, is a widely known renal cell carcinoma risk factor as in the dialysis patient as in KTR. In ACKD patients, risk of RCC is increased 30- to 40- fold over its incidence in the general population [91].

According to US data, prevalence of ACKD affects one third or more of long-term ($\geq$3 yr) hemodialysis patients up to 90% in patients with ESRD with longer than 10 years of dialysis [92]. Progressive destruction of functional renal mass causes the accumulation of non-dialyzable mitogenic factors (especially Epidermal Growth Factor, EGF, and Platelet Derived Growth Factors, PDGF) in the remaining functional nephrons, leading to hypertrophic and hyperplasic growth of epithelial cells. For this reason, after KT higher risk of RCC is associated with a longer time on dialysis, and consequently all recipients, but especially in those patients, should have regular ultrasonography of their native kidneys [93].

Another risk factors for the development of RCC (and other transitional cell carcinomas in various parts of the urinary tract) is analgesic nephropathy, an injury of the kidney caused by excessive use of combinations of analgesic medications such as aspirin, phenacetin, and paracetamol [91].

RCC arising from the donated organ can be present but inadvertently transplanted with the organ, be undetectable and develop after transplantation or result after a malignant transplantation in the donated organ in the long follow-up (median time of diagnosis 5 years) [91]. Development of *de novo* RCC in a renal allograft is of the greatest clinical concern on the transplant recipients.

If RCC is early diagnosed, nephron-sparing surgery or cryoablation are good treatment options, however when a minimally invasive approach is not possible, radical nephrectomy is the treatment of choice and in the presence of metastatic disease, chemotherapy with adjustment or cessation of immunosuppressive therapy is required.

Other Solid Tumours

The most frequently occurring malignant tumours in the general population, carcinomas of the bronchus, prostate, and breast are not seen more frequently after KT [2]. A possible explanation is that the origin of these tumours is not related to immunosuppression and/or control of oncogenic viruses.

The incidence of colorectal carcinoma after transplant was initially thought to be similar to that in the general population, but recent reports have shown up a 2-fold increased risk when compared to general population [10]. As is true for most malignancies in the general population, survival after colorectal cancer correlates closely with tumor stage, but unfortunately, stage for stage, prognosis in transplant recipients is by far worse than in the general population [94].

It is not clear if this increased risk has to be associated to the consequence of prolonged immunosuppression or major prevalence in these populations of persons with predisposing factors, but an explanation, at least of some lesions, has been given by recent findings of the association of colorectal cancer with infection or re-activation of EBV and CMV infections [95].

Among other form of cancers possibly related to viral infection, recently is under discussion if papillomaviruses, which predominantly associate with anal, vulvar and penile cancer, all of them found with increased frequency after KT, could be also responsible for some forms of lung or oropharyngeal squamous cell-carcinoma [96].

CONCLUSIONS

The incidence of post-transplant malignancies is greatly increased in KTR compared to the general population, but this risk is mainly concentrated in viral-related cancers such as PTLD or Kaposi's Sarcoma and skin cancers. Moreover, the prognosis of all post-transplant cancers is worse than in the general population, with an aggressive course and a lower survival; also with the progressive ageing of transplanted patients, malignancies would become the most significant cause of mortality in transplanted patients. Immunosuppressive therapy is an important risk factor and higher level of immunosuppression is directly correlated with an augmented risk of PTM development.

With the intent to reduce the problem of PTM, transplant physicians should be familiar with the types of malignancies that may occur in their patient. The intensity of immunosuppressive regimens should be lowered to the minimum compatible with a good allograft function.

Prophylactic measures should be adopted, radically treating any precancerous lesions and carefully follow-up patients after transplantation and look for any symptoms and sign that enable any early identification and treatment, hopefully at a curable stage, of any cancer. When high-risk patients (such as those with polyps or inflammatory bowel disease) are identified, closer interval screenings are essential.

Given the importance of oncogenic viruses in PTM development, a more accurate pre-transplant screening and post-transplant monitoring of viral activity should be adopted at least to defined high risk patients to be more intensively screened after transplant.

REFERENCES

[1] Australian and New Zealand dialysis and transplant registry. The twenty eight report, 2005.

[2] Wong G, Chapman JR. Cancers after renal transplantation. Transplant Rev., 2008, 22: 141-149.

[3] Doll R, Kinlen L. Immunosurveillance and cancer: epidemiological evidence. Br Med J 1970; 4: 420-422.

[4] Murray JE, Gleason R, Bartholomay A. Fourth report of the Human Kidney Transplant Registry: 16 September 1964 to 15 March 1965. Transplantation 1965; 3: 684-699.

[5] McKhann CF. Primary malignancy in patients undergoing immunosuppression for renal transplantation. Transplantation 1969; 8: 209-212.

[6] Penn I, Hammond W, Brettschneider L, Strarzl TE. Malignant lymphomas in transplant patients. Transplant Proc 1969; 1: 106-112.

[7] http://www.ipittr.org.

[8] Dal Maso L, Serraino D, Franceschi S. Epidemiology of AIDS-related tumours in developed and developing countries. Eur J Cancer 2001; 37: 1188-1201.

[9] Trofe J, Beebe TM, Buell JF, *et al.* Posttransplant malignancy. Prog Transplant 2004; 14: 193-200.

[10] Buell JF, Gross TG, Woodle ES. Malignancy after transplantation. Transplantation 2005; 80: S254-S264.

[11] International Agency for Research on Cancer (IARC). Epstein-Barr virus and Kaposi's sarcoma herpesvirus/human herpesvirus 8. Lyon (France): IARC. 1997, 375-494.

[12] Yarchoan R, Little R. Immunosuppression-related malignancies. In: DeVita VT , Hellman S , Rosenberg SA , eds. Cancer Principles and Practice of Oncology, 7th ed. Philadelphia, Pa: Lippincott; 2005, pp. 2247-2263.

[13] Yamashita N, Kimura H, Morishima T. Virological aspects of Epstein-Barr virus infections. Acta Med Okayama 2005; 59: 239-246.

[14] Wensing B, Farrell PJ. Regulation of cell growth and death by Epstein-Barr virus. Microbes Infect 2000; 2: 77-84.

[15] Everly MJ, Bloom RD, Tsai DE, Trofe J. Posttransplant lymphoproliferative disorder. Ann Pharmacother 2007; 41: 1850-1858.

[16] Hoshida Y, Aozasa K. Malignancies in organ transplant recipients. Pathol Int 2004; 54: 649-658.

[17] Dukers NHTM, Rezza G. Human herpesvirus 8 epidemiology: what we do and do not know. AIDS 2003; 17: 1717-1730.

[18] Hoshida Y, Li T, Dong Z, *et al.* Lymphoproliferative disorders in renal transplant patients in Japan. Int J Cancer 2001; 91: 869-875.

[19] Ramsay HM, Fryer AA, Hawley CM, *et al.* Non-melanoma skin cancer risk in the Queensland renal transplant population. Br J Dermatol 2002; 147: 950-956.

[20] Euvrard, S., Kanitakis, J., Claudy, A. Skin Cancers after Organ Transplantation. N Engl J Med 2003; 348: 1681-1691.

[21] Maitra, SK, Gallo H, Rowland-Payne C, *et al.* Second primary cancers in patients with squamous cell carcinoma of the skin. Br J Cancer 2005; 9: 570-571.

[22] Webb MC, Compton F, Andrews PA, Koffman CG. Skin tumours posttransplantation: a retrospective analysis of 28 years' experience at a single centre. Transplant Proc 1997; 29: 828-830.

[23] Martinez JC, Otley CC, Stasko T, *et al.* Transplant-Skin Cancer Collaborative. Defining the clinical course of metastatic skin cancer in organ transplant recipients: a multicenter collaborative study. Arch Dermatol 2003; 139: 301-306.

[24] Mehrany K, Otley CC, Weenig RH, *et al.* A meta-analysis of the prognostic significance of sentinel lymph node status in Merkel cell carcinoma. Dermatol Surg 2002; 28: 113-117.

[25] Grulich AE, van Leeuwen MT, Falster MO, Vajdic CM. Incidence of cancers in people with HIV/AIDS compared with immunosuppressed transplant recipients: a meta-analysis. Lancet 2007; 370: 59–67.

[26] van Leeuwen MT, Grulich AE, McDonald SP, *et al.* Immunosuppression and other risk factors for lip cancer after kidney transplantation. Cancer Epidemiol Biomarkers Prev 2009; 18: 561-569.

[27] Kyllönen L, Pukkala E, Eklund B. Cancer incidence in a kidney-transplanted population. Transpl Int 1994;7 Suppl 1:S350-2.

[28] Adami J, Gäbel H, Lindelöf B, *et al.* Cancer risk following organ transplantation: a nationwide cohort study in Sweden. Br J Cancer 2003; 89: 1221-1227.

[29] Arends MJ, Benton EC, McLaren KM, *et al.* Renal allograft recipients with high susceptibility to cutaneous malignancy have an increased prevalence of human papillomavirus DNA in skin tumours and a greater risk of anogenital malignancy. Br J Cancer 1997; 75: 722-728.

[30] Harwood CA, Surentheran T, McGregor JM, *et al.* Human papillomavirus infection and non-melanoma skin cancer in immunosuppressed and immunocompetent individuals. J Med Virol 2000; 61: 289-297.

[31] Martinez JC, Otley CC, Stasko T, *et al.* Transplant-Skin Cancer Collaborative. Defining the clinical course of metastatic skin cancer in organ transplant recipients: a multicenter collaborative study. Arch Dermatol 2003; 139: 301-306.

[32] Rubel JR, Milford EL, Abdi R. Cutaneous neoplasms in renal transplant recipients. Eur J Dermatol 2002; 12: 532-535.

[33] Geisller EK, Schlitt HJ. The relation between immunosuppressive agents and malignancy. Curr Opin Org Transp 2004; 9:394-399.

[34] Morath C, Arns W, Schwenger V, *et al.* Sirolimus in renal transplantation. Nephrol Dial Transplant 2007; 22: viii61-viii65.

[35] Gutiérrez-Dalmau A, Campistol JM. The role of proliferation signal inhibitors in post-transplant malignancies. Nephrol Dial Transplant 2007; 22: i11-i16.

[36] Monaco AP. The role of mTOR inhibitors in the management of post-transplant malignancy. Transplantation 2009; 87: 157-163.

[37] Loren AW, Tsai DE. Post-transplant lymphoproliferative disorder. Clin Chest Med 2005; 26: 631-645.

[38] Taylor AL, Marcus R, Bradley JA. Post-transplant lymphoproliferative disorders (PTLD) after solid organ transplantation. Crit Rev Oncol Hematol 2005; 56: 155-167.

[39] Paya CV, Fung JJ, Nalesnik MA, *et al.* Epstein-Barr virus-induced posttransplant lymphoproliferative disorders. ASTS/ASTP EBV-PTLD Task Force and The Mayo Clinic Organized International Consensus Development Meeting. Transplantation 1999; 68: 1517-1525.

[40] Jaffe ES, Harris NL, Stein H, Vardiman JW, editors. World Health Organization classification of tumours: pathology and genetics of tumours of haematopoietic and lymphoid tissues. Lyon, IARC Press, 2001.

[41] Preiksaitis JK. New developments in the diagnosis and management of posttransplantation lymphoproliferative disorders in solid organ transplant recipients. Clin Infect Dis 2004; 39: 1016-1023.

[42] Dror Y, Greenberg M, Taylor G, *et al.* Lymphoproliferative disorders after organ transplantation in children. Transplantation 1999; 67: 990–998.

[43] Burns DM, Crawford DH. Epstein-Barr virus-specific cytotoxic T lymphocytes for adoptive immunotherapy of post-transplant lymphoproliferative disease. Blood Rev 2004; 18: 193–209.

[44] Tran H, Nourse J, Hall S, *et al.* Immunodeficiency-associated lymphomas. Blood Reviews 2008; 22: 261-281.

[45] Nelson BP, Nalesnik MA, Bahler DW, *et al.* Epstein-Barr virus-negative post-transplant lymphoproliferative disorders: a distinct entity? Am J Surg Pathol 2000;24: 375-385.

[46] Niller HH, Salamon D, Ilg K, *et al.* EBV-associated neoplasms: alternative pathogenetic pathways. Med Hypotheses 2004; 62: 387-391.

[47] Gao SZ, Chaparro SV, Perlroth M, *et al.* Post-transplantation lymphoproliferative disease in heart and heart-lung transplant recipients: 30-year experience at Stanford University. J Heart Lung Transplant 2003; 22: 505–514.

[48] Opelz G, Dohler B. Lymphomas after solid organ transplantation: a collaborative transplant study report. Am J Transplant 2004; 4: 222–230.

[49] Bustami RT, Ojo AO, Wolfe RA, *et al.* Immunosuppression and the risk of post-transplant malignancy among cadaveric first kidney transplant recipients. Am J Transplant 2004; 4: 87-93.

[50] Birkeland SA, Hamilton-Dutoit S. Is posttransplant lymphoproliferative disorder (PTLD) caused by any specific immunosuppressive drug or by the transplantation *per se*? Transplantation 2003; 76: 984–988.

[51] Cherikh WS, Kauffman HM, McBride MA, *et al.* Association of the type of induction immunosuppression with posttransplant lymphoproliferative disorder, graft survival, and patient survival after primary kidney transplantation. Transplantation 2003; 76: 1289-1293.

[52] Dharnidharka VR, Sullivan EK, Stablein DM, *et al.* North American Pediatric Renal Transplant Cooperative Study (NAPRTCS). Risk factors for posttransplant lymphoproliferative disorder (PTLD) in pediatric kidney transplantation: a report of the North American Pediatric Renal Transplant Cooperative Study (NAPRTCS). Transplantation 2001; 71: 1065-1068.

[53] Tsai DE, Hardy CL, Tomaszewski JE, *et al.* Reduction in immunosuppression as initial therapy for posttransplant lymphoproliferative disorder: analysis of prognostic variables and long-term follow-up of 42 adult patients. Transplantation 2001; 71: 1076-1088.

[54] Orjuela M, Gross TG, Cheung YK, *et al.* A pilot study of chemoimmunotherapy (cyclophosphamide, prednisone, and rituximab) in patients with post-transplant lymphoproliferative disorder following solid organ transplantation. Clin Cancer Res 2003; 9: 3945S–3952S.

[55] Choquet S, Oertel S, LeBlond V, *et al.* Rituximab in the management of post-transplantation lymphoproliferative disorder after solid organ transplantation: proceed with caution. Ann Hematol 2007; 86: 599–607.

[56] Pascual, J. Post-transplant lymphoproliferative disorder--the potential of proliferation signal inhibitors. Nephrol Dial Transplant 2007, 22, i27-35.

[57] Caillard S, Agodoa LY, Bohen EM, Abbott KC. Myeloma, Hodgkin disease, and lymphoid leukemia after renal transplantation: characteristics, risk factors and prognosis. Transplantation 2006; 81: 888-895.

[58] Penn I, Porat G. Central nervous system lymphomas in organ allograft recipients. Transplantation 1995; 59: 240-244.

[59] Oriel JD. Moritz Kaposi (1837-1902). Int. J. S.T.D. AIDS., 1997; 8: 715-717.

[60] Antman, K., Chang, Y. Kaposi's sarcoma. N Engl J Med 2000; 342: 1027-1038.

[61] Lebbé C, Legendre C, Francès C. Kaposi sarcoma in transplantation. Transplant Rev 2008; 22: 252-261.

[62] Du MQ, Bacon CM, Isaacson PG. Kaposi sarcoma-associated herpesvirus/human herpesvirus 8 and lymphoproliferative disorders. J Clin Pathol 2007; 60: 1350-1357.

[63] Soulier J, Grollet L, Oksenhendler E, *et al.* Kaposi's sarcoma-associated herpesvirus-like DNA sequences in multicentric Castleman's disease. Blood 1995; 86: 1276-1280.

[64] Kasiske BL, Snyder JJ, Gilbertson DT, Wang C. Cancer after kidney transplantation in the United States. Am J Transplant 2004; 4: 905-913.

[65] Piselli P, Busnach G, Citterio F, *et al.* Immunosuppression and Cancer Study Group. Risk of Kaposi sarcoma after solid-organ transplantation: multicenter study in 4,767 recipients in Italy, 1970-2006. Transplant Proc 2009 41: 1227-1230.

[66] Zavos G, Bokos J, Papaconstantinou I, *et al.* Clinicopathological aspects of 18 Kaposi's sarcoma among 1055 Greek renal transplant recipients. Artif Organs 2004; 28: 595-599.

[67] García-Astudillo LA, Leyva-Cobián F. Human herpesvirus-8 infection and Kaposi's sarcoma after liver and kidney transplantation in different geographical areas of Spain. Transpl Immunol 2006; 17: 65-69.

[68] Qunibi WY, Barri Y, Alfurayh O, *et al.* Kaposi's sarcoma in renal transplant recipients: a report on 26 cases from a single institution. Transplant Proc 1993; 25: 1402-1405.

[69] Nafar M, Einollahi B, Hemati K, *et al.* Development of malignancy following living donor kidney transplantation. Transplant Proc 2005; 37: 3065-3067.

[70] Berber I, Altaca G, Aydin C, *et al.* Kaposi's sarcoma in renal transplant patients: predisposing factors and prognosis. Transplant Proc 2005; 37: 967-968.

[71] El-Agroudy AE, El-Baz MA, Ismail AM, *et al.* Clinical features and course of Kaposi's sarcoma in Egyptian kidney transplant recipients. Am J Transplant 2003; 3: 1595-1599.

[72] Shepherd FA, Maher E, Cardella C, *et al.* Treatment of Kaposi's sarcoma after solid organ transplantation. J Clin Oncol 1997; 15: 2371-2377.

[73] Mbulaiteye SM, Engels EA. Kaposi's sarcoma risk among transplant recipients in the United States (1993–2003). Int J Cancer 2006; 119: 2685–2691.

[74] Euvrard S, Kanitakis J, Cochat P, Claudy A. Skin cancers following pediatric organ transplantation. Dermatol Surg 2004; 30: 616-621.

[75] Allen U. Human herpesvirus type 8 infections among solid organ transplant recipients. Pediatr Transplant 2002; 6: 187-192.

[76] Moore PS. The emergence of Kaposi's sarcoma-associated herpesvirus (human herpesvirus 8). N Engl J Med 2000; 343: 1411-1413.

[77] Hudnall SD, Rady PL, Tyring SK, Fish JC. Serologic and molecular evidence of human herpesvirus 8 activation in renal transplant recipients. J Infect Dis 1998; 178: 1791-1794.

[78] Mendez JC, Procop GW, Wspy MJ, *et al.* Relationship of HHV8 replication and Kaposi's sarcoma after solid organ transplantation. Transplantation 1999;67: 1200-1201.

[79] Francès C, Mouquet C, Calvez V. Human Herpesvirus 8 and Renal Transplantation. N Eng J Med 1999; 340: 1045-1046.

[80] Andreoni M, Goletti D, Pezzotti P, *et al.* Prevalence, incidence and correlates of HHV8/KSHV infection and Kaposi's sarcoma in renal and liver transplant recipients. J Infect 2001; 3: 195-199.

[81] Serraino D, Piselli P, Scuderi M, *et al.* Studio Italiano Trapianti e Infezioni. Screening for human herpesvirus 8 antibodies in Italian organ transplantation centers. Clin Infect Dis, 2005; 40: 203-205.

[82] Luppi M, Barozzi P, Guaraldi G, *et al.* Human herpesvirus 8-associated diseases in solid-organ transplantation: importance of viral transmission from the donor. Clin Infect Dis 2003; 37: 606-607.

[83] Barozzi P, Luppi M, Facchetti F, *et al.* Post-transplant Kaposi sarcoma originates from the seeding of donor-derived progenitors. Nat Med 2003; 9: 554-561.

[84] Poli F, Sirchia G, Gao SJ, *et al.* Risk of Kaposi's sarcoma-associated herpes virus transmission from donor allografts among Italian posttransplant Kaposi's sarcoma patients. Blood 1997; 90: 2826-2829.

[85] Parravicini C, Scalamogna C, Calattini S, *et al.* KSHV reactivation in post-transplant Kaposi sarcoma. Nat Med 2003; 9: 986.

[86] Shepherd FA, Maher E, Cardella C, *et al.* Treatment of Kaposi's sarcoma after solid organ transplantation. J Clin Oncol 1997; 15: 2371-2377.

[87] Koehl GE, Schlitt HJ, Geissler EK. Rapamycin and tumor growth: mechanisms behind its anticancer activity. Transplant Rev 2005; 19: 20–31.

[88] Montaner S. Akt/TSC/mTOR activation by the KSHV G protein-coupled receptor: emerging insights into the molecular oncogenesis and treatment of Kaposi's sarcoma. Cell Cycle 2007; 6: 438-443.

[89] Boratyńska M, Zmonarski SC, Klinger M. Recurrence of Kaposi's sarcoma after increased exposure to sirolimus. Int Immunopharmacol 2006; 6: 2018-2022.

[90] Kliem V, Kolditz M, Behrend M, *et al.* Risk of renal cell carcinoma after kidney transplantation. Clin Transplant 1997; 11: 255-258.

[91] Penn I. Primary kidney tumors before and after renal transplantation. Transplantation, 1995; 59: 480-485.

[92] Scandling JD. Acquired cystic kidney disease and renal cell cancer after transplantation: time to rethink screening? Clin J Am Soc Nephrol 2007; 2: 621-622.

[93] Bisceglia M, Galliani CA, Senger C, *et al.* Renal cystic diseases: a review. Adv Anat Pathol 2006; 13: 26-56.

[94] Papaconstantinou HT, Sklow B, Hanaway MJ, *et al.* Characteristics and survival patterns of solid organ transplant patients developing *de novo* colon and rectal cancer. Dis. Colon Rectum 2004; 47: 1898-1903.

[95] Adani GL, Baccarani U, Lorenzin D, *et al. De novo* gastrointestinal tumours after renal transplantation: role of CMV and EBV viruses. Clin Transplant 2006; 20: 457-460.

[96] Rezazadeh A, Laber DA, Ghim SJ, *et al.* The role of human papilloma virus in lung cancer: a review of the evidence. Am J Med Sci 2009; 338: 64-67.

CHAPTER 21

Post-Transplant Cancer: Diagnostic and Therapeutic Management

Giuseppe Giuffrida*, **Daniela Corona and Massimiliano Veroux**

Department of Surgery, Transplantation and Advanced Technologies, Vascular Surgery and Organ Transplant Unit, University Hospital of Catania, Italy

Abstract: Increasing success in organ transplantation, longer graft and patient survival malignancies are becoming a major burden in transplantation medicine.

There is now convincing evidence to confirm a 3- to 5-fold increase in overall cancer incidence.

Duration and intensity of immunosuppression have been linked to the increased incidence of malignancies and the choice of immunosuppressive therapy could also play a role in the development of cancer.

It is mandatory to understand how and when the tumoral process began and if a screening program could be established. Considering the poor outcome of transplanted patients that develop a tumour process, immunosuppression dose reduction or withdrawal is sometimes necessary to control the progression of life-threatening malignancies maintaining, when possible, graft function.

A conversion from CNI to PSI, although is not curative, could be potentially helpful to prolong survival in some patients. Transplant recipients with evidence of cancer should be offered the best medical and surgical oncology treatment in addition to the choice of immunosuppressive therapy.

Those patients in whom the neoplastic process is advanced and life expectance is really poor probably could not have any clinical advantage reducing or stopping immunosuppressive therapy, adding at cancer disease the risk of acute rejection and graft loss.

Keywords: Calcineurin Inhibitors, Immunosuppression, PSI, Kaposi, Cancer, Post-Transplant Cancer, Sirolimus, Post-Transplant Screening, Everolimus, Lymphoproliferative Disorders.

INTRODUCTION

In the early days of transplantation medicine the most important problems that clinician had to face were represented by fulminant acute rejection episodes and severe infections that often led to the loss of the graft and to death of the recipient. Due to short term survival of transplantation malignancy represented only a minor problem.

Increasing success in organ transplantation, longer graft and patient survival, due to improvements in transplantation technology and immunosuppressant medications, and older donors (as well as recipients), long term complications, such as malignancies, are becoming a major burden in transplantation medicine and a limiting factor for graft and patient survival.

Prolonged use of modern immunosuppression, which leads to alteration of immune function and immune surveillance, is associated with increased cancer risk. There is now convincing evidence from observational studies and registry data to confirm a 3- to 5-fold increase in overall cancer incidence [1, 2].

Indeed, the incidence of death as a result of malignancies is increasing, although this is partly a result of lower incidence of deaths related to cardiovascular disease and infection. Over the next 10-20 years, it is possible that deaths from malignancy in renal transplant recipients will exceed those related to cardiovascular disease [1, 2].

***Address correspondence to Giuseppe Giuffrida:** Department of Surgery, transplantation and Advanced Technologies, Vascular surgery and Organ Transplant Unit, University Hospital of Catania, *Via* Santa Sofia, 83, 95123 Catania, Italy; Tel: + 39 0953782306; E-mail: giuffrida.giuseppe@gmail.com

Although duration and intensity of immunosuppression have been linked to the increased incidence of malignancies, also the choice of different type of immunosuppressive therapy could play a fundamental role in the development of neoplastic disease.

Considering the poor outcome and life expectance of transplanted patients that develop a tumoral process, a tailored management of immunosuppressive therapy seems mandatory.

The role of immunosuppressive therapy in the development of post-transplant malignancies was elucidated in several early clinical reports showing an association between reduction/discontinuation of immunosuppressive drug therapy and the regression of tumours [3].

Moreover, several series demonstrated also that different types of immunosuppressive drugs are associated with different type of cancer and different tumoral risk [3-6].

CALCINEURIN INHIBITORS

The immunosuppressive power of cyclosporine is attributed to two different mechanisms: the bind to the immunophillin cyclophilin A and the inhibition of calcineurin phosphatase and subsequently the block of nuclear factor of activated T cells (NFAT) translocagy into the nucleus.

Cyclosporine also increases transforming growth factor (TGF)-β, a potent inhibitor of interleukin (IL)-2 fondamental to T-cell proliferation [7].

The oncogenic effects of cyclosporine were attributed to the inhibition of T-lymphocyte-mediated immune surveillance. However, cyclosporine increases TGFβ expression, and that TGFβ promotes tumour cell invasion and metastasis. Hojo *et al.* demonstrated that cyclosporine induced an invasive phenotype in nontransformed adenocarcinoma cells *via* a TGFβ- dependent mechanism [8].

In a randomized controlled trial was also observed relationship between CyA use and incidence of cancer post transplantation between normal and low dose cyclosporine use [9].

Despite more frequent acute rejection episodes, the overall incidence of cancers was significantly lower in the low-dose group than the normal-dose one. The risk of viral-related neoplasms was also greater in the normal-dose population than the low-dose arm.

Others studies showed that similarly, tacrolimus, which have similar immunosuppressive effects as CyA by inactivating calcineurin through the same binding site, enhanced the expression of TGFβ both *in vitro* and *in vivo* and promoted renal cancer cell pulmonary metastases in both immunocompetent and immunodeficient mice [10]. In another study, tacrolimus was shown to increase proliferation rate of human hepatoma cells [11].

Others *in vivo* studies have shown that CyA also promote angiogenesis and increase expression of vascular endothelial growth factor (VEGF) enhancing tumour growth particularly in colon adenocarcinoma [12].

Cyclosporine has also been shown to upregulate IL-6, a cytokine that promotes B-cell activation and growth of EBV-transformed B cells. IL-6 may be involved in the development of post-transplant lymphoproliferative disease (PTLD) [13].

Evidence from observational studies and registry data suggested a higher risk of PTLD after renal transplant in recipients treated with tacrolimus when compared with CyA [14].

CORTICOSTEROIDS

Corticosteroids are largely used in transplant recipients in combination with other immunosuppressive agents, and for this reason is hard to define a specific oncogenetic role of this class of drugs.

When evaluating the risk of corticosteroid use without other confounding immunosuppressive agents, patients were at higher risk of developing malignancy, especially skin cancers [15, 16].

ANTIMETABOLITES

Azathioprine

Azathioprine is a purine analogue that inhibits purine synthesis and interferes with RNA metabolism and synthesis.

The carcinogenic potential of azathioprine is probably related to impaired cellular DNA mismatch repair and microsatellite DNA instability within functioning noncancerous cells [17].

Although there are not many epidemiological studies confirming the pro oncogenic effect of azathioprine, there is evidence for an increase in post-transplant malignancy associated with azathioprine in the pre-cyclosporine era from the Penn Registry [18].

Certainly, azathioprine has been shown not to be as potent a pro-oncogenic agent as the calcineurin inhibitors (CNIs) [19, 20].

Moreover azathioprine treatment can lead to increased photosensitivity to UVA [21] reducing the period for tumour development and increasing the number of skin cancers [6].

There are also some reports showing the role of azathioprine in the development of Non-Hogdkin lymphoma (NHL), both in transplant recipients and in patients treated for immunological disorders such as Wegener's Granulomatosis or Crohn's disease [22].

Mycophenolate Mofetil

Mycophenolate Mofetil (MMF) is a prodrug of Mycophenolic Acid (MPA) a potent immunosuppressive antimetabolite. MMF is an inhibitor of *de novo* guanine nucleotide synthesis through inhibition of inosine monophosphate dehydrogenase, which is essential for T and B lymphocyte proliferation.

Few epidemiological studies showed an increased risk of malignancy in patients on MMF and in contrast to azathioprine, MMF and MPA, appeared to be protective to the development of post-transplant cancer, although some data suggest that MMF may increase tumour cell invasiveness [23], and may prevent adhesion receptor-dependent tumour progression [24].

In vitro and *in vivo* studies had confirmed the apoptotic and antiproliferative effects of MPA in lymphomas and multiple myeloma cells [25].

INDUCTION AGENTS (BIOLOGICAL AGENTS)

The incidence of PTLD, most commonly, B cell and EBV related and skin cancers, is increased among renal transplant recipients who have used induction agents, such as OKT3/ATG, as part of their immunosuppression regimen.

Data extrapolated from approximately 200,000 solid organ transplant recipients of the Collaborative Transplant Study Group database, showed an at least 2-fold increase in excess risk of PTLD with OKT3/ATG as induction and/or antirejection therapy. This incidence is higher during the first year after transplantation and decreases thereafter [26].

Analysis using data from the UNOS-OPTN database showed a 72% increase risk in developing PTLD with monoclonal lymphocyte-depleting polyclonal antibodies as induction therapy [27].

Monoclonal antibodies activity is restricted to activated T cells and monocytes/macrophages. This mechanism reduces the number of circulating T lymphocytes expressing IL-2 receptors, leaving unaffected the number of total lymphocytes [28].

Comparing to the polyclonal antibodies there are several series that indicate that thymoglobulin may have higher relative risk of malignancy than the ATG [29].

MAMMALIAN TARGET OF RAPAMYCIN INHIBITORS (MTOR), PROLIFERATION SIGNAL INHIBITORS (PSI)

PSI, Sirolimus and Everolimus, are macrocylic fermentation products of Streptomyces hygroscopicus, originally isolated from the soil in Easter Island, initially discovered as an antifungal antibiotic, was recognized to have anticancer activity (at high doses) in murine models [30].

These molecules interact with the same binding protein (KFBP12) as tacrolimus but with no effect on calcineurin phosphatise. They also bind with high affinity to the mammalian target of rapamycin (mTOR). PSI control the phosphatidylinositol-3-kinase (PI3K)/Akt signalling pathway, which plays a pivotal role in cell growth and survival.

Inhibition of mTOR by sirolimus or its derivatives temsirolimus and everolimus downregulates p70S6 kinase activity and subsequent translation of specific mRNAs required for cell-cycle progression from the G1 to S phase, effectively blocking IL-2 stimulation of proliferation [31-33].

As well as an immunosuppressive effect, sirolimus was found to have a striking antitumour effect in experimental models of renal cell carcinoma.

In several murine models sirolimus has been shown to delay renal cancer cells growth and metastatic progression and prolong survival, even in the presence of cyclosporine therapy [34].

In contrast to CNI, PSI had been shown to have an antiangiogenic effect, *via* downregulation of VEGF [12] as well as an antiangiogenetic effect, which may contribute to its antineoplastic action through an indirect mechanism [35].

Everolimus, by reducing IL-10, has been shown to have an immunosuppresant effect on EBV-transformed B lymphocytes secretion. This mechanism is potentially helpful in the prevention or treatment of PTLD [36].

CANCER SCREENING IN POTENTIAL RECIPIENT, POTENTIAL DONOR AND TRANSPLANTED POPULATION

Cancer screening in general population is a standard practice that allows detecting tumour at an early stage reducing mortality and morbidity.

Patients that received an organ solid transplant represent a high-risk population for cancer developing, so that seems mandatory to understand how and when the tumour process began and if a screening program could be established.

Malignancy after transplantation can develop in three different ways:

1. *De novo* occurrence in the recipient.
2. Recurrent malignancy in the recipient.
3. Transmission of malignancy from the donor.

To reduce the incidence of cancer, or at least detect the tumour process in early preclinical phase, a careful clinical and instrumental evaluation is necessary.

Dosage of tumour markers, research of HHV8, HPV and EBV, that are often associated with Kaposi sarcoma, uterine cancer and PLTD respectively, may represent the first step to detect patients who are at higher risk to develop this kind of cancer.

Ultrasound exam of neck, upper and lower abdomen, gastroscopy and sigmoidoscopy, and X-Ray examination of chest are the basic instrumental investigations that all patients need to perform to recognize a preclinical cancer disease.

Female patients had to undergo annually to a cervical cytological cancer screening and pelvic examination once sexually active.

Women older than 40 years had to perform annually a mammography.

Male potential renal transplant recipients older than 50 years should undergo prostate ultrasound, prostate digital rectal examination (DRE) and PSA measurement (Free fraction and Ratio) every year.

Patients with polycystic disease need a careful examination of their native kidney, doing the higher risk of developing a cancer in polycystic kidneys and the likely higher levels of tumoral markers in these patients.

Magnetic resonance imaging represents the best instrumental exam to analyze polycystic kidneys and could be useful to detect early renal cancer. After transplantation MRI could give us information about the evolution of the cysts especially in patients that use PSI in their immunosuppressive regimen (several studies demonstrate reduction on number and dimension of cysts in transplanted patients treated with PSI).

In absence of clear signs of tumoral disease and if the patients is on dialysis treatment and had no urine output anymore, a prophylactic nephrectomy should be performed before transplantation, deserving the contralateral nephrectomy at the time of transplantation. If the patient has a residual functionality, the polycystic kidney nephrectomy should be delayed at the time of transplant. In case of tumoral disease discovered during the first nephrectomy is mandatory to perform the second one as soon as possible to avoid tumoral diffusion.

History of malignant disease could be not an absolute contraindication to renal transplantation depending of type, site, aggressiveness and diffusion of the cancer.

There is consensus that of 3 years waiting period should be interposed between the complete eradication of the cancer and the inclusion of the patient on the waiting list.

Low malignity cancer, like incidentally discovered renal cell carcinoma, any type of *in situ* carcinoma, and basal cell carcinoma of the skin don't require a waiting period.

Patients whit history of malignant melanoma, breast cancer and colorectal carcinoma or cancer with high invasiveness, need longer waiting period and accurate cancer screening.

In a retrospective study of 1297 renal allograft recipients with a history of malignancy, recurrence for tumours diagnosed and treated before transplantation was 21%. For tumours diagnosed and treated after transplantation recurrence rate was 33% [37].

Although these patients had to be considered "healed" from the tumoral disease , they must be considered at high-risk, and should require a tailored immunosuppression.

In transplant population there is scarcity of data about the effectiveness, benefits, and harms of cancer screening despite the increased risk.

One published study argued against routine cancer screening because of low cost effectiveness rate due to reduced expected survival benefits in this population [38].

Anyway recommendations for cancer screening in the renal transplant recipient were mostly extrapolated from the general population.

History and physical examination, with attention to symptoms suggesting organ involvement by malignant process should be performed every three months during the first year after transplantation and at least yearly thereafter.

All the patients should have cancer markers dosage each three months, and every year they have to perform chest X-Ray examination and abdomen and neck ultrasonography (every six month in high-risk individuals).

Some studies suggest also colorectal annual faeces occult blood test (FOBT) and/or 5-yearly flexible sigmoidoscopy for individuals older than 50 years [39, 41].

Self-skin examination, with emphasis on sun-exposed areas, should be performed monthly [40, 41] and every 6-12 months a total body skin examination performed by expert physicians and dermatologists (overall in patients with HHV8 positivity, or recurrence of skin cancer).

Transmission of a tumour *via* micrometastases of an undiagnosed malignancy in the donor is rare. Data from the Organ Procurement and Transplantation Network/UNOS showed a total of 21 (0.02%) donor-related malignancies on 108,062 transplant recipients [42].

The evaluation of the potential organ donor (dosage of tumoral markers, CT scan and ultrasound) is sufficient to detect cancer even in preclinical stage.

Accurate examination of the skin and evaluation of thoracic and abdominal organs had to be done by surgeons during the organ procurement. Small lesions of liver, lungs, bowel, prostate or uterus, and kidneys, could be visually evaluated by the surgeon and eventually biopsied. A second evaluation of the graft had to be done during the bench surgery, to detect small lesions under the Gerota capsule.

If one kidney is affected by low grade renal cell carcinoma, smaller then 2 cm, the contralatreral organ could be considered suitable for transplantation.

The recipient of this graft had to be informed of the potential risk, although low, to develop a kidney cancer and had to undergone to a tailored screening program and an appropriate immunosuppressive therapy.

THERAPY MANAGEMENT

Management of recipients with cancers after transplantation is complex and difficult.

Immunosuppression dose reduction or withdrawal, proposed by expert opinions and retrospective observational studies, is sometimes necessary to control the progression of life-threatening malignancies (Table **1**).

This approach has the aims to recover recipients' defective immune system but may lead to fulminant rejection, which could potentially lead to graft failure and loss.

Retrospective analyses of the Organ Procurement and Transplantation Network/United Network for Organ Sharing (OPTN/UNOS) registry has suggested that CNIs (cyclosporine/tacrolimus), that are the most commonly used immunosuppressive agents, have been implicated in the etiology of post-transplant tumors.

Table 1: Role of immunosuppression and therapy management in *de novo* post-transplant cancer

Immunosuppressive Agents	**Cancer Risk**	**Cancer Management**
Cyclosporine	Increases overall cancer risk Increase non melanoma skin cancer	Withdrawal/reduction in dose
Tacrolimus	Increases overall cancer risk Risk of PTLD > CyA	Withdrawal/reduction in dose
Induction therapy OKT3/ATG	Increases risk of PTLD	Avoid use as induction therapy
Azathioprine	May increase risk for some cancers	Withdrawal/reduction in dose Switch to other antimetabolites such as MMF
Mycophenolate (MMF/MPA)	May reduce risk of PTLD Increase risk of Kaposi Sarcoma	Potential antioncogenic and antiproliferative role
PSIs (everolimus and sirolimus)	May reduce overall cancer risk	Potential antioncogenic and antiproliferative role Evidence of tumor regression for recipients with Kaposi sarcoma treated with Sirolimus

Sirolimus and everolimus, while less frequently used, have been shown to have potent immunosuppressive activity, protecting the graft from immunological rejection, as well as exhibiting significant antineoplastic properties [1].

In high risk class patients such as patients with clinical history of cancer or patients receiving a kidney from donor affected of contralateral low grade renal cell carcinoma is preferable to use *de novo* therapeutic protocol involving mTOR inhibitors, taking advantage of the antineoplastic power of this class of drugs, in association with low dose of CNI or MMF.

Obviously in these patients an appropriate and tailored cancer screening program had to be settled Fig. **1**.

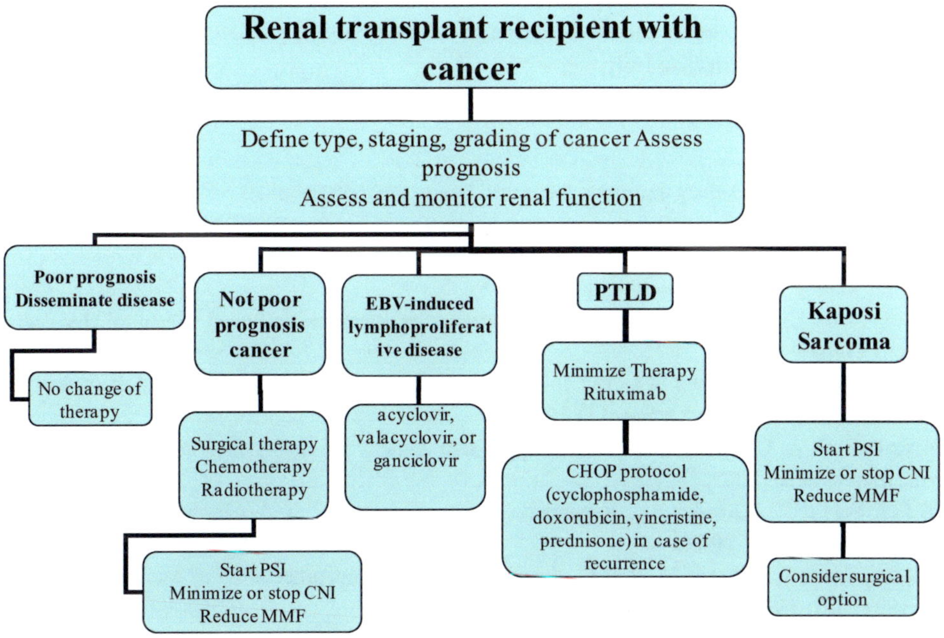

Figure 1: Diagnostic and therapeutic algorithm in post-transplant cancer.

In patients with polycystic disease is also appropriate to use mTOR inhibitors, due to the suggested potential to decrease the number and dimension of cysts due to a specific antiproliferative action on renal cells, combined with good immunosuppressant action.

A conversion from CNI to PSI, although is not curative, could be potentially helpful to prolong survival in some patients, maintaining renal function.

Transplant recipients with evidence of cancer should be offered the best medical and surgical oncology treatment in addition to the choice of immunosuppressive therapy.

Surgical treatment of cancer should include, when possible, total excision of the neoplasm and accurate lymphadenectomy, followed by appropriate radio and chemotherapy.

The therapeutic strategy is represented by the minimization of immunosuppressive therapy maintaining, when possible, graft function.

When immunosuppression is changed, decreased or even stopped, particularly early after transplantation, closer follow up of graft function is mandatory, to avoid the acute rejection with graft loss.

Potential role of mTOR inhibitors in the management of post-transplant malignancies could be based both on direct anti-oncogenic activity and indirectly through the minimization or elimination of CNIs. Considering Kaposi carcinoma and skin cancer, usually detected in an early stage, the most used and effective management of the immunosuppressive therapy consist on the conversion from CNI to PSI. Several series showed a complete regression of Kaposi's sarcoma lesions while maintaining kidney graft function in renal transplant patients, after the conversion to CNI [43, 44] .

Therapeutic strategy of PTLD in transplant population requires reduction of immunosuppression. It is increasingly common to include in PTLD treatment the use of local or systemic administration of specific anti-CD20, CD21 and CD24 (rituximab) as first line therapy followed by chemotherapy using CHOP protocol (cyclophosphamide, doxorubicin, vincristine, prednisone) in case of recurrence [45, 46].

Good results were also obtained combining rituximab and conversion from CNIs to PSI [47, 48].

There are also reports of successful antiviral treatment with acyclovir, valacyclovir, or ganciclovir in EBV-induced lymphoproliferative disease [49].

REFERENCES

[1] Kapoor A. Malignancy in kidney transplant recipients. Drugs. 2008;68 Suppl 1:11-19.

[2] Wong G, Chapman JR. Cancers after renal transplantation. Transplant Rev 2008;22:141-149.

[3] Kauffman HM, Cherikh WS, McBride MA, *et al.* Post-transplant *de novo* malignancies in renal transplant recipients: the past and present. Transplant Int 2006; 19: 607-620.

[4] Dantal J, Pohanka E. Malignancies in renal transplantation: an unmet medical need. . Nephrol Dial Transplant 2007; 22:(Suppl 1): i4-i10.

[5] Gutierrez-Dalmau Á. Campistol JM. The role of proliferation signal inhibitors in post transplant malignancies. Nephrol Dial Transplant 2007; 22:(Suppl 1): i11-i16.

[6] Gutierrez-Dalmau Á. Campistol JM. Immunosuppressive therapy and malignancy in organ transplant recipients: a systemic review. Drugs 2007; 67: 1167-1198.

[7] Koehl GE, Schlitt HJ, Geissler EK. Rapamycin and tumor growth: mechanisms behind in anticancer activity. Transplant Rev 2005; 19 : 20-31.

[8] Hojo M, Morimoto T, Maluccio M, *et al.* Cyclosporine induces cancer progression by a cell-autonomous mechanism. Nature 1999 ; 397: 530-534.

[9] Dantal J, Hourmant M, Cantarovich D, *et al.* Effect of long-term immunosuppression in kidney-graft recipients on cancer incidence: randomised comparison of two cyclosporin regimens. Lancet 1998; 351:623-628.

[10] Maluccio M, Sharma V, Lagman M, *et al.* Tacrolimus enhances transforming growth factor-beta1 expression and promotes tumor progression. Transplantation 2003; 76: 597-602.

[11] Schumacher G, Oidtmann M, Rosewicz S, *et al.* Sirolimus inhibits growth of human hepatoma cells in contrast to tacrolimus which promotes cell growth. Transplant Proc 2002; 34 1392-1393.

[12] Guba M, von Breitenbuch P, Steinbauer M *et al.* Rapamycin inhibits primary and metastatic tumor growth by antiangiogenesis: involvement of vascular endothelial growth factor. Nat Med 2002; 8: 128-135.
[13] Walz G, Zanker B, Melton LB, *et al.* Possible association of the immunosuppressive and B cell lymphoma-promoting properties of cyclosporine. Transplantation 1990; 49: 191-194.
[14] Caillard S. Dharnidharka V, Agodoa L, *et al.* Posttransplant lymphoproliferative disorders after renal transplantation in the United States in era of modern immunosuppression. Transplantation 2005; 80: 1233-1243.
[15] Sørensen HT, Mellemkjaer L, Nielsen GL, *et al.* Skin cancers and non-Hodgkin lymphoma among users of systemic glucocorticoids: a population-based cohort study. J Natl Cancer Inst 2004; 96): 709-711.
[16] Karagas MR, Cushing Jr GL, Greenberg ER, *et al.* Non-melanoma skin cancers and glucocorticoid therapy. Br J Cancer 2001; 85 : 683-686.
[17] Swann PF,Waters TR, Moulton DC, *et al.* Role of postreplicative DNA mismatch repair in the cytotoxic action of thioguanine. Science 1996; 273:1109-1111.
[18] Penn I. Malignant tumors in organ transplant recipients. Berlin: Springer, 1970.
[19] McGeown MG, Douglas JF, Middleton D. One thousand renal transplants at Belfast City Hospital: post-graft neoplasia 1968-1999, comparing azathioprine only with cyclosporin- based regimes in a single centre. Clin Transpl 2000, 202.
[20] Hiesse C, Rieu P, Kriaa F, *et al.* Malignancy after renal transplantation: analysis of incidence and risk factors in 1700 patients followed during a 25-year period. Transplant Proc 1997; 29: 831-833.
[21] O'Donovan P, Perrett CM, Zhang X *et al.* Azathioprine and UVA light generate mutagenic oxidative DNA damage. Science 2005; 309: 1871-1874.
[22] Patel P, Moazzam N, Potti A, Mehdi SA. Azathioprine induced Hodgkin lymphoma: a case report and review of literature. Am J Clin Oncol 2005; 28: 427-428.
[23] Chui AK, Herbertt K, Wang LS, *et al.* Risk of tumor transmission in transplantation from donors with primary brain tumors: an Australian and New Zealand registry report. Transplant Proc 1999;31:1266-1267.
[24] Chapman JR, Webster AC. Australian and New Zealand Dialysis and Transplant Registry (ANZDATA) The 25th Annual Report (2002) Chapter 10; 2003.
[25] Vegso G, Sebestyen A, Paku S, *et al.* Antiproliferative and apoptotic effects of mycophenolic acid in human B-cell non-Hodgkin lymphomas. Leuk Res 2007;31:1003-1008.
[26] Opelz G, Dohler B. Lymphomas after solid organ transplantation: a collaborative transplant study report. Am J Transplant 2004;4:222-230.
[27] Cherikh WS, Kauffman HM, McBride MA, *et al.* Association of the type of induction immunosuppression with posttransplant lymphoproliferative disorder, graft survival, and patient survival after primary kidney transplantation. Transplantation 2003;76:1289-1293.
[28] Chapman TM, Keating GM. Basiliximab: a review of its use as induction therapy in renal transplantation. Drugs 2003; 63: 2803-2835.
[29] Ducloux D, Kazory A, Challier B, *et al.* Long-term toxicity of antithymocyte globulin induction may vary with choice of agent: a single-center retrospective study. Transplantation 2004; 77: 1029-1033.
[30] Eng CP, Sehgal SN, Vezina C. Activity of rapamycin (AY-22,989) against transplanted tumors. J Antibiot (Tokyo) 1984; 37: 1231-1237.
[31] Andrassy J, Graeb C, Rentsch M, *et al.* mTOR inhibition and its effect on cancer in transplantation. Transplantation 2005; 80: S171-174.
[32] Koehl GE, Schlitt HJ, Geissler EK. Rapamycin and tumor growth: mechanisms behind its anticancer activity. Transplant Rev 2005; 19: 20-31.
[33] Guba M, Graeb C, Jauch KW, *et al.* Pro- and anti-cancer effects of immunosuppressive agents used in organ transplantation. Transplantation 2004; 77 : 1777-1782.
[34] Luan FL, Hojo M, Maluccio M, *et al.* Rapamycin blocks tumor progression: unlinking immunosuppression from antitumor efficacy. Transplantation 2002; 73 : 1565-1572.
[35] Guba M, Yezhelyev M, Eichhorn ME, *et al.* Rapamycin induces tumor-specific thrombosis *via* tissue factor in the presence of VEGF. Blood 2005; 105 : 4463-4469.
[36] Majewski M, Korecka M, Kossev P, *et al.* The immunosuppressive macrolide RAD inhibits growth of human Epstein-Barr virus-transformed B lymphocytes *in vitro* and *in vivo*: a potential approach to prevention and treatment of posttransplant lymphoproliferative disorders. Proc Natl Acad Sci U S A 2000; 97: 4285-4290.
[37] Penn I: Evaluation of transplant candidates with pre-existing malignancies. Ann Transplant 2: 14-17, 1997.

[38] Kiberd BA, Keough-Ryan T, Clase CM. Screening for prostate, breast and colorectal cancer in renal transplant recipients. Am J Transplant 2003;3:619-625.

[39] EBPG Expert Group on Renal Transplantation. European best practice guidelines for renal transplantation. Section IV: long-term management of the transplant recipient. IV.6.3. Cancer risk after renal transplantation. Solid organ cancers: prevention and treatment. Nephrol Dial Transplant 2002;17:(Suppl 4):32, 34-36.

[40] EBPG Expert Group on Renal Transplantation. European best practice guidelines for renal transplantation. Section IV: long-term management of the transplant recipient. IV.6.2. Cancer risk after renal transplantation. Skin cancers: prevention and treatment. Nephrol Dial Transplant 2002;17(Suppl 4):31-36.

[41] Kasiske BL, Vazquez MA, Harmon WE, *et al.* Recommendations for the outpatient surveillance of renal transplant recipients. American Society of Transplantation.

[42] Myron Kauffman H, McBride MA, Cherikh WS, Spain PC, Marks WH, Roza AM: Transplant tumor registry: donor related malignancies. Transplantation 2002; 74: 358-362.

[43] Campistol JM, Gutierrez-Dalmau A, Torregrosa JV. Conversion to sirolimus: a successful treatment for posttransplantation Kaposi's sarcoma. Transplantation 2004; 77 : 760-762.

[44] Stallone G, Schena A, Infante B, *et al.* Sirolimus for Kaposi's sarcoma in renal-transplant recipients. N Engl J Med 2005; 352: 1317-1323.

[45] Knoop C, Kentos A, Remmerlink M *et al.* Post-transplant lymphoproliferative disorder after lug transplantation: first-line treatment with rituximab may induce complete remission. Clin transplant 2006; 20: 179-187.

[46] Elstrom RL, Andreadis C, Aqui NA *et al.* Treatment of PTLD with rituximab and chemotherapy. Am J Transplant 2006; 6: 569-576.

[47] Garcia VD, Bonamigo Filho JL, Neumann J, *et al.* Rituximab in association with rapamycin for post-transplant lymphoproliferative disease treatment. Transpl Int 2003; 16 : 202-206.

[48] Sierka K, Kumar MSA, Heifets M, *et al.* Successful minimization of immunosuppression (IM) and conversion to sirolimus (SLR) in kidney transplants recipients with post transplant lymphoproliferative disease (PTLD) and *de novo* nonskin antithymocyte malignancies (DNSM). Am J Transplant 2004; Suppl. 8: 523.

[49] Pirsch JD, Stratta RJ, Sollinger HW, Hafez GR, D'Alessandro AM, Kalayoglu M, Belzer FO: Treatment of severe Epstein-Barr virus-induced lymphoproliferative syndrome with ganciclovir: two cases after solid organ transplantation. Am J Med 1989;86: 241-244.

CHAPTER 22

Cardiovascular Disease and Renal Transplantation

Emily P. McQuarrie[1], Alan G. Jardine[1,*], Bengt C. Fellström[2] and Hallvard Holdaas[3]

[1]*Department of Nephrology, University of Glasgow, UK,* [2]*Department of Nephrology, University of Uppsala, Sweden and* [3]*Department of Nephrology, University of Oslo, Norway*

Abstract: Cardiovascular disease in renal transplant recipients is a major cause of graft loss and patient mortality. It is only in recent years that it has become understood that the mechanisms underlying coronary events in these patients differ from the general population. Patients with renal disease are more likely to suffer a fatal cardiovascular event than a non-fatal event and simply addressing conventional risk factors, which relate to atheromatous coronary artery disease, is insufficient in this population, where uraemic cardiomyopathy and graft specific factors uniquely increase risk. We discuss known epidemiological data relating to cardiovascular risk in these patients, consider traditional risk factors such as smoking, hypertension, diabetes and lipids, as well as graft-specific factors such as immunosuppressive therapies, and graft dysfunction. Management of cardiovascular risk in renal transplant recipients is necessarily multi-factorial but strong prospective evidence is lacking.

Keywords: Lipids, Hypertension, Mortality, Epidemiology, Kidney Transplantation, Cardiovascular Complication, Statins, Endovascular Procedures, Invasive Diagnosis.

INTRODUCTION

End stage renal failure is associated with a cardiovascular mortality risk 20-fold greater than the general population [1]. The best available treatment for this increased risk is renal transplantation [2]. Despite this, cardiovascular risk in renal transplant recipients remains 3-5 times greater than the general population [3, 4]. This risk is likely to relate to factors associated with chronic uraemia in the pre-transplant phase, as well as factors specific to transplantation, such as immunosuppressive therapies and complications of transplantation. In the general population, cardiovascular disease (CVD) is synonymous with atheromatous coronary artery disease (CAD), with a variety of known modifiable and non-modifiable cardiovascular risk factors. Atheroma leads to functional narrowing of the coronary vessels and consequent myocardial ischaemia, causing the patient to present with angina, generally on exertion. Acutely, when a plaque ruptures and the lipid rich core is exposed, thrombus forms on the surface of the plaque, occluding the coronary vasculature, leading to myocardial infarction. This may be followed by recovery, the development of progressive ischaemic heart failure, or sudden death (either as a consequence of pump failure or the development of arrhythmias). In patients with renal transplants, however, it has become increasingly apparent that the pattern of CV disease differs from the general population, a feature we have been slow to appreciate. Whilst CAD may co-exist, it is heart failure and sudden cardiac death that are the major manifestations of cardiovascular disease in this population. Table **1** illustrates these differing cardiovascular risks amongst 3 populations at "high CV risk" – normal individuals with high cardiovascular risk (4S study [5]), patients on maintenance haemodialysis (AURORA [6], 4D study [7]) and renal transplant recipients (ALERT [8]). Although the absolute levels of risk, and event rates, reflect the inclusion criteria for these studies, the figures illustrate that patients with CAD (4S study [5]) are three times as likely to have a non-fatal myocardial infarction (MI) as a fatal cardiac event. This pattern is completely reversed in the dialysis patients (AURORA [6], 4D study [7]) who are three times more likely to have a fatal as a non-fatal cardiac event; whereas transplant recipients have an equal risk of fatal and non-fatal cardiac events. The "take home message" is that renal disease is associated with an increased risk of cardiac death rather than non-fatal MI. As such, applying pathophysiological concepts, screening and therapeutic evidence from the general population is likely to be flawed in this particular group of patients.

***Address correspondence to Alan G. Jardine:** Department of Nephrology University of Glasgow, Glasgow, UK. Phone: +44 141 330 2705, Fax: +44 141 330 6972 ; E-mail: a.g.jardine@clinmed.gla.ac.uk

Massimiliano Veroux and Pierfrancesco Veroux (Eds)

In this chapter we plan to describe the nature of cardiovascular disease in renal transplant recipients, discuss potential interventions and available evidence for treatment including data from the ALERT study, the first and only published large-scale study of cardiovascular intervention and outcomes in renal transplant patients [8, 9] and address the issue of pre-transplant screening.

Table 1: Cardiovascular endpoints in different at risk populations

	CD (%)	AMI (NF) (%)	Non-CVD (%)
4S	8.5	22.6	2.2
ALERT	5.1	6.3	6.2
4D	23	12	25
AURORA	23.4	7.7	19.4

CD = sudden cardiac death; AMI (NF) = Acute myocardial infarction, non-fatal; Non-CVD = non-cardiac death. 4S[9] = patients at conventional risk; ALERT [8] = renal transplant recipients; 4D[7] and AURORA[6] = maintenance haemodialysis. Renal transplant recipients are at risk that is intermediate between patients receiving dialysis and the general population.

EPIDEMIOLOGICAL STUDIES AND RISK FACTOR IDENTIFICATION

Longitudinal Cohort Studies

Informing our understanding of the epidemiology of cardiovascular disease in renal transplant recipients, there have been a number of retrospective or longitudinal follow-up studies [3, 10, 11]. These have often been single centre studies or registry analyses. One of the drawbacks of these studies has been the tendency to pool cardiovascular event (CVE), with the incorrect assumption that such CVE will have common determinants. Predominant amongst these studies, are the works of Kasiske in Minnesota. Over the last 15 years, Kasiske and colleagues have reported longitudinal follow-up of over 1000 renal transplant recipients, in their single centre, in whom they have recorded mortality and cardiovascular events [10, 11]. These studies have demonstrated a high prevalence of cardiovascular events and mortality and have focused our view and our research interest on cardiovascular disease in this population. They have been consistent in identification of some conventional risk factors for pooled cardiovascular events. Specifically, age, gender and the presence of diabetes mellitus are strong risk factors for cardiovascular outcomes in patients with functioning renal transplants [12]. Thus, for each year of life the risk of a cardiovascular event is increased by 3-5%, male gender is associated with an approximate doubling of cardiovascular risk, and the presence of diabetes (either pre-existing or post-transplant diabetes) is associated with an approximate doubling of overall risk. However, demonstration of a relationship between hyperlipidaemia and cardiovascular events has proved more difficult.

In his earlier study [10] Kasiske was unable to identify any significant relationship between post-transplant levels of triglycerides, total cholesterol or LDL cholesterol and cardiovascular events, although a small relationship between HDL cholesterol and outcome was evident. Moreover, and very surprisingly, there was no clear and obvious relationship between cigarette smoking and outcome. The major risk factors for outcome were pre-existing disease, *i.e.* pre-existing coronary artery disease, peripheral vascular disease or cerebral vascular disease, which were associated with a 3-9 fold risk in the development of subsequent events. These observations are of major importance, demonstrating that the strongest determinants of long-term transplant cardiovascular event are pre-existing and non-remediable disease or risk factors. In addition, Kasiske identified additional risk factors that do not apply in the general population, specifically, presence or history of acute rejection episodes and splenectomy. A later study by Kasiske, in a larger population [12] confirmed the relationship with non-remediable risk factors – age, gender and diabetes, but did for the first time note a relationship between cigarette smoking and major cardiovascular events (relative risk 2.14, 95% CI 1.49-3.08) [12] and hyperlipidaemia and outcome (in that very elevated total cholesterol was associated with an increased risk of long term cardiovascular events) [11].

Studies by other investigators including Abbott [13] and Rigatto [13, 14] have corroborated these findings. The studies by Abbot followed patients at two centres and, uniquely, divided the outcomes into those patients developing heart failure and those suffering cardiovascular mortality. They were able to demonstrate additional risk factors including graft dysfunction, specifically graft failure, being associated with an approximately three fold increased risk of cardiovascular events including heart failure. In addition, anaemia proved to be a risk factor for the development of heart failure. Overall, these studies show the importance of good graft function in preserving the health of the patient, and specifically the risks of cardiovascular events. In fact, it is possible to model cardiovascular outcomes in this patient population by the use of a two compartment model where graft failure (or patients on maintenance haemodialysis) has an overall cardiovascular risk that is three times that of patients with a functioning transplant [15].

Kasiske subsequently expanded on his earlier single centre findings with the PORT study [16]. In this retrospective observational study, data from 14 centres in Northern America, New Zealand, Japan and Europe were collected. From these data cardiovascular risk models were constructed for the risk of suffering a cardiovascular event (fatal or nonfatal MI, coronary revascularisation or sudden death). Pooling these events was probably necessary due to the retrospective nature of the study and to allow sufficient statistical power, however again it impairs analysis of the impact of different risk factors on individual endpoints. Conventional risk factors such as recipient age, sex, history of diabetes and pre-existing CVD were again identified as important predictors. Transplant specific factors such as years from first End-stage renal disease (ESRD) treatment to transplant, occurrence of delayed graft function, acute rejection and impaired graft function were also shown to predict risk. However other traditional risk factors such as hyperlipidaemia and smoking were not shown to be independently predictive, probably due to the pooling of cardiovascular events which precludes more detailed analysis of the impact of risk on differing endpoints.

Table 2: Univariate Cox analysis of risk factors for sudden cardiac death (upper Panel) and myocardial infarction (Lower panel) from the ALERT study in RTR [8, 10, 19]

	HR	**CI**	**p**
Sudden cardiac death			
Age	1.03	1.02-1.08	0.01
Diabetes	2.82	1.62-4.91	0.01
Smoking	1.55	0.86-2.8	0.15
CHD	3.6	1.96-6.63	0.01
LDL	1.28	0.99-1.65	0.06
SBP	1.01	1.0-1.03	0.05
PP	1.01	1.0-1.03	0.01
LVH	2.08	1.11-3.89	0.01
ST-T	3.59	2.07-6.21	0.01
Myocardial infarction			
Age	1.03	1.0-1.05	0.02
Diabetes	2.36	1.42-3.04	0.01
Smoking	2.31	1.78-5.63	0.01
CHD	3.17	2.08-5.18	0.01
LDL	1.41	1.12-1.77	0.01

HR= Hazard ratio; CI = Confidence interval; p = p-value. CHD = pre-existing coronary artery disease; LDL = mmol/l LDL; SBP and PP – systolic and pulse pressure per mmHg; LVH = left ventricular hypertrophy; ST-T = ischaemic changes on ECG.

Randomised Trial end-Points

In the ALERT study [8, 9], unlike registry data and single centre longitudinal follow-up studies, the end-points were validated by an independent end-point committee who were blinded to treatment allocation. This provides high fidelity information that may be used to derive information on risk factors and individual cardiovascular outcomes. Thus, the end-point committee reported on non-fatal myocardial infarction, fatal cardiac events and also on other events including stroke. The study recruited 2100 patients with functioning renal transplants of over six months duration that were randomised to receive fluvastatin 40-80 mg/day or placebo. The main study followed patients for a median of 5½ years, following which there was an open label extension study where all patients were offered fluvastatin and followed for a further 2 years. Thus, there is information on 2100 patients followed for almost 8 years with validated, independently verified end-points. Statin therapy was associated with a reduction in myocardial infarction but, overall, the study failed to show a significant reduction in the chosen composite cardiovascular endpoint (major adverse cardiac events, non-fatal myocardial infarction, cardiovascular death and stroke) over the 5½ years of the initial study. This composite cardiac end-point was, however, significant at the end of 7½ years of follow-up.

Risk factor analysis in the placebo arm [17, 18] revealed, for the first time, the differential impact of conventional cardiovascular risk factors on cardiovascular end-points (Table **2**). Thus, if we look first at non-fatal myocardial infarction, a relatively uncommon end-point in this population, we see that lipid subfractions are major determinants of this end-point. For each mmol of total or LDL cholesterol at baseline, the risk of a subsequent myocardial infarction was increased 30-40%. Increased HDL was associated with a benefit, such that for every mmol increase, the risk of a subsequent cardiac event was reduced by approximately one third. Baseline triglycerides were also associated with increased risk of myocardial infarction. These data show that myocardial infarction in renal transplant recipients is dependant on lipids in the same way as myocardial infarction is in the general population, or in patients recruited to cardiovascular prevention studies. The absence of such associations in the studies of Kasiske is likely a reflection of the decision to pool cardiovascular outcomes. Since myocardial infarction is proportionately less common in pooled cardiovascular outcomes in transplant recipients than in the general population, this masks the impact of lipids on cardiovascular outcomes.

In contrast, cardiovascular death, a consequence of heart failure or arrhythmias, in the ALERT study was determined by lipids to a lesser extent and was instead highly dependent on the consequences of high blood pressure, with a 1% increase in risk for each 1mmHg increase in systolic blood pressure. The presence of complications of hypertension were also strongly associated *i.e.* left ventricular hypertrophy, particularly when associated with strain, on the baseline electrocardiogram, as well as impaired renal function. Thus, cardiac death is determined by blood pressure and its consequences (specifically left ventricular hypertrophy (LVH)) and so called uraemic cardiomyopathy [19]. Uraemic cardiomyopathy, the principle manifestation of which is LVH, is a highly prevalent condition in patients starting dialysis programmes, and is associated with poor outcome [20, 21]. It is associated with myocardial fibrosis and electrophysiological markers of arrythmogenicity (such as abnormal microvolt T wave alternans and increased QT dispersal [19]), suggesting it may be a determinant of sudden death. The factors associated with the development of LVH in this condition are predominantly systolic blood pressure and pulse pressure [22]. The less common manifestation of dilated cardiomyopathy (with systolic dysfunction) may be a sequel of LVH or may be associated with (often silent) CAD.

The key message is that cardiovascular outcomes in renal transplant recipients are the same as the general population but that the balance is shifted so that non-fatal myocardial infarction is less common than fatal cardiac events. Whilst non-fatal myocardial infarction is dependant on lipids, suggesting that the underlying pathophysiology is similar to the general population, with cholesterol rich atheromatous plaques, cardiac death is more determined by structural changes in the left ventricle and their determinants, specifically blood pressure (Fig. **1**).

HYPERTENSION AND ANTI-HYPERTENSIVE THERAPY

Hypertension is an almost invariable accompaniment of renal transplantation. The vascular changes seen consequent to chronic renal failure and dialysis contribute to the persistence of hypertension even after successful transplantation and improvement in GFR. Secondly, although transplantation improves wellbeing it does not normalise GFR, thus contributing to persistence of hypertension, and lastly the immunosuppressive agents in common usage cause hypertension, even in patients without primary renal disease. The primary agents that cause hypertension are corticosteroids and calcineurin inhibitors. The mechanism by which corticosteroids cause hypertension is still not completely understood however there are two principle components. The first is retention of salt and water due to actions of corticosteroids on the kidney, involving to some extent the mineralocorticoid receptor. The major influence however is likely to be through enhanced autonomic function, and vascular tone, contributing to the development of hypertension, even when patients are salt restricted [23]. Similarly, the hypertensive effects of calcineurin inhibitors are poorly understood. Nephrotoxicity may contribute through diminution of renal function, but there are also direct effects, again mediated by salt and water retention in the kidney, and enhanced vasoconstrictor tone and vasomotor function [24]. Overall, over 80% of patients in our own centre require anti-hypertensive agents, with the majority requiring more than one anti-hypertensive agent [25], despite which levels of blood pressure control are relatively poor. Whilst compliance may be an issue in patients with renal transplants that require polypharmacy, it is likely that hypertension in this setting is relatively resistant to therapy, and there is also a tendency to avoid effective agents like angiotensin converting enzyme (ACE) inhibitors and angiotensin receptor blockers [26], because of the risk of renal artery stenosis in the transplanted kidney.

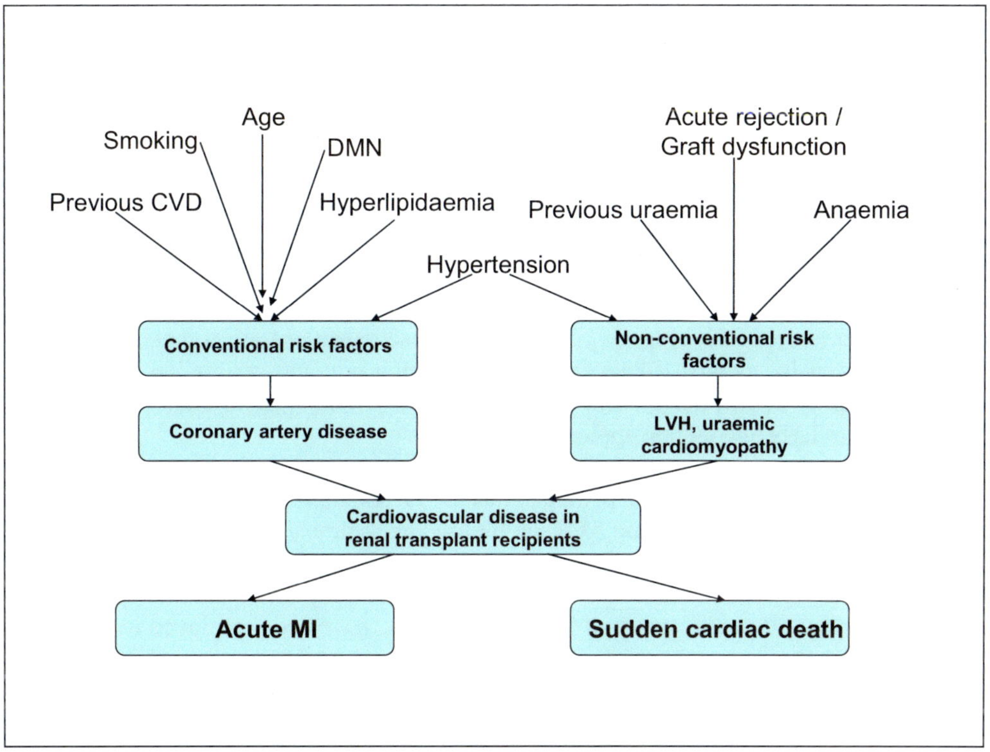

Figure 1: Cardiac risk factors in renal transplant recipients; CVD: Cardiovascular disease; DMN: Diabetes mellitus; LVH: Left ventricular hypertrophy; Acute MI: acute myocardial infaction.

The impact of hypertension has not been studied prospectively. However, Opelz and colleagues performed a retrospective analysis of the European Registry [27]. They took blood pressure measurements recorded at outpatient clinics and patients with a functioning transplant one year after transplantation. These data show that blood pressure, albeit not independent from graft function, is a major determinant of long-term patient and graft survival. Moreover, this effect is seen even at levels below which one would label the patient as being hypertensive such that patients with a systolic blood pressure of 130mmHg, had a substantially worse graft outcome than patients with a systolic blood pressure of 120mmHg. In the ALERT study blood pressure was not an independent risk factor for myocardial infarction, but was associated with cardiac death, and stroke [18].

The relationship with sudden death is of major importance. Blood pressure is the major determinant of left ventricular hypertrophy [22], and both left ventricular hypertrophy and specifically left ventricular hypertrophy with strain, were the strongest determinants of cardiac death within the ALERT study [18]. The likely pathophysiological mechanism is that left ventricular hypertrophy, particularly when associated with subendocardial ischaemia, is associated with myocardial fibrosis. Fibrosis is associated with increased QT dispersal (a marker of spontaneous arrhythmias), and also predisposes to chaotic conduction within the heart. It is this pattern that predisposes to sudden death in this population, either due to spontaneous arrhythmias or as a consequence of minor ischaemic episodes. Moreover, it identifies a potentially remediable risk factor for the major cardiovascular outcome in this patient population.

There are no interventional studies of blood pressure lowering in the transplant communities. However, a carefully conducted retrospective analysis from Austria performed by Oberbauer and colleagues [28] showed that patients treated with ACE inhibitors or angiotensin receptor blockers fared better both in respect to graft function and patient survival. A similar analysis performed by Opelz [29], on a highly selected subgroup of the European Renal Registry, failed to show a similar trend. However, the findings of Oberbauer are consistent with short-term studies that show beneficial effects on proteinuria and blood pressure in transplant recipients [30]. Thus, future studies of blood pressure lowering in the transplant population should involve agents that block the renin angiotensin system, should explore whether blood pressure targets derived from the general population are appropriate in this population, and should look at surrogate measures of long-term outcomes – specifically reversal of proteinuria, a marker of chronic allograft nephropathy and graft failure, and left ventricular hypertrophy, a marker of the severity of hypertension and the strongest risk factor for cardiac death.

An unresolved issue is whether modification of immunosuppressive therapy should also be employed in the management of hypertension in this population. Studies involving minimisation or withdrawal of steroids [31] and minimisation of calcineurin inhibitors, switching from cyclosporine to tacrolimus [32] or stopping calcineurin inhibitors and switching to sirolimus [33], have all been shown to result in a substantial reduction in blood pressure, of the order of 10/5 mmHg. These reductions are comparable to the effects of individual anti-hypertensive agents. However, just as switching immunosuppression has failed to engage the transplant community in the management of hyperlipidaemia, modifying immunosuppression to control blood pressure is a similarly uncommon approach.

Finally, exploring the underlying cause of hypertension, for example the identification of renal artery stenosis, is often performed before starting ACE inhibitors. This is probably a council of perfection, bearing in mind that intervention in renal artery stenosis is of no proven benefit in this population, nor in any other population where atheromatous disease is the underlying cause [34]. More radical approaches, such as embolisation or laparoscopic nephrectomy of the native kidneys, have been employed in extreme cases and may be effective. However, in our experience they do little to improve blood pressure in patients with long standing hypertension, although, nephrectomy prior to transplantation may be associated with improved long term blood pressure control.

LIPIDS AND LIPID LOWERING THERAPY

Dyslipidaemia is an almost invariable accompaniment of renal transplantation. The pattern comprises elevated total and LDL cholesterol, triglycerides and HDL. Moreover, there are increased concentrations of intermediate lipoproteins, including small dense LDL, which are potentially extremely atherogenic [26]. The mechanisms behind this dyslipidaemia are multi-factorial. Firstly, there is the impact of reduced renal function, given that even a well functioning graft is unlikely to give a GFR of much more than 60 ml/min. Secondly, and predominantly, are the influences of immunosuppressive agents.

Individual anti-rejection agents have variable, but often synergistic effects of serum lipids. Corticosteroids cause an increase in total and LDL cholesterol, triglyceride, and HDL cholesterol. This is well known, and is a feature of steroid therapy with normal renal function and in patients with functional corticosteroid excess such as Cushing's syndrome. The impact of steroids is clearly seen in the early post-transplant period [35] where the initiation of anti-rejection therapy, associated with normalisation of renal function, increased appetite and changes in diet are associated with an average 1.5 mmol/L increase in total cholesterol, 1 mmol/L increase in LDL cholesterol and approximately 0.5 mmol/L in HDL cholesterol. Calcineurin inhibitors (cyclosporine and tacrolimus) also cause dyslipidaemia however, their use is more associated with increases in total and LDL cholesterol. Finally, TOR inhibitors (TORi) such as sirolimus and everolimus, have a dramatic, dose dependent effect on lipids. This comprises an increase in total and LDL cholesterol, but also a potentially protective effect through an increase in HDL cholesterol [26]. It is worth commenting that the dyslipidaemia caused by immunosuppressive agents has not been proven specifically to cause cardiovascular disease.

A number of studies have investigated the short term impact of modification of immunosuppressive therapy on hyperlipidaemia in transplant recipients. Artz and colleagues [36] studied the switch from a cyclosporine containing immunosuppressive triple therapy regime to tacrolimus containing triple therapy. This was associated with a reduction in total and LDL cholesterol of approximately 1 mmol/L. Similarly, studies of steroid withdrawal have shown beneficial reductions in all cholesterol subfractions [37]. The only study to compare modification of immunosuppression with the initiation of lipid lowering therapy is the study of Abramovich and colleagues [38]. In this study, patients were switched from cyclosporin based therapy to tacrolimus based therapy, and this was compared to the addition to atorvastatin. Although tacrolimus based therapy was associated with a reduction in total, LDL cholesterol and triglycerides, patients on cyclosporin and atorvastatin had comparable lipid levels as those on tacrolimus and atorvastatin. Thus, it may be more effective to add a lipid lowering agent than to consider changing immunosuppression, with the attendant – albeit small- risks of precipitating a rejection episode. Moreover, the impact is far from clear given the fact that both atherogenic lipid subfractions, and potentionally protective subfractions (HDL cholesterol) are increased. Nonetheless, modification of immunosuppressive agents is a relatively unexplored and underused strategy to modify the dyslipidaemia associated with transplantation. Given these uncertainties, and the dramatic increases in cardiovascular disease that are associated with renal transplantation, interventional studies have, and will be necessary to explore the impact of lipid lowering therapy in this population. Although, registry studies [39] have noted that statin use is both increasing and is associated with reduced mortality and cardiovascular mortality in transplant recipients, these associations prove little.

The only published interventional study is the ALERT trial [8]. As described above, this study randomised patients to fluvastatin or placebo and followed them for almost 8 years. Although, as explained above, the composite primary end-point was not statistically significant in the first instance, the risk of myocardial infarction was reduced by approximately 30% by therapy. This is comparable to the reduction in myocardial infarction seen in cardiovascular preventive studies in the general population and, specifically, those patients at high risk of coronary artery disease. Thus, just as we have unravelled the complexity of the pathophysiology of cardiovascular disease in the transplant population, it is clear that coronary artery disease is both dependant on lipids, and preventable by statin therapy, just as it is in the general population.

An additional observation, unique to this population of renal transplant recipients, relates to a well established relationship of lipid levels and graft dysfunction. Many of the features of chronic allograft nephropathy (CAN) are similar to the pathophysiological mechanisms that cause atherosclerosis in the general population. Thus, there is deposition of lipid within the kidney, and glomerulus in particular, associated with proliferation of vascular smooth muscle cells and the related, mesangial cells within the glomerulus. This leads to excessive matrix production by mesangial cells and vascular smooth muscle cells, that contribute both to vascular damage, interstitial fibrosis, and glomerulosclerosis, the hallmarks of CAN.

It would be reasonable to postulate therefore that modification of hyperlipidaemia, by the use of statins or alternative lipid lowering therapy, may slow progression of chronic kidney disease. Indeed, this has been proven in experimental models of glomerulonephritis, and also of chronic allograph nephropathy [40]. However, studies in humans have been less effective. Notably, in the ALERT study, although renal impairment was a major risk factor for progressive loss of renal function, all cause mortality and cardiovascular events, and lipid levels were associated with the rate of decline of renal function, randomised allocation to fluvastatin or placebo had no impact on the rate of decline of renal function. Thus, it appears that although glomerulosclerosis may be dependant on lipids, this is not a modifiable risk factor in the progressive loss of renal function associated with CAN.

OTHER CARDIOVASCULAR RISK FACTORS

Cigarette Smoking

In the general population cigarette smoking is highly associated with the development cardiovascular disease. Remarkably, some of the earlier studies in renal transplant recipients [10] failed to show any association with cigarette smoking. However, subsequent studies have shown that smoking is associated with all cause mortality, and with cardiovascular events [41]. Moreover, cigarette smoking appears to be associated with graft loss and more rapid progression of chronic allograft nephropathy. In the ALERT study, cigarette smoking was sub-grouped into non-smokers, current smokers, and ex-smokers. The relationship was difficult to interpret, but it appeared that ex-smokers retained the risk associated with smoking [17, 18]. Whether or not this represented a true effect, or inconsistent reporting of smoking cessation, remains to be established. Regardless, patients with progressive renal disease, end-stage renal failure and transplant recipients should be advised to stop smoking in the same way as one would advise any member of the general population [4].

Allograft Dysfunction

Other potentially remediable risk factors include renal allograft dysfunction. This is akin to the impact of reduced eGFR in the general population [42]. The most extreme example is graft failure, where there is an established increased risk of sudden cardiac death, heart failure and all cause mortality failure [13, 43, 44]. In the ALERT study, we observed that renal dysfunction had a progressive impact on the development of cardiovascular events. However, in contrast to lipids, the major impact of renal dysfunction was on the risk of stroke and of sudden cardiac death. Again, this is likely to be mediated through the development of left ventricular hypertrophy and it's impact on arrhythmogenicity.

Diabetes

A further mechanism that promotes premature CVD in RTR is the development of diabetes. Post transplant diabetes mellitus (PTDM) is a recognised complication of transplantation [45, 46]. It is more common in older patients, in patients who are overweight, patients of African or Asian origin, and in patients who have experienced stress-induced diabetes previously (associated with surgery, steroids or pregnancy). It is likely that transplantation merely accelerates the underlying predisposition to develop diabetes in susceptible individuals. The main contributory factor is the use of corticosteroids which cause insulin resistance. Minimisation of steroid dose reduces the risk of PTDM and may reverse diabetes, restoring insulin sensitivity [37, 46] . CNI can also contribute to the development of diabetes; tacrolimus being considerably more diabetogenic than ciclosporine. This reflects the role of tacrolimus specific, intracellular FK-binding proteins on insulin secretion [37]. Minimisation of corticosteroids or tacrolimus; or switching from tacrolimus to cyclosporine; are both appropriate therapeutic measures [46], although despite this many patients require insulin or oral hypoglycaemic agents. An alternative strategy is to avoid tacrolimus and/ or steroids in patients at high risk for the development of PTDM [47, 48]. This strategy may be of particular relevance in older patients where rejection is less of an issue [48]. Such an approach has few advocates, largely as a consequence of the availability of management strategies for diabetes and the failure to recognise the long-term consequences of PTDM. Previously viewed as a nuisance, PTDM has been shown to have long-term implications for patients, and is associated with a 2-3 fold increase in all cause mortality and CV events. Emerging evidence suggests that PTDM has a greater impact on patient outcomes than acute rejection. Thus, strategies to limit the incidence and impact of PTDM have emerged as a major target in the fight against CVD [46, 49].

SCREENING

Clearly, with cardiovascular disease in renal transplant recipients being a common cause of morbidity, mortality and graft loss post-transplant and with considerations relating to ethical distribution of organs, substantial interest has focussed on screening patients for cardiovascular disease prior to transplantation. The aims of this approach being to optimise the patients' cardiovascular status, but also to refuse organs to those deemed to be at highest risk. Whilst this approach may appear reasonable, it is difficult to formulate a suitable screening program, as there is a reliance on utilising tests which predominantly assess for atheromatous coronary artery disease, in a group of patients whose cardiac disease is multi-factorial and not necessarily well predicted by the presence, or indeed absence, of obstructive coronary artery disease.

As such, there is no unified approach to cardiovascular screening. Some centres undertake invasive coronary angiography as standard pre-transplant work up. Others perform selected non-invasive stress testing in high risk patients and undertake further investigation dependent on the results of that. Clearly, as this is a screening program, patients are generally asymptomatic and there is an understandable reluctance in the cardiology community to perform percutaneous coronary intervention, a procedure not without risk, in patients who are asymptomatic and undergoing the procedure in an almost prophylactic setting, particularly in the absence of any proven survival benefit [50].

Lastly, introducing a further burden to transplant listing can be detrimental to the patient in that they are delayed from receiving the one treatment proven to reduce their cardiovascular risk and overall mortality, transplantation.

In our centre [51] we undertook cardiovascular assessment in patients deemed at high risk prior to inclusion onto the transplant waiting list. Assessment involved exercise testing, ECG and cardiac MRI. One third had positive findings and underwent coronary angiography, of which one third had obstructive coronary artery disease. Overall 5.6% were treated with percutaneous coronary intervention, which was not associated with a survival benefit. In the absence of a randomised controlled trial, it seems reasonable that patients who are at high risk of underlying cardiovascular disease, such as diabetics with peripheral vascular disease, undergo non-invasive stress testing pre-operatively. They should receive advice regarding risk factor optimisation and any invasive intervention should be a joint decision between the transplant team, cardiologist and patient, based on each individual case.

CONCLUSIONS

It can therefore be seen that the cause of cardiovascular disease in renal transplant recipients is multi-factorial. Patients carry with them the burden of long-standing chronic kidney disease and possibly dialysis therapy, with the attendant hypertension and chronic vascular changes, leading to left ventricular hypertrophy, uraemic cardiomyopathy, aberrant conduction and sudden cardiac death. The immunosuppressive medication used in renal transplantation is itself pro-atherogenic and similarly, they have the same risks for atheromatous coronary artery disease as the general population and therefore the same risk factors of age, diabetes, smoking and lipids. Any cardiovascular intervention will need to be multi-factorial to address the complex risk profile in this population. However, at present there are few randomised controlled trials to inform practice. The only randomised controlled trial in this area is of statin therapy, which clearly will impact only on those end-points that are dependent on circulating cholesterol levels. The ALERT study demonstrated a reduction in the risk of myocardial infarction by approximately a third. However, since myocardial infarction only represents a relatively small proportion of cardiovascular end-points in the transplant population, compared with the general population, the overall impact of statins was less. What these data reveal however, is the risk factor profile when the impact of cholesterol on cardiovascular outcomes is effectively annulled by statin therapy (unpublished data from the ALERT trial), unmasking or shifting the emphasis towards other risk factors, including left ventricular hypertrophy with strain, blood pressure, and renal dysfunction (see Table **3**). The key message is that to address the range of cardiovascular risks in this population, statin use must be combined with effective anti-hypertensive therapy, regression of left ventricular hypertrophy, and optimisation of graft function. Whether this need can be met through additional medication or will require cardiovascular risk factor management that includes modification of immunosuppression remains to be established in prospective controlled trials.

Table 3: Risk factors for myocardial infarction in renal transplant recipients receiving statin therapy and those without [19]

	Placebo		Fluvastatin	
Risk factor	**HR (CI)**	**P**	**HR (CI)**	**p**
Age at baseline (y)	1.03 (1.00-1.05)	0.02	1.04 (1.01-1.06)	0.01
Age at transplant (y)	1.03 (1.01-1.05)	0.03	1.03 (1.00-1.05)	0.03
Female	0.74 (0.44-1.26)	0.27	0.61 (0.33-1.14)	0.12
Diabetes	2.36 (1.42-3.94)	0.01	4.2 (2.47-71.4)	0.01
BMI	1.04 (0.99-1.09)	0.11	0.96 (0.90-1.03)	0.24
CHD	3.17 (1.78-5.16)	0.01	4.36 (2.43-7.80)	0.01
Smoking (ever)	2.31(1.37-3.91)	0.02	1.60(0.72-2.62)	0.33
SBP	1.01(0.99-1.02)	0.40	1.02(1.00-1.03)	0.01
DBP	0.98(0.96-1.01)	0.15	0.98(0.95-1.01)	0.13
LVH	0.88(0.42-1.84)	0.73	2.81(1.58-0.50)	0.01
ST-T	1.36(0.76-2.41)	0.30	4.38(2.57-7.47)	0.01
Ct	1.01(0.96-1.06)	0.65	1.00(1.00-1.01)	0.06
TC	1.40(1.14-1.71)	0.01	1.10(1.87-1.39)	0.42
LDL	1.41(1.12-1.77)	0.01	1.23(0.95-1.58)	0.12
HDL	0.72(0.40-1.29)	0.27	0.67(0.36-1.25)	0.21
TG	1.12(1.02-1.22)	0.01	1.00(0.80-1.25)	0.99

HR= Hazard ratio; CI = Confidence interval; p = p-value. BMI = Body mass index, g/m2; CHD = pre-existing coronary artery disease; SBP and DBP – systolic and diastolic pressure per mmHg; LVH = left ventricular hypertrophy; ST-T = ischaemic changes on ECG; Ct = serum creatinine (mg/mmol);TC = Total cholesterol mmol/l; LDL = low density lipoprotein mmol/l; HDL = High density lipoprotein mmol/l; TG = Triglycerides mmol/l.

REFERENCES

[1] Go AS, Chertow GM, Fan D, *et al.* Chronic kidney disease and the risks of death, cardiovascular events, and hospitalization. N Engl J Med 2004; 351:1296-1305.

[2] Wolfe RA, Ashby VB, Milford EL, *et al.* Comparison of mortality in all patients on dialysis, patients on dialysis awaiting transplantation, and recipients of a first cadaveric transplant. N Engl J Med 1999; 341:1725-1730.

[3] Baigent C, Burbury K, Wheeler D. Premature cardiovascular disease in chronic renal failure. Lancet 2000; 356:147-152.

[4] KDIGO clinical practice guideline for the care of kidney transplant recipients. Am J Transplant 2009;9 Suppl 3:S1-155.

[5] Randomised trial of cholesterol lowering in 4444 patients with coronary heart disease: the Scandinavian Simvastatin Survival Study (4S). Lancet 1994; 344:1383-1389.

[6] Fellstrom BC, Jardine AG, Schmieder RE, *et al.* Rosuvastatin and cardiovascular events in patients undergoing hemodialysis. N Engl J Med 2009;360:1395-1407.

[7] Wanner C, Krane V, Marz W, *et al.* Atorvastatin in patients with type 2 diabetes mellitus undergoing hemodialysis. N Engl J Med 2005;353:238-248.

[8] Holdaas H, Fellstrom B, Cole E, *et al.* Long-term cardiac outcomes in renal transplant recipients receiving fluvastatin: the ALERT extension study. Am J Transplant 2005; 5:2929-2936.

[9] Holdaas H, Fellstrom B, Jardine AG, *et al.* Effect of fluvastatin on cardiac outcomes in renal transplant recipients: a multicentre, randomised, placebo-controlled trial. Lancet 2003; 361:2024-2031.

[10] Kasiske BL, Guijarro C, Massy ZA, *et al.* Cardiovascular disease after renal transplantation. J Am Soc Nephrol 1996; 7:158-165.

[11] Kasiske BL, Chakkera HA, Roel J. Explained and unexplained ischemic heart disease risk after renal transplantation. J Am Soc Nephrol 2000;11:1735-1743.

[12] Kasiske BL, Klinger D. Cigarette smoking in renal transplant recipients. J Am Soc Nephrol 2000; 11:753-759.

[13] Abbott KC, Hypolite IO, Hshieh P, *et al.* Hospitalized congestive heart failure after renal transplantation in the United States. Ann. Epidemiol. 2002; 12:115-122.

[14] Rigatto C, Parfrey P, Foley R, *et al.* Congestive heart failure in renal transplant recipients: risk factors, outcomes, and relationship with ischemic heart disease. J Am Soc Nephrol 2002; 13:1084-1090.

[15] McLean DR, Jardine AG. A simulation model to investigate the impact of cardiovascular risk in renal transplantation. Transplant Proc 2005; 37:2135-2143.

[16] Israni AK, Snyder JJ, Skeans MA, *et al.* Predicting coronary heart disease after kidney transplantation: Patient outcomes in renal transplantation (PORT) study. Am J Transplant 2010;10:338-353.

[17] Jardine AG, Fellstrom B, Logan JO, *et al.* Cardiovascular risk and renal transplantation: post hoc analyses of the Assessment of Lescol in Renal Transplantation (ALERT) Study. Am J Kidney Dis 2005;46:529-536.

[18] Jardine AG, Holdaas H, Fellstrom B, *et al.* Fluvastatin prevents cardiac death and myocardial infarction in renal transplant recipients: post-hoc subgroup analyses of the ALERT Study. Am J Transplant 2004;4:988-995. ----

[19] Stewart GA, Gansevoort RT, Mark PB, *et al.* Electrocardiographic abnormalities and uremic cardiomyopathy. Kidney Int 2005; 67:217-226.

[20] Foley RN, Parfrey PS, Harnett JD, *et al.* The prognostic importance of left ventricular geometry in uremic cardiomyopathy. J Am Soc Nephrol 1995; 5:2024-2031.

[21] Mark PB, Johnston N, Groenning BA, *et al.* Redefinition of uremic cardiomyopathy by contrast-enhanced cardiac magnetic resonance imaging. Kidney Int 2006; 69:1839-1845.

[22] Patel RK, Oliver S, Mark PB, *et al.* Determinants of left ventricular mass and hypertrophy in hemodialysis patients assessed by cardiac magnetic resonance imaging. Clin J Am Soc Nephrol 2009; 4:1477-1483.

[23] Walker BR. Glucocorticoids and cardiovascular disease. Eur. J Endocrinol 2007;157:545-559.

[24] Zhang R, Leslie B, Boudreaux JP, *et al.* Hypertension after kidney transplantation: impact, pathogenesis and therapy. Am J Med Sci 2003; 325:202-208.

[25] Tutone VK, Mark PB, Stewart GA, *et al.* Hypertension, antihypertensive agents and outcomes following renal transplantation. Clin Transplant 2005; 19:181-192.

[26] Holdaas H, Kobashigawa JA, Fellstrom B, Jardine AG. Special Transplant Populations: Transplant recipients. In: Clinical Lipidology, 1 edn. , edited by Ballantyne CM, Elsevier, Philadelphia, 2008, pp 486-499.

[27] Opelz G, Wujciak T, Ritz E. Association of chronic kidney graft failure with recipient blood pressure. Collaborative Transplant Study. Kidney Int 1998;53:217-222.

[28] Heinze G, Mitterbauer C, Regele H, *et al.* Angiotensin-converting enzyme inhibitor or angiotensin II type 1 receptor antagonist therapy is associated with prolonged patient and graft survival after renal transplantation. J Am Soc Nephrol 2006; 17:889-899.

[29] Opelz G, Zeier M, Laux G, *et al.* No improvement of patient or graft survival in transplant recipients treated with angiotensin-converting enzyme inhibitors or angiotensin II type 1 receptor blockers: a collaborative transplant study report. J Am Soc Nephrol 2006; 17:3257-3262.

[30] Philipp T, Martinez F, Geiger H, *et al.* Candesartan improves blood pressure control and reduces proteinuria in renal transplant recipients: results from SECRET. Nephrol Dial Transplant 2010; 25:967-976

[31] Vanrenterghem Y, van Hooff JP, Squifflet JP, *et al.* Minimization of immunosuppressive therapy after renal transplantation: results of a randomized controlled trial. Am J Transplant 2005;5:87-95.

[32] Srinivas TR, Meier-Kriesche HU. Minimizing immunosuppression, an alternative approach to reducing side effects: objectives and interim result. Clin J Am Soc Nephrol 3 2008;Suppl 2:S101-S116.

[33] Johnson RW, Kreis H, Oberbauer R, *et al.* Sirolimus allows early cyclosporine withdrawal in renal transplantation resulting in improved renal function and lower blood pressure. Transplantation 2001; 72:777-786.

[34] Wheatley K, Ives N, Gray R, *et al.* Revascularization versus medical therapy for renal-artery stenosis. N Engl J Med 2009; 361:1953-1962.

[35] Holdaas H, Jardine AG, Wheeler DC, *et al.* Effect of fluvastatin on acute renal allograft rejection: a randomized multicenter trial. Kidney Int 2001;60:1990-1997.

[36] Artz MA, Boots JM, Ligtenberg G, *et al.* Randomized conversion from cyclosporine to tacrolimus in renal transplant patients: improved lipid profile and unchanged plasma homocysteine levels. Transplant Proc2002; 34:1793-1794.

[37] Knight SR, Morris PJ. Steroid avoidance or withdrawal after renal transplantation increases the risk of acute rejection but decreases cardiovascular risk. A meta-analysis. Transplantation 2010; 89:1-14.

[38] Wissing KM, Unger P, Ghisdal L, *et al.* Effect of atorvastatin therapy and conversion to tacrolimus on hypercholesterolemia and endothelial dysfunction after renal transplantation. Transplantation 2006; 82:771-778.

[39] Cosio FG, Pesavento TE, Pelletier RP, *et al.* Patient survival after renal transplantation III: the effects of statins. Am J Kidney Dis 2002; 40:638-643.

[40] Zhang W, Liu M, Wu Y, *et al.* Protective effects of atorvastatin on chronic allograft nephropathy in rats. J Surg. Res2007; 143:428-436.

[41] Kasiske BL, Klinger D. Cigarette smoking in renal transplant recipients. J Am Soc Nephrol 2000;11:753-759.

[42] Zoccali C. Traditional and emerging cardiovascular and renal risk factors: an epidemiologic perspective. Kidney Int 2006;70:26-33.

[43] Fellstrom B, Holdaas H, Jardine AG, *et al.* Risk factors for reaching renal endpoints in the assessment of Lescol in renal transplantation (ALERT) trial. Transplantation 2005;79:205-212.

[44] Soveri I, Holdaas H, Jardine A, *et al.* Renal transplant dysfunction--importance quantified in comparison with traditional risk factors for cardiovascular disease and mortality. Nephrol Dial Transplant 2006; 21:2282-2289.

[45] Balla A, Chobanian M. New-onset diabetes after transplantation: a review of recent literature. Curr. Opin. Organ Transplant 2009; 14:375-379.

[46] Wilkinson A, Davidson J, Dotta F, *et al.* Guidelines for the treatment and management of new-onset diabetes after transplantation. Clin Transplant 2005;19:291-298.

[47] Cosio FG, Kudva Y, van der Velde M, *et al.* New onset hyperglycemia and diabetes are associated with increased cardiovascular risk after kidney transplantation. Kidney Int 2005;67:2415-2421.

[48] Joss N, Staatz CE, Thomson AH, Jardine AG. Predictors of new onset diabetes after renal transplantation. Clin Transplant 2007; 21:136-143.

[49] Cole EH, Johnston O, Rose CL, Gill JS. Impact of acute rejection and new-onset diabetes on long-term transplant graft and patient survival. Clin J Am Soc Nephrol 2008;3:814-821.

[50] De Lima JJ, Gowdak LH, de Paula FJ, *et al.* Treatment of Coronary Artery Disease in Hemodialysis Patients Evaluated for Transplant-A Registry Study. Transplantation 2010;89: 845-850.

[51] Patel RK, Mark PB, Johnston N, *et al.* Prognostic value of cardiovascular screening in potential renal transplant recipients: a single-center prospective observational study. Am J Transplant 2008;8:1673-1683.

CHAPTER 23

Glomerulonephritis After Kidney Transplantation

Bela Ivanyi[1,*], Dejan Dobi[1], Eva Kemeny[1] and Edit Szederkenyi[2]

[1]*Department of Pathology,* [2]*Renal Transplantation Unit, Clinics of Surgery, University of Szeged, Szeged, Hungary*

Abstract: The prevalence, impact and main clinicopathological aspects of recurrent and *de novo* glomerulonephritis are reviewed, with the use of unpublished data of the authors. The prevalence in Hungarian recipients was investigated in 697 biopsies obtained for cause and analyzed by light microscopy and an expanded panel of immunofluorescence. Electron microscopy was performed if there were symptoms of glomerular disease or the histological alterations or immunfluorescent findings indicated. Glomerular disease was recorded in 199 biopsies (28.5%): chronic rejection-induced transplant glomerulopathy in 155 biopsies (22.2%), post-transplantation glomerulonephritis (recurrent, *de novo* or undetermined) in 39 (5.5%) biopsies, and systemic disease affecting the glomeruli in 8 biopsies (1.1%). Membranous nephropathy (17), IgA nephritis (9), focal-segmental glomerulosclerosis (8), mesangial proliferative glomerulonephritis, (3) IgM nephropathy (1) and type I membranoproliferative glomerulonephritis (1) were identified. Transplant glomerulopathy frequently coincided with membranous nephropathy. Unusual combinations of histological patterns and/or immunofluorescent findings were occasionally observed, such as mesangial proliferation with mesangial and peripheral immune deposits, or epimembranous and mesangial deposits, or mesangial proliferation and subperimesangial deposits of solely IgM. Post-transplantation GN, more frequent in males, unfavorably influenced graft survival. Our results and the literature data indicate that post-transplantation glomerulonephritis relatively rarely involves the white race. Male gender, non-white ethnicity, younger age and biopsy-proven glomerulonephritis in the native kidney are predictors of post-transplantation glomerulonephritis. Post-transplantation glomerulonephritis contributes significantly to late allograft loss; through elevated serum creatinine levels and proteinuria, it precipitates the cardiovascular mortality and morbidity of the recipient. Limited evidence is available on the management of post-transplantation glomerulonephritis.

Keywords: *De novo* Glomerulonephritis, Epidemiology, Kidney Transplant, Recurrent Glomerulonephritis, Plasmapheresis, Rituximab, Steroids, Immunosuppression, Kidney Biopsy, Membranous Nephropathy.

INTRODUCTION

Up to 43% of kidney allograft recipients develop proteinuria of more than 1 g/24 h, which may reach the nephritic range in up to 13% of these individuals [1, 2]. Chronic antibody-mediated rejection-induced transplant glomerulopathy, calcineurin inhibitor toxicity, and recurrent and *de novo* (new-onset) glomerulonephritis (GN) all produce proteinuria, and differentiation between these conditions can be achieved only by morphological evaluation of the allograft tissue. GN is defined as recurrent when the same form of GN as in the native kidney recurs in the transplanted kidney, whereas it is *de novo* when the type of GN is different from that which existed in the patient before transplantation. In general, most recurrences tend to develop in the first few weeks after transplantation (though in a wide range of from days to years), whereas *de novo* diseases usually appear years after transplantation. The present chapter reviews the prevalence, pathogenesis, main histopathological features, clinical correlates and effects on graft outcome of recurrent and *de novo* GNs in kidney allografts. Some unpublished data of the authors on the clinicopathologic features of post-transplantation GN are presented. Treatment options are briefly outlined.

The prevalence of recurrent and *de novo* GN is not accurately known, for at least four reasons. First, there is a lack of consensus regarding the clinical approach to an allograft dysfunction occurring more than 12

***Address correspondence to Bela Ivanyi:** Department of Pathology, University of Szeged, Allomas utca 2, Szeged H-6720, Hungary; Tel: +36-62-545148; Fax: +36-62-545 868; E-mail: ivanyi@patho.szote.u-szeged.hu

Massimiliano Veroux and Pierfrancesco Veroux (Eds)

months after transplantation. Urinalysis may not be performed routinely during outpatient surveillance or prior biopsy; recipients who display proteinuria, hematuria and/or an increased serum creatinine level are evaluated differently; and the proteinuria is frequently viewed as a consequence of transplant glomerulopathy, and biopsy is not carried out. Second, there is a marked interlaboratory variance in the handling and processing of renal transplant biopsies. In view of cost and benefit concerns, some laboratories evaluate the biopsies only with special light microscopic stainings and immunohistochemical staining of complement 4d (C4d) to detect antibody-mediated rejection, and do not consider details of glomerular pathology not related to rejection. Others supplement this protocol with a panel of antibodies to identify immunoglobulins and various complement components, and regularly sample kidney tissue for electron microscopy, rendering the diagnosis of recurrent or *de novo* GN possible. Some laboratories routinely apply this expanded protocol from the beginning of the post-transplantation period, while others do so only from the first year after transplantation, and yet others do so only if the recipient displays substantial proteinuria before the biopsy. The third factor influencing the prevalence data is the situation that the native glomerular disease is not verified by biopsy in a significant proportion of patients who present with contracted kidneys, and the biopsy-proven GN that develops after transplantation in these patients may therefore be either recurrent or *de novo*. As a result, some investigators do not distinguish between the data for these two types of disease, referring simply to 'post-transplantation' GN. The fourth reason limiting a clear-cut picture of prevalence is the uncertainty concerning the inclusion or exclusion of recipients with systemic diseases involving the glomeruli/metabolic glomerulopathies [3].

The impact of post-transplantation GN on graft survival is not easy to determine either, because recurrent or *de novo* GN may itself rarely cause graft failure. In the majority of cases, acute and/or chronic rejection and/or chronic calcineurin inhibitor toxicity coexist with post-transplantation GN, and the conditions together contribute to graft loss. *Via* elevated serum creatinine levels and proteinuria, post-transplantation GN contributes significantly to cardiovascular morbidity and mortality of the recipient [4, 5].

RECURRENT AND *DE NOVO* GLOMERULAR DISEASES: EXPERIENCE FROM A SINGLE CENTER

Material and Methods

In the Department of Pathology, University of Szeged, Hungary, the standard procedures for the evaluation of kidney transplant biopsies involve the combination of light microscopy (hematoxylin and eosin, periodic acid-Schiff, Masson's trichome, acid fuchsin orange G, methenamine silver and elastin) and immunofluorescence (antibodies to IgG, IgA, IgM and C3; and C4d and HLA-DR from the year 2000), and the fixation and embedding of samples for optional electron microscopy in each case. The ultrastructural examination of glomeruli is carried out if the light microscopic morphology of the glomeruli is abnormal, or the immunofluorescence reveals positivity, or the patient displays symptoms of glomerular disease. The protocol allows the identification of post-transplantation GN even if glomerular manifestations of acute or chronic rejection coincide. Between January 1, 1990 and August 1, 2009, 697 biopsy samples carried out for cause were sent to our department. Both donors and recipients were almost exclusively Caucasians, and almost all grafts were obtained from deceased donors. A few recipients were romas. The vast majority of the recipients were immunosuppressed with cyclosporine and steroids between 1990 and 1998, and with tacrolimus or cyclosporine, mycophenolate mofetil and steroids from 1998. Post-transplantation GN was diagnosed on the basis of the characteristic light microscopic, immunofluorescence and electron microscopic features. Post-transplantation GN occurred either alone or with other causes of allograft dysfunction, such as chronic antibody-mediated or T-cell-mediated rejection, and/or acute T-cell-mediated rejection grades IA or IB, and/or borderline changes, and/or calcineurin inhibitor nephrotoxicity. The latter conditions were diagnosed as described in the Banff consensus papers [6, 7] and standard textbooks.

The cases were retrieved from the registry of the nephropathological laboratory. The interval between the time of transplantation and the biopsy diagnosis, the presence of proteinuria and/or hematuria, and the estimated GFR (eGFR) at the time of diagnosis were collected from the patients' records. The degree of proteinuria was determined with the dipstick method. The eGFR values were calculated by using the 4-variable Modification of Diet in Renal Disease formula. The impact of post-transplantation GN on the 10-year graft survival was studied in the case group (GN-positive group) matched with a selected series of controls (GN-negative group). The latter comprised 91 patients who were transplanted between January 1, 1998 and December 31, 2002, and were on a triple immunosuppressive regimen, and who underwent biopsy because of a graft dysfunction. The evaluation revealed chronic antibody-mediated or T-cell-mediated rejection, and/or acute T-cell mediated rejection of grade IA or IB, and/or borderline changes, and/or calcineurin inhibitor nephrotoxicity, and/or interstitial fibrosis and tubular atrophy, with no evidence of any specific etiology. Loss of graft function was defined as the point at which dialysis had to be restarted. None of the groups included patients who died with a functioning graft. Since the case group comprised a relatively low number of recipients, the gender, the mean eGFR values, and the duration of graft survival were compared with the controls without separation of the case group into specific glomerular diseases.

Statistics

Gender predominance was tested with the χ^2-probe. Differences in mean eGFR values at the time of the biopsy were compared by means of Student's t-test. Graft survival was investigated by using Kaplan-Meier Survival Analysis.

Results

Lesions indicative of glomerular disease were observed in 199 biopsies (28.5%): transplant glomerulopathy in 155 biopsies (22.2%), post-transplantation GN in 39 (5.5%), and systemic disease affecting the glomeruli in 8 (1.1%). Some pertinent features of post-transplantation GN are presented in Table **1**. Post-transplantation GN and transplant glomerulopathy coincided in 11 cases. New-onset hyaline arteriolopathy with or without peripheral nodular protein deposits indicative of chronic calcineurin inhibitor nephrotoxicity was recorded in cases with membranous nephropathy (MNP) on 4 occasions, in IgA nephritis (IGAN) on 4 occasions, in *de novo* focal-segmental glomerulosclerosis (FSGS) on 2 occasions, and in the case with undetermined FSGS. Post-transplantation GN occurred more frequently in males (not plotted; p=.012), the mean eGFR values at biopsy were significantly lower in the GN-positive group (Fig. **1**; p=.0056), and the graft survival proved significantly worse in the GN-positive group (Fig. **2**; p=.011). Glomerular involvement of systemic disease included a case of recurrent diabetic nephropathy, a case of recurrent kappa-light chain deposition disease in a patient with myeloma, a case of recurrent Fabry's disease, a case of recurrent anti-tubular basement membrane nephritis and MNP, a case of *de novo* pauci-immune segmental necrotizing GN, and 3 cases of thrombotic microangiopathy (TMA; acute antibody-mediated rejection and calcineurin inhibitor toxicity were excluded).

Table 1: Clinicopathologic features of post-transplantation GN in the biopsy series of University of Szeged, Hungary

	Recurrent	***De novo***	**Undetermined**
Membranous NP N=17		17 cases; 68 months (7-156) PU 3+: 12; 2+: 1; 1+: 1; n.a.: 3 HCV-pos. 1 Purely membranous 8 With TxG 5 With TxG and crescents (50%) 1 With IgM deposits and TxG 1 With mesangial IgG deposits and mesangial proliferation 2	
IgAN N=9	5 cases; 67 months (49-102) Microhematuria and PU 3+: 1; 2+: 2, 1+: 1 Only PU 2+: 1 Mesangial proliferation 3 With TxG 2	1 case; 109 months Microhaematuria and PU 3+ Mesangial proliferation 1	3 cases; 66 months (48-84) Microhaematuria and PU 2+: 2; n.a.: 1 Mesangial proliferation 2 With CyA-induced TMA 1

Table 1: cont….

FSGS N=8	5 cases; 54 months (3-74) PU 3+: 4; 2+: 1 NOS type 4 Cellular type 1	2 cases; 141 months (139-144) PU 3+: 1; 2+:1 *Post-transplantation diabetes, hypertension, extreme obesity and HbsAg-pos. NOS type 1 *Perihilar type 1	1 cases; 12 months PU 2+ Cellular type
Mesangial proliferative GN N=3	1 case; 28 months PU 1+ Mesangial IgG, IgM, and C3; mild mesangial proliferation	1 case; 40 months PU 1+ Mesangial, subendothelial and intramembranous IgG, IgM, C3, and C1q; mesangial proliferation	1 case; 72 months PU 3+ and microhematuria Mesangial and subendothelial IgG, IgA, and C3; mesangial proliferation, TxG, crescents (10%) and secondary FSGS
IgMNP N=1		1 case; 33 months PU 3+; HBsAg-pos. Mild mesangial expansion, subperimesangial electron-dense IgM deposits, no C3	
MPGN type I N=1	1 case; 36 months PU 3+ and microhematuria Mesangial and subendothelial IgG and C3; MPGN with segmental glomerular sclerosis		

Abbreviations: N – the number of cases with the diagnosed condition; months – the interval between engraftment and diagnosis (mean and range); PU – proteinuria determined by the dipstick method and expressed as as 1+, 2+ or 3+; n.a.: not available; TxG – antibody-mediated rejection-induced transplant glomerulopathy; CyA-induced TMA – cyclosporine-induced thrombotic microangiopathy; HBsAg – hepatitis B surface antigen, HCV – hepatitis C virus; pos. – positive; C3 - complement 3 factor.

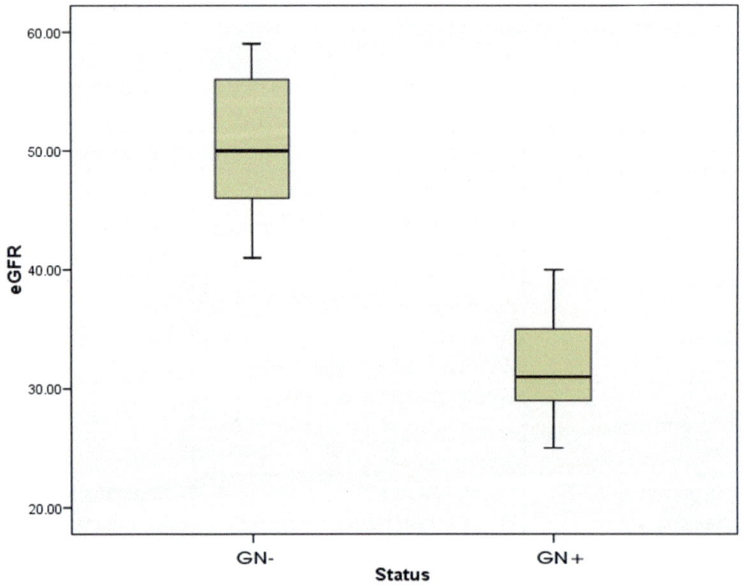

Figure 1: Box diagram of eGFR values in the group with post-transplantation GN (GN+) and the group without glomerular disease (GN-). The group with post-transplantation GN had significantly worse renal function at the time of the biopsy.

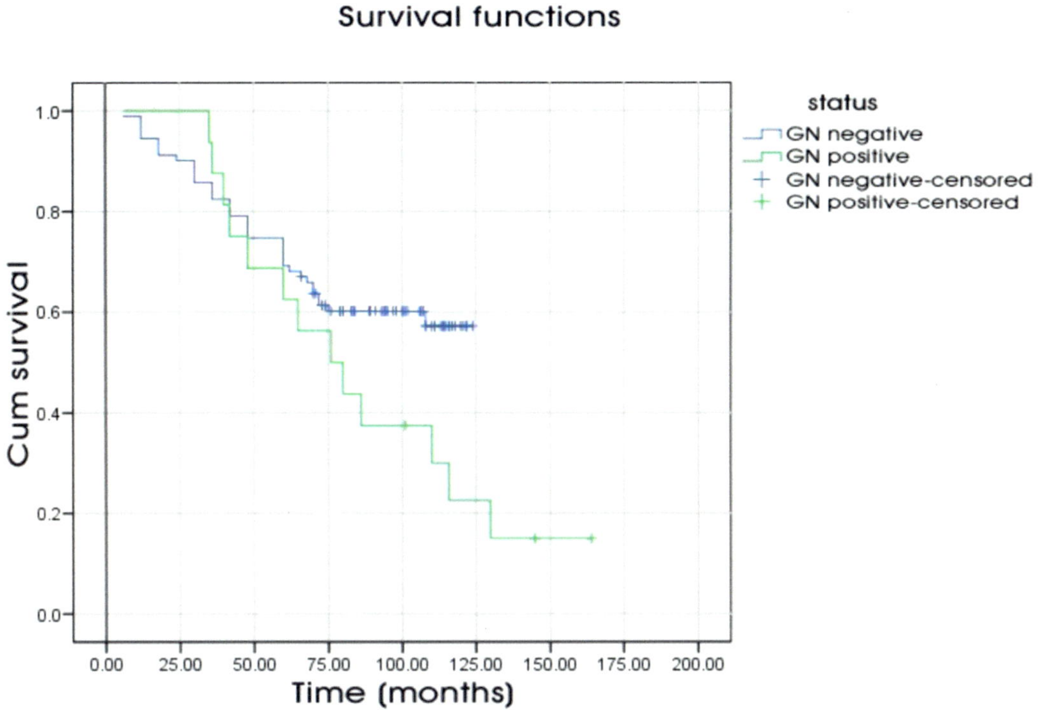

Figure 2: Graft survival in the group with post-transplantation GN (bottom line) and the group without post-transplantation GN (upper line). The survival was significantly worse in the post-transplantation GN group.

PREVALENCE, PREDICTORS AND OUTCOME OF POST-TRANSPLANTATION GLOMERULONEPHRITIS

The most common glomerular lesion in our material was transplant glomerulopathy, occurring in a similar range as in other series: 20-25% of long-surviving renal allografts [8]. The lesion is alloantibody-mediated [9, 10], characterized light microscopically by double-contoured glomerular capillary loops, and is associated with proteinuria and a declining graft function. It must be differentiated from membranoproliferative GN (MPGN), TMA, or cryoglobulinemic G/hepatitis C virus-related GN, which do not pose a problem if tissue for immunofluorescence and electron microscopy is available. Post-transplantation GN occurred relatively infrequently (5.5%) in our series. Males were affected more frequently, and post-transplantation GN *per se* influenced the graft survival unfavourably. Literature data indicate that geographic and ethnic differences exist in the prevalence of post-transplantation GN. The Caucasian population in Eastern Europe, for example, seems to be affected by post-transplantation GN relatively rarely, since, similarly to our experience from Hungary, a low prevalence of post-transplantation GN was reported from Poland [11]. By contrast, in the series of the Renal Allograft Disease Registry/USA, post-transplantation GN occurred in 13.2% of the cases [12, 13]. In a recent Canadian study, male gender, non-white ethnicity, younger age, and biopsy-proven GN in the native kidney predicted post-transplantation GN [14]. Children have a greater prevalence than adults [15]. Our results confirm the earlier observations that post-transplantation GN results in a reduced graft survival, and post-transplantation GN *per se* is an independent contributor to late allograft loss [14, 16].

Series on recurrent GN reveal a prevalence of 1.8% to 19%, which increases with the duration of the follow-up [12, 13, 17-20]. In an Australian study, recurrent GN was responsible for 8.4% of all graft losses at 10 years after transplantation [19]. The recurrence rates and graft losses due to recurrence are listed in Table **2**.

Table 2: Overview of recurrence and recurrence related graft loss [3]

	Clinical Recurrence Rate (% of Recipients)	Graft Loss After 5-10 Years (% of Recipients)
FSGS	20-30	50
Membranous NP	10-30	50
MPGN type 1	20-33	high
MPGN type 2	67-100	high
Anti-GBM nephritis	uncommon	probably low
ANCA-pos. crescentic GN	7-20	0-7
IgA nephritis	7-58	3-26
Idiopathic D⁻HUS	33-56	90

Immunosuppressive regimens, including steroids, do not influence the rate of histologic recurrence or graft loss [14, 19, 20]. Treatment with an angiotensin-converting enzyme inhibitor or an angiotensin II type 1 receptor antagonist decreases the progression of native kidney diseases, but for unclear reasons, this renoprotective effect could not be demonstrated in a series involving more than 17000 kidney transplants [21]. Only limited evidence is available on the management of post-transplantation GN, and clinical practice is based on non-randomized and uncontrolled case series. In the following paragraphs, the most important types of post-transplantation GN will be reviewed, beginning with those observed in our own biopsy material.

Membranous Nephropathy (MNP)

MNP, the most common cause of nephrotic syndrome in Caucasian adults, is characterized by the accumulation of immune deposits on the outer aspect of the glomerular basement membrane (GBM), leading to thickening of the capillary loops. In the past few years, two antigens have been identified in human MNP. The first is the type-M phospholipase A2 receptor, which has proved to be the autoantigen in the majority of adult MNP cases [22], and the second is neutral endopeptidase, involved in the very rare neonatal form of MNP [23]. These antigens are expressed on the podocyte surface, where they serve as targets for circulating antibodies (often IgG4), leading to *in situ* immune complex formation, and generation of the membrane attack complex of complement C5b-9. The membrane attack complex seems to be formed in sublytic quantities that activate the podocytes to the production of oxygen radicals and matrix metalloproteinase-9 and the peroxidation of lipids, which in turn damage the GBM and proteinuria ensues [23].

De novo MNP

This is the most frequent *de novo* GN in kidney transplants [8], an observation that held true for our own biopsy series. In the majority of our cases, it was associated with nephrotic-range proteinuria, diagnosed at a mean of 68 months post-transplantation. In our experience, the morphological manifestation of the disease may differ from that observed in the native kidneys: MNP may coincide with transplant glomerulopathy, or the membranous lesion may associate with some other pattern(s) of glomerular injury, or the deposits may prove unusual. Accordingly, coincidence with transplant glomerulopathy was encountered in more than one-third of the cases. We noted 2 patients in whom the subepithelial IgG deposits were associated with mesangial deposits of IgG and mesangial cell proliferation (lupus nephritis was excluded after biopsy), and one patient in whom the subepithelial deposits were positive for IgM, but not for IgG as seen earlier in his native kidneys. This case also exhibited coexisting transplant glomerulopathy. We also experienced a particular case involving a mixture of MNP, transplant glomerulopathy and cellular crescents in half of the glomeruli. The common association of *de novo* MNP with transplant glomerulopathy, similarly observed in other series worldwide, raises the possibility that *de novo* MNP is a special manifestation of chronic antibody-mediated rejection, possibly mediated by the *in situ* formation of immune deposits through antibodies directed to transplantation antigens. Indeed, donor-specific antibodies can be detected at the time of the biopsy in a significant number of patients with *de novo* MNP [24]. Besides rejection, hepatitis C virus infection has been considered as an etiological factor for *de novo* MNP [25]. The prognosis is dismal: 40-60% of the patients lose their grafts within 3-6 years after the diagnosis.

Recurrent MNP

Recent publications identified two patterns: early and late recurrence [25, 26]. Recurrence is usually heralded by proteinuria, often in the nephrotic range. Half of the cases progress to end-stage renal failure a decade later [27]. In a series of protocol biopsies, the initial clinical manifestations of recurrent MNP were mild or absent [28] indicating that heavy proteinuria may not be an immediate consequence of immune complex formation along the glomerular capillary loops.

Treatment

Anti-CD20 antibody (rituximab) was recently demonstrated to reduce proteinuria effectively in small series of patients with recurrent MNP [26, 29, 30].

IgA nephritis (IgAN)

IgAN is defined by the presence of dominant or codominant mesangial deposits of IgA on immunofluorescence microscopy. The glomeruli display a broad spectrum of histologic changes, related in part to the differences in the indication for the biopsy by the referring nephrologist. The pathogenesis is not fully known. Mucosal antigenic exposure, in genetically susceptible individuals, results in the production of nephritogenic polymeric IgA molecules of the IgA1 subclass lacking galactose and sialic acid-containing residues in some of the 5-9 glycan side-chains in the hinge region. The polymeric galactose-deficient IgA1 autoantigen and a glycan-specific oligoclonal IgG1 autoantibody form circulating immune complexes and eventually deposits in the mesangium, perhaps by interaction with IgA receptors (such as the transferring receptor, CD71) located on the surface of mesangial cells, and induce inflammation [31-33]. In some patients, IgA1 deposition is not followed by inflammation (hidden or 'lanthanic' deposits, usually without the co-deposition of IgG or C3); in others, the inflammation resolves without fibrosis; and in the remainder, progressive glomerular injury ensues.

In our series, post-transplantation IgAN was manifested clinically by microhematuria and proteinuria of various degrees in all but one patient, and by moderate proteinuria alone in one patient with recurrent disease; thus, the presentation was similar to that in the native kidneys. All cases displayed mesangial proliferative GN on light microscopy, in 2 cases coincident with transplant glomerulopathy, and in one case with cyclosporine-induced TMA. Literature data indicate that the histologic recurrence rate depends on the length of the follow-up and the biopsy policy. In 30-50% or even more of the recipients, the disease will recur if followed for more than 5 years. Recurrent IgAN fortunately contributes to a significant graft dysfunction or loss of only between 3% and 26% of the cases [17, 34-40]. The risk factors for recurrence are not known. The data from the Australia & New Zealand Dialysis and Transplant Registry demonstrated that IgAN recurred more frequently among recipients from living donors if there were no HLA mismatches. However, there was no difference in graft survival between zero and ≥1 HLA-mismatched living donor recipients [37].

Treatment

Clear-cut therapeutic recommendations are not available. The use of anti-lymphocyte induction regimens, followed by the conventional post-transplant maintenance immunosuppression treatment protocol, may exert a slight adverse effect on the risk of recurrence [33]. Tonsillectomy with or without steroid pulse therapy may lead to a reduction of proteinuria in an appreciable proportion of patients with recurrent IgAN [4, 41].

Focal Segmental Glomerulosclerosis (FSGS)

The lesion of FSGS is characterized histologically by variable amounts of sclerosis, hypercellularity and hyalin deposition, all of which affect some (but not all) of the glomeruli and involve only segments of each glomerulus. The 'Columbia classification' distinguishes five morphologic variants of primary FSGS in native kidneys: classic, cellular, diffuse mesangial hypercellularity, collapsing, and tip lesion [42].

Recurrent FSGS

The majority of FSGS cases are non-hereditary. A circulating albuminuric factor has been at the focus of interest as concerns the pathogenesis since 1984, when rats infused with serum from a patient with recurrent FSGS developed proteinura [43]. Attempts have been made to determine the nature of this putative permeability factor [44], but its molecular characterization has remained elusive. In hereditary FSGS, mutations have been identified in genes encoding podocyte proteins, including WT1, NPHS2, ACTN4, CD2AP and TRPC6. Mutations in the NPHS2 gene (which encodes podocin) are the most common cause of hereditary FSGS, and may occur in some patients with sporadic nephrotic syndrome [45, 46]. The rate of recurrence in NPHS2 homozygous or compound heterozygous mutation carriers (two pathogenic mutations in the NPHS2 gene) is below 10%. By contrast, patients with the rarer heterozygous mutations (affected by only one NPHS2 mutation) display a recurrence rate of more than 30% [47, 48], comparable to that in non-hereditary FSGS. Although the circulating permeability factor has been demonstrated in some patients with one pathogenic NPHS2 mutation [49], elucidation of the exact relationship between the heterozygous mutation of NPHS2 and the circulating permeability factor awaits further studies.

The onset of proteinuria in patients with recurrence is frequently observed within weeks after kidney transplantation, and 80% of the patients become nephrotic. A significant number of patients also undergo acute renal failure; hypertension and hematuria are common. Recurrence leads to graft loss within 5 years in 50% of the cases. Risk factors for recurrence include childhood FSGS (a recurrence rate of 50-80% under the age of 6 years), a rapid progression (within 3 years) from diagnosis to end-stage renal failure, white race, diffuse mesangial hypercellularity in the native kidney biopsy, and recurrence in a previous allograft [50-53]. In a recent multicenter study, 81% of the cases recurred in the same pattern as for the original disease [54], while in another study, the variant type observed in the native kidneys was not predictive of either recurrence or the type of FSGS seen on the allograft [55]. Our series comprised 5 cases of recurrent FSGS. Unfortunately, not all the FSGS cases in the native kidney were diagnosed in our department, and, we could therefore not compare the subtype of FSGS in the native kidney and in the allograft.

Treatment

Prior to transplantation, it is suggested that FSGS should be treated with non-steroidal anti-inflammatory drugs, with or without angiotensin blockade, and the degree of proteinuria should be reduced to below 1 g/day in order to detect the recurrence of significant proteinuria as early as possible after transplantation. Plasmapheresis plus cyclosporine prior to transplantation may prevent recurrent FSGS in high-risk patients. The avoidance of living donor kidney transplantation is recommended if risk factors for recurrence are present [51]. Bilateral nephrectomy might be considered if conventional anti-proteinuric treatment proves ineffective. Following transplantation, the recipient should be monitored daily for proteinuria until discharge, then weekly for 4 weeks, and monthly for 1 year, and a diagnostic kidney biopsy should be performed if the 24-h urine protein level is equal to or exceeds 2 g. The full-blown histologic lesion of FSGS may not be observed up to 4-6 weeks after transplantation, but electron microscopic evaluation of the glomeruli reveals diffuse effacement of the foot processes. Well-designed clinical trials of the treatment of recurrent FSGS are lacking. Prolonged and repeated courses of plasmapheresis or immunoadsorption are conventionally carried out, usually in combination with some other form of treatment, such as cyclophosphamide, an increased dosage of cyclosporine in children, rituximab, angiotensin converting enzyme inhibitors or indomethacin [51, 53, 56, 59, 60]. Plasmapheresis combined with rituximab may result in prolonged remission of proteinuria [52, 57]. However, nonresponsiveness may occur [57, 58]. Plasmapheresis, increased immunosuppression, and the administration of anti-TNFalpha treatment induced a decrease of proteinuria in a case of early recurrent FSGS [61].

De novo FSGS

The pathogenesis is unclear. It develops later than recurrent FSGS, also noted in our series, and it might be related somehow to chronic cyclosporine nephrotoxicity [1, 62, 63]. Indeed, both patients in our material had received cyclosporine as part of the immunosuppressive regimen, and the biopsy evaluation revealed either FSGS of NOS type or FSGS of perihilar type, and chronic calcineurin inhibitor nephrotoxicity. The patient with perihilar FSGS had other factors influencing the glomerular morphology: post-transplantation diabetes, hypertension, and morbid obesity. The FSGS lesion may also be encountered in cases with 'chronic allograft nephropathy' and chronic rejection-induced transplant glomerulopathy, but also in the absence of these conditions. In the series of Ohio State University, FSGS was observed in 30% of the cases with 'chronic allograft nephropathy' at a mean of 57 months post-transplantation. 24% of the patients with FSGS on biopsy exhibited the nephrotic syndrome. At 5 years after diagnosis, recipients with *de novo* FSGS had a graft survival of 40%, as compared with 60% in those with 'chronic allograft nephropathy' alone [63].

Collapsing FSGS may occur in HIV-infected individuals or as an idiopathic form, characterized clinically by heavy proteinuria, a progressive renal insufficiency and rapid evolution to end-stage renal disease. In one study, the majority of cases of collapsing FSGS in kidney transplants occurred *de novo*. Both *de novo* and recurrent collapsing FSGS displayed a higher rate of graft loss relative to non-collapsing variants of FSGS [64]. No reliable data exist on the rates of or clinical correlates of other variants of *de novo* FSGS that occur after transplantation.

Mesangial Proliferative GN and IgM Nephropathy

These entities are not well documented in the literature. Their reported incidences would probably be higher if immunofluorescence and electron microscopy were performed routinely on all allograft biopsies. In our series, the category of mesangial proliferative GN included a recurrent case, and 2 cases with a mixture of mesangial and peripheral immune deposits, and mesangial proliferation. We recall that 2 cases were classified as *de novo* MNP, in which the subepithelial deposits codeposited with mesangial immune deposits. These unusual combinations indicate that in the kidney allograft a small fraction of GN cannot be assigned to any well-established category of GN. Clinically, the recurrent and the *de novo* case of mesangial proliferative GN displayed only mild proteinuria, whereas heavy proteinuria and microhematuria were noted in the undetermined case. The proteinuria in the latter case could be related to coincident transplant glomerulopathy.

As concerns IgM nephropathy, similar cases were reported from Canada: a total of 118 consecutive renal allograft biopsies were studied by light microscopy, immunofluorescence and electron microscopy, and 4 patients showed IgM-positive mesangial electron-dense deposits, with or without C3 positivity [65]. One patient had IgAN in the native kidney (but IgA was negative in the graft biopsy), and 3 patients displayed current viral infection (BK, cytomegalovirus, and hepatitis C and B). The etiology of post-transplantation IgM nephropathy remains unclear, but the morphologic features suggest that it should be regarded as a separate clinicopathological entity.

Membranoproliferative Glomerulonephritis (MPGN)

The histologic features include mesangial hypercellularity and expansion, giving rise to the lobular appearance of the glomeruli, and thickening of the capillary loops because of mesangial cell interposition and duplication of the GBM. Three clinico-pathologic types are distinguished, all of which affect mainly children and young adults. Type 1 (subendothelial deposits) and type 3 (subendothelial and subepithelial deposits) have an immune complex pathogenesis. Type 2 is a very rare disorder, characterized by the presence of C3 nephritic factor, activation of the alternate complement pathway, persistent systemic hypocomplementemia, C3 deposition along the GBMs, a membranoproliferative pattern on light microscopy and electron-dense transformation of the lamina densa of the GBM (dense deposit disease). The membranoproliferative lesion in a renal allograft raises the possibility of recurrent or *de novo* MPGN, acute transplant glomerulitis, transplant glomerulopathy and TMA. Immunofluorescence and electron microscopy are essential in the differential diagnosis, since immune deposits are not present in the last three of these conditions [8].

Type 1 MPGN frequently recurs in graft recipients, and no form of treatment has proved effective. In our patient, the disease recurred 3 years after transplantation with nephrotic range proteinuria and microhaematuria. Graftectomy was carried out 1 year later, and the evaluation revealed MPGN with cellular crescents in 37% of the glomeruli. Recurrence may start without clinical symptoms, as documented in protocol biopsies [66]. Type 2 MPGN, with a high recurrence rate, presents with hematuria and heavy proteinuria during the first year after transplantation, accompanied by a slowly declining renal function. Again, no effective therapy is known. In a report on type 2 MPGN, the severity of mesangial proliferation was less than that observed in the native kidneys, and the recurrent disease was the cause of graft failure in 14.7% of the patients. Kidneys from living related donor had a significantly better 5-year survival rate (65.9%) as compared with kidneys from deceased donors (34.1%) [67]. In an Irish study, a younger age at the initial diagnosis, and the presence of crescents in the original biopsy proved to be risk factors for recurrence, and the authors concluded that the renal survival and the recurrence risk are determined by the severity of the primary MPGN, rather than the MPGN type [68].

Anti-GBM Nephritis

Anti-GBM nephritis is an uncommon disorder characterized by the formation of autoantibodies to the non-collagenous domain (NC1) of the α3 chain of type IV collagen, necrotizing-crescentic GN and a rapidly progressive GN syndrome. A significant proportion of the patients develop end-stage renal disease. Renal transplantation is usually delayed until the patients have been anti-GBM antibody-negative for at least 12 months. Recurrence, which is infrequent [69], may be manifested years after transplantation [70, 71], either as acute renal failure or as rapidly progressive GN. The allograft can be saved by methylprednisolone pulse therapy, with or without the administration of cyclosphosphamide, together with plasma exchange.

Pauci-Immune Crescentic GN

The anti-neutrophil cytoplasmic antibody (ANCA)-associated vasculitides, *i.e.* Wegener's granulomatosis, microscopic polyangitis, Churg-Strauss syndrome and idiopathic necrotizing crescentic GN, lead to segmental/global necrotizing inflammation of the glomeruli with the formation of crescents, the absence or paucity of glomerular immunoglobulins or complement, and usually a rapidly progressive GN syndrome.

Recurrence may develop even years after the transplantation [18, 72-74]. Clinically, there is a rapid rise in the serum creatinine level, accompanied by an active urine sediment, with or without symptoms of vasculitis involving other organs. The pre-transplantation disease course, the cANCA or pANCA specificity, the disease subtype and the ANCA titer in the absence of clinically active disease are not predictive of recurrence [72, 75]. Kidney transplantation should be delayed until the disease is inactive. Relapses are likely to respond to cyclophosphamide combined with plasmapheresis, with or without intravenous immunoglobulin administration. Refractory cases may be treated with rituximab [76]. In a report on 35 recipients with ANCA-associated vasculitis and immunosuppressed with antibody induction, corticosteroid, mycophenolate mofetil and tacrolimus, renal recurrence was not observed during a 5-year follow-up [77].

Alport syndrome

Three genetic forms exist: X-chromosome-linked (85%; XLAS), autosomal recessive (15%; ARAS) and autosomal dominant (5%; ADAS). XLAS arises from mutations in the COL4A5 gene, which encodes the type IV collagen α5 chain [α5(IV)]. ARAS results from mutations affecting both alleles of the COL4A3 or COL4A4 gene, which encode the type collagen IV α3(IV) chain and α4(IV) chain. The mutations block the developmental switch from the embryonic α1α1α2(IV) collagen network to the adult α3α4α5(IV) network. The kidney disease is characterized histologically by nonspecific segmental/global glomerulosclerosis, scattered interstitial fibrosis and tubular atrophy and interstitial foam cells, and electron microscopically by splitting, splintering, a basket weave appearance and thinning of the GBMs. Males with XLAS have childhood-onset microhematuria, and progressively worsening proteinuria, starting some years later than the hematuria, with 50% reaching the end-stage renal disease by the age of 25, 80% by the age of 40, and 100% by the age of 60. Females with XLAS are microhematuric, and the risk of end-stage renal disease is lower. In ARAS, the patients lack a family history of renal disease, and are haematuric, and females are affected as frequently as males. Progression to the end-stage renal disease before the age of 30 years is the rule. The heterozygous carriers of the COL4A3 and COL4A4 mutations are either asymptomatic or display microhematuria. For unreason reasons, a small number of these individuals follow a slowly progressive course and develop end-stage renal disease in middle age. These patients are considered to have ADAS [78].

Approximately, 5% of Alport patients develop post-transplantation anti-GBM nephritis [78], this being mediated by alloantibodies to the α5NC1domain in XLAS, and to the α3NC1 and α4NC1 domains in ARAS. The onset generally occurs within the first year following transplantation, and irreversible graft failure usually develops within a few weeks to months after the diagnosis. The clinical presentation is commonly a picture of rapidly progressive GN or occasionally a delayed graft function. Efforts with anti-T-cell therapy, pulse methylprednisolone and cyclophosphamide, longer-term plasmapheresis and the administration of mycophenolate mofetil have proved of only limited benefit. The accelerated development of post-transplantation anti-GBM nephritis has been observed in subsequent allografts [79]. There is a low risk of anti-GBM nephritis after transplantation among females with XLAS and patients who retain some GBM expression of α3α4α5 (IV) trimers because of missense mutations.

Hemolytic-Uremic Syndrome/Thrombotic Microangiopathy (HUS/TMA)

HUS is a rare disease manifested as microangiopathic hemolytic anemia, thrombocytopenia and acute renal failure. Histologically, the lesions of TMA are observed: the glomeruli are bloodless because of occlusion of the capillary tufts by subendothelial/endothelial swelling and mesangial cell interposition, and by microthrombi; the interlobular arteries and afferent arterioles exhibit fibrinoid necrosis and intimal hyperplasia, and are often occluded by thrombi. The majority of HUS cases occur in children and are triggered by *Shiga* toxin-producing *Escherichia coli* infection, with a manifestation of watery or bloody diarrhea (D^+ HUS). Other cases are not associated with diarrhea (D^- HUS), and mutations may be identified in one of the complement control proteins: factor H, factor I or membrane cofactor protein. These cases involve uncontrolled complement activation, which generally leads to end-stage renal disease [80]. Infrequently, familial HUS appears. The triggering factors of HUS in adults include pregnancy, exposure to drugs (*e.g.,* calcineurin inhibitors, oral contraceptives, mytomycin-C, quinine, ticlopidine and clopidogrel), bacterial or viral infections, and malignancies. Certain cases do not seem to be associated with any obvious etiologic factors and are regarded as idiopathic HUS [81].

Recurrent HUS

Whereas D^+ HUS and D^- HUS secondary to pregnancy, drugs, *etc.* usually do not recur, idiopathic D^- HUS has a significant recurrence rate [82]. In patients with a factor H or factor I mutation, a high recurrence rate was observed, whereas in patients with a membrane cofactor protein mutation, the recurrence rate proved low [83-86], indicating that membrane cofactor protein mutations are associated with a better prognosis. Recurrent HUS may be observed in the early postoperative period. Microangiopathic anemia, thrombocytopenia and renal failure are the leading sysmptoms; neurologic abnormalities and fever are infrequent. The diagnosis is difficult in routine biopsy practice, because TMA induced by recurrent HUS, acute antibody-mediated rejection, calcineurin inhibitor toxicity, bacterial or viral infection, or anticardiolipin antibodies cannot be differentiated on the basis of the morphology alone. C4d-positivity along the peritubular capillaries is a diagnostic marker of antibody-mediated rejection, and pronounced arterial intimal changes are not typical of calcineurin inhibitor-induced TMA.

Treatment

It is advised to avoid calcineurin inhibitors, mTOR antagonists and OKT3 in patients at high risk of recurrence. In the event of recurrence, plasma exchange and intravenous immunoglobulins should be administered until remission. If a response is not achieved, rituximab may be attempted [84]. The prognosis is dismal, however, in a significant number of cases [82]. The anti-complement monoclonal antibody eculizumab that binds to C5 and thus prevents generation of C5a and the membrane attack complex is a promising new therapeutic option in patients with a factor H mutation [87, 88].

De novo TMA

The most important risk factors are calcineurin inhibitors and mTOR drugs, which may amplify the endothelial lesions caused by ischemia-reperfusion injury, viral infection and/or rejection. *De novo* TMA usually occurs in the early post-transplant period [89]. The clinical picture is variable: some patients may present mild clinical and laboratory features of HUS, while others display a progressive graft dysfunction, often associated with arterial hypertension. The differential diagnosis is essentially the same as detailed above. Although therapeutic guidelines for *de novo* TMA are not well defined, withdrawal of the offending calcineurin inhibitor is important. The prognosis is less severe than with recurrent HUS. It is recommended not to start with a drug potentially involved in the etiology of a previous TMA [90].

Minimal Change Nephropathy (MCN)

De novo MCN is a rare cause of post-transplantation nephrotic syndrome, which may develop immediately after transplantation or later. MCN in the native kidney may be related to undetermined circulating permeability factors, probably lymphokines, secreted by T-lymphocytes [91], and this presumed pathogenesis may also be operative after transplantation. This diagnosis should be made if the glomeruli are normal or display mild focal segmental mesangial sclerosis and/or hypercellularity on light microscopy and the immunostainings are negative except for scattered mesangial IgM and/or C3. In a study of 5 MCN cases, electron microscopy of the podocytes revealed segmental effacement of the foot processes. Remission was achieved with elevated doses of steroids [92].

CONCLUDING REMARKS

Death with a functioning graft, chronic rejection, chronic calcineurin inhibitor toxicity and post-transplantation GN are the most frequent causes of late kidney allograft loss at 10 years. The prevalence of post-transplantation GN is not known precisely because not all cases are diagnosed. An important factor in the underdiagnosis is the lack of consensus as to how to evaluate kidney transplant recipients who exhibit a slow deterioriation of the graft function. A significant number of such recipients never undergo allograft biopsy, and a diagnosis of 'chronic rejection/chronic allograft nephropathy' is presumed. Routine evaluation of kidney allograft biopsies with similar methodology as for native kidney biopsies would increase the reported prevalence of post-transplantation GN. White people throughout in Europe develop post-transplantation GN relatively infrequently indicating that ethnic and geographic differences have a non-negligible impact on the prevalence. Although both short and long-term graft survival rates have improved markedly during the past 20 years, the immunosuppressive regimens applied have not influenced the natural history of post-transplantation GN. All forms of glomerular disease can recur after transplantation, but differences are observed in the recurrence rates. FSGS, MPGN, and idiopathic diarrhoea-negative HUS recur frequently. MNP, FSGS, anti-GBM nephritis in Alport patients, and drug-induced TMA are the most common *de novo* diseases. Although there have been numerous uncontrolled reports of successful interventions for recurrent and *de novo* GNs, multicenter studies on how to treat post-transplantation GN are clearly needed [93].

ACKNOWLEDGEMENT

Supported by a grant to B. I: (TÁMOP-4.2.1/B-09/1/KONV-2010-0005, Budapest, Hungary).

REFERENCES

[1] Yakupogly U, Baranowska-Daca E, Rosen D, *et al.* Post-transplant nephrotic syndrome: A comprehensive clinicopathologic study. Kidney Int 2004; 65: 2360-2370.

[2] Chung J, Park SK, Park JS, *et al.* Glomerulonephritis is the major cause of proteinuria in renal transplant recipients: histopathologic findings of renal allografts with proteinuria. Clin Transpl 2000; 14: 499-504.

[3] Ivanyi B. A primer on recurrent and *de novo* glomerulonephritis in renal allografts Nature Clin Pract Nephrol 2008; 4: 446-457.

[4] Meier-Kriesche HU, Baliga R, Kaplan B. Decreased renal function is a strong risk factor for cardiovascular death after renal transplantation. Transplantation 2003; 75: 1291-1295.

[5] Fernández-Fresnedo G, Plaza JJ, Sánchez-Plumed J, *et al.* Proteinuria: a new marker of long-term graft and patient survival in kidney transplantation. Nephrol Dial Transplant 2004; 19(Suppl 3): iii47-iii51

[6] Racusen LC, Solez K, Colvin RB, *et al.* The Banff 97 working classification of renal allograft pathology. Kidney Int 1999; 55: 713-723.

[7] Solez K, Colvin RB, Racusen LC, *et al.* Banff 07 classification of renal allograft pathology: updates and future directions. Am J Transplant 2008; 8: 753-760.

[8] Nadasdy T, Satoskar A, Nadasdy Gy. Pathology of renal transplantation. In: Zhou XJ, Laszik Z, Nadasdy T, D'Agati V, Silva FG, eds. Silva's diagnostic renal pathology. Cambridge University Press, 2009; pp. 522-567.

[9] Einicke G, Sis B, Reeve J, *et al.* Antibody-mediated microcirculation injury is the major cause of alte kidney transplant failure. Am J Transplant 2009; 9: 2520-2531.

[10] Loupy A, Suberbielle-Boissel C, Hill GS, *et al.* Outcome of subclinical antibody-mediated rejection in kidney transplant recipients with preformed donor-specific antibodies. Am J Transplant 2009; 9: 2561-2570.

[11] Ostrowska J, Pazik J, Lewandowski Z, *et al.* Posttransplantation glomerulonephritis: risk factors associated with kidney allograft loss. Transplant Proc 2007; 39: 2751-2753.

[12] Hariharan S, Ram Peddi V, Savin VJ, *et al.* Recurrent and *de novo* renal diseases after renal transplantation: a report from the Renal Allograft Disease Registry. Am J Kidney Dis 1998; 31: 928-931.

[13] Hariharan S, Adams MB, Brennan DC, *et al.* Recurrent and *de novo* glomerular disease after renal transplantation: a report from Renal Allograft Disease Registry (RADR). Transplantation 1999; 68: 635-641.

[14] Chailimpamontree W, Dmitrienko S, Li G, *et al.* Probability, predictors, and prognosis of posttransplantation glomerulonephritis. J Am soc Nephrol 2009; 20: 843-851.

[15] Cochat P, Fargue S, Mestrallet G, *et al.* Disease recurrence in paediatric renal transplantation. Pediatr Nephrol 2009; 24: 2097-2108.

[16] Reguiao-Moura LR, Moscoso-Solorzano GT, Franco MF, *et al.* Prognostic factors associated with poor graft outcomes in renal recipients with post-transplant glomerulonephritis. Clin Transplant 2007; 21: 363-370.

[17] Chadban S. Glomerulonephritis recurrence in the renal graft. J Am Soc Nephrol 2001; 12: 394-402.

[18] Briganti EM, Russ GR, McNeil JJ, *et al.* Risk of renal allograft loss from recurrent glomerulonephritis. N Engl J Med 2002; 347: 103-109.

[19] Ibrahim H, Rogers T, Casingal V, *et al.* Graft loss from recurrent glomerulonephritis is not increased with a rapid steroid discontinuation protocol. Transplantation 2006; 81: 214-219.

[20] Mulay AV, van Walraven C, Knoll GA. Impact of immunosuppressive medication on the risk of renal allograft failure due to recurrent glomerulonephritis. Am J Transplant 2009; 9: 804-811.

[21] Opelz G, Zeier M, Laux G, *et al.* No improvement of patient or graft survival in transplant recipients treated with angiotensin-converting enzyme inhibitors or angiotensin II type 1 receptor blockers: a collaborative transplant study report. J Am Soc Nephrol 2006; 17: 3257-3262.

[22] Beck LH, Boniego RG, Lambeau G, *et al.* M-type phospholipase A2 receptor as target antigen in idiopathic membranous nephropathy. N Eng J Med 2009; 361: 11-21.

[23] Ronco P, Debiec H. Molecular pathomechanisms of membranous nephropathy: from Heymann nephritis to alloimmunization. J Am Soc Nephrol 2005; 16: 1205-1213.

[24] Honda K, Horita S, Toki D, *et al.* *De novo* membranous nephropathy and antibody-mediated rejection in transplanted kidney. Clin Transplant 2010 DOI: 10.1111/j.1399-0012.2010.01213.x

[25] Aline-Fardin A, Rifle G, Martin L, *et al.* Recurrent and *de novo* membranous glomerulopathy after kidney transplantation. Transplant Proc 2009; 41: 669-671.

[26] Sprangers B, Lefkowitz GI, Cohen SD, *et al.* Beneficial effect of rituximab in the treatment of recurrent idiopathic membranous nephropathy after kidney transplantation. Clin J Am Soc Nephrol 2010; 5: 790-797.

[27] Cosyns JP, Couchoud C, Pouteil-Noble C, *et al.* Recurrence of membranous nephropathy after renal transplantation: probability, outcome and risk factors. Clin Nephrol 1998; 50: 144-153.

[28] Dabade TS, Grande JP, Norby SM, *et al.* Recurrent idiopathic membranous nephropathy after kidney transplantation: a surveillance biopsy study. Am J Transplant 2008; 8: 1318-1322.

[29] El-Zoghby ZM, Grande JP, Fraile MG, *et al.* Recurrent idiopathic membranous nephropathy: early diagnosis by protocol biopsies and treatment with anti-CD20 monoclonal antibodies. Am J Transplant 2009 9: 2800-2807.

[30] Bomback AS, Derebail VK, McGregor JG, *et al.* Rituximab therapy for membranous nephropathy: a systematic review. Clin J Am Soc Nephrol 2009; 4: 734-744.

[31] Roufosse CA, Cook TH. Pathological predictors of prognosis in immunoglobulin A nephropathy: a review. Curr Op Nephrol Hypertens 2009; 18: 212-219.

[32] Suzuki H, Fan R, Zhang Z, *et al.* Aberrantly glycosylated IgA1 in IgA nephropathy patients is recognized by IgG antibodies with restricted heterogeneity. J Clin Invest 2009; 119: 1668-1677.

[33] Coppo R, Feehally J, Glassock RJ. IgA nephropathy at two score and one. Kidney Int 2010; 77: 181-186.

[34] Bumgardner GL, Amend WC, Ascher NL, *et al.* Single center long-term results of renal transplantation for IgA nephropathy. Transplantation 1998; 65: 1053-1060.

[35] Jeong HJ, Huh KH, Kim YS, Kim SI. IgA nephropathy in renal allografts -recurrence and graft dysfunction. Yonsei Med J 2004; 45: 1043-1048.

[36] Chacko B, George JT, Neelakantan N, *et al.* Outcomes of renal transplantation in patients with immunoglobulin A nephropathy in India. J Postgrad Med 2007; 53: 92-95.

[37] McDonald S, Russ GR. Recurrence of IgA nephropathy among renal allograft recipients from living donors is greater among those with zero HLA mismatches. Transplantation 2006; 82: 759-762.

[38] NG YS, Vathsala A, Chew ST, *et al.* Long term outcome of renal allografts in patients with immunoglobulin a nephropathy. Med J Malaysia 2007; 62: 109-113.

[39] Jeong HJ, Park S-K, Cho YM, *et al.* Progression of renal allograft histology after renal transplantation in recurrent and nonrecurrent immunoglobulin A nephropathy. Hum Pathol 2008; 39: 1511-1518.

[40] Kennoki T, Ishida H, Yamaguchi Y, Tanabe K. Proteinuria-reducing effects of tonsillectomy alone in IgA nephropathy recurring after kidney transplantation. Transplantation 2009; 88: 935-941.

[41] Tsuchiya T, Ito S, Yamaguchi Y, *et al.* Tonsillectomy and steroid pulse therapy for recurrent IgA nephropathy in renal allograft. Clin Nephrol 2010; 73: 68-71.

[42] D'Agati VD, Fogo AB, Bruijn JA, Jenette JCh. Pathologic classification of focal segmental glomerulosclerosis: a working proposal. Am J Kidney Dis 2004; 43: 368-382.

[43] Zimmerman SW. Increased urinary protein excretion in the rat produced by serum from a patient with recurrent focal glomerular sclerosis after renal transplantation. Clin Nephrol 1984; 22: 32-38.

[44] Bruneau S, Le Berre L, Hervé C, *et al.* Potential role of soluble ST" protein in idiopathic nephritic syndrome recurrence following kidney transplantation. Am J Kidney Dis 2009; 54: 522-532.

[45] Caridi G, Bertelli R, Scolari F, *et al.* Podocin mutations in sporadic focal-segmental glomerulosclerosis occurring in adulthood. Kidney Int 2003; 64: 365.

[46] Caridi G, Bertelli R, Di Duca M, *et al.* Broadening the spectrum of diseases related to podocin mutations. J Am Soc Nephrol 2003; 14: 1278-1286.

[47] Ruf RG, Lichtenberger A, Karle SM, *et al.* Patients with mutations in NPHS2 (podocin) do not respond to standard steroid treatment of nephrotic syndrome. J Am Soc Nephrol 2004; 15: 722-732.

[48] Weber S, Gribouval O, Esquivel EL, *et al.* NPHS2 mutation analysis shows genetic heterogeneity of steroid-resistant nephrotic syndrome and low post-transplant recurrence. Kidney Int 2004; 66: 571-579.

[49] Carraro M, Caridi G, Bruschi M, *et al.* Serum glomerular permeability activity in patients with podocin mutations (NPHS2) and steroid-resistant nephrotic syndrome. J Am Soc Nephrol 2002; 13: 1946-1952.

[50] Douglas Briggs J, Jones E. Recurrence of glomerulonephritis following renal transplantation. Nephrol Dial Transplant 1999; 14: 564-565.

[51] Newstead CG. Recurrent disease in renal transplants. Nephrol Dial Transplant 2003; 18(Suppl 6): vi68-74.

[52] Hickson LJ, Gera M, Amer H, *et al.* Kidney transplantation for primary focal segmental glomerulosclerosis: outcomes and response to therapy for recurrence. Transplantation 2009; 87: 1232-1239.

[53] Moroni G, Gallelli B, Quaglini S, *et al.* Long-term outcome of renal transplantation in adults with focal segmental glomerulosclerosis. Transpl Int 2010; 23: 208-216.

[54] IJpelaar DHT, Farris AB, Goemaere N, *et al.* Fidelity and evolution of recurrent FSGS in renal allografts. J Am Soc Nephrol 2008; 19: 2219-2224.

[55] Canaud G, Dion D, Zuber J, *et al.* Recurrence of nephritic syndrome after transplantation in a mixed population of children and adults: course of glomerualr lesions and value of the Columbia classification of histological variants of focal and segmental glomerulosclerosis (FSGS). Nephrol Dial Transplant 2010; 25: 1321-1328.

[56] Weber S, Tönshoff B. Recurrence of focal-segmental glomerulosclerosis in children after renal transplantation: clinical and genetic aspects. Transplantation 2005; 80: S128-S134.

[57] Dello Strogolo L, Guzzo I, Laurenzi C, *et al.* Use of rituximab in focal glomerulosclerosis relapses after renal transplantation. Transplantation 2009; 88: 417-420.

[58] Rodrígez-Ferrero M, Ampuero J, Anaya F. Rituximab and chronic plasmapheresis therapy of nephrotic syndrome in renal transplantation patients with recurrent focal segmental glomerulosclerosis Transplant Proc 2009; 41: 2406-2408.

[59] Canaud G, Zuber J, Sberro R, *et al.* Intensive and prolonged treatment of focal and segmental glomerulosclerosis recurrence in adult kidney transplant recipients: a pilot study. Am J Transplant 2009; 9: 1081-1086.

[60] Cara Fuentes GM, Meseguer CG, Carrion AP, *et al.* Long-term outcome of focal segmental glomerulosclerosis after pediatric renal transplantation. Pediatr Nephrol 2010; 25: 529-534.

[61] Leroy S, Guigonis V, Bruckner D, *et al.* Succesful anti-TNFalpha treatment in a child with posttransplant recurrent focal segmental glomerulosclerosis. Am J Transplant 2009; 9: 858-861.

[62] Morozumi K, Takeda a, Uchida K, Mihatsch MJ. Cyclosporine nephrotoxicity: how does it affect renal allograft function and transplant morphology? Transplant Proc 2004; 36(Suppl 2S): 251S-256S.

[63] Cosio FG, Frankel WL, Pelletier RP, *et al.* Focal segmental glomerulosclerosis in renal allografts with chronic nephropathy: implications for graft survival. Am J Kidney Dis 1999; 34: 731-738.

[64] Swaminathan S, Lager DJ, Qian X, *et al.* Collapsing and non-collapsing focal segmental glomerulosclerosis in kidney transplants. Nephrol Dial Transplant 2006; 21: 2607-2614.

[65] Gough J, Yilmaz A, Yilmaz S, Benediktsson H. Recurrent and *de novo* glomerular immune-complex deposits in renal transplant biopsies. Arch Pathol Lab Med 2005; 129: 231-233.

[66] Lorenz EC, Sethi S, Leung N, *et al.* Recurrent membranoproliferative glomerulonephritis after kidney transplantation. Kidney Int 2010; 77:721-728.

[67] Braun MC, Stablein DM, Hamiwka LA, *et al.* Recurrence of membranoproliferative glomerulonephritis type II in renal allografts: the North American Pediatric Renal Transplant Cooperative Study Experience. J Am Soc Nephrol 2005; 16: 2225-2233.

[68] Little MA, Dupont P, Campbell E, *et al.* Severity of primary MPGN, rather than MPGN type, determines renal survival and post-transplantation recurrence risk. Kidney Int 2006; 69: 504-511.

[69] Levy JB, Turner N, Rees AJ, *et al.* Long-term outcome of anti-glomerular basement membrane antibody disease treated with plasma exchange and immunosuppression. Ann Intern Med 2001; 134: 1033-1042.

[70] Khandelwal M, McCormick BB, Lajoie G, *et al.* Recurrence of anti-GBM disease 8 years after renal transplantation. Nephrol Dial Transplant 2004; 19: 491-494.

[71] Borza DB, Chedid MF, Colon S, *et al.* Recurrent Goodpasture's disease secondary to a monoclonal IgA1-kappa antibody autoreactive with the alpha1/alpha2 chains of type IV collagen. Am J Kidney Dis 2005; 45: 397-406.

[72] Nachman PH, Segelmark M, Westman K, *et al.* Recurrent ANCA-associated small vessel vasculitis after transplantation: a pooled analysis. Kidney Int 1999; 56: 1544-1550

[73] Elmedhem A, Adu D, Savage COS. Relapse rate and outcome of ANCA-associated small vessel vasculitis after transplantation. Nephrol Dial Transplant 2003; 18: 1001-1004.

[74] Tabata H, Honda K, Moriyama T, *et al.* Two cases of ANCA-associated vasculitis in post-transplant kidney: relapse and *de novo*. Clin Transplant 2009; Suppl 20: 49-53.

[75] Choy BY, Chan TM, Lai KN, *et al.* Recurrent glomerulonephritis after kidney transplantation. Am J Transpl 2006; 6: 2535-2542.

[76] Geetha D, Seo P, Specks U, Fervenza FC. Successful induction of remission with rituximab for relapse of ANCA-associated vasculitis post-kidney transplant: report of two cases. Am J Transplant 2007; 7: 2821-2825.

[77] Gera M, Griffin MD, Specks U, *et al.* Recurrence of ANCA-associated vasculitis following renal transplantation in the modern era of immunosupression. Kidney Int 2007; 71: 1296-1301.

[78] Kashtan CE. Renal transplantation in patients with Alport syndrome. Pediatr Transplantation 2006; 10: 651-657.

[79] Browne G, Brown PAJ, Tomson CRV, *et al.* Retransplantation in Alport post-transplant anti-GBM disease. Kidney Int 2004; 65: 675-681.

[80] Licht C, Fremeaux-Bacchi V. Hereditary and acquired complement dysreglation in membranoproliferative glomerulonephritis. Thromb Haemost 2009; 101: 271-278.

[81] Noris M, Remuzzi G. Hemolytic uremic syndrome. J Am Soc Nephrol 2005; 16: 1035-1050.

[82] Artz MA, Steenbergen EJ, Hoitsma AJ, *et al.* Renal transplantation in patients with hemolytic uremic syndrome: high rate of recurrence and increased incidence of acute rejections. Transplantation 2003; 76: 821-826.

[83] Caprioli J, Noris M, Brioschi S, *et al.* Genetics of HUS: the impact of MCP, CFH, and IF mutations on clinical presentation, response to treatment and outcome. Blood 2006; 108: 1267-1279.

[84] Ponticelli C, Banfi G. Thrombotic microangiopathy after kidney transplantation. Transplant Int 2006; 19: 789-794.

[85] Sellier-Leclerc A, Fremeaus-Bacchi V, Dragon-Durey M, *et al.* Differential impact of complement mutations on clinical characteristics in atypical hemolytic uremic syndrome. J Am Soc Nephrol 2007; 18: 2392-2400.

[86] Bresin E, Daina E, Noris M, *et al.* Outcome of renal transplantation in patients with non-Shiga toxin-associated hemolytic uremic syndrome: prognostic significance of genetic background. Clin J Am Soc Nephrol 2006; 1: 88-99.

[87] Benz K, Amann K. Thrombotic microangiopathy: new insights. Curr Opin Nephrol Hypertens 2010; 19: 242-247.

[88] Davin JC, Gracchi V, Bouts A, *et al.* Maintenance of kidney function following treatment with eculizumab and discontinuation of plasma exchange after a third kidney transplant for atypical haemolytic uremic syndrome associated with a CFH mutation. Am J Kidney Dis 2010; 55: 708-711.

[89] Reynolds JC, Agodoa LY, Yuan CM, Abott KC. Thrombotic microangiopathy after renal transplantation in the United States. Am J Kidney Dis 2003; 42: 1058-1068.

[90] Schwimmer J, Nadasdy TA, Spitalnik PF, *et al. De novo* thrombotic microangiopathy in renal transplant recipients: a comparison of haemolytic uremic syndrome with localized renal thrombotic microangiopathy. Am J Kidney Dis 2003; 41: 471-479.

[91] Androgue HE, Borillo J, Torres L, *et al.* Coincident activation of Th2 T cells with onset of the disease and differential expression of GRO-gamma in peripheral blood leukocytes in minimal change disease. Am J Nephrol 2007; 27: 253-261.

[92] Zafarmand AA, Baranowska-Daca E, Ly PDC, *et al. De novo* minimal change disease associated with reversible post-transplant nephrotic syndrome. A report of five cases and review of literature. Clin Transplant 2002; 16: 350-361.

[93] Matas A. Recurrent disease after kidney transplantation – it is time to unite to address this problem! Am J Transplant 2006; 6: 2527-2528.

CHAPTER 24

Chronic Renal Allograft Dysfunction

Roberto Marcén*

Department of Nephrology. Ramon y Cajal Hospital. University of Alcalá de Henares, Spain

Abstract: Chronic allograft nephropathy (CAN) and death with graft function have been the leading causes of late kidney graft loss in the last 20 years. The term CAN substituted the old term "chronic allograft rejection" and designs a poorly understood condition characterized by a progressive decline of graft function often associated with hypertension and proteinuria and non-specific histologic changes affecting all kidney compartments. As CAN includes many specific chronic diseases caused by different etiopathogenic mechanisms, workers attending the 8th Banff Conference on Allograft Nephropathy decided to eliminate and to replace the term CAN by "interstitial fibrosis and tubular atrophy without evidence of any specific etiology". The implications of this change in the future could probably be of paramount importance and contribute to a better understanding and treatment of the different entities included in the term CAN. In the present chapter, the different conditions associated with a progressive decline of graft function such as interstitial fibrosis and tubular atrophy, transplant glomerulopathy, chronic T-cell mediated rejection and calcineurin inhibitor toxicity are described, with special emphasis on the clinical course, the possible etiopathogenic mechanism, the diagnostic criteria and the different therapeutical options.

Keywords: Kidney Transplantation, Graft Dysfunction, Immunosuppression, Chronic Allograft Vasculopathy, Interstitial Fibrosis, Tubular Atrophy, Transplant Glomeruolpathy, Calcineurin Inhibitors, Calcineurin Toxicity, Kidney Biopsy.

INTRODUCTION

The term chronic allograft nephropathy (CAN) was coined in the early 90s as a more generic alternative to the then popular term "chronic allograft rejection". It was considered that the new term was better than chronic rejection because the chronic changes may result from different forms of immunologically and nonimmunologically mediated injury mechanisms to the allograft. Since then, CAN has designed a poorly understood condition clinically characterized by progressive allograft dysfunction and graft failure, usually associated with hypertension and proteinuria after three or six post-transplant months and nonspecific histopathologic changes involving the vascular, glomerular and tubulointerstitial compartments of the kidneys [1, 2]. CAN was, after death with a functioning graft, the leading cause of graft loss and of lack of improvement of long-term graft survival rates [3, 4]. As CAN included many specific chronic diseases such as chronic calcineurin inhibitor (CNI) toxicity, chronic rejection, recurrrent and *de novo* glomerulonephritis, chronic hypertension, chronic obstruction, bacterial pyelonephritis and viral infections, caused by different etiologies and through different pathophysiologic mechanisms [5], workers attending the 8th Banff Conference on Allograft Pathology decided to replace the term CAN by "interstitial fibrosis and tubular atrophy without evidence of any specific etiology" [6]. However, as kidney graft biopsies are not routinely performed in patients with declining graft function, chronic allograft dysfunction (CAD) is the term used when CAN is presumed to be the most likely cause of progressive renal graft dysfunction in the absence of renal graft biopsy. The present chapter highlights the causes of chronic graft dysfunction emphasizing the different pathological pictures, the diagnostic methods, and the treatment.

CHRONIC ALLOGRAFT DYSFUNCTION

Clinical Picture

The causes of graft loss after the first post-transplant year are death with a functioning graft and loss of

***Address correspondence to Roberto Marcén:** Servicio de Nefrología, Hospital Ramón y Cajal, Ctra Colmenar Viejo s/n 28034 Madrid. Spain; Tel: +34 91 336 90 17; Fax: +34 91 336 88 00; E-mail: rmarcen.hrc@salud.madrid.org

Massimiliano Veroux and Pierfrancesco Veroux (Eds)

graft function. Each one is responsible for around 50% of graft losses. Several studies have shown that graft function progressively declines over time and this change is approximately linear [7-9]. The rate of decline is variable and may start at any time after transplant. It is frequently accompanied by variable proteinuria, from 0.5 g/day to nephrotic range, and hypertension. In many cases proteinuria may appear before graft function deterioration. Until now, CAN was considered the leading cause of graft deterioration and consequent graft loss. However as the term was used as a wastebasket, attempts should be made to identify the predominant pathologic lesion.

Causes of Chronic Allograft Dysfunction

The causes of chronic kidney allograft dysfunction are expressed in Table **1**. The Banff's classification distinguishes different entities which were generally included in the old term CAN [6, 10].

Table 1: Causes of chronic kidney allograft dysfunction

Interstitial fibrosis and tubular atrophy, with no evidence of any specific etiology
Late/chronic antibody related rejection
Chronic active T-cell mediated rejection
CNI toxicity
Glomerulonephritis: recurrent and *de novo*
Chronic hypertension
Chronic obstruction
Viral infection
Unclassified changes

Interstitial Fibrosis and Tubular Atrophy

Interstitial fibrosis and tubular atrophy (Fig. **1**) are frequently detected in patients with deteriorating graft function as well as in protocol biopsies early after transplantation in well functioning grafts [11]. Both are a common finding in graft biopsies from patients with chronic non-immune conditions such as chronic hypertension, CNI toxicity, chronic obstruction, bacterial pyelonephritis and viral infection and with chronic immune injury: transplant glomerulopathy and chronic T-cell mediated rejection [6]. It has been reported that their incidence increased with the length of follow-up, they were present in 94.2% of grafts at 1 year and at 10 years their presence was universal in patients mostly on cyclosporine therapy [12]. Another study has reported an incidence of 40% to 50% in standard dose tacrolimus in combination with mycophenolate mofetil (MMF) and prednisone at two years [13]. The 8th Banff conference established a new entity "interstitial fibrosis and tubular atrophy without evidence of any specific etiology" which replaced the term CAN. The presence of fibrosis has been correlated with graft loss [14] and the extention of interstitial fibrosis using quantitative assessment with graft survival and time to renal failure [15].

It was thought that interstitial fibrosis and tubular atrophy were the consequence of inflammation, ischemia, subclinical rejection and CNI nephrotoxicity. The decrease in the incidence of acute and subclinical rejection makes the link between rejection and fibrosis more unlikely. The role of CNI is also questioned as the incidence of fibrosis at one year was similar in patients on tacrolimus as in those on a tacrolimus avoidance regimen [16]. Gene expression studies suggest the presence of an ongoing exaggerated inflammatory proccess in allografts with fibrosis [17, 18]. A critical mechanism for interstitial fibrosis and tubular atrophy in kidney allografts appears to be epithelial-mesenchimal transformation (EMT). In this proccess, some cells are transformed into fibroblast with myocyte-like properties within the interstitium. Studies in animals and in humans have implicated growth factors such as transforming growth factor beta (TGF-β) and connective tissue growth factor (CTGF) as important molecules in the provision of powerful signals for EMT. Allograft kidneys destinated to develop tubular atrophy and fibrosis have significant expression for TGF-β and CTGF mRNA and other molecules related to fibrogenesis prior to histologically detectable graft fibrosis [19].

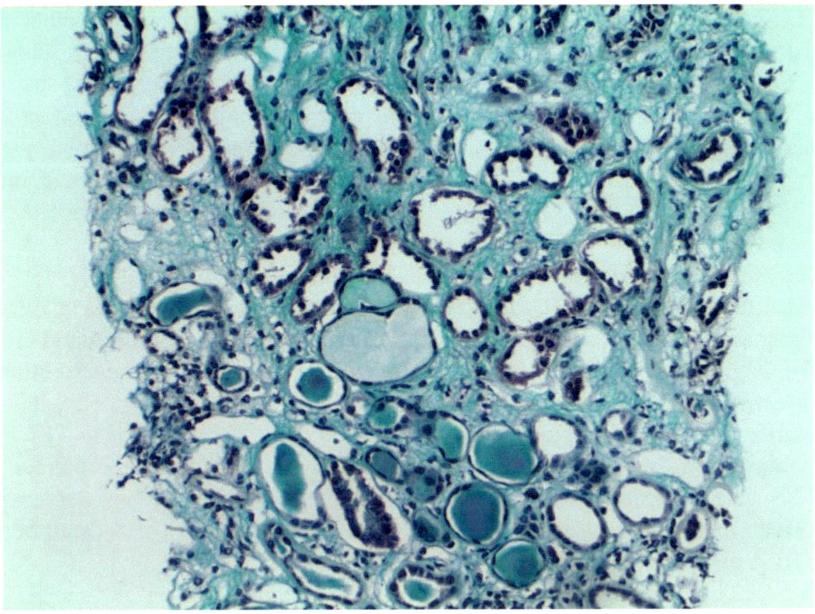

Figure 1: Renal allograft biopsy (Masson staining) showing moderate interstitial fibrosis and tubular atrophy (loss of tubular height and increased luminal size) associated with a chronic inflammatory infiltrate and two sclerosed glomeruli. (From Dr Ana Saiz, Department of Pathology. Ramon y Cajal Hospital).

Transplant Glomerulopathy

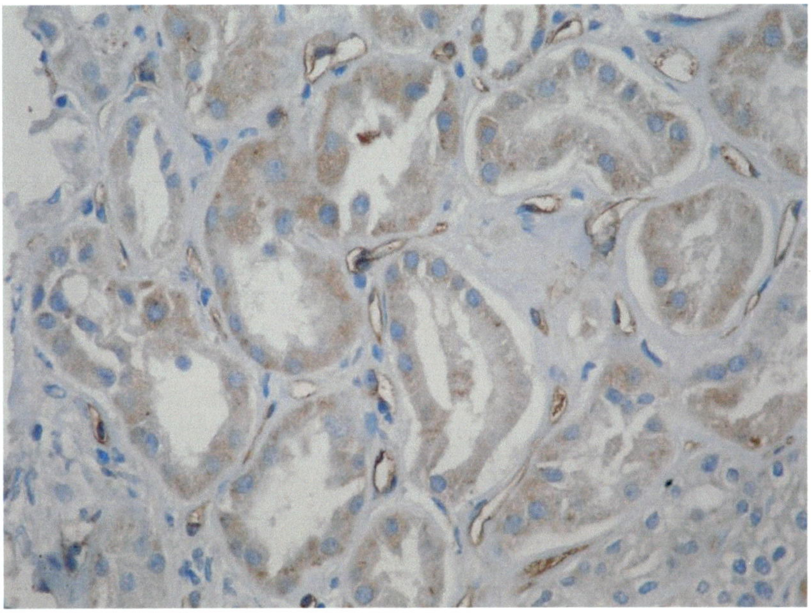

Figure 2: Renal allograft biopsy showing C4d deposition (in brown) in peritubular capillaries. (From Dr Ana Saiz, Department of Pathology. Ramon y Cajal Hospital).

Considered as a variant of CAN of unknown origin, interstitial fibrosis and tubular atrophy is now recognized as a new entity. Transplant glomerulopathy is a condition characterized by duplication of glomerular capillary basement membranes, "double contours", mesangial matrix expansion and mesangial cell interposition [20]. Fibrosis and tubular atrophy are commonly seen but their severity is mild and does not correlate with the degree of severity of transplant glomerulopathy. Immunofluorescence is typically negative or may show nonspecific IgM and C3 deposits. C4d staining in peritubular capillaries (Fig. **2**) and/or glomerular capillaries is observed in about one third of the patients [21]. Electron microscopy shows multilamination in the peritubular capillary basement membrane. Longitudinal studies have shown that ultrastructural changes occur very early, from 1 month in patients destined for subsequent transplant glomerulopathy. Early changes suggest endothelial cell activation characterized by vacuolation and hypertrophy and interdigitation of the endothelial cell processes within the subendothelial space [22]. Transplant glomerulopathy, diffuse C4d deposition, multilamination of peritubular capillaries and the presence of donor specific antibodies constitute the diagnostic tetrad of chronic antibody-mediated rejection.

The clinical manifestations of transplant glomerulopathy are decreased graft function and proteinuria usually higher than 1 000 mg/day. The disease has a poor prognosis and about 50% of the patients with this entity have lost the graft or have reduced GFR by 50% after 36 months of follow-up [11]. The incidence is variable. When the diagnosis was only in biopsies performed for unexplained renal function deterioration or proteinuria, the incidence of transplant glomerulopathy was around 3% to 7% [20, 21, 23]. In protocol biopsies the incidence increases with the length of follow-up from 3% at 1 year to 11.5 % at 5 years, but when additional biopsies performed for clinical dysfunction were considered the incidence reached up to 20% at 5 years [24]. The variables associated with transplant glomerulopathy are acute rejection, hepatitis C antibody positivity before transplantation, prior transplantation and HLA antibodies at transplant specially against HLA class II antigens [24].

The presence of positive C4d staining in the biopsy and anti-HLA donor antibodies suggests that transplant glomerulopathy is a clinical entity strongly associated with alloantibody mediated injury. In the cases of C4d negative transplant glomerulonephritis its pathogenesis is unclear and several hypothesis have been proposed as sampling error, residual injury from previous episodes of antibody mediated rejection, T-cell mediated transplant glomerulonephritis and non-alloimmune causes of transplant glomerulonephritis [6].

Chronic Active T-Cell-Mediated Rejection

In the past, chronic rejection was the term used to design chronic allograft dysfunction, it was often confused with CAN and the two terms were frequently interchanged. The Banff classification made the distinction between chronic active antibody-mediated rejection (transplant glomerulopathy) and chronic active T-cell mediated rejection. In this classification, the chronic vascular changes suggested to be due to "chronic rejection" are disruption of elastica and inflammatory cells in the fibrotic intima. Other features are proliferation of myofibroblasts in the expanded intima and formation of a second "neointima" [10]. Vascular changes are graded based on the extent of occlusion of the most severely affected vessels [10]. Chronic rejection is uncommon in transplant recipients on treatment with CNI, and histological changes suggesting chronic rejection have been found in around 6% of patients [12].

Calcineurin Inhibitor (CNI) Toxicity

The CNIs, cyclosporine and tacrolimus, both share the same immunosuppressive mechanism of action and both are nephrotoxic. The nephrotoxicity of cyclosporine has been well known since the first trials. It has been demonstrated with the improvement of graft function and long term graft survival after early withdrawal [25]. The nephrotoxicity of tacrolimus was observed in phase III trials, in which no differences were observed between those receiving tacrolimus or cyclosporine in protocol biopsies obtained at 2 years [26].

The hallmark of chronic CNI toxicity is an arteriolopathy which has been considered to be a variant of thrombotic microangiopathy with a slow subclinical course. The initial lesion consists of vacuolization of endothelial and smooth muscle cells in afferent arterioles with later replacement of the necrotic smooth muscle cells by nodular hyaline deposits in the outer media of the arterioles leading to thickening of vessel walls (Fig. **3**). The vascular changes of CNI toxicity have a special lesion scoring in the Banff schema and are classified as mild, moderate or severe according to the intensity and distribution of the lesion [10]. As reproducibility using the Banff score was poor a new system was proposed in which the severity of CNI arteriolopathy was quantified according to the presence of circular or noncircular involvement and the number of involved arterioles [27]. In some studies its application improved the inter-observer reproductibility [28]. This arteriolopathy with the narrowing of the vascular lumen leads to hypoxia and tissue damage and to development of fibrosis, tubular atrophy and glomeruloesclerosis. Focal segmental glomerulosclerosis lesions accompanied by arteriolopathy in absence of other causes represent a new transplant glomerulopathy associated with cyclosporine therapy [27]. The onset of the first lesion of CNI toxicity is around six months. The incidence is variable, Nankivell *et al.* [29] found that CNI toxicity occurred in 90.5% of patients by 5 years and 100% by 10 years after transplantation. Other studies have observed that CNI toxicity was present in around 16% to 20 % of recipients at 2 years [17, 26].

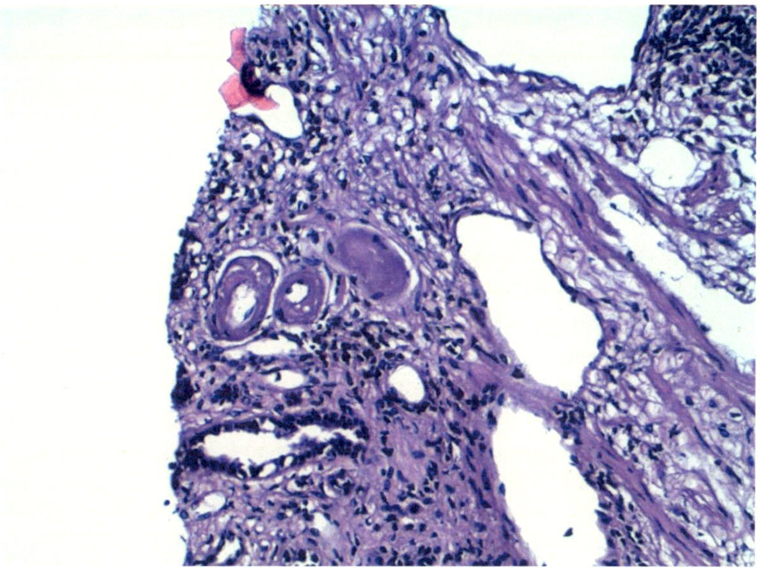

Figure 3: Renal allograft biopsy showing arteriolar hyalinosis (PAS staining). (From Dr Ana Saiz, Department of Pathology. Ramon y Cajal Hospital).

Chronic CNI toxicity has been considered one important cause of late graft failure and of no improvement of allograft long-term survival rates in the last decade. The etiology of CNI nephrotoxicity is probably multi-factorial and its intimal pathogenic mechanisms are not well understood [30]. CNIs cause local vasoconstriction through an imbalance of prostaglandin E_2 and thromboxane A_2 and prolonged vasoconstriction may lead to tubulointerstitial injury. They also are potential inducers of the vasoconstrictor endothelin-1. Cyclosporine may interfere with production of nitric oxide which plays an important role in maintaining renal vascular tone. Both CNIs, but mainly cyclosporine, are associated with increased expression of transforming growth factor beta-1 (TGF-β1) which is implicated in the development of interstitial fibrosis [30, 31]. Recent studies indicate that P-glycoprotein and the cytochrome P450 drug metabolizing enzyme CYP 3A4 expression or activity could be involved in promoting CNI nephrotoxicity [32].

Other Disease Processes

There are a number of other disease processes that could produce changes in the renal parenchyma and graft function deterioration and they must be considered in the differential diagnosis with the previous entities: recurrent and *de novo* glomerulonephritis, long-term uncontrolled hypertension, chronic obstruction, chronic pyelonephritis, viral infection mostly by BK polyoma virus and unclassifiable changes. Recurrence of glomerulonephritis increases as grafts and patients survive longer. Focal segmental glomerular sclerosis, mesangicapillary glomerulonephritis, IgA nephropathy and membranous glomerulonephritis are those with the highest risk of recurrence [33]. In a series of 1505 patients with both native and graft biopsies, recurrent glomerulonephritis was the third cause for graft loss 10 years after transplant [34]. BK virus nephropathy, affecting about 5% of recipients, manifests as an asymptomatic gradual rise in serum creatinine that results in allograft loss or permanent dysfunction in about 50% of cases [35, 36]. Immunosuppression with tacrolimus and MMF was considered the most important risk factor of infection [37].

DIAGNOSIS OF CHRONIC ALLOGRAFT DYSFUNCTION

Graft Function

Routine biochemical parameters lack the specificity to detect early structural damage. Serum creatinine (SCr) levels and estimated glomerular filtration rate (eGFR) are the most common measurement methods of graft function and both have been used for clinical decision making. However, SCr level increases and GFR decreases when significant structural damage has been established and they are a poor marker of the early ongoing disease. On the other hand, renal allografts may develop chronic lesions despite a stable or optimal graft function [11]. Proteinuria, another marker of kidney damage, is common in renal transplant recipients. About 50% of them have proteinuria above 150 mg/day at one year [38] but the incidence decreases to 20% when higher than 1000 mg/day [39]. Low levels of proteinuria are not associated with specific pathologies but most patients with proteinuria higher than 1500 mg/day have glomerular pathology in biopsy, including transplant glomerulopathy [40].

Histological Studies

Only protocol biopsies can discover early graft injury and may define graft prognosis and identify those recipients at risk of graft function deterioration and graft loss. There are two main systems to evaluate graft histology: the chronic allograft damage index (CADI) and the Banff schema. The first one is the sum of six histological parameters, including interstitial inflammation and fibrosis, tubular atrophy, mesangial matrix increase and sclerosis of the glomeruli and intimal proliferation of the blood vessels [41]. The Banff schema is more complex, establishes 6 diagnostic categories and semiquantitative grading of changes of acute/active rejection and chronic/sclerosing allograft nephropathy [6, 10]. However, both methods have the problem of reproductibility with important inter- and intra-observer variations. Several modifications have been done in order to improve reproductibility through the evaluation of quantitative parameters such as morphometry, image-analysis based for the CADI scoring [42], computerized image analysis of sirius red-stained biopsies [15], immunohistochemistry or molecular biology techniques. Moreover despite kidney biopsy being the gold standard in the diagnosis of graft dysfunction, it is an invasive diagnosis procedure. The information obtained is limited by the quality of the sample (Banff 97 classification requires ten glomeruli and two arteries to provide an adequate core sample) and by the fact that biopsy material is only a small part of the kidney.

HLA Antibodies

The utility of alloantibody testing as a routine diagnostic tool in the diagnosis of chronic allograft dysfunction is not well defined. Antibodies directed against human leukocyte antigens (HLA), donor-specific and non-donor-specific, appear after transplantation in a variable percentage of kidney transplant recipients, ranging from 16 to 60%, according to the characteristics of the population studied and the techniques used for HLA antibodies screening [43-47]. Pretransplant immunization, HLA-DR matching and acute rejection episodes are among the variables related with the production of antibodies [43]. Post-transplant detection of HLA antibodies, mostly during the first year, was associated with poor graft outcome, graft dysfunction and the onset of proteinuria [43-46, 48]. It has been suggested that chronic allograft losses are always preceded by HLA alloreactivity [46]. In patients with chronic graft dysfunction, donor specific antibodies were detected in 75% of patients with capillary C4d deposition [49] and morphological findings of transplant glomerulonephritis provided the definitive proof of antibody mediated rejection. However, patients with normal allograft function may maintain stable graft function post-transplantation for large periods of time, despite detectable circulating alloantibodies [50]. These findings suggest that testing HLA-antibodies seems to be useful in the evaluation of graft dysfunction and proteinuria as an additional tool in the identification of the causative process but in patients with normal graft function at the time of testing, the value of reactivity may not necessarily predict a poor graft outcome.

Other Procedures

Finding a reproducible and non-invasive procedure to assess the state of the allograft seems essential. Molecular markers in serum, peripheral cells, urine and graft are now under investigation. This approach has been successful in the case of acute cellular rejection, for which urine levels of ganzyme B and FOXP3 transcripts have diagnostic and prognostic value. Gene expression studies and proteomic approaches are the most promising tools for non-invasive investigation of late graft injury and transplant outcomes as well as for studying the beneficial and toxic effects of the immunosuppressive agents. For example Tribbles homolog 1 (TRIB1), a gene that regulates mitogen-activated protein kinase signalling and controls proliferation and chemotaxis of smooth muscle cells, increases in the blood and in the graft of kidney transplant patients with chronic antibody mediated rejection *versus* other clinical diagnoses [51]. Kidney injury molecule-1 (KIM-1) is a specific marker for diagnosing early tubular injury. In kidney allograft biopsies, KIM-1 staining was associated with kidney epithelial cell injury even when there were no detectable changes on histologic examination, and correlated with renal dysfunction [52]. Urinary KIM-1 levels also predicted graft loss independently of creatinine clearance, proteinuria or donor age [53].

TREATMENT

General Measures

Chronic allograft dysfunction has to be considered as a type of chronic kidney disease and treatment should follow similar principles. Blood pressure, cholesterol levels, anaemia and diabetes have to be maintained at the target recommended by the clinical guidelines [54, 55]. A suggested algorithmic treatment approach is shown in Fig. **4**.

Hypertension

Hypertension is a very common complication after transplantation and some longitudinal studies have shown litle improvement in the blood pressure control in the most recent eras [56]. Data from cross-sectional studies which included an important number of recipients have shown that despite the recommendations about 70% to 80% of recipients have blood pressure higher than 130/80 mm Hg [57-60]. High blood pressure has been considered as a risk factor of progressive graft dysfunction and controlling hypertension even several years after transplantation could improve graft outcome [61, 62]. Adequate control of blood pressure seems to be mandatory as it helps to preserve graft function and to improve long-term outcome. Most of the even thoughany antihypertensive agent is absolutely contraindicated in kidney transplant recipients. Angiotensin-converting enzime inhibitors (ACEIs) and angiotensin receptor blockers (ARB) have been associated with reduced proteinuria and intragraft TGF-β expression [63] and improvement in the slope of decline in reciprocal serum creatinine [64]. Recent studies support the hypothesis that ACEI/ARB might have a protective effect on the interstitial fibrosis/tubular atrophy progression as angiotensin II and ischemia can induce CTGF a powerful signal for EMT [13]. However, the beneficial effects of ACEI/ARBs are not definitively established [65-67] and a meta-analysis concluded that there were not sufficient data to determine the effect on patient or graft survival [68]. Calcium channel blockers are effective in controlling hypertension and may ameliorate the vasoconstriction associated with calcineurin therapy and improve GFR [69, 70]. The superiority of ACEI/ARB over calcium channel blockers has not been definitively demonstrated. When comparing calcium channel blockers with ACEIs, blood pressure control was similar but GFR was better in the calcium channel blockers [71], although this has not been a consistent finding.

Hyperlipidemia

Hyperlipidemia defined as a total cholesterol >200 mg/dl (6 mmol/L) or LDL-cholesterol > 100 mg/dl (3.5 mmol/L) or triglycerides >150 mg/dl was present in approximately 60% of renal transplant recipients [57, 59, 60]. Both hypertriglyceridemia and hypercholesterolemia have been identified as a risk factor of graft loss [72, 73)]. Randomized control trials in the general population have suggested that treatment with statins may have a protective effect on renal function [74]. Studies in patients with coronary artery disease or myocardial infaction treated with simvastatin or pravastatin showed a reduced decline rate of eGFR [75, 76]. Moreover, atorvastatin prevented the decline in renal function in patients with cardiac events [77] and glomerulonephritis [78] and the effects seemed to be dosage related [77, 78]. The clinical guidelines suggest treating hyperlipidemia in order to keep the cholesterol within the recommended limits in the assumption that, as in the general population, these measures could reduce cardiovascular morbidity and mortality and taking into consideration the previous reports could also ameliorate the CKD progression. The results of the Assessment of Lescol in renal Transplantation (ALERT) study, the only randomized study of statin therapy in renal transplant recipients, did not support this statement, as treatment with statins (fluvastatin) had no effect on graft function [79]. Other retrospective studies failed to demonstrate a beneficial effect in graft survival [80].

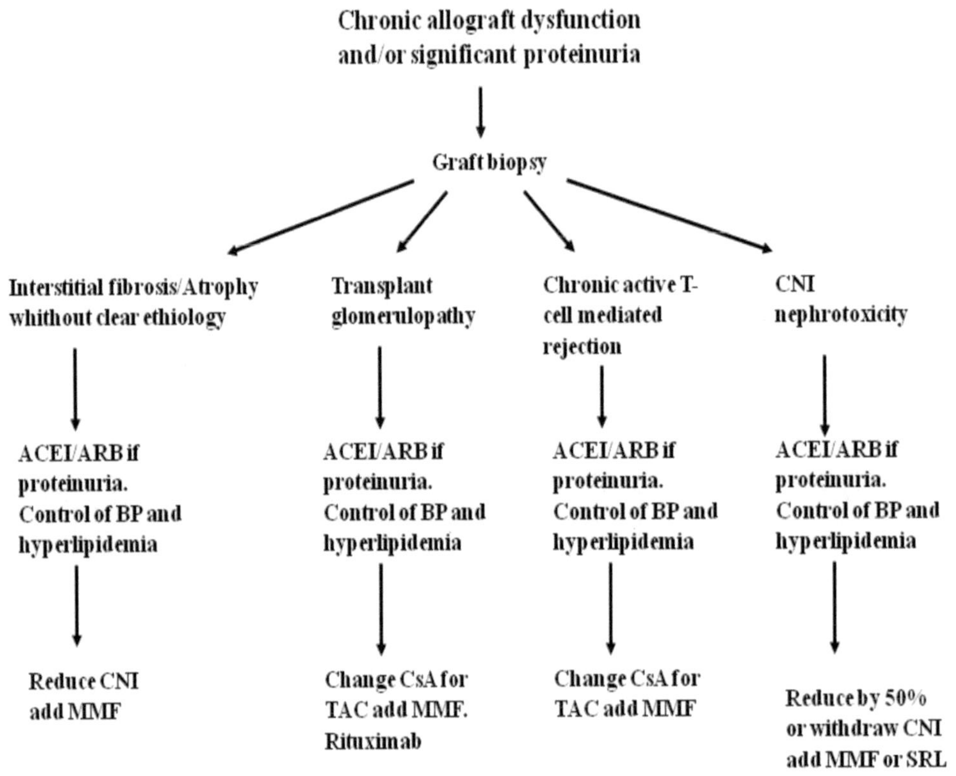

Figure 4: Suggested treatment algorithmic approach to chronic allograft dysfunction. ACEI/ARB= Angiotensin-converting enzime inhibitors/angiotensin receptor blockers BP= Blood Pressure. CNI=Calcineurine inhibitors. CsA=cyclosporine. MMF=Mycophenolate mofetil. SRL=Sirolimus. TAC=Tacrolimus.

Diabetes

Post-transplant diabetes is an increasing complication in kidney transplant recipients. Its incidence is variable according to the diagnosis criteria. When diagnosed following the American Diabetes Association recommendations, the incidence of diabetes was 39% at one year [81]. Among the immunosuppressive agents, tacrolimus is more diabetogenic than cyclosporine [82]. Post-transplant diabetes is a risk factor of late graft loss and cardiovascular diseases [83, 84]. An adequate control of this complication could ameliorate its impact on graft outcome.

Proteinuria

Proteinuria is a risk factor of progression of renal disease and its reduction provides nephroprotection in many nephropathies. As stated before, proteinuria is a common complication after renal transplantation. It is a risk factor of graft loss independently of graft function or histological findings [39]. Treatment includes control of blood pressure (<130/80 mm Hg) using the maximum tolerable dose of either ACEI/ARB or a combination of both, lipids control with statins, maintenance of ideal body weight and sirolimus discontinuation [40].

Immunosuppression

As stated before, CNIs, cyclosporine and tacrolimus, are very potent immunosuppressive agents but both are nephrotoxic. This adverse effect could overcome the beneficial effect of reducing acute rejection incidence and of improving long-term graft outcomes. There is not consensus about the best treatment of CNI nephrotoxicity. Two main strategies of treatment have been used, conversion from one CNI-based immunosuppressive regimen to another without CNI, or addition of a new immunosuppressive agent to patients in two agent regimens with or without reduction of CNI agents.

Conversion Studies

In most conversion studies, CNI agents, cyclosporine or tacrolimus, are withdrawn and substituted by non-nephrotoxic agents such as mycophenolic acid or mTOR inhibitors, sirolimus or everolimus. The rational of this therapeutical approach is based on the findings of the protocol biopsies in which late changes such as arteriolar hyalinosis, ischemic glomerulosclerosis and interstitial fibrosis have been associated with long-term CNI nephrotoxicity.

In control trials in which patients on treatment with CNI were randomized for the addition of MMF to CNI regimen or MMF addition followed by CNI withdrawal, renal function improved and blood pressure decreased significantly in the MMF/CNI withdrawal group [85, 86]. In patients with declining graft function "creeping creatinine" on CsA treatment, CsA stepwise withdrawal following MMF introduction improved graft function when compared with patients remaining in their existing regimen, CsA monotherapy, CsA/steroids, or CsA/AZA/steroids [87]. There are several studies in which patients with CNI toxicity were converted to sirolimus, the introduction of sirolimus with CNI withdrawal improved graft survival, the progression of chronic allograft injury and vascular damage and reduced the expression of genes of renal damage when compared with CNI reduction plus MMF [88, 89]. This beneficial effect on graft survival persisted at 5-year follow-up in patients without proteinuria [90]. Similar results have been observed in tacrolimus-based regimens. So, in patients with moderate to severe renal dysfunction on tacrolimus/MMF therapy conversion to sirolimus was associated with a sustained improvement of eGFR in 74% of patients. No beneficial effects were observed in those patients with eGFR <20 ml/min/1.73m2 at the time of conversion therapy [91]. But conversion to sirolimus had some adverse effects such as increases in cholesterol and triglycerides blood levels [92]. It appears that CNI withdrawal is safe and could be an alternative for treatment of graft function deterioration. However both medications, MMF and sirolimus, have important adverse effects that preclude their generalized administration.

Although both CNI agents, cyclosporine and tacrolimus, are nephrotoxic, the effect of switching from cyclosporine to tacrolimus on chronic allograft failure has also been investigated with different results. Some studies did not show any benefit or the results were similar to those obtained by reducing cyclosporine doses [93]. In others, cyclosporine withdrawal was associated with improvement of graft function and cardiovascular risk factors, and with a reduction in the occurrence of new-onset cardiac events [94, 95].

Addition Studies

In the addition studies there are two different approaches: adding a new agent to the previous CNI immunosuppressive regimen without modifying it or reducing the CNI dose after adding the new agent. The addition of myophenolate mofetil to CNI therapy improved graft function and graft outcomes independently of the blood levels of cyclosporine [96], which suggests that MMF could have nephroprotective properties. In patients on cyclosporine, the reduction to half dose cyclosporine and the addition of MMF improved graft function without increasing the risk of rejection and decreased triglycerides levels when compared with patients on a cyclosporine-based regimen [97]. These findings are supported by histological studies in which the association of MMF with cyclosporine and/or tacrolimus decreased the incidence of fibrosis in protocol biopsies when compared with azathioprine [98]. On the other hand, the addition of rapamycin with dose reduction of cyclosporine did not improve graft function or molecular or histological outcome when compared with reduction alone [99].

Other Treatments

The previous therapies try to control chronic kidney disease complications and CNI nephrotoxicity. The better understanding of the mechanisms and early diagnosis of graft injury may allow treatment of the causes of the injury. The new treatment targets should be directed against the development of fibrosis and tubular atrophy. TGF-β has also important immunomodulary propierties in suppressing inflammation and acute rejection that makes CTGT a more suitable target for the future management of graft fibrosis [100]. Several approaches have been used in animal models such as blockade of prolyl-4-hydroxylase that limits the collagen biosynthesis [101], inhibition of matrix metalloproteinase enzymes [102], retinoids that have antiinflammatory properties [103], and hepatocyte growth factor disruption of epithelial-mesenchimal transformation [104].

Transplant glomerulopathy is an entity mediated by alloantibodies that could benefit from treatment with Rituximab. This immunosuppressive agent has been used for treating several glomerulopathies after kidney transplantation. In a pilot experience, Rituximab therapy (4 injections of 375 mg/m2 week) in kidney transplant recipients with transplant glomerulopathy was associated with allograft function stabilization in 50% of cases [105]. The treatment of BK virus nephropathy includes reduction and/or discontinuation of immunosuppressive agents and administration of cidofovir, leflunomide, or quinolones [106-108].

ACKNOWLEDGEMENTS

The author thanks Mary Harper for her assistance in preparing the English version of this article and Dr Ana Saiz for preparing the histological figures. Conflicts of interest: none.

REFERENCES

[1] Paul LC. Chronic renal transplant loss. Kidney Int 1995; 47: 1491-1499.

[2] Hariharan S. Long-term kidney transplant survival. Am J Kidney Dis 2001; 38(suppl6): S44-S50.

[3] Matas AJ, Humar A, Gillingham KJ, *et al.* Five preventable causes of kidney graft loss in the 1990s: A single-center analysis. Kidney Int 2002; 62: 704-714.

[4] Excerpts from the United States Renal Data System 2008 annual data report. Am J Kidney Dis 2009; 53(suppl 1): S227-S237.

[5] Colvin RB. Chronic allograft nephropathy. N Engl J Med 2003; 349: 2288-2290.

[6] Solez K, Colvin, Racusen F, *et al.* Banff'05 meeting report: differential diagnosis of chronic allograft injury and elimination of chronic allograft nephropathy ('CAN'). Am J Transplant 2007; 7: 518-526.

[7] Gourishankar S, Hunsicker LG, Jhangri GS, *et al.* The stability of the glomerular filtration rate after transplantation is improving. J Am Soc Nephrol 2003; 14: 2387-2394.

[8] Gill JS, Tonelli M, Mix CH, Pereira BJG. The change in allograft function among long-term kidney transplant recipients. J Am Soc Nephrol 2003; 14: 1636-1642.

[9] Gera M, Slezak JM, Rule AD, *et al.* Assessment of changes in kidney allograft function using creatinine-based estimates of glomerular filtration rate. Am J Transplant 2007; 7: 880-887.

[10] Racusen LC, Solez K, Colvin RB, *et al.* The Banff 97 working classification of renal allograft pathology. Kidney Int 1999; 55: 713-723.

[11] Serón D, Moreso F, Bover J, *et al.* Early protocol renal allograft biopsies and graft outcomes. Kidney Int 1997; 51: 310-316.

[12] Nankivell BJ, Borrows RJ, Fung CL-S, *et al.* The natural history of chronic allograft nephropathy. N Engl J Med 2003; 349: 2326-2333.

[13] Rush DN, Cochkfield SM, Nickerson PW, *et al.* Factors associated with progression of interstitial fibrosis in renal transplant recipients receiving tacrolimus and mycophenolate mofetil. Transplantation 2009; 88: 897-903.

[14] Cosio FG, Grande JP, Wadei H, *et al.* Predicting subsequent decline in kidney allograft function from early surveillance biopsies. Am J Transplant 2005; 5: 2464-2472.

[15] Grimm PC, Nickerson P, Gough P, *et al.* Computerized image analysis of Sirius Red-stained renal allograft biopsies as a surrogate marker to predict long-term allograft function. J Am Soc Nephrol 2003; 14: 1662-1668.

[16] Larson TS, Dean PG Stegall MD. Complete avoidance of calcineurin inhibitors in renal transplantation: A randomized trial comparing sirolimus and tacrolimus. Am J Transplant 2006; 6: 514-522.

[17] Flechner SM, Kurian SM, Solez K, *et al. De novo* kidney transplantation without use of calcineurin inhibitors preserves renal structure and function at two years. Am J Transplant 2004; 4: 1776-1785.

[18] Park W, Griffin M, Grande JP, *et al.* Molecular evidence of injury and inflammation in normal and fibrotic renal allografts one year posttransplant. Transplantation 2007; 83: 1466-1476.

[19] Cheng O, Thuillier R, Sampson E, *et al* Connective tissue growth factor is a biomarker and mediator of kidney allograft fibrosis. Am J Transplant 2006; 6: 2297-2306.

[20] Suri DL, Tomlanovich SJ, Olson JL, Meyer W. Transplant glomerulopathy as a cause of late graft loss. Am J Kidney Dis 2000; 35: 674-680.

[21] Sis B, Campbell PM, Mueller T, *et al.* Transplant glomerulopathy, late antibody-mediated rejection and the ABCD tetrad in kidney allograft biopsies for cause. Am J Transplant 2007; 7: 1743-1752.

[22] Wavamunno MD, O´Connell PJ, Vitalone M, *et al.* Transplant glomerulopathy: ultrastructural abnormalities occur early in longitudinal analysis of protocol biopsies. Am J Transplant 2007; 7: 2757-2768.

[23] Bunnag S, Eiinecke G, Reeve J, *et al.* Molecular correlates of renal function in kidney transplant biopsies.J Am Soc Nephrol 2009; 20: 1149-1160.

[24] Gloor JM, Sethi S, Stengall MD, *et al* Transplant glomerulopathy: subclinical incidence and association with alloantibody. Am J Transplant 2007; 7: 2124-2132.

[25] Gallagher M, Jardine M, Perkovic V, *et al.* Cyclosporine withdrawal improves long-term graft survival in renal transplantation. Transplantation 2009; 87: 1877-1883.

[26] Solez K, Vincenti F, File R. Histopathologic findings from 2-ýear protocol biopsies from US multicenter kidney transplant trial comparing tacrolimus *versus* cyclosporine. Transplantation 1998; 66: 1736-1740.

[27] Morozumi K, Takeda A, Uchida K, Mihatsch MJ. Cyclosporine nephrotoxicity: how does it affect renal allograft function and transplant morphology?. Transplant Proc 2004; 36(suppl 2S): 251S-256S.

[28] Sis B, Dadras F, Khoshjou F, *et al.* Reproductibility studies on arteriolar hyaline thickening scoring in calcineurin inhibitors-treated renal allograft recipients. Am J Transplant 2006; 6: 1444-1450.

[29] Nankivell BJ, Borrows RJ, Fung CL, *et al.* Calcineurin inhibitor nephrotoxicity: longitudinal assessment by protocol histology. Transplantation 2004; 78: 557-565.

[30] Naesens M, Kuypers DRJ, Sarwal M. Calcineurin inhibitor nephrotoxicity. Clin J Am Soc Nephrol 2009; 4: 481-508.

[31] Olyaei AJ, de Mattos AM, Bennett WM. Nephrotoxicity of immunosuppressive drugs: new insight and preventive strategies. Curr Op Crit Care 2001; 7: 384-389.

[32] Joy MS, Hogan SL, Thompson BD, *et al.* Cytochrome P450 3A5 expression in the kidney of patients with calcineurin inhibitor nephrotoxicity. Nephrol Dial Transplant 2007; 22: 1963-1968.

[33] Hariharan S, Peddi VR, Jonhson CP, *et al.* Recurrent and *de novo* renal diseases after renal transplantation: a report from the renal allograft disease registry. Am J Kidney Dis 1998; 31: 928-931.

[34] Briganti EM, Epi MC, Russ GR, *et al.* Risk of renal allograft loss from recurrent glomerulonephritis. N Eng J Med 2002; 347: 103-109.

[35] Hirsch HH, Knowles W, Dickerman M, *et al.* Prospective study of polyoma virus type BK replication and nephropathy in renal-transplant recipients. N Engl J Med 2002; 347: 488-496.

[36] Hariharan S. BK virus nephritis after renal transplantation. Kidney Int 2006; 69: 655-662.

[37] Dall A, Hariharan S. BK nephritis after renal transplantation. Clin J Am Soc Nephrol 2008; 3: S68-S75.

[38] Amer H, Fidler ME, Myslak M, *et al.* Proteinuria after kidney transplantation, relationship to allograft histology and survival. Am J Transplant 2007; 7: 2748.

[39] Halimi J-M, Laouad I, Buchler M, *et al* Early low-grade proteinuria; causes, short-term evolution and long-term consequences in renal transplantation. Am J Transplant 2005; 5: 2281-2288.

[40] Amer H, Cosio FG. Significance and management of proteinuria in kidney transplant recipients. J Am Soc Nephrol 2009; 20: 2490-2492.

[41] Isoniemi HM, Krogerus L, von Willebrand E, *et al.* Histopathological findings in well-functioning, long-term renal allografts. Kidney Int 1992; 41: 155-160.

[42] Lauronen J, Häyry P, Paavonen T. An image analysis-based method for quantification of chronic allograft damage index parameters. APMIS 2006; 114: 440-448.

[43] Hourmant M, Cesbron –Gautier A, Terasaki PI, *et al.* Frequency and clinical implications of development of donor-specific and non-donor-specific HLA antibodies after kidney transplantation. J Am Soc Nephrol 2005; 16: 2804-2812.

[44] Lee PC, Terasaki PI, Takemoto SK, *et al.* All chronic rejection failures of kidney transplants were preceded by the development of HLA antibodies. Transplantation 2002; 74: 1192-1194.

[45] Terasaki PI, Ozawa A. Predictive value of HLA antibodies and serum creatinine in chronic rejection: results of a 2-year prospective trial. Transplantation 2005; 80: 1194-1197.

[46] Worthington JE, Martin S, Al-Husseini DM, *et al.* Posttransplantation production of donor HLA-specific antibodies as a predictor of renal transplant outcome. Transplantation 2003 : 75 : 1034-1040.

[47] Mizutami K, Terasaki P, Rosen A, *et al.* Serial ten-year follow-up of HLA and MICA antibody production prior to kidney graft failure. Am J Transplant 2005; 5: 2265-2272.

[48] Lee PC, Zhu L, Terasaki PL, Evely MJ. HLA-specific antibodies developed in the first year posttransplant are predictive of chronic rejection and renal graft loss. Transplantation 2009; 88: 568-574.

[49] Scornik JC, Guerra G, Schold JD, *et al.* Value of posttransplant antibody tests in the evaluation of patients with renal graft dysfunction. Am J Transplant 2007; 7: 1806-1814.

[50] Bartel G, Regele H, Wahrmann M, *et al.* Posttransplant HLA alloreactivity in stable kidney transplant recipients-incidences and impact on long-term allograft outcomes. Am J Transplant 2008; 8: 2652-2660.

[51] Ashton-Chess J, Giral M, Mengel M, *et al.* Tribbles-1 as a novel biomarker of chronic antibody mediated rejection. J Am Soc Nephrol 2008; 19: 116.

[52] Zhang PL, Rothblum LI, Han WK, *et al.* Kidney injury molecule-1 expression in transplant biopsies is a sensitive measure of cell injury. Kidney Int 2008 ; 73 : 608-614.

[53] Van Timmeren MM, Vaidya VS, van Ree RM, *et al.* High urinary excretion of kidney injury molecule-1 is an independent predictor of graft loss in renal transplant recipients. Transplantation 2007; 84: 1625-1630.

[54] EDTA-ERA: European best practice guidelines. Nephrol Dial Transplant 2000; 15 (suppl 4): 1-67.

[55] K/DOQI clinical practice guidelines for chronic kidney disease: evaluation, classification, and stratification. Am J Kidney Dis 2002; 39(suppl 1): S1-S266.

[56] Kasiske BL. Anjum S, Shah R, *et al.* Hypertension after kidney transplantation. Am J Kidney Dis 2004; 43: 1071-1081.

[57] Karthikeyan V, Karpinski J, Nair RC, Knoll G. The burden of chronic kidney disease in renal transplant recipients. Am J Transplant 2003; 4(2): 262-269.

[58] Marcén R, Pascual J, Tenorio M, *et al.* Chronic kidney disease in renal transplant recipients. Transplant Proc 2005; 37: 3718-3720.

[59] Ansell D, Udayaraj UP, Steenkamp R, Dudley CRK. Chronic renal failure in kidney transplant recipients. Do they receive optimum care?: data from the UK renal registry. Am J Transplant 2008; 7: 1167-1176.

[60] Marcén R, Del Castillo D, Capdevila L, *et al.* Achieving kidney disease treatment targets in renal transplant recipients: results from a cross sectional study in Spain. Transplantation 2009; 87: 1340-1346.

[61] Opelz G, Döhler B for the Collaborative Transplant Study. Improved long-term outcomes after renal transplantation associated with blood pressure control. Am J Transplant 2005; 5: 2725-2731.

[62] Arias M, Fernández-Fresnedo G, Rodrigo E, *et al.* Non-immunologic intervention in chronic allograft nephropathy. Kidney Int 2005; 68(suppl 99): S118-S123.

[63] Heize G, Mitterbauer C, Regele H, *et al.* Angiotensin-converting enzyme inhibitor or angiotensin II type 1 receptor antagonist therapy is associated with prolonged patient and graft survival after renal transplantation J Am Soc Nephrol 2006; 17: 89-999.

[64] Opelz G, Zeier M, Laux G, *et al.* No improvement of patients or graft survival in transplant recipients treated with angiotensin-converting enzyme inhibitors or angiotensin II type 1 receptor blockers: a collaborative transplant study report. J Am Soc Nephrol 2006; 17: 3257-3262.

[65] Amara AB, Sharma A, Alexander JL, *et al* Randomized controlled trial: lisinopril reduces proteinuria, ammonia and renal polypeptide tubular catabolism in patients with chronic allograft nephropathy. Transplantation 2010; 89: 104-114.

[66] Mas VR, Alvarellos T, Maluf DG, *et al.* Molecular and clinical response to angiotensin II receptor antagonist in kidney transplant patients with chronic allograft nephropathy. Transpl Int 2004; 17: 540-544.

[67] Zaltzman JS, Nash M, Chiu R, Prasad R. The benefits of renin-angiotensin blockade in renal transplant recipients with biopsy proven allograft nephropathy. Nephrol Dial Transplant 2004; 19: 940-944.

[68] Hiremath S, Fergusson D, Doucette S, *et al.* Renin angiotensin blockade in kidney transplantation: a systematic review of the evidence. Am J Transplant 2007: 7: 2350-2360.

[69] Van Riemsdijk IC, Mulder PG, de Fijter JW, *et al.* Addition of isradipine (Lomir) results in a better renal function after kidney transplantation; a double-blind, randomized, placebo-controlled, multi-center study. Transplantation 2000; 70: 122-126.

[70] Madsen JK, Sorensen SS, Hansen HE, Pedersen EB. The effect of felodipine on renal function and blood pressure in cyclosporin-treated renal transplant recipients during the first three months after transplantation. Nephrol Dial Transplant 1998; 13: 2327-2334.

[71] Midtvedt K, Hartmann A, Foss A, *et al.* Sustained improvement of renal graft function for two years in hypertensive renal transplant recipients treated with nifedipine as compared to lisinopril. Transplantation 2001; 72: 1787-1792.

[72] Carvalho MF, Soares V. Hyperlipidemia as a risk factor of renal allograft function impairment. Clin Transplant 2001; 15: 48-52.

[73] Wissing KM, Abramowicz D, Broeders N, Vereerstraeten P. Hypercholesterolemia is associated with increased kidney graft loss caused by chronic rejection in male patients with previous acute rejection. Transplantation 2000; 70: 464-472.

[74] Fried LF, Orchard TJ, Kasiske BL. Effect of lipid reduction on the progression of renal disease: a meta-analysis. Kidney Int 2001; 59: 260-269.

[75] Collins R, Armitage J, Parish S, *et al.* MRC/BHF Heart Protection Study of cholesterol-lowering with simvastatin in 5963 people with diabetes: a randomized placebo-controlled trial. Lancet 2003; 361: 2005-2016.

[76] Tonelli M, Moye L, Sacks FM, Cole T, Curhan GC. Effect of pravastatin on loss of renal function in people with moderate chronic renal insufficiency and cardiovascular disease. J Am Soc Nephrol 2003; 14: 1605-1613.

[77] Shepherd J, Kastelein JJP, Bittner V, *et al.* for the Treating to New Targets Investigators. Effect of intensive lipid lowering with atorvastatin on renal function in patients with coronary heart disease: the Treating to New Targets (TNT) study. Clin J Am Soc Nephrol 2007; 2: 1131-1139.

[78] Bianchi S, Bigazzi R, Caiazza A, Campese VM. A controlled, prospective study of the effects of atorvastatin on proteinuria and progression of kidney disease. Am J Kidney Dis 2003; 41: 565-570.

[79] Holdaas H, Fellström B, Jardine AG, *et al.* Effect of fluvastatin on cardiac outcomes in renal transplant recipients: a multicentre, randomised, placebo-controlled trial. Lancet 2003; 361: 2024-2031.

[80] Wiesbauer F, Heinze G, Mitterbauer C, *et al.* Statin use is associated with prolonged survival of renal transplant recipients. J Am Soc Nephrol 2008; 19: 2211-2218.

[81] Hur KY, Kim MS, Kim YS, *et al* Risk factors associated with the onset and progression of posttransplantation diabetes in renal allograft recipients. Diabetes Care 2007; 30: 609-615.

[82] Vincenti F, Friman S, Scheuermann E, *et al* on behalf of the DIRECT investigators. Results of an international, randomised trial comparing glucose metabolism disorders and outcome with cyclosporine *versus* tacrolimus. Am J Transpl 2007; 7: 1-9.

[83] Kasiske BL, Snyder JJ, Gilbertson D, Matas AJ. Diabetes mellitus after kidney transplantation in the United States. Am J Transplant 2003; 3: 178-185.

[84] Cosio FG, Kudva Y, van der Velde M, *et al.* New onset hyperglycemia and diabetes are associated with increased cardiovascular risk after kidney transplantation. Kidney Int 2005; 67: 2415-2421.

[85] Abramowicz D, Del Carmen Rial M, Vitko S, *et al.* Cyclosporine withdrawal from a mycophenolate mofetil – containing immunosuppressive regimen: results of a five years, prospective, randomized study. J Am Soc Nephrol 2005; 16: 2234-2240.

[86] Suwelack B, Gerhardt U, Hohage H. Withdrawal of cyclosporine or tacrolimus after addition of mycophenolate mofetil in patients with chronic allograft nephropathy. Am J Transplant 2004; 4: 655-662.

[87] Dudley C, Prohanka E, Riad H, *et al.* for the Mycophenolate mofetil "Creeping creatinine" Study Group. Mycophenolate mofetil substitution for cyclosporine A in renal transplant recipients with chronic progressive allograft dysfunction: the "Creeping Creatinine" study. Transplantation 2005; 79: 466-475.

[88] Watson CJE, Firth J, Williams PF, *et al.* A randomized controlled trial of late conversion from CNI-based to sirolimus-based immunosuppression following renal transplantation. Am J Transplant 2005; 5: 2496-2503.

[89] Stallone G, Infante B, Schena A, *et al.* Rapamycin for treatment of chronic allograft nephropathy in renal transplant patients. J Am Soc Nephrol 2005; 16: 3755-3762.

[90] Diekman F, Budde K, Slowinski T, *et al.* Conversion to sirolimus for chronic allograft dysfunction: long-term results confirm predictive value of proteinuria. Transpl Int 2008; 21: 152-155.

[91] Wali RK, Mohanlal V, Ramos E, *et al.* Early withdrawal of calcineurin inhibitors and rescue immunosuppression with sirolimus-based therapy in renal transplant recipients with moderate to severe renal dysfunction. Am J Transplant 2007; 7: 1572-1583.

[92] Mulay AV, Cockfield S, Stryker R, *et al.* Conversion from calcineurin inhibitors to sirolimus for chronic renal allograft dysfunction: a systematic review of the evidence. Transplantation 2006; 82: 1153-1162.

[93] Tang SC, Chan KW, Tang CS, *et al.* Conversion of ciclosporin A to tacrolimus in kidney transplant recipients with chronic allograft nephropathy. Nephrol Dial Transplant 2006; 21: 3243-3251.

[94] Meier M, Nitschke M, Weidtmann B, *et al.* Slowing progression of chronic allograft nephropathy by conversion from cyclosporine to tacrolimus: a randomized control trial. Transplantation 2006; 81: 1035-1040.

[95] Shihab FS, Waid TH, Conti DJ, *et al* for the CRAF study group. Conversion from cyclosporine to tacrolimus in patients at risk for chronic renal allograft failure: 60-months results of the CRAF study. Transplantation 2008; 85: 1261-1269.

[96] Gonzalez- Molina M, Serón D, García del Moral R, *et al.*Mycophenolate mofetil reduces deterioration of renal function in patients with chronic allograft nephropathy. A follow-up study by the Spanish Cooperative Study Group of Chronic Allograft Nephropathy. Transplantation 2004; 77: 215-219.

[97] Frimat L, Cassuto-Viguier E, Charpentier B, *et al.* Impact of cyclosporine reduction with MMF: a randomized trial in chronic allograft dysfunction. The ´reference´study. Am J Transplant 2006; 6: 2725-2734.

[98] Merville P, Bergé F, Deminière C, *et al.* Lower incidence of chronic allograft nephropathy at 1 year post-transplantation in patients treated with mycophenolate mofetil. Am J Transplant 2004; 4: 1769-1775.

[99] Saunders RN, Bicknell GR, Nicholson ML. The impact of cyclosporine dose reduction with or without the addition of rapamycin on functional, molecular, and histological markers of chronic allograft nephropathy. Transplantation 2003; 75: 772-780.

[100] Djamali A, Samaniego M. Fibrogenesis in kidney transplantation: potential targets for prevention and therapy. Transplantation 2009; 88: 1149-1156.

[101] Franceschini N, Cheng O, Zhang X, *et al.* Inhibition of propyl-4-hydrolase ameliorates chronic rejection of mouse kidney allografts. Am J Transplant 2003; 79: 355-360.

[102] Lunz J, Yao Y, Song E, *et al.* Inhibition of matrix metalloproteinases during chronic allograft nephropathy in rats. Transplantation 2005; 79: 655-661.

[103] Kiss E, Adams J, Grone HJ, Wagner J. Isotrenoin ameliorates renal damage in experimental acute renal allograft rejection. Transplantation 2003; 76: 480-489.

[104] Azuma H, Takahara S, Matsumoto K, *et al.* Hepatocyte growth factor prevents the development of chronic allograft nephropathy in rats. J Am Soc Nephrol 2001; 12: 1280-1292.

[105] Rostaig L, Guilbeau-Frugier C, Fort M, *et al.* Treatment of symptomatic transplant glomerulopathy with rituzimab. Transplant Int 2009; 22: 906-913.

[106] Hariharan S. BK virus nephritis after renal transplantation. Kidney Int 2006; 69: 655-662.

[107] Vasudev B, Hariharan S, Hussian SA, *et al.* BK virus nephritis: risk factors, timing and outcomes in renal transplant recipients. Kidney Int 2005; 68: 1834-1839.

[108] Trofe J, Hirsch HH, Ramos E. Polyomavirus-associated nephropathy: update of clinical management in kidney transplant patients. Transplant Infect Dis 2006; 8: 76-85.

CHAPTER 25

Pregnancy and Kidney Transplantation

Lisa A. Coscia, Carolyn H. McGrory and Vincent T. Armenti*

Department of Surgery, Thomas Jefferson University, Philadelphia, PA, USA

Abstract: The National Transplantation Pregnancy Registry (NTPR) was established in 1991 to study the outcomes of pregnancies in female transplant recipients as well as pregnancies fathered by male transplant recipients. Data from the NTPR along with publications of smaller experiences have endorsed the concepts that successful pregnancies are possible in the solid-organ transplant population. The largest cohort among the organ transplant population studied by the NTPR continues to be the kidney transplant recipient group. Data collected over the last twenty years by the NTPR have addressed a myriad of issues, thus providing a variety of additional information for healthcare providers in caring for transplant recipients of childbearing age. Preconception guidelines proposed in 1976 have undergone some refinement over the years, however most remain applicable today. Outcomes of the children of transplant recipients have been encouraging with few negative effects identified, but ongoing surveillance is still important. This article will provide a review of the historical literature regarding pregnancy in the kidney transplant population, recent studies conducted by the NTPR, and a brief review of the current literature regarding pregnancy after kidney transplantation.

Keywords: Kidney Transplant, Pregnancy, High-Risk, Quality of Life, Immunosuppression, Tacrolimus, Cyclosporine, Fetal Malformations, Sirolimus, Mycophenolate Mofetil.

INTRODUCTION

Kidney graft survival has reached 95% for living related kidney transplants in the United States, allowing an increased number of female kidney transplant recipients to contemplate parenthood [1]. The issues faced by female transplant recipients considering pregnancy today vary dramatically when compared to those of the first recipient whose pregnancy occurred more than 50 years ago. In the first case reported by Murray *et al.* there was more concern for the kidney itself and whether it would be affected by the gravid uterus than concern regarding immunosuppression or comorbid diseases in the recipient, as is the case in the modern era of transplantation. This recipient, who received a living donor kidney from her identical twin, went on to deliver a healthy infant and two years later delivered another healthy infant [2]. A celebration of the 50th anniversary of this first post-transplant birth was commemorated by recipients, their families and NTPR staff on March 10, 2008 in Philadelphia.

Since this first report of a pregnancy in a female kidney recipient, thousands of such pregnancies have been noted *via* single case reports, transplant center reports and registry data [3-36]. There have been numerous advances in transplantation and immunosuppression since that first report of pregnancy after kidney transplantation.

Nearly twenty years ago, the National Transplantation Pregnancy Registry (NTPR) was established at Thomas Jefferson University to study the outcomes of female transplant recipients who have had pregnancies and those pregnancies fathered by male transplant recipients. The number of recipients enrolled in the registry as of September 2010 is listed in Tables **1** and **2**.

The NTPR collects information on all types of solid-organ recipients who have had pregnancies and all of their outcomes, whether livebirth, stillbirth, spontaneous abortions, therapeutic abortions and ectopic pregnancies. As noted in the tables, the number of pregnancies is greater than the number of recipients, as

***Address correspondence to Vincent T. Armenti:** Thomas Jefferson University, 1025 Walnut Street, Suite 605, Philadelphia, PA 19107, USA; Tel: 215-955-4482; Fax: 215-923-1420; E-mail: Vincent.Amenti@jefferson.edu

Massimiliano Veroux and Pierfrancesco Veroux (Eds)

some have had more than one pregnancy. The number of pregnancy outcomes is greater than the number of pregnancies due to multiple births, some of these are a result of *in vitro* fertilization.

Table 1: Pregnancies in female transplant recipients reported to the NTPR as of September 2010

Organ	Recipients	Pregnancies	Outcomes*
Kidney	880	1395	1442
Liver	160	281	287
Liver-Kidney	4	6	7
Small-Bowel	1	1	1
Pancreas-Kidney	43	77	79
Pancreas alone	1	4	5
Heart	55	94	96
Heart-Lung	5	5	5
Lung	21	30	32
Totals	**1170**	**1893**	**1954**

*Includes twins and triplets.

Table 2: Pregnancies fathered by male transplant recipients reported to the NTPR as of September 2010

Organ	Recipients	Fathered Pregnancies	Outcomes*
Kidney	595	905	921
Liver	63	101	107
Liver-Kidney`	2	4	4
Liver-Heart-Kidney	1	1	1
Liver-Intestine-Kidney	1	2	2
Pancreas-Kidney	33	41	42
Heart	105	152	155
Heart-Lung	1	2	2
Heart-Lung-Kidney	1	2	2
Lung	3	3	3
Total	**805**	**1213**	**1239**

*Includes twins and triplets.

Consent allows for the NTPR to collect data *via* questionnaires, hospital records and phone interviews.

The largest cohort in the NTPR is the kidney transplant recipient population. This article will review historical cases of pregnancy after kidney transplantation, reexamine data from the NTPR, and provide a brief literature review of current issues relating to pregnancy after kidney transplantation.

PRECONCEPTION GUIDELINES

Published in 1976, Davison and colleagues published a review of the literature at that time, and along with their clinical experience, formulated guidelines for counseling the female kidney transplant recipient contemplating pregnancy. The original list consisted of the following eight guidelines: (1) good general health for at least two years since the transplant, (2) stature compatible with good obstetric outcome, (3) no proteinuria, (4) no significant hypertension, (5) no evidence of renal rejection, (6) no evidence of pelvicalceal distention on a recent excretory urogram, (7) plasma creatinine of 2 mg/dL (180μmol/L) or less, and (8) drug therapy: prednisone 15 mg/day or less, azathioprine 3 mg/kg/day or less. For the most part, these guidelines for counseling kidney recipients in large part remain applicable today [37].

Before Cyclosporine

Hume *et al.* reported the first case of pregnancy in a recipient receiving immunosuppression during pregnancy. The recipient conceived shortly after transplant and delivered a healthy infant while on azathioprine 125 mg and prednisone 10 mg, both daily [38]. Since that report, thousands of successful post-transplant pregnancies have occurred in kidney transplant recipients during the azathioprine era. The spontaneous abortion rate was approximately 14%, and the therapeutic abortion rate was approximately 20%. Of pregnancies that continued beyond the first trimester, more than 90% were successful. Renal impairment occurred in approximately 15% of women, and hypertension complicated approximately 30% of pregnancies. Preterm delivery was common, affecting 45% to 60% of pregnancies, with fetal growth restriction occurring in approximately 20% [39].

Cyclosporine Era

Reports in the late 1980s demonstrated that the use of cyclosporine (CsA) during pregnancy may be associated with intrauterine growth restriction [40, 41]. An NTPR study compared outcomes of those pregnancies with cyclosporine exposure and/or prednisone and azathioprine (156), to those pregnancy outcomes with exposure to azathioprine and prednisone (249). Significant variables included: mean birthweight (CsA-group lower), drug-treated hypertension (CsA-group higher), diabetes (CsA-group higher), and rejection (CsA-group higher) [11].

Another early NTPR study in the CsA group analyzed prepregnancy predictors of adverse outcomes. Those recipients starting pregnancies with poorer allograft function (*i.e.* serum creatinine > 1.5 mg/dL) had a greater likelihood of allograft dysfunction during and after pregnancy [12]. Additionally, if there was an increase in serum creatinine during pregnancy, it was more likely to be associated with an adverse graft outcome, as well as poorer newborn outcomes. An upward trend in serum creatinine during pregnancy however, should not be attributed to pregnancy alone, so this should warrant prompt investigation. Since serum creatinine normally decreases during pregnancy due to increased glomerular filtration rate, therefore, during gestation, renal allograft rejection may be signaled by only a minor rise in serum creatinine. In a case controlled study, kidney recipients with no graft loss during or after pregnancy reported a prepregnancy mean serum creatinine of 1.3 mg/dL, compared to those where graft loss was reported in whom prepregnancy mean serum creatinine was 1.6 mg/dL. Similarly, mean birth weight and gestational age correlated with the degree of graft function; children of better graft function recipients had a mean birth weight of 2428 g and mean gestational age of 36 weeks, in contrast to 1949 g and 33.9 weeks for those with poorer function [12].

NTPR: CURRENT PREGNANCY OUTCOMES AND STUDIES IN KIDNEY RECIPIENTS

With the kidney cohort comprising the largest data set in the NTPR, many studies have been conducted in this group. Overall outcomes of kidney recipients on different types of immunosuppression are shown in Table **3** [35].

Table 3: NTPR: Pregnancy outcomes in female kidney transplant recipients with CsA, Neoral® and Prograf® exposure during pregnancy

	CsA	**Neoral®**	**Prograf®**
Maternal Factors (n=pregnancies)	**(514)**	**(199)**	**(190)**
Mean transplant to conception interval (yrs)	3.5 ± 2.8	5.8 ± 3.9	4.1 ± 2.9
Hypertension during pregnancy	62%	68%	52%
Diabetes during pregnancy	12%	2%	9%
Infection during pregnancy	23%	19%	24%
Preeclampsia	29%	28%	31%
Rejection episode during pregnancy[1]	1%	3%	3%

Table 3: cont….

Mean serum creatinine (mg/dl)			
Before pregnancy	1.4 ± 0.5	1.3 ± 0.4	1.2 ± 0.4
During pregnancy	1.4 ± 0.7	1.4 ± 0.5	1.3 ± 1.0
After pregnancy	1.6 ± 0.97	1.5 ± 0.6	1.4 ± 0.9
Graft loss within 2 yrs of delivery	11%	8%	10%
Outcomes (n)*	**(526)**	**(211)**	**(194)**
Therapeutic abortions	8%	1%	1%
Spontaneous abortions	12%	18%	24%
Ectopic	0.6%	0.5%	0.5%
Stillborn	3%	1%	2%
Livebirths	76%	80%	72%
Livebirths (n)	**(401)**	**(168)**	**(140)**
Mean gestational age (wks)	36 ± 3.4	36 ± 3.0	35 ± 3.7
Premature (<37 wks)	52%	48%	54%
Mean birthweight	2490 ± 755 g	2536 ± 700 g	2422 ± 869 g
Low birthweight (<2500 g)	46%	43%	48%
Cesarean section	53%	42%	61%
Newborn complications	41%	42%	50%
Neonatal deaths n (%) (within 30 days of birth)	4 (1%)	4 (2%)**	4 (3%)

[1] biopsy-proven acute rejection only.
[*] includes twins, triplets, quadruplets.
** quadruplet 24 wk pregnancy; all newborn died.
CsA - Sandimmune® brand cyclosporine (338 recipients, 514 pregnancies).
Neoral® brand cyclosporine (132 recipients, 199 pregnancies).
Prograf® (126 recipients, 190 pregnancies).

The outcomes are shown in 3 different categories: pregnancies exposed to cyclosporine (Sandimmune®), cyclosporine USP modified (Neoral®) and tacrolimus (Prograf®). Overall pregnancy outcomes are similar among the groups, and the majority of the recipients do well if the recipient has adequate stable graft function prior to pregnancy. There continues to be a high incidence of hypertension and preeclampsia during pregnancy among kidney recipients.

Some recipients may have had more than one pregnancy on a different calcineurin inhibitor. Not included in this table are those recipients on other regimens or where regimen could not be determined.

Recent NTPR studies performed among the female kidney recipient cohort have included: analyses of potential predictors of early postpartum graft loss, the association between an increase in serum creatinine during pregnancy and kidney transplant survival after delivery; the effects of successive pregnancies in kidney recipients on newborn and maternal outcomes, and comparison of pregnancy outcomes in recipients who received a kidney transplant from a live donor (LD) *versus* recipients of a deceased donor (DD) kidney transplant. As the studies were performed at different times, the numbers will not reflect the overall numbers in Table **1**. The studies are reviewed below.

We evaluated the association between early postpartum graft dysfunction (defined as the need for a biopsy and/or treatment of acute rejection within 3 months postpartum) and several potential predictors: type of immunosuppressive therapy, hypertension before and during pregnancy, diabetes mellitus before and during pregnancy, preeclampsia, serum creatinine (Cr) increase during pregnancy; prepregnancy Cr $\geq$ 1.4 mg/dl and transplant to conception interval. A total of 508 pregnancies were analyzed. Preeclampsia, Cr increase during pregnancy of 0.2 mg/dl and prepregnancy Cr $\geq$ 1.4 mg/dl were independent predictors of early postpartum graft dysfunction (Table **4**) [42].

Table 4: NTPR: Predictors of early postpartum graft dysfunction in kidney transplant recipients

	Adjusted OR	95% CI	P value
Preeclampsia	**2.67**	**1.20-5.97**	**0.016**
Creatinine increase during pregnancy (0.2 mg/dl)	**1.19**	**1.06-1.33**	**0.004**
Prepregnancy Creatinine ≥ 1.4 mg/dl	**5.39**	**2.14-13.55**	**<0.001**

Overall, an increase in Cr of 0.2 mg/dl had the highest sensitivity and specificity in predicting early postpartum graft dysfunction and was most predictive in recipients with a prepregnancy Cr ≥ 1.4 mg/dl. Preeclampsia, Cr increase during pregnancy of 0.2 mg/dl and prepregnancy Cr ≥ 1.4 mg/dl are all independent predictors of early postpartum graft dysfunction. These results suggest that kidney transplant recipients with any of the above described risk factors require close attention to graft function and immunosuppressive monitoring in the early postpartum months.

An NTPR analysis studied the association between serum creatinine during pregnancy and graft loss (GL) at any time after delivery [43]. A total of 488 pregnancies were analyzed in kidney transplant recipients. The graft survival for those with any increase in serum creatinine during pregnancy and those without an increase in serum creatinine were compared using the Kaplan-Meier method and the log-rank test. Graft survival was significantly lower among the recipients who experienced an increase in serum creatinine during pregnancy. After adjusting for immunosuppressive therapy, hypertension before and during pregnancy, preeclampsia, and graft survival remained significantly different between the two groups (p=0.001). Mean prepregnancy serum creatinine was 1.3 ± 0.4 mg/dl in the kidney recipients without GL, and 1.5 ± 0.6 mg/dl in those who had GL after delivery, while mean serum creatinine during pregnancy was 1.2 ± 0.4 mg/dl in the recipients without GL, and 1.7 ± 0.9 mg/dl for the GL group. The data suggest that kidney transplant recipients with any increase in serum creatinine during pregnancy require appropriate diagnostic and therapeutic intervention early after delivery, given the higher risk of deterioration in graft function [43].

The NTPR also analyzed the effects of successive pregnancies in female kidney transplant recipients on newborn and maternal outcomes (Table **5**) [44].

Table 5: NTPR: Subsequent pregnancies in female kidney recipients

	1st Pregnancy	2nd Pregnancy	3rd Pregnancy	4th Pregnancy	5th Pregnancy	p value#
No. of recipients	478	189	68	19	6	
Age at conception (yrs)	29±5	30.2±5.1	31.3±4.8	32.8±4.4	31.2±4.5	
Pregnancy outcomes*	495	191	70	20	6	
Livebirths	78%	72%	83%	65%	67%	NS
Spontaneous abortions	13%	19%	13%	20%	17%	NS
Stillbirths	3%	3%	1%	10%	0	NS
Therapeutic abortions	6%	6%	3%	5%	0	NS
Mean gestational age (wks)	35.6±3.4	36±3.4	36.6±3	36.8±2.5	37.6±1.3	0.01
Prematurity (<37 wks)	54.7%	48.5%	46.4%	41.7%	25%	0.01
Mean birthweight (g)	2426±772	2578±749	2613±752	2646±816	3076±831	0.002
Low birthweight (<2500 g)	49.7%	40.2%	39.7%	30.8%	25%	0.001
Rejection during pregnancy	1.5%	1.6%	4.5%	0	0	NS
Graft loss within 2 yrs after delivery	8%	7.5%	7.4%	5.3%	0	NS

*Includes twins, triplets; #linear trends; NS=not significant.

There were 782 outcomes of 760 pregnancies, including twins and triplets. Of 478 renal recipients who had a first pregnancy, 189 had between one and four subsequent pregnancies. The proportion of livebirths was not statistically different among the groups. With successive pregnancies there was a trend towards increased gestational age. Female kidney recipients with successive pregnancies had similar rejection rates during each pregnancy, and no difference in graft loss within 2 years after delivery. Successive pregnancies in kidney transplant recipients are not associated with adverse fetal outcomes and/or increased maternal graft loss. Transplant recipients with adequate allograft function who wish to have more than one pregnancy should not be discouraged to conceive [44].

Another NTPR analysis compared pregnancy outcomes in female recipients who received a kidney transplant from a live donor (LD) *versus* recipients of a deceased donor (DD) kidney transplant (Table **6**) [45].

Table 6: NTPR: Pregnancy outcomes after live donor *vs.* deceased donor kidney transplantation

	Live donor	**Deceased donor**	**P value**
Recipients	148	111	
Pregnancies	240	165	
Pregnancy outcomes*	251	170	
Maternal Conditions			
Transplant to conception interval (yrs)	5.2 ± 3.5	5.2 ± 3.7	NS
Hypertension during pregnancy	56%	63%	NS
Preeclampsia	28%	35%	NS
Infections during pregnancy	21%	22%	NS
Rejection during pregnancy	2%	2%	NS
Serum creatinine before pregnancy (mg/dl)	1.3 ±0.4[1]	1.2 ±0.4	<0.01
Serum creatinine during pregnancy (mg/dl)	1.4 ±0.5	1.2 ±0.95	0.03
Serum creatinine after pregnancy (mg/dl)	1.5 ±0.6[2]	1.3 ±0.8	<0.01
Graft loss within 2 yrs of delivery	8%	7%	NS
Neonatal Outcomes			
Livebirths	77%	74%	NS
Gestational age (wks)	35.5 ±3.7	35.8 ±3.2	NS
Birthweight (g)	2470 ± 809	2501 ±765	NS

* Includes twins; 1 *vs.* 2 $p<0.01$; NS=not significant.

All recipients were maintained on a calcineurin inhibitor based regimen during pregnancy. Mean serum creatinines before, during and after pregnancy were analyzed in those pregnancies with complete data (LD n=166 and DD n=123). Among the LD group is a subset of recipients who had received their husbands' kidney and went on to become pregnant. There were 9 recipients who had 15 pregnancies after receiving a LD kidney from their husband. The incidence of rejection during pregnancy was low in both groups (2%), and graft loss within 2 years after pregnancy was 8% in LD group and 7% in the DD group. Mean serum creatinine was slightly higher after pregnancy in each group, this difference reaching statistical significance only in LD group. Based on this analysis, evaluation of recipient and newborn variables does not reveal significant differences in the outcomes of pregnancies in LD *versus* DD kidney transplant recipients, except slightly higher serum creatinine in the LD group before and after pregnancy. The high incidences of hypertension, preeclampsia and infection during pregnancy underscore the high-risk nature of pregnancy in kidney transplant recipients irrespective of donor source [45].

With the increase in kidney graft survival there are many recipients who were transplanted under the age of 21 and went on to have a pregnancy. Outcomes are listed in Table **7** [46]. Trends are similar to that of the overall kidney group.

Table 7: NTPR: Outcomes in female kidney pediatric recipients (age<21 years at time of transplant)

Maternal Factors	**CsA**	**Neoral**	**Tacrolimus**
Mean transplant to conception interval	4.2 yrs	7.1 yrs	4.3 yrs
Hypertension during pregnancy	57%	65%	53%
Diabetes during pregnancy	2%	3%	5%
Infection during pregnancy	27%	27%	41%
Rejection episode during pregnancy	2%	0%	11%
Pre-eclampsia	27%	52%	21%
Mean serum creatinine (mg/dL)			
Before pregnancy	1.4	1.3	1.2
During pregnancy	1.4	1.3	2.0
After pregnancy	1.7	1.4	1.7
Graft loss within 2 yrs of delivery	13%	0%	25%
Outcomes (n)[1]	(150)	(37)	(19)
Therapeutic abortions	9%	0%	0%
Spontaneous abortions	10%	11%	16%
Ectopic	1%	0%	0%
Stillborn	5%	3%	11%
Livebirths	77%	87%	74%
Livebirths (n)	(114)	(32)	(14)
Mean gestational age	36 wks	37 wks	36 wks
Premature (<37 wks)	49%	50%	36%
Mean birthweight	2493 gms	2531 gms	2575 gms
Low birthweight (<2500 gms)	46%	47%	43%
Cesarean section	54%	48%	50%
Newborn complications	39%	28%	50%
Neonatal deaths n (%) (within 30 days of birth)	1 (1)	0	0

[1]includes twins, triplets;CsA - Sandimmune brand cyclosporine (90 recipients, 147 pregnancies);Neoral brand cyclosporine (29 recipients, 35 pregnancies);Tacrolimus-Prograf (16 recipients, 19 pregnancies).

Pregnancies resulting from *in vitro* fertilization (IVF) have been reported. Six kidney recipients reported using IVF for conception with 6 pregnancies resulting in 8 outcomes (two sets of twins). There were 7 livebirths and 1 spontaneous abortion. Immunosuppression at conception included: tacrolimus and prednisone (n=1), Neoral®, azathioprine and prednisone (n=2), Neoral® and azathioprine (n=1), Sandimmune® and prednisone (n=1) and azathioprine and prednisone (n=1). All 6 recipients reported drug-treated hypertension during pregnancy and one recipient reported preeclampsia (twin pregnancy). None of the recipients reported gestational diabetes or transplant rejection during pregnancy. The mean gestational age of the infants was 33.6 ± 2.6 weeks and the mean birthweight was 1624 ± 687 g. At last follow-up, all 7 children were reported healthy and developing well, however one child was diagnosed with a heart murmur and had a small periorbital hemangioma removed. One recipient reported loss of kidney function 1.5 years postpartum and one recipient reported poor function 11 years postpartum. These preliminary data support the use of assisted reproductive technologies following kidney transplantation and warrant the further study of IVF following other solid organ transplants.

Mycophenolic Acid Products (Mpa)

Of recent concern are those pregnancies exposed to MPA, specifically mycophenolate mofetil (MMF, CellCept® and others) and mycophenolic acid (Myfortic®). There have been reports to the NTPR and in the literature describing a risk of a phenotypic pattern of craniofacial dysmorphology in the offspring of those pregnancies exposed to MPA [47-70].

In October 2007, the FDA pregnancy category of MPA products was changed from category C to D, based on registry and post-marketing data [47, 48]. Package inserts recommend discontinuation of MPA 6 weeks prior to conception. The European Best Practice Guidelines also have the same recommendation regarding MPA [70]. In this section, all exposures to MPA reported to the NTPR are described including those in extra-renal recipients [49]. There are 68 (44 kidney, 5 pancreas-kidney (P/K), 9 liver and 10 heart) recipients who have reported 97 pregnancies (98 outcomes, includes one set of twins) with exposure to MPA products (n=95 MMF; n= 2 EC-MPS, enteric-coated mycophenolate sodium). Maternal dosage varied greatly and ranged from 250 mg daily to 1500 mg bid (MMF) and from 180 mg bid to 720 mg bid (EC-MPS). Upon discovery of pregnancy, in some cases the dose was decreased, discontinued or switched to another immunosuppressive, usually azathioprine. Pregnancy outcomes included: 48 (49%) livebirths, 48 (49%) spontaneous abortions and 2 stillbirths (2%). There were 59 pregnancies in kidney, 8 P/K, 14 liver, and 16 heart recipients.

Of the 48 livebirths, structural birth defects were described in 11 livebirths, for an incidence of 22.9%. Multiple anomalies were reported in one stillbirth. Birth defects included: hypoplastic nails and shortened fifth fingers n=1, cleft lip and palate and microtia n=1, microtia n=1, syndactyly and ear malformations n=1, facial malformations n=1, duodenal atresia, atrioventricular canal defect and Tetralogy of Fallot n=1, total anomalous pulmonary venous return n=1, and 4 infants had multiple anomalies and died [49]. Prior to MPA, birth defect incidences in the newborn of transplant recipients ranged from 4-5%, similar to that of the general population (3-5%).

In addition to the cases reported to the NTPR, there is a growing body of literature regarding MPA use during pregnancy [49-70]. The cases reported in the literature review include transplant recipients and those patients treated with MPA for other diagnoses such as systemic lupus erythematosus and other autoimmune disorders. Many of these cases are also included in NTPR data. The first case described in the literature with exposure to MPA was in 1996 [51]. Since this report there has been numerous reports regarding MPA [52-63]. Some of the more recent cases are described below.

One article describes in greater detail a case reported by the NTPR in 2006 [50]. Parisi *et al.* report the first case of congenital diaphragmatic hernia after exposure to MMF [64]. The kidney recipient was treated with MMF 250 mg twice daily, tacrolimus 3 mg in the morning and 2 mg at night and prednisone 5 mg daily. A 35 week 2163 g infant was delivered. Birth defects, in addition to the congenital diaphragmatic hernia, included tracheoesophageal fistula, cleft lip, heart defects, microtia, and hypoplastic toenails. The infant died the day after birth. Initially the authors hypothesized that this was a case of Fryns syndrome, a genetic syndrome. Upon further evaluation and as more data appeared in the literature, the authors suggest that MMF exposure can produce a phenocopy of a genetic syndrome.

Dei Malatesta, from Italy, describes a kidney transplant recipient who became pregnant 6 months after azathioprine was switched to MMF (500 mg daily) due to rejection [65]. Additionally the recipient was administered tacrolimus and prednisone. The MMF was continued due to the recent rejection. At 15 weeks the ultrasound revealed a normal fetus with no malformations. At 37 weeks a healthy 2850 g infant was delivered. The recipient observed that the infant's right eye was smaller than the left and the iris was abnormal. Upon further evaluation, ocular fundoscopy demonstrated a choroidal colomba involving the optic disc.

Anderka *et al.* report MMF exposure during pregnancy in a patient with lupus nephritis [66]. The mother was treated with 1000 mg twice daily of MMF for 11-12 weeks gestation along with prednisone. At 31 weeks the patient delivered a 980 g infant. The patient was induced due to fetal growth restriction. The infant was noted to have bilateral microtia.

Five pregnancies with exposure to MMF in 5 patients with systemic lupus erythematosis (SLE) were described in an abstract [67]. MMF exposure ranged from 21-37 days gestation. Of the 5 pregnancies, 3 resulted in livebirths, spontaneous abortion at 6.5 weeks and a fetal demise at 22 weeks (active nephritis). There were no structural malformations reported. The authors concluded that there were a high number of pregnancy losses in their cohort. They also recommended more stringent counseling and monitoring for effective contraception in patients taking MMF.

An additional case from Spain described an SLE patient who conceived while being treated with MMF 1500 mg/day and deflazacort 90 mg/day. The pregnancy was discovered at 8 weeks. Due to the patient's severe kidney disease, medical therapy was not altered. The infant was delivered at 31 5/7 weeks due to preeclampsia. The neonate was noted to have microretrognathia and complete cleft palate. The authors did note that at 2 years of age the infant had normal neurocognitive development [70].

Reports to the NTPR continue to reveal an increased incidence of birth defects in recipients with exposure to MPA products during pregnancy when compared to those recipients not maintained on those agents. Structural birth defects consisting of microtia (ear deformity) and facial defects suggest a pattern of malformations. Evaluation of the higher incidence of non-viable outcomes requires further study in this cohort.

There continue to be many challenges ahead as this class of medication is utilized in young women. Continuing reports in the literature and reports to the NTPR will help to formulate additional preconception and pregnancy guidelines for recipients taking this medication.

NTPR: Sirolimus and Everolimus

Reports of pregnancy outcomes with exposure to sirolimus remain limited and in two cases there was also exposure to MMF. There are 10 kidney recipients reporting 11 pregnancies with exposure to sirolimus (9 livebirths, 2 spontaneous abortions). Birth defects were reported in 2 of the 9 liveborn and included: cleft lip, cleft palate and microtia (initial MMF exposure with late pregnancy exposure to sirolimus, previously reported) [50] and in the second case Tetralogy of Fallot (no concomitant MMF). Among 2 liver recipients, 2 pregnancies were reported (1 normal livebirth, 1 spontaneous abortion). There was one P/K recipient who reported a spontaneous abortion. There were two heart recipients who reported 2 pregnancies; one livebirth with facial malformations (maternal immunosuppression was Gengraf®, MMF, and sirolimus at conception), and one spontaneous abortion [35]. There are only a limited number of case reports with exposure to sirolimus during pregnancy as well [72-74]. To date there have been no pregnancies reported to the NTPR with exposure to everolimus.

Breastfeeding

This topic remains controversial and reports continue to be individual case-based [35, 75-79]. The number of recipients in the NTPR who choose to breastfeed continues to increase. There have been no specific problems reported in the children who were breastfed. In the NTPR, there are 51 kidney recipients have reported breastfeeding their 64 children.

Some believe that any immunosuppressive drug exposure to the infant could potentially exceed the threshold for safety, but the relatively small amount of drug transferred and the lack of reported adverse effects together with the documented benefits of breastfeeding may outweigh the theoretical risks of this exposure. Continued study and case reports in this area are warranted, especially in regard to infant drug exposure and immunological development.

NTPR: Offspring of Kidney Transplant Recipients

The largest cohort among the kidney recipients is the Sandimmune®-treated group. This group was analyzed for the incidence of structural malformations among their offspring (502 pregnancies, 391 live births) [80]. Other immunosuppressive agents used in these recipients included azathioprine and/or prednisone, not MPA products. In the liveborn, there were 19 (4.9%) birth defects reported without a predominant pattern of malformations (Table **8**). This incidence of structural malformations is comparable with the general population, which ranges from 3-5% [81].

Table 8: Structural birth defects in kidney transplant recipients by maintenance immunosuppression reported to the NTPR

	Sandimmune®	Neoral®	Tacrolimus*
Total # of pregnancies	502	174	102
Total # of livebirths	391	143	72
Total # of liveborn with birth defects	19	4	3
Incidence of birth defects	4.9 %	2.8%	4.2%

*without adjunctive use of mycophenolate mofetil (MMF).

Follow-up of the children of transplant recipients is one of the goals of the NTPR. There were 304 female kidney recipients on cyclosporine-based immunosuppression who had 456 pregnancies delivered between March 1983 and November 1999, identified. Of these, 133 female recipients were contacted for information on their 175 children. In this group, 71 of the children were older than five years, and eight (11%) of these had been diagnosed with attention deficit/hyperactivity disorder (ADHD) [82]. Two years subsequent to this initial survey, 114 of the 133 recipients were again contacted and detailed information was gathered on 147 children. At follow-up, the mean age of the children was 6.5±2.8 years. The rate of ADHD was similar to that found in the general population. It was concluded that even though significant comorbidity exists among kidney recipients, developmentally the offspring of kidney transplant recipients did not appear to be adversely affected with regard to learning disabilities.

A follow-up study of 187 kidney recipients on Sandimmune® included a detailed questionnaire evaluating 249 offspring [83]. Special consideration was afforded to structural malformations, kidney function, neurocognitive development and the immune system. The 249 children had a mean birth weight of 2554 ± 739 g and a mean gestational age of 36 ± 3.2 weeks. Structural malformations were reported in 4% of the offspring. The parents reported that renal problems possibly attributed to maternal disease had occurred in nine of their children, and twelve others had mild kidney problems. ADHD was diagnosed in 5.2% of the children (compared to 6-7% of all U.S. children in the general population) and 4% had neurocognitive problems; no immune deficits were reported. Forty-six percent of the parents who stated concerns about parenting also expressed apprehension regarding the possibility of long-term effects on the children's immune system or their general health. The mean age at follow-up was 11 years old ranging from 1.6 to 18.6 years. This analysis of offspring in the cyclosporine cohort did not reveal a particular pattern, an increased risk of birth defects, or significant problems with renal function, ADHD, neurocognitive or immune development. This study substantiates that, in the cyclosporine cohort where there are available data on the long-term outcome of the children, while there are concerns that require continued surveillance, there has not been a predominance of problems among these offspring. Continued surveillance and long-term follow-up of offspring is warranted.

Literature Review

Authors continue to report pregnancy outcomes after kidney transplant *via* case reports, single transplant center data and registry data [19-36, 84-100]. A majority of the articles published originate from outside the United States. Many publications are reviews of the current literature [84-90].

The American Society of Transplantation organized a consensus conference on women's health and the group subsequently published consensus guidelines [101]. An additional recommendation of the conference was for the transplant community to participate in active pregnancy registries that could assist in formulating more definitive guidelines.

Contemporary publications have confirmed previous reports [102-104] that when compared to a matched non-pregnant population, long-term graft function has not been statistically different among the kidney recipients who were pregnant [105, 106].

Recently, two studies analyzed the pregnancy rate and livebirth rate in kidney transplant recipients using large healthcare databases [33, 34]. The first by Gill *et al.* used the United States Renal Data System to examine pregnancy outcomes in the first 3 years post transplant [33]. Using ICD-9 codes they identified 530 pregnancies in 483 female transplant recipients. One of the primary conclusions of the paper was that the pregnancy rate in kidney transplant recipients was lower and decreased more rapidly over time compared to the general US population.

Levidiotis *et al.* used data from the Australian and New Zealand Dialysis and Transplant (ANZDATA) Registry to study pregnancy and maternal outcomes in kidney recipients [34]. As with previous studies, no difference was seen in graft survival when comparing kidney recipients who had a pregnancy to control recipients without a pregnancy. As with the Gill paper, the ANZDATA Registry study demonstrated a r more recent trend toward a reduced and decreasing fertility rate in kidney recipients. Both studies add information to the increasing number of studies performed regarding pregnancy after transplantation.

Others have been able to tabulate data from their entire country due to access to a national healthcare system. This was done in Sweden, Italy, and Japan. The overwhelming tone of the reports is that pregnancies post kidney transplant are possible and successful, although they should be considered high-risk and managed in coordination with the transplant team and high-risk obstetricians.

It would be beneficial to the reader to review a number of articles regarding the health of the offspring of kidney transplant recipients [18, 82, 107, 108]. Also suggested are articles focusing on the management of any high-risk pregnancy and on the ethical issues and dilemmas facing all concerned. A number of articles have emphasized the high-risk nature of pregnancies after transplantation and the myriad of issues surrounding these pregnancies. All published reports continue to provide a valuable resource to this field.

Management

Guidelines for management of the pregnant transplant recipient are listed in Table **9**. Additional publications contain suggested guidelines for the management of pregnant transplant recipients [6, 37, 85, 101-110]. Pregnancies after transplantation should be considered high-risk and require diligent maternal and fetal surveillance and teamwork among all healthcare providers involved.

Summary

The field of pregnancy post transplantation is ever expanding with experience gained through continued case reports, center reports, and registry data. The NTPR maintains an ongoing active database to study the safety of pregnancy and includes the outcomes of female transplant recipients as well as of male recipients who father pregnancies. Analyses are ongoing and include long-term follow-up of recipients' graft status and of their offspring.

For kidney recipients, guidelines proposed in 1976 for counseling recipients during pregnancy remain applicable [37]. Recipients should be in general good health, and graft function should be stable and, ideally, rejection free. There should be optimal control of comorbid conditions such as hypertension and diabetes prior to conception. While the shortest safe interval from transplant to conception has not been established, one year is a reasonable milestone, given the prerequisites of stable, adequate graft function and maintenance level immunosuppression. During pregnancy, maintenance medication regimens should be continued with vigilant monitoring for effective drug levels and drug side effects with appropriate dose adjustment. These pregnancies are high-risk and require close maternal and fetal surveillance through coordinated care among maternal-fetal medicine specialists and transplant personnel.

With 20 years of experience, the NTPR remains an active resource for the transplant community. All transplant centers should encourage their recipients to participate in the NTPR. The continued recording of data in registries such as the NTPR is essential for assessing the safety of pregnancy in solid organ transplant recipients. Key benefits of the NTPR are the personal contact between registry staff and participants, the wide range of pregnancy-related variables that are analyzed, and the opportunity for health-care providers to obtain information that helps them care for transplant recipients on a case-by-case basis.

Table 9: Pregnancy after transplantation: Evaluations and management options

Prepregnancy
Patients should defer conception for at least 1 year after transplantation, with adequate contraception
Assessment of graft function (organ specific): • Maintenance immunosuppression options • Recent biopsy • Proteinuria • Hepatitis B & C status • CMV, toxoplasmosis, herpes simplex status
The effect of comorbid conditions, (*i.e.* diabetes, hypertension) should be considered and their management optimized; non-renal recipients should have their baseline kidney function assessed
Vaccinations should be given if needed (*i.e.* rubella, *etc.*)
Explore etiology of original disease; discuss genetic issues if relevant
Discuss the effect of pregnancy on renal allograft function
Discuss the risks of intrauterine growth restriction, prematurity, low birthweight
Prenatal
Accurate early diagnosis and dating of pregnancy
Clinical and laboratory monitoring of functional status of transplanted organ and immunosuppressive drug levels every 4 weeks until 32 weeks, then every 2 weeks until 36 weeks, and then weekly until delivery
Monthly urine culture
Surveillance for rejection with biopsy if it is suspected
Surveillance for bacterial or viral presence, *i.e.* CMV, toxoplasmosis, hepatitis
Fetal surveillance
Monitor for hypertension and nephropathy
Surveillance for preeclampsia
Screening for gestational diabetes
Labor and Delivery
Vaginal delivery is optimal; cesarean delivery for obstetric reasons
For heart/heart-lung/lung recipients: Vigilance for poor or absent cough reflex, the need for airway protection, unpredictable response to vasoactive medications; judicious use of intravenous fluids
Postnatal
Monitor immunosuppressive drug levels for at least 1 month postpartum, especially if dosages increased during pregnancy
Surveillance for rejection with biopsy if it is suspected
Breastfeeding discussion
Contraception counseling

ACKNOWLEDGEMENTS

The NTPR acknowledges the cooperation of transplant recipients and over 200 centers in North America who have contributed their time and information to the registry. The NTPR is supported by grants from Novartis Pharmaceuticals Corp., Astellas Pharma US, Inc., Genentech, Inc., Pfizer Inc, Teva Pharmaceuticals USA and Sandoz Inc.

To contact the NTPR:

National Transplantation Pregnancy Registry (NTPR), Thomas Jefferson University, Department of Surgery, 605 College Building, 1025 Walnut Street, Philadelphia, PA 19107, 215-955-4820; Toll-free 877-955-6877; E-mail NTPR.Registry@jefferson.edu; http://www.tju.edu/ntpr/

REFERENCES

[1] http://optn.transplant.hrsa.gov/latestData/rptStrat.asp; Accessed September 7, 2010.

[2] Murray JE, Reid DE, Harrison JH, Merrill JP. Successful pregnancies after human renal transplantation. N Engl J Med. 1963;269:341-343.

[3] Rudolph J, Schweizer RT, Bartus SA. Pregnancy in renal transplant patients. Transplantation 1979; 27:26-29.

[4] Penn I, Makowski EL, Harris P. Parenthood following renal and hepatic transplantation. Transplantation. 1980;30:397-400.

[5] Davison JM, Lindheimer MD. Pregnancy in renal transplant recipients. J Reprod Med. 1982;27:613.

[6] Hou S. Pregnancy in transplant recipients. Med Clin North Am 1989; 73: 667-683.

[7] Muirhead N, Sabharwal AR, Rieder MJ, *et al.* The outcome of pregnancy following renal transplantation –The experience of a single center. Transplantation. 1992;54;429-432.

[8] Rizzoni G, Ehrich JHH, Broyer M, *et al.* Successful pregnancies in women on renal replacement therapy: Report from the EDTA Registry. Nephrol Dial Transplant 1992; 7: 279-287.

[9] Bumgardner GL and Matas AJ. Transplantation and pregnancy. Transplantation Reviews. 1992; 6: 139-162.

[10] Salmela KT, Kyllonen LEJ, Holmberg C, *et al.* Impaired renal function after pregnancy in renal transplant recipients. Transplantation 1993; 56: 1372-1375.

[11] Armenti VT, Ahlswede KM, Ahlswede BA, *et al.* National Transplantation Pregnancy Registry - Outcomes of 154 pregnancies in cyclosporine-treated female kidney transplant recipients. Transplantation. 1994; 57: 502-506.

[12] Armenti VT, Ahlswede KM, Ahlswede BA, *et al.* Variables affecting birthweight and graft survival in 197 pregnancies in cyclosporine-treated female kidney transplant recipients. Transplantation 1995;59:476-479.

[13] Jimenez E, Gonzalea-Carabello Z, Morales-Otero L, *et al.* Triplets born to a kidney transplant recipient. Transplantation. 1995;59:435-436.

[14] Ehrich JHH, Loirat C, Davison JM, *et al.* Repeated successful pregnancies after kidney transplantation in 102 women (Report by the EDTA Registry). Nephrol Dial Transplant 1996; 11: 1314-1317.

[15] Kozlowska-Boszko B, Lao M, Gaciong Z, *et al.* Chronic rejection as a risk factor for deterioration of renal allograft function following pregnancy. Transplant Proc 1997; 29: 1522-1523.

[16] Resch B, Mache CJ, Windhager T, *et al.* FK506 and successful pregnancy after renal transplantation. Transplant Proc 1998; 30: 163-164.

[17] Toma H, Kazunari T, Tokumoto T, *et al.* Pregnancy in women receiving renal dialysis or transplantation in Japan: a nationwide survey. Nephrol Dial Transplant 1999;14:1511-1516.

[18] Willis FR, Findlay CA, Gorrie MJ, *et al.* Children of renal transplant recipient mothers. J Paediatr Child Health 2000; 36: 230-235.

[19] Oz BB, Hackman R, Einarson T, Koren G. Pregnancy outcome after cyclosporine therapy during pregnancy: a meta-analysis. Transplantation 2001;71(8):1051-1055.

[20] Scott JR, Branch DW, Holman J. Autoimmune and pregnancy complications in the daughter of a kidney transplant patient. Transplantation 2002; 73: 815-816.

[21] Thompson BC, Kingdon EJ, Tuck SM, *et al.* Pregnancy in renal transplant recipients: the Royal Free Hospital experience. Q J Med 2003; 96: 837-844.

[22] Jain AB, Shapiro R, Scantlebury VP, *et al.* Pregnancy after kidney and kidney-pancreas transplantation under tacrolimus: a single center's experience. Transplantation. 2004; 77(6):897-902.

[23] Källèn B, Westgren M, Aberg A, Olausson PO. Pregnancy outcome after maternal organ transplantation in Sweden. BJOG: An International Journal of Obstetrics & Gynaecology 2005;112:904-909.

[24] Miniero R, Tardivo I, Curtoni ES, *et al.* Outcome of pregnancy after organ transplantation: a retrospective survey in Italy. Transplant Int 2005;17(11):724-729.

[25] Ghanem ME, El-Baghdadi LA, Badawy AM, *et al.* Pregnancy outcome after renal allograft transplantation: 15 years experience. Europ J Obstet, Gyne, & Repro Biology 2005; 121:178-181.

[26] Goshorn J, Youell TD. Darbepoetin alfa treatment for post-renal transplantation anemia during pregnancy. Am J Kidney Dis 2005 46:e8-16.

[27] Saito K, Suzuki K, Yamagishi T, *et al.* Hydronephrosis in the early stages of pregnancy after renal transplantation. Int J Urology 2006;13:809-810.

[28] Naqvi R, Noor H, Ambareen S, *et al.* Outcome of pregnancy in renal allograft recipients: SIUT experience. Transplant Proc 2006;38:2001-2002.

[29] Sibanda N, Briggs JD, Davison JM, *et al.* Pregnancy after organ transplantation: a report from the UK Transplant pregnancy registry. Transplantation 2007;83:1301-1307.

[30] Kim HW, Seok HJ, Kim TH, *et al.* The experience of pregnancy after renal transplantation: pregnancies even within postoperative 1 year may be tolerable. Transplantation 2008;85:1412-1419.

[31] Ghafari A, Sanadgol H. Pregnancy after renal transplantation: ten-year single-center experience. Transplant Proc 2008;40: 251-252.

[32] Nicovani V, Poblete H, Toro J,*et al.* Successful multiple pregnancy (triplets) in a kidney transplant recipient: a case report. Transplant Proc 2009; 41:2688-2690.

[33] Gill JS, Zalunardo N, Rose C, Tonelli M. The pregnancy rate and live birth rate in kidney transplant recipients. Am J Transplant 2009;9:1541-1549.

[34] Levidiotis V, Chang S, McDonald S. Pregnancy and maternal outcomes among kidney transplant recipients. J Am Soc Nephrol 2009; 20: 2433-2440.

[35] Coscia LA, Constantinescu S, Moritz MJ, *et al.* Report from the National Transplantation Pregnancy Registry (NTPR): Outcomes of Pregnancy after Transplantation. In: Clinical Transplants 2009. Cecka J.M. and Terasaki P.I. (Eds), UCLA Terasaki Foundation Laboratory, Los Angeles, CA, 113-122, 2010.

[36] Gorgulu N, Yelken B, Caliskan Y, *et al.* Does pregnancy increase graft loss in female renal allograft recipients? Clin Exp Nephrol 2010;14:244-247.

[37] Davison JM, Lind T, Uldall PR. Planned pregnancy in a renal transplant recipient. Br J Obstet and Gynaecol 1976; 83:518-527.

[38] Board JA, Lee HM, Draper DA, Hume DM. Pregnancy following kidney homotransplantation from a non-twin. Report of a case with concurrent administration of azathioprine and prednisone. Obstet & Gynecol 1967;29:318-323.

[39] Davison JM. Pregnancy in renal allograft recipients: problems, prognosis and practicalities. In: Lindheimer MD, Davison JM, editors. Balliere's Clin Obstet Gynaecol. 8. London (UK): Bailliere Tindall, 1994: 501-527.

[40] Pickrell MD, Sawers R, Michael J. Pregnancy after renal transplantation: Severe intra-uterine growth retardation during treatment with cyclosporin A. BMJ. 1988;296:825.

[41] Fein A, Vechoropoulos M, Nebel L. Cyclosporin-induced embryotoxicity in mice. Biol Neonate. 1989; 56:165-173.

[42] Seibel-Seamon J, Leiby B, Constantinescu S, *et al.* Predictors of postpartum graft dysfunction in kidney transplant recipients. Presented at the Society for Maternal-Fetal Medicine 29th Annual Meeting 2009.

[43] Seibel-Seamon J, Berghella V, Constantinescu S, *et al.* Creatinine increase during pregnancy is associated with decreased graft survival after delivery in kidney recipients. Am J Transplant 2009;S2: 277A.

[44] Constantinescu S, Silva P, Khan SS, *et al.* Outcomes of subsequent pregnancies in female kidney transplant recipients. Am J Transplant 2007;S2: 555A.

[45] Constantinescu S, Coscia LA, Gitman L, *et al.* Pregnancy Outcomes after Live Donor *vs.* Deceased Donor Kidney Transplantation. Am J of Transplant 2010;S4:128.

[46] Armenti VT, Moritz MJ, Davison JM. Pregnancy. In: Pediatric Solid Organ Transplantation, 2nd Edition, Blackwell Publishing, Ltd. Malden, MA, 425-436, 2007.

[47] Roche Laboratories. Mycophenolate mofetil package insert. Nutley, NJ: Roche Laboratories, 2009.

[48] Novartis Pharmaceuticals Corp. Mycophenolic acid package insert. East Hanover, NJ: Novartis Pharmaceuticals, 2009.

[49] Sifontis NM, Coscia LA, Nguyen TD, *et al.* Pregnancy Outcomes with Exposure to Mycophenolic Acid Products. Am J Transplant 2010;10(S4):169.

[50] Sifontis NM, Coscia LA, Constantinescu S, *et al.* Pregnancy outcomes in solid organ transplant recipients with exposure to mycophenolate mofetil or sirolimus. Transplantation 2006;82:1698-1702.

[51] Pérgola PE, Kancharla A, Riley DJ. Kidney transplantation during the first trimester of pregnancy: immunosuppression with mycophenolate mofetil, tacrolimus and prednisone. Transplantation 2001;71:994-997.

[52] Le Ray C, Coulomb A, Elefant E, *et al.* Mycophenolate mofetil in pregnancy after renal transplantation: a case of major fetal malformations. Obstet & Gyn 2004;103: 1091-1094.

[53] Tjeertes IFA, Bastiaans DET, van Ganzewinkel CJLM, Zegers SHJ. Neonatal anemia and hydrops fetalis after maternal mycophenolate mofetil use. J Perinatol 2007;27:62-64.

[54] Perez-Aytes A, Ledo A, Boso V, *et al.* In utero exposure to mycophenolate mofetil: A characteristic phenotype? Am J Med Genet Part A 2008;146A:1-7.

[55] El Sebaaly A, Charpentier B, Snanoudj R. Fetal malformations associated with mycophenolate mofetil. Nephrol Dial Transplant 2007;22:2722.

[56] Velinov M, Zellers N. The mycophenolate mofetil syndrome. Clin Dysmorphol 2008;17:77-78.

[57] Schoner K, Steinhard J, Figiel J, Rehder H. Severe facial clefts in acrofacial dysostosis: a consequence of prenatal exposure to mycophenolate mofetil? Obstet & Gynecol 2008;111(2 Pt 2):483-86.

[58] Huang SY, Chueh HY, Shaw SW, Shih JC, Cheng PJ. Sonographic diagnosis of fetal malformations associated with mycophenolate mofetil exposure in utero. Am J of Obstet & Gynecol 2008;199(2):e6-8.

[59] Ang GS, Simpson SA, Reddy AR. Mycophenolate mofetil embryopathy may be dose and timing dependent. Am J Med Genet 2008;146A:1963-1966.

[60] Koren G. Mycophenolate mofetil: emerging as a potential human teratogen. Can Fam Physician 2008;54:1112-1113.

[61] Vento M, Perez Aytes A, Ledo A, *et al.* Mycophenolate mofetil during pregnancy: some words of caution. Pediatrics 2008;122:184-185.

[62] Carey JC. "Where observation is concerned, chance favors only the prepared mind". Obstet Gynecol 2008 111(2 Pt 2):479-480.

[63] Pisoni CN, D'Cruz DP. The safety of mycophenolate mofetil in pregnancy. Expert Opin Drug Saf 2008;7:219-222.

[64] Parisi MA. Zayed H. Slavotinek AM. Rutledge JC. Congenital diaphragmatic hernia and microtia in a newborn with mycophenolate mofetil (MMF) exposure: phenocopy for Fryns syndrome or broad spectrum of teratogenic effects? Am J Med Genet. Part A. 2009;149A:1237-1240.

[65] Dei Malatesta MF, Rocca B, Gentile T. A case of coloboma in a newborn to a woman taking mycophenolate mofetil in pregnancy after kidney transplantation. Transplant Proc 2009; 41:1407-1409.

[66] Anderka MT, Lin AE, Abuelo DN, *et al.* Reviewing the evidence for mycophenolate mofetil as a new teratogen: case report and review of the literature. Am J Med Genet. Part A 2009;149A:1241-1248.

[67] Ortiz EC, Torralba KD, Evelyn CM, Quismorio FP. Fetal and maternal outcomes with mycophenolate mofetil (MMF) exposure during the first trimester in patients with systemic lupus erythematosus. Arthritis & Rhem 2009:60:S591.

[68] Jackson P, Paquette L, Watiker V, *et al.* Intrauterine exposure to mycophenolate mofetil and multiple congenital anomalies in a newborn: possible teratogenic effect. Am J of Med Genet Part A 2009;149A:1231-1236.

[69] Merlob P, Stahl B, Klinger G. Tetrada of the possible mycophenolate mofetil embryopathy: a review. Reproductive Toxicology 2009;28(1):105-8.

[70] Ruiz-Campillo CW, Castillo F, Perapoch J, Salcedo S. Mycophenolate mofetil use for lupus nephritis during pregnancy: Report of a case of fetal malformations and literature update. Internet J Gynecol Obstet 2009;11(2).

[71] EBPG Expert Group on Renal Transplantation. European best practice guidelines for renal transplantation. Section IV. Long-term management of the transplant recipient. IV.10. Pregnancy in renal transplant recipients. Nephrol Dial Transplant 2002;17(Suppl.):50–55.

[72] Jankowska I, Oldakowska-Jednyak U, Jabiry-Zieniewicz Z, *et al.* Absence of teratogenicity of sirolimus used during early pregnancy. Transplant Proc 2004;36:3232-3233.

[73] Guardia O, del Rial MC, Casadei D. Pregnancy under sirolimus immunosuppression. Transplantation 2006;81:636.

[74] Chu SH, Liu KL, Chiang YJ, *et al.* Sirolimus used during pregnancy in a living related renal transplant recipient: a case report. Transplant Proc 2008;40:2446-2448.

[75] Nyberg G, Haljamäe U, Frisenette-Fich C, *et al.* Breast-feeding during treatment with cyclosporine. Transplantation. 1998; 65: 253-255.

[76] Thiru Y, Bateman D, Coulthard M. Successful breast-feeding while mother was taking cyclosporin. BM J. 1997;23:463.

[77] Thiagarajan KD, Easterling T, Davis C, *et al.* Breast-feeding by a cyclosporine–treated mother. Obstet Gynecol 2001;97:816-818.

[78] Moretti M, Sgro M, Johnson D, *et al.* Cyclosporine excretion into breast milk. Transplantation. 2003;75:2144-2146.

[79] Gardiner S, Begg E. Breastfeeding during tacrolimus therapy. Obstet Gynecol 2006; 107:453-455.

[80] Coscia LA, Constantinescu S, Moritz MJ, *et al.* Report from the National Transplantation Pregnancy Registry (NTPR): Outcomes of Pregnancy after Transplantation. In: Clinical Transplants 2007. Cecka J.M. and Terasaki P.I. (Eds), UCLA Terasaki Foundation Laboratory, Los Angeles, CA, 29-42, 2008.

[81] Finnell RH. Teratology: General considerations and principles. J Allergy Clin Immunol 1999;103:337-342.

[82] Stanley CW, Gottlieb R, Zager R, *et al.* Developmental well-being in offspring of women receiving cyclosporine post-renal transplant. Transplant Proc 1999;31:241-242.

[83] Lavelanet AF, Coscia LA, Moritz MJ, Armenti VT. Long-term follow-up in the offspring of Sandimmune treated female kidney recipients. Am J Transplant 2006;S164.

[84] McKay DB, Josephson MA. Pregnancy in recipients of solid organs- Effects on mother and child. N Engl J Med 2006;354:1281-1293.

[85] Josephson JA, McKay DB. Considerations in the medical management of pregnancy in transplant recipients. Adv Chronic Kidney Dis 2007;14:156-167.

[86] Watnick S, Rueda J. Reproduction and contraception after kidney transplantation. Curr Opin Obstet Gynecol 2008;20:308-312.

[87] McKay DB, Josephson MA. Pregnancy after kidney transplantation. CJASN. 2008;3 Suppl 2:S117-125.

[88] Mastrobattista JM, Gomez-Lobo V. Society for Maternal-Fetal Medicine. Pregnancy after solid organ transplantation. Obstetr Gynecol 112;2008:919-932.

[89] Wielgos M, Pietrzak B, Bobrowska K, *et al.* Pregnancy after organ transplantation. Neuroendocrinology Letters 2009;30(1):6-10.

[90] Zachariah MS. Tornatore KM. Venuto RC. Kidney transplantation and pregnancy. Curr Opin Organ Transplant 2009;14:386-391.

[91] Al Duraihimh H, Ghamdi G, Moussa D, *et al.* Outcome of 234 pregnancies in 140 renal transplant recipients from five middle eastern countries. Transplantation 2008 85:840-843.

[92] Oliveira LG, Sass N, Sato JL, Ozaki KS, Medina Pestana JO. Pregnancy after renal transplantation – a five yr single center experience. Clin Transplant 2007;21:3014.

[93] Abe T, Ichimaru N, Okumi M, *et al.* Pregnancy after renal transplantation: A single-center experience. Int J Urol 2008;15:587-592.

[94] Guazzelli CA, Torloni MR, Sanches TF, *et al.* Contraceptive counseling and use among 197 female kidney transplant recipients. Transplantation 2008;86:669-672.

[95] Areia A, Galvao A, Pais MSJ, *et al.* Outcome of pregnancy in renal allograft recipients. Arch Gynecol Obstet 2008;279:273-277.

[96] Alfi AY, Al-essawy MA, Al-lakany M, *et al.* Successful pregnancies post renal transplantation. Saudi J Kidney Dis Transpl 2008;19:746-750.

[97] Karkar A. Pregnancy and contraceptive issues in renal transplant recipients. Saudi J Kidney Dis Transpl 2008;19:165-173.

[98] Gutièrrez MJ, Gonzalez P, Delgado I, *et al.* Renal allograft function and cardiovascular risk in recipients of kidney transplantation after successful pregnancy. Transplant Proc 2009;41:2399-2402.

[99] Bouattar T, Hakim H, Rhou H, *et al.* Pregnancy in renal transplant recipients. Transplant Proc 2009; 41:1586-1588.

[100] Khedmat H, Alavian SM, Taheri S. Pregnancy after renal transplantation: prospects and concerns. Ann Transplant 2009;14:55-60.

[101] McKay DB, Josephson MA, Armenti VT, *et al.* Women's Health Committee of the American Society of Transplantation. Reproduction and transplantation: report on the AST Consensus Conference on Reproductive Issues and Transplantation. Am J Transplant 2005;5:1592-1599.

[102] Sturgiss SN, Davison JM. Effect of pregnancy on long-term function renal allografts. Am J Kidney Dis 1992; 19: 167-172.

[103] Sturgiss SN, Davison JM. Effect of pregnancy on the long-term function of renal allografts: An update. Am J Kidney Dis 1995;26:54-56.

[104] First MR, Combs CA, Weiskittel P, *et al.* Lack of effect of pregnancy on renal allograft survival or function. Transplantation 1995;59:472–476.

[105] Fischer T, Neumayer HH, Fischer R, *et al.* Effect of pregnancy on long-term kidney function in renal transplant recipients treated with cyclosporine and with azathioprine. Am J Transplant 2005; 5:2732-2739.

[106] Rahamimov R, Ben-Haroush A, Wittenberg C, *et al.* Pregnancy in renal transplant recipients: Long-term effect on patient and graft survival. A single-center experience. Transplantation 2006;81:660-664.

[107] Di Paolo S, Schena A, Morrone L, *et al.* Immunologic evaluation during the first year of life of infants born to cyclosporine-treated kidney transplant recipients: Analysis of lymphocyte subpopulation and immunoglobulin serum levels. Transplantation 2000; 69: 2049-2054.

[108] Giudice PL, Dubourg L, Hadj-Aïssa A, *et al.* Renal function of children exposed to cyclosporine in utero. Nephrol Dial Transplant 2000; 15: 1575-1579.

[109] Ross LF. Ethical considerations related to pregnancy in transplant recipients. NEJM 2006;354:1313-1316.

[110] del Mar Colon M, Hibbard JU. Obstetric considerations in the management of pregnancy in kidney transplant recipients. Adv Chronic Kidney Dis 2007;14:168-177.

CHAPTER 26

Clinical Tolerance in Kidney Transplantation

Tatsuo Kawai* **and A. Benedict Cosimi**

Massachusetts General Hospital, Transplant Center, Harvard Medical School, Boston, USA

Abstract: Induction of donor specific tolerance has been the ultimate goal in organ transplantation. Recent application of approaches to the induction of allograft tolerance in human kidney transplant recipients has been based upon preclinical studies in nonhuman primates, including 1) profound T cell depletion by powerful anti-T cell antibodies, 2) use of total lymphoid irradiation, 3) costimulatory blockade, 4) infusion of anergic cells 5) donor bone marrow (DBM) infusion without anticipation of engraftment and 6) DBM transplantation leading to Mixed Chimerism. Mixed Chimerism following DBM transplantation has to date been the most successful approach for induction of renal allograft tolerance in clinical kidney transplantation trials.

Keywords: Tolerance, Mixed Chimerism, Kidney Transplantation, Immunosuppression, Central Tolerance, Peripheral Tolerance, Prope Tolerance, Costimulatory Blockade, T-Cells Depletion, Blood Marrow Infusion.

INTRODUCTION

Since the advent of calcineurin inhibitors and other potent immunosuppressive medications, a significant improvement has been achieved in short-term survival rates following organ transplantation over the past two decades. However, longer-term results have been less satisfactory [1], mainly due to chronic rejection and the toxicities of chronically administered immunosuppressive drugs [2]. Therefore, induction of specific immunologic tolerance remains an important goal of organ transplantation. Although numerous tolerance induction strategies have been developed in rodent models, only a limited number of these approaches have been successfully translated to nonhuman primates (NHP) and even fewer to humans.

PRECLINICAL (NHP) STUDIES

Strategies that have successfully induced renal allograft tolerance in NHP include 1) profound depletion of recipient T cells, 2) total lymphoid irradiation (TLI), 3) costimulatory blockade, 4) infusion of anergic cells, 5) donor bone marrow (DBM) infusion and 6) DBM transplantation.

1) Profound T cell depletion: Knechtle *et al.* investigated the use of anti-CD3 immunotoxin (IT) for prolongation of renal allograft survival. In their experiments, all monkeys treated with anti-CD3 IT had significantly prolonged allograft survival [3]. However, the production of anti-donor alloantibody was not consistently prevented with anti-CD3 IT resulting in late alloantibody-mediated glomerular and arterial damage of the kidney allografts [4]. Although the use of immunotoxins with this strategy has not entered clinical trials, numerous attempts to withdraw conventional immunosuppressive medications after T-cell depletion have been undertaken (see "Prope" Tolerance below).

2) TLI: Tolerance induction using TLI was extensively tested in the1980s in several large animal models (dogs and NHP). The Stanford group applied TLI with a cumulative dose of 2800-4500 cGy in their canine experiments [5]. Myburgh *et al.* subsequently demonstrated prolonged renal or liver allograft survival in baboons with a reduced cumulative TLI dose of

***Address correspondence to Tatsuo Kawai:** Associate Professor of Surgery, Harvard Medical School Transplant Surgery, Massachusetts General Hospital Surgical Director, Dialysis Access Program MGH, White 510 55 Fruit St., Boston MA 02114, USA; Tel: +1 -617-726-0289; Fax: + 1 617-726-9322; E-mail: tkawai@partners.org

Massimiliano Veroux and Pierfrancesco Veroux (Eds)

1600 cGy [6]. DBM was also infused in some recipients, but prolonged survival was achieved even in recipients without DBM infusion. Based upon these observations, clinical trials of this strategy have been undertaken (see below).

3) Costimulatory blockade: Among the co-stimulatory signals that have been identified, the CD28 or CTLA4 (CD152)/CD80, CD86 and the CD40/CD40 ligand (CD154) pathways have been determined to be of central importance for T-cell activation or long-term kidney allograft survival [7, 8]. Several nonhuman primate tolerance models have been designed to evaluate the effect of blocking these critical pathways. Kirk *et al.* evaluated co-stimulatory blockade using humanized anti-CD154 mAb (hu5C8) in rhesus monkeys and achieved long-term kidney allograft survival [7, 8]. However, as with many tolerance induction protocols in large animals and man, these recipients eventually developed chronic rejection with alloantibody production. Kirk also tested a combination of CD154 blockade, sirolimus and donor specific transfusion in rhesus monkeys and, again, achieved long-term renal allograft survival in 3/5 recipients with specific acceptance of even skin allografts in two [9]. More recently Haanstra reported long-term stable renal allograft tolerance in two of four rhesus monkeys treated with a combination of anti-CD40 and anti-CD86 mAbs, followed by a 12-week course of CyA [10]. These encouraging observations led to some of the earliest clinical trials of tolerance induction as detailed below. Blocking the counter molecule of CD154, CD40, has also been tested in the NHP kidney transplant model. Blocking CD40 did not promote tolerance, but it significantly prolonged renal allograft survival without side effects [11]. This approach has not yet been extended to humans.

4) Infusion of anergic cells: Bashuda *et al.* reported successful induction of renal allograft tolerance in 3/6 monkey recipients who received adoptive transfer of anergic T cells induced by coculture with donor alloantigen in the presence of anti-CD80/CD86 antibody [12]. Although all three long-term survivors eventually succumbed to chronic rejection (personal communication), this is the first approach by adoptive transfer of regulatory cells tested in NHP.

5) DBM infusion: This strategy consists of host T-cell depletion, usually with antithymocyte globulin (ATG) or Alemtuzumab (Campath-1H), followed by DBM infusion. Although DBM engraftment, induction of macrochimerism (typically >1% of donor cells clearly detectable by flow cytometry), is not required in this approach, temporary functional activity of specific BM components has been cited as a possible mechanism leading to the prolonged allograft survival achieved in some recipients [13, 14]. With this regimen, graft survival has exceeded one year in approximately 50% of monkeys, and specific suppression of anti-donor CTL responses was demonstrated in long-term survivors. However, the production of anti-donor alloantibody could not be prevented and most recipients eventually succumbed to chronic rejection [14, 15]. This approach to tolerance induction has undergone extensive clinical evaluation.

6) DBM transplantation/Mixed chimerism: This approach requires at least transient DBM engraftment leading to mixed hematopoietic chimerism. The mechanism of tolerance induced in murine recipients has been defined as central resulting from migration of donor cells to the thymus and clonal deletion of donor-reactive cells [16]. Based on earlier rodent studies on mixed chimerism [16, 17], we developed a clinically relevant non-myeloablative preparative regimen that permits the induction of mixed chimerism and renal allograft tolerance following DBM transplantation in MHC fully-mismatched cynomolgus monkeys [18, 19]. With this approach, approximately 60% of recipients of MHC mismatched kidney allograft acquired tolerance, with the longest survival exceeding 16 years. However, different from the mixed chimerism observed in rodent models, chimerism induced in these monkeys has been transient, typically becoming undetectable within 2 months. Therefore, the mechanism of tolerance in these monkeys is considered the requirement of both peripheral and central processes. Supporting this hypothesis is evidence of involvement of T regulatory cells in the maintenance of tolerance, which has recently been demonstrated (manuscript in preparation).

CLINICAL ATTEMPTS FOR INDUCTION OF ALLOGRAFT TOLERANCE

As summarized in Table **1**, many attempts to induce clinical tolerance have been made, but successful allograft tolerance in a consecutive series of recipient has been achieved only by DBM transplantation to date.

Table 1: Clinical trials for induction of allograft tolerance

Protocol	Refs.
Profound T cell depletion by Campath-1H or Thymoglobulin	[20-27]
TLI	[28-30]
Costimulatory blockade/anti-CD154 mAb	[31-33]
Infusion of anergic cells	[12]
DBM infusion	[34-38]
DBMT/Mixed or Full Chimerism –HLA identical	[39-42]
DBMT/Mixed Chimerism –HLA mismatch	[43-45]

TLI: total lymphoid irradiation; DBM: donor blood marrow.

Profound T Cell Depletion

Calne *et al.* first reported a condition described as "Prope (almost) tolerance", in which low rejection rates of renal allografts were achieved with low dose cyclosporine monotherapy after peri-transplant alemtuzumab [20]. Alemtuzumab (Campath-1H) is a humanized monoclonal antibody that binds CD52, which is expressed on multiple hematopoietic cell populations, including T cells, B cells, monocytes, natural killer (NK) cells and dendritic cells. Rapid and profound lymphocyte depletion is achieved with only two doses of this antibody. Starzl *et al.* reported 90 clinical kidney transplant recipients who were treated with Alezutumab (Campath-1H) or rabbit thymoglobulin [21]. In these studies, subsequent planned weaning of conventional immunosuppressants was then undertaken but, unlike their experience in recipients of liver transplants, complete withdrawal of maintenance therapy (tolerance) was not achieved in renal recipients. Long-term follow-up revealed no improvement in patient or graft survival in these recipients compared with historic controls, and chronic allograft nephropathy (CAN) progressed at the same rate [22]. Kirk *et al.* added deoxyspergualine (DSG) to alemtuzumab to test a similar strategy that had been developed in NHP by Thomas [23]. Despite profound T-cell depletion and therapeutic DSG dosing, all alemtuzumab/DSG patients developed reversible rejection that was similar to that seen in patients treated with alemtuzumab alone [24]. Knechtle *et al.* have modified the protocol by using rapamycin monotherapy following the profound lymphocyte depletion by alemtuzumab [25]. Again, stable allograft function was observed in patients receiving only low-dose immunosuppression (drug minimization); but complete withdrawal (tolerance) was not attempted [26]. Thus, there remains little evidence that alemtuzumab promotes tolerance. It, therefore, continues to be used off-label as an induction agent to minimize maintenance immunosuppression [27].

Total Lymphoid Irradiation (TLI)

The Stanford group initially applied TLI in clinical kidney transplantation with a cumulative dose of 2000 cGy. Although successful discontinuation of immunosuppression was reported in three patients [28], two of these three patients eventually lost their graft function due to ureteral stenosis and chronic rejection [29]. One-year renal graft survival of patients receiving this regimen was 76% [30], which was inferior at that time to graft survival with conventional immunosuppression. The complexity of the regimen as well as failure to show an advantage in graft survival limited the enthusiasm for further studies with this approach. More recently, however, the same investigators have resumed their clinical studies of TLI in confirmation with donor stem cell infusion (see below).

Costimulatory Blockade

Despite the encouraging NHP observations with stimulatory blockade treatment, the initial clinical trials of anti-CD154 mAb in kidney transplantation were suspended because of unacceptable thromboembolic complications in the first few patients [31]. The precise mechanisms of thrombophilia associated with anti-CD154 monoclonal antibody (mAb) treatment have not been clarified. However, in our monkey studies, we have found that Ketorolac, a non-steroidal anti-inflammatory drug, is markedly effective for preventing such thromboembolic complications. This suggests involvement of platelet activation as one of the causes of thrombosis [32]. Although continuing preclinical studies indicate that CD154 blockade is a promising approach, clinical application of currently available anti-CD154 mAbs appears unlikely in view of the previously encountered thromboembolic complications. CTLA4Ig has also shown promising costimulatory blockade effects in both NHP and humans. Recently, a modified version of CTLA4Ig, LEA29Y or Belatacept, in which two amino acids were substituted to provide slower dissociation rates from both CD80 and CD86 ligands has been tested in human renal allograft recipients. In this clinical trial, Belatacept proved to be as effective and safe as conventional pharmacologic immunosuppression and renal function was better preserved [33]. No attempts have yet been reported to completely discontinue immunosuppressive therapy in patients treated with Belactacept.

Infusion of Anergic Cells

Based on their study in NHP [12], the Japanese group has started a clinical trial to induce tolerance in HLA mismatched living donor kidney transplant recipients. Anergic cells induced in MLR by blocking CD80/CD86 with monocloncal antibody were infused back to the recipient after treatment with cyclophosphamide. Ten patients have been enrolled into this study to date. Immunosuppression has not been discontinued completely in any of these patients (personal communication).

Donor Blood Marrow (DBM) Infusion

In 1991, Barber *et al.* reported a clinical trial in renal allograft recipients of DBM combined with ALG. Although significantly better allograft survival was observed in recipients treated with DBM, immunosuppression was not completely discontinued in any of these recipients [34]. In 1992, Starzl *et al.* reported seminal observations of 30 recipients of livers or kidneys with long-term stable graft function. With sensitive cytostaining and PCR techniques, small numbers of donor leukocytes (microchimerism) were identified in one or more peripheral recipient locations in all 30 patients [35, 36]. It was hypothesized that responses of coexisting donor and recipient cells can result in reciprocal clonal exhaustion, followed by peripheral clonal deletion [37]. To enhance such "microchimerism" state after organ transplantation, groups in Pittsburgh and Miami evaluated DBM infusion with conventional immunosuppression in various organ transplants. In these studies, although superior graft survival with less incidence of acute or chronic rejection was reported, clear evidence of tolerance induction has not been demonstrated [38]. Several groups have also attempted tolerance induction by profound lymphocyte depletion.

DBM Transplantation/Mixed Chimerism

HLA Identical Kidney Transplant Recipients

In HLA matched kidney transplant recipients, more durable chimerism has been reported. The Stanford group has reported successful induction of stable mixed chimerism and renal allograft tolerance using TLI and donor peripheral stem cell transplantation in a patient receiving an HLA identical kidney transplant [39]. The recipient was conditioned with TLI (80 cGy X 10, days 1-14), anti-rabbit thymocyte globulin (1.5 mg/kg X 5, days 0-4), and received HLA matched peripheral blood stem cells on day 14. Triple immunosuppressive therapy (mycophenolate mofetil, prednisone and cyclosporine) was continued after transplantation, but all immunosuppressive medications were slowly tapered off over 6 months. The patient has been doing well with normal kidney function with stable mixed chimerism for more than 28 months without immunosuppression. An advantage of this approach, if it can be extended to recipients of non HLA matched allografts, would be applicability to deceased donor transplantation, since all treatments in the regimen are initiated after organ transplantation.

At Massachusetts General Hospital (MGH), a total of seven patients with renal failure secondary to multiple myeloma have received HLA identical combined kidney and bone marrow transplantation (CKBMT) following conditioning with a non-myeloablative regimen. The preparative regimen consisted of cyclophosphamide (60mg/kg X2), local thymic irradiation 700 cGy, horse ATG and a 60-day course of post-transplant cyclosporine administration [40-42]. All recipients developed mixed hemopoietic chimerism which, however, became undetectable by day 100 after CKBMT in four of seven patients: two developed stable full chimerism and one developed stable mixed chimerism after additional donor lymphocyte infusions (DLI), administered in the attempt to improve the graft versus lymphoma (GVL) effect. Remission of the myeloma was observed in three of the four patients with transient chimerism, suggesting a GVL effect despite loss of chimerism. Immunosuppression was successfully withdrawn in all four recipients with transient chimerism with the longest kidney allograft survival exceeding 10 years. One of the recipients with full chimerism achieved complete remission of his myeloma but has been on mycophenolate mofetil and steroids to prevent GVHD. The other patient with full chimerism lost her renal function due to myeloma recurrence. The seventh patient developed stable mixed chimerism and normal renal function for longer than 3 years without immunosuppression. These observations demonstrate that CKBMT with a non-myeloablative regimen from an HLA-matched donor can be an excellent option for patients with renal failure secondary to myeloma, for which other treatment options, including stem cell autotransplantation, have been less effective.

HLA Mismatched Kidney Transplant Recipients

The Stanford group also attempted peripheral blood stem cell transplantation with a TLI-based regimen for induction of renal allograft tolerance in HLA mismatched kidney transplantation [43]. In this clinical trial, three of four recipients developed transient multilineage chimerism but rejection developed when immunosuppression withdrawal was attempted. These investigators concluded that this protocol did not induce allograft tolerance in HLA mismatched recipients [44].

At MGH, based on the encouraging nonhuman primate results and initial clinical trial on HLA identical transplantation for myeloma, we developed a regimen for induction of mixed chimerism and renal allograft tolerance in HLA mismatched human KTx recipients (NKD03) in collaboration with the Immune Tolerance Network (ITN) [45]. The perioperative preparative conditioning regimen consisted of 60 mg/kg/d of cyclophosphamide administered I.V. on days –5 and –4; 0.6 mg/kg/dose humanized anti-CD2 mAb on days -2, -1, 0 and +1; and thymic irradiation (700 cGy) on day –1. On day 0, recipients underwent kidney transplantation, followed by I.V. infusion of donor bone marrow (DBM). Oral CyA was continued postoperatively at 8 to 12 mg/kg/d with target blood levels of 250-350 ng/ml, then tapered and discontinued over 9-14 months. The protocol was modified slightly after the development of antibody-mediated rejection in the third patient. Rituximab 375 mg/m²/dose was added on days -7 and -2; and prednisone, 2 mg/kg/d starting was started on day 0 and then tapered over the next 10 days post-operatively (Fig. **1**).

All five recipients developed transient mixed chimerism, lasting up to 21 days. Except for the third patient, who developed acute humoral rejection, immunosuppression was successfully discontinued at 9-14 months following the transplant in the other four recipients. All showed donor-specific unresponsiveness by *in vitro* assays but the mechanism responsible for stable graft function without exogenous immunosuppression in these recipients remains under investigation. These 4 recipients continue to be stable with normal kidney function off all immunosuppression for 4-7 years (Table **2**). Two of these recipients developed anti-donor HLA class II antibody shortly after immunosuppression discontinuation, but have had no functional impairment, nor evidence of rejection on sequential protocol biopsies. An adverse event observed to varying degrees in all of these patients was spontaneously reversible derangement of renal function between days 10-20. This has been attributed to cytokine release (engraftment syndrome) associated with DBM engraftment and/or loss of donor hematopoietic cells [46].

Since January 2009, an expanded, multi-center clinical trial for tolerance induction following HLA mismatched kidney transplantation has been underway. In this protocol, CyA has been replaced with tacrolimus, two additional doses of rituximab are administered and the steroid regimen has been extended to day 20 in the effort to further mitigate the engraftment syndrome. The study is currently in progress, but immunosuppression has been successfully discontinued in the first two recipients at 8 months after transplantation.

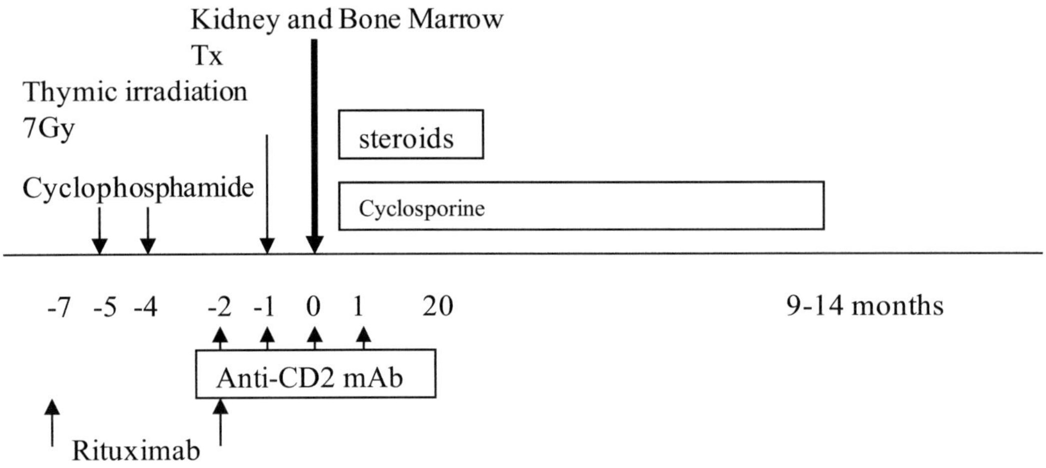

Figure 1: Preparative conditioning regimen for induction of mixed chimerism and renal allograft tolerance: The nonmyeloablative conditioning regimen consisted of 60 mg/kg/d of cyclophosphamide administered I.V. on days –5 and –4; 0.6 mg/kg/dose humanized anti-CD2 mAb on days -2, -1, 0 and +1; and thymic irradiation (700 cGy) on day –1. On day 0, recipients underwent kidney transplantation, followed by I.V. infusion of donor bone marrow (DBM). Oral CyA was continued postoperatively at 8 to 12 mg/kg/d with target blood levels of 250-350 ng/ml, then tapered and discontinued over 9-14 months. The protocol was subsequently modified to add Rituximab (days -7 and -2) and prednisone (day 0-day10).

Table 2: Results of the first clinical trial for tolerance induction

Age	Sex	Donor	Immunosuppression Discontinuation	Kidney Survival (years)	Current Serum Creatinine
22	F	Mother	OFF (day 240)	> 7.4 yrs	1.2
22	M	Father	OFF (day 422)	> 6.7 yrs	1.6
39	M	Sister	-	10	- *
25	M	Mother	OFF (day 244)	>5 yrs	1.6
46	M	Sister	OFF (day 276)	> 4 yrs	2.0

* underwent second kidney transplantation and currently doing with creatinine 1.6 mg/dl with conventional immunosuppression.

REFERENCES

[1] Meier-Kriesche HU, Schold JD, Srinivas TR, Kaplan B. Lack of improvement in renal allograft survival despite a marked decrease in acute rejection rates over the most recent era. Am J Transplant 2004; 4 : 378-383.

[2] Pascual M, Theruvath T, Kawai T, *et al.* Strategies to improve long-term outcomes after renal transplantation. N Engl J Med 2002; 346: 580-590.

[3] Knechtle SJ, Vargo D, Fechner J, *et al.* FN18-CRM9 immunotoxin promotes tolerance in primate renal allografts. Transplantation 1997; 63: 1-6.

[4] Knechtle SJ, Kirk AD, Fechner JH, Jr., *et al.* Inducing unresponsiveness by the use of anti-CD3 immunotoxin, CTLA4-Ig, and anti-CD40 ligand. Transplant Proc 1999; 31: 27S-28S.

[5] Slavin S, Gottlieb M, Strober S, *et al.* Transplantation of bone marrow in outbred dogs without graft-versus-host disease using total lymphoid irradiation. Transplantation 1979; 27: 139-142.

[6] Myburgh JA, Smit JA, Stark JH, Browde S. Total lymphoid irradiation in kidney and liver transplantation in the baboon: prolonged graft survival and alterations in T cell subsets with low cumulative dose regimens. J Immunol 1984; 132: 1019-1025.

[7] Kirk AD, Harlan DM, Armstrong NN, *et al.* CTLA4-Ig and anti-CD40 ligand prevent renal allograft rejection in primates. Proc Natl Acad Sci U S A 1997; 94: 8789-8794.

[8] Kirk AD, Burkly LC, Batty DS, *et al.* Treatment with humanized monoclonal antibody against CD154 prevents acute renal allograft rejection in nonhuman primates. Nat Med 1999; 5 : 686-693.

[9] Preston EH, Xu H, Dhanireddy KK, *et al.* IDEC-131 (anti-CD154), sirolimus and donor-specific transfusion facilitate operational tolerance in non-human primates. Am J Transplant 2005; 5: 1032-1041.

[10] Haanstra KG, Sick EA, Ringers J, *et al.* Costimulation blockade followed by a 12-week period of cyclosporine A facilitates prolonged drug-free survival of rhesus monkey kidney allografts. Transplantation 2005; 79: 1623-1626.

[11] Aoyagi T, Yamashita K, Suzuki T, *et al.* A human anti-CD40 monoclonal antibody, 4D11, for kidney transplantation in cynomolgus monkeys: induction and maintenance therapy. Am J Transplant 2009; 9: 1732-1741.

[12] Bashuda H, Kimikawa M, Seino K, *et al.* Renal allograft rejection is prevented by adoptive transfer of anergic T cells in nonhuman primates. J Clin Invest 2005; 115: 1896-1902.

[13] Thomas JM, Carver FM, Cunningham P, *et al.* Veto cells induce long-term kidney allograft tolerance in primates without chronic immunosuppression. Transplant Proc 1991; 23 (1 Pt 1): 11-13.

[14] Thomas JM, Carver FM, Kasten-Jolly J, *et al.* Further studies of veto activity in rhesus monkey bone marrow in relation to allograft tolerance and chimerism. Transplantation 1994; 57: 101-115.

[15] Thomas J, Kasten-Jolly J, Verbanac K, *et al.* Requirement for DR sharing in stable kidney allograft tolerance induced by donor bone marrow in rhesus monkeys. Transplant Proc 1995; 27: 686.

[16] Tomita Y, Khan A, Sykes M. Role of intrathymic clonal deletion and peripheral anergy in transplantation tolerance induced by bone marrow transplantation in mice conditioned with a nonmyeloablative regimen. J Immunol 1994; 153: 1087.

[17] Sharabi Y, Sachs DH. Mixed chimerism and permanent specific transplantation tolerance induced by a nonlethal preparative regimen. J Exp Med 1989; 169:493-502.

[18] Kawai T, Cosimi AB, Colvin RB, *et al.* Mixed allogeneic chimerism and renal allograft tolerance in cynomolgus monkeys. Transplantation 1995; 59: 256-262.

[19] Kawai T, Sogawa H, Boskovic S, *et al.* CD154 blockade for induction of mixed chimerism and prolonged renal allograft survival in nonhuman primates. Am J Transplant 2004; 4: 1391-1398.

[20] Calne R, Friend P, Moffatt S, *et al.* Prope tolerance, perioperative campath 1H, and low-dose cyclosporin monotherapy in renal allograft recipients. Lancet 1998; 351: 1701-1702.

[21] Starzl TE, Murase N, Abu-Elmagd K, *et al.* Tolerogenic immunosuppression for organ transplantation. Lancet 2003; 361: 1502-1510.

[22] Shapiro R, Basu A, Tan H, *et al.* Kidney transplantation under minimal immunosuppression after pretransplant lymphoid depletion with Thymoglobulin or Campath. J Am Coll Surg 2005; 200: 505-515.

[23] Thomas JM, Contreras JL, Jiang XL, *et al.* Peritransplant tolerance induction in macaques: early events reflecting the unique synergy between immunotoxin and deoxyspergualin. Transplantation 1999; 68: 1660-1673.

[24] Kirk AD, Mannon RB, Kleiner DE, *et al.* Results from a human renal allograft tolerance trial evaluating T-cell depletion with alemtuzumab combined with deoxyspergualin. Transplantation 2005; 80: 1051-1059.

[25] Bloom DD, Hu H, Fechner JH, Knechtle SJ. T-lymphocyte alloresponses of Campath-1H-treated kidney transplant patients. Transplantation 2006; 81: 81-87.

[26] Knechtle SJ, Pascual J, Bloom DD, *et al.* Early and limited use of tacrolimus to avoid rejection in an alemtuzumab and sirolimus regimen for kidney transplantation: clinical results and immune monitoring. Am J Transplant 2009; 9: 1087-1098.

[27] Agarwal A, Shen LY, Kirk AD. The role of alemtuzumab in facilitating maintenance immunosuppression minimization following solid organ transplantation. Transpl Immunol 2008; 20: 6.11.

[28] Strober S, Dhillon M, Schubert M, *et al.* Acquired immune tolerance to cadaveric renal allografts. A study of three patients treated with total lymphoid irradiation. N Engl J Med 1989; 321: 28-33.

[29] Strober S, Benike C, Krishnaswamy S, *et al.* Clinical transplantation tolerance twelve years after prospective withdrawal of immunosuppressive drugs: studies of chimerism and anti-donor reactivity. Transplantation 2000; 69 : 1549-1554.

[30] Saper V, Chow D, Engleman ED, *et al.* Clinical and immunological studies of cadaveric renal transplant recipients given total-lymphoid irradiation and maintained on low-dose prednisone. Transplantation 1988; 45: 540-546.

[31] Kawai T, Andrews D, Colvin RB, *et al.* Thromboembolic complications after treatment with monoclonal antibody against CD40 ligand. Nat Med 2000; 6: 114.

[32] Koyama I, Kawai T, Andrews D, *et al.* Thrombophilia associated with anti-CD154 monoclonal antibody treatment and its prophylaxis in nonhuman primates. Transplantation 2004; 77: 460-462.

[33] Vincenti F, Larsen C, Durrbach A, *et al.* Costimulation blockade with belatacept in renal transplantation. N Engl J Med 2005; 353: 770-781.

[34] Barber WH, Mankin JA, Laskow DA, *et al.* Long-term results of a controlled prospective study with transfusion of donor-specific bone marrow in 57 cadaveric renal allograft recipients. Transplantation 1991; 51: 70-75.

[35] Starzl TE, Demetris AJ, Trucco M, *et al.* Systemic chimerism in human female recipients of male livers. Lancet 1992; 340: 876-877.

[36] Starzl TE, Demetris AJ, Trucco M, *et al.* Cell migration and chimerism after whole-organ transplantation: the basis of graft acceptance. Hepatology 1993; 17: 1127-1152.

[37] Starzl TE. Chimerism and tolerance in transplantation. Proc Natl Acad Sci U S A 2004; 101 Suppl 2: 14607-14614.

[38] Tryphonopoulos P, Tzakis AG, Weppler D, *et al.* The role of donor bone marrow infusions in withdrawal of immunosuppression in adult liver allotransplantation. Am J Transplant 2005; 5: 608-613.

[39] Scandling JD, Busque S, Dejbakhsh-Jones S, *et al.* Tolerance and chimerism after renal and hematopoietic-cell transplantation. N Engl J Med 2008; 358 : 362-368.

[40] Spitzer TR, Delmonico F, Tolkoff-Rubin N, *et al.* Combined histocompatibility leukocyte antigen-matched donor bone marrow and renal transplantation for multiple myeloma with end stage renal disease: the induction of allograft tolerance through mixed lymphohematopoietic chimerism. Transplantation 1999; 68: 480-484.

[41] Buhler LH, Spitzer TR, Sykes M, *et al.* Induction of kidney allograft tolerance after transient lymphohematopoietic chimerism in patients with multiple myeloma and end-stage renal disease. Transplantation 2002; 74: 1405-1409.

[42] Fudaba Y, Spitzer TR, Shaffer J, *et al.* Myeloma responses and tolerance following combined kidney and nonmyeloablative marrow transplantation: *in vivo* and *in vitro* analyses. Am J Transplant 2006; 6: 2121-2133.

[43] Millan MT, Shizuru JA, Hoffmann P, *et al.* Mixed chimerism and immunosuppressive drug withdrawal after HLA-mismatched kidney and hematopoietic progenitor transplantation. Transplantation 2002; 73: 1386-1391.

[44] Millan MT SJ, Shizuru J, Lowsky R, Strober S. Studies of tolerance and chimerism after combined blood stem cell and kidney transplantation in humans. Am J Transplant 2005; 5 (suppl 11): 544.

[45] Kawai T, Cosimi AB, Spitzer TR, *et al.* HLA-mismatched renal transplantation without maintenance immunosuppression. N Engl J Med 2008; 358: 353-361.

[46] Spitzer TR. Engraftment syndrome following hematopoietic stem cell transplantation. Bone Marrow Transplant 2001; 27: 893-898.

CHAPTER 27

Xenotransplantion: Perspectives on the Future

Burcin Ekser[1,2,*]

[1]*Department of Surgery and Organ Transplantation, University of Padua, Padua, Italy, and* [2]*Thomas E. Starzl Transplantation Institute, University of Pittsburgh Medical Center, Pittsburgh, PA, USA*

Abstract: Xenotransplantation using pig organs as source for transplant has the potential to overcome the severe shortage of human donor organs. Wide utilization of genetically-engineered pigs is enabling progress to be made in pig-to-nonhuman primate experimental models. Novel, non-nephrotoxic immunosuppressive regimens have largely overcome T cell rejection and a T cell-dependent elicited antibody response. Recent advances in understanding of the biology of xenograft rejection and zoonotic infections and the generation of alpha1,3-galactosyltransferase-gene knockout pigs have moved this approach closer to the clinical application. However, inter-species coagulation dysregulation is proving a major hurdle. Progress in islet xenotransplantation has been more encouraging controlling diabetes in nonhuman primates up to 6 months, though this has usually been achieved using immunosuppressive protocols that might not be clinically applicable. Further advances are required to overcome the remaining barriers.

Keywords: Xenotransplantation, Coagulation Dysregulation, Pig, Genetically-Engineered, Nonhuman Primate, Tolerance, Knock-Out, Hyperacute Rejection, Immunosuppression, Xenozoonosis.

INTRODUCTION

Clinical transplantation is the only effective therapy for end-stage organ failure. However, there is a well-known shortage of organs and tissues from deceased human donors for the purposes of clinical organ and cell transplantation. Although there are >100, 000 patients waiting for a donor organ of one sort or another in the USA today, the number of donor organs that will become available during the current year will be <30, 000 [1]. The discrepancy between available transplantable organs and patients on the waiting list grows each year and due to the lack of transplantable organs more than 6, 500 patients on the waiting list have died every year in the last 5 years. Despite successful introduction of living-related donors for kidney and liver transplantation, marginal (extended criteria) deceased donors, and donation after cardiac death, it remains exceedingly unlikely that human organs will fulfill the needs of those who require organ transplantation.

The situation is even worse for patients in need of cell transplantation, such as islet transplantation for those affected by diabetes mellitus. Many of the 2-3 million patients with Type 1 diabetes in the USA would benefit from pancreatic islet transplantation, but clearly the number of deceased human donors available each year (<7, 000) will not resolve this problem. Indeed, the potential supply of islets from human donors will never be sufficient to treat the millions of patients with diabetes.

Despite recent advances in stem cell biology and tissue engineering, the clinical application of these techniques realistically remains in the distant future. This supply-demand imbalance could be corrected by the ability to transplant organs, tissues and cells from other species (xenografts) into humans. A readily available animal source of organs, tissues, and cells for clinical transplantation (cross-species transplantation or 'xenotransplantation') would resolve the problem. There have been a small number of clinical attempts to use animal organs for transplantation during the past century (reviewed by Taniguchi and Cooper 1997) [2]. In the majority of cases, nonhuman primates were the sources of organs. The results were generally poor, though a baboon liver functioned in a human recipient for 70 days and a chimpanzee kidney supported life of good quality for almost 9 months. Clinical experience with pigs as the source of organs or cells has been very limited, and the results have been extremely poor.

***Address correspondence to Burcin Ekser:** Kidney and Pancreas Transplantation Unit, Department of Surgery and Organ Transplantation, University of Padua, *Via* Giustiniani, 2 35128 Padua, Italy; Tel: +1-412-624-1402; Fax: +1-412-624-1172; E-mail: burcinexer@yahoo.com

Massimiliano Veroux and Pierfrancesco Veroux (Eds)

Although non-human primates are phylogenetically closer than other species to humans, they are not considered to be suitable source animals for clinical xenotransplantation because of ethical issues, the high risk of cross-species transmission of infections to humans, difficulties in breeding, organ size disparities and other impracticalities [3, 4]. The pig is now the preferred source animal. The advantages and disadvantages of the pig have been debated: in addition to similarities in pig organ size and physiology to humans, the ability to breed pigs rapidly makes them particularly amenable to genetic modifications that could enhance their use as an organ source [3-5]. Pigs could also be source animals for the clinical transplantation of islets of Langerhans in humans, as pigs maintain blood glucose levels that are similar to those of humans, and porcine insulin is effective in humans.The advantages are many, but the primate immune response to transplanted pigs organs and cells has been a significant barrier that may not yet have been fully overcome [6].

In this chapter, the current status, the major remaining obstacles of xenotransplantation shall be briefly summarized and discussed. Since the most relevant experimental model is pig-to-nonhuman primate xenotransplantation, the attention will be concentrated on it.

BRIEF HISTORY OF CLINICAL XENOTRANSPLANTATION

More than 100 years ago, before the introduction of clinical allotransplantation, there were some reports of the transplantation of animal tissues into human recipients with organ failure. In 1905, Princeteau *et al.* [7] implanted slices of rabbit kidney into a uremic child. The author claimed improvement of renal function before the child's death from pneumonia. Almost 50 years ago, in the 1960s, some success was obtained in human after the transplantation of chimpanzee kidney [8]. Different immunosuppression treatments were used including local irradiation of the organ. The patient survived for 9 months and died due to infection rather than renal failure.

In the closer past, in 1984, Bailey *et al.* [9] performed orthotopic baboon heart transplantation in a human neonate and the baboon heart functioned for 20 days. In 1993, Starzl *et al.* [10] transplanted a baboon liver into terminal liver failure patient and patient survived 70 days. There was evidence of hepatic function and coagulation, however patient died from overwhelming sepsis and infection with little histological features of rejection.

IMMUNOLOGICAL OBSTACLES TO PIG-TO-NONHUMAN PRIMATE TRANSPLANTATION

Hyperacute Rejection

In initial experiments, when wild-type pig organs were transplanted into nonhuman primates, the complement cascade was activated through the binding of natural (preformed) antibodies to the pig vascular endothelium [11, 12]. The endothelial cells of the graft responded to the immune activation by converting from an anticoagulant to a procoagulant phenotype [13, 14]. The result of activation of the complement and coagulation systems was hyperacute rejection.

Acute Humoral Xenograft Rejection

When hyperacute rejection was partly overcome, *e.g.*, by the depletion of anti-pig antibodies or complement from the nonhuman primate serum [12-15], a delayed form of antibody-mediated rejection occurred, known variously as acute humoral xenograft rejection (AHXR), acute vascular rejection, or delayed xenograft rejection [16]. Natural antibody binding and complement activation resulted in vascular endothelial cell activation and injury caused by the complement and cellular components of the innate immune system. Despite the administration of pharmacologic immunosuppressive agents AHXR may occur, and it is believed that it is seen particularly following the development of a T cell-dependent elicited antibody response. Natural killer (NK) cells play a role in AHXR [17-19] as do macrophages [20], but their exact importance remains unclear.

Acute Cellular Rejection

Acute cellular rejection can be mainly prevented by intense immunosuppressive regimens (*i.e.* T and B cell infiltration of the graft and T cell activation) and a T cell-dependent elicited antibody response, even though the T cell response is believed to be stronger than the allo response [21, 22]. This is possibly because T cell activation leads to a rapid antibody response that results in AHXR before significant T cell infiltration occurs in the graft. Acute cellular rejection is therefore typically not seen with intense immunosuppressive drug regimens [23-26]. Costimulation blockade agents, such as an anti-human CD154 monoclonal antibody, have been found particularly effective in preventing T cell activation in the xenotransplant setting, however side effects, such as increased thromboembolic events and stroke prevent their use in clinical approaches [27].

Chronic Rejection

In grafts that survive for more than a few weeks, features of chronic vasculopathy may develop, similar to the chronic rejection seen in long-surviving allografts. Its causative factors remain not fully understood.

GENETICALLY-ENGINEERED PIGS

The introduction of genetically-engineered pigs was an important step in the field of xenotransplantation. The most significant advances to date have been the production of pigs expressing a human complement-regulatory protein, *e.g.*, human decay-accelerating factor (CD55), membrane cofactor protein (CD46), or CD59 [28-32], and pigs in which the gene for α1, 3-galactosyltransferase has been knocked out (GTKO pigs) [33-36].

With the presence of a complement-regulatory protein on the surface of vascular endothelial cells in the pig, the grafts were mainly protected from hyperacute rejection. Of interest is the suggestion that over-expression of a pig complement-regulatory protein might be as effective as the expression of a human complement-regulatory protein in protecting the pig cell from lysis [37], though this theory has never been tested in an *in vivo* model.

The gene for α1, 3-galactosyltransferase enables this enzyme to add Galα1, 3Gal (Gal) oligosaccharides to various underlying glycoproteins and glycolipids in the pig [38, 39]. Gal is the major target for human and nonhuman primate anti-pig antibodies [33, 40] (reviewed in [41]), and its deletion from pigs has greatly reduced the incidence of hyperacute rejection of pig grafts in nonhuman primates [42-44]. GTKO pigs additionally transgenic for a human complement-regulatory protein provide increased benefit over either modification alone [45].

Genetically-engineered pig hearts placed heterotopically in baboons have functioned for periods of 3-6 months [42, 43, 46, 47], life-supporting kidneys for periods approaching 3 months [24, 44, 48], livers for a matter of days [49, 50] (reviewed in [51]), and lungs for a matter of hours [52, 53]. Progress during the past 20 years or so can be illustrated by the prolongation of survival or pig hearts transplanted heterotopically into baboons using wild-type or genetically-modified pigs and various immunosuppressive protocols [54].

Although the availability of GTKO pigs has been a major step forward, there are well-documented other natural antibodies to nonGal antigens, namely nonGal antibodies, in humans and nonhuman primates [18, 55, 56], the nature of which remains unknown. Although there were reasons to believe these may be directed to nonGal oligosaccharides [57, 58]. It has been known for some time that antibodies in humans directed to N-glycolylneuraminic acid (NeuGc) may play a role in pig graft destruction [59, 60]. NeuGc is expressed on the vascular endothelium of all mammals with the exception of humans; even chimpanzees express this oligosaccharide. In pig-to-nonhuman primate transplantation models, therefore, other antigens must be the targets for anti-nonGal antibodies. These anti-nonGal antibodies, whether directed to NeuGc or other antigens, are weaker and less destructive than anti-Gal antibodies, but nevertheless can be associated with hyperacute rejection or AHXR [61].

Genetic modifications to inhibit NK cell activity [62-64] and macrophage activity [65, 66] are possible, but have not yet been tested in a pig-to-nonhuman primate model. Despite the absence of hyperacute rejection and classic AHXR, survival of pig organ grafts in nonhuman primates is currently limited by either the development of a thrombotic microangiopathy [67, 68] or a consumptive coagulopathy or both [69-70]. These are clearly features of coagulation dysregulation between pig and primate, and this barrier has not yet been overcome. Following GTKO pig heart transplantation in baboons, thrombotic microangiopathy is the predominant feature, with subsequent consumptive coagulopathy in some cases. However, after GTKO/CD46 pig kidney xenotransplantation, consumptive coagulopathy occurs relatively early in the absence of obvious features of thrombotic microangiopathy [71]. Following GTKO/CD46 pig liver xenotransplantation, thrombocytopenia develops within minutes and, although most coagulation parameters appear to remain within the normal ranges, the lack of platelets leads to spontaneous internal hemorrhage within days [50]. Increasing experimental evidence suggests that the classic immune response is no longer the major problem, but physiologic incompatibilities between the coagulation systems of pig and primate are more problematic.

COAGULATION DYSREGULATION

Today, coagulation dysregulation between species remains not fully understood and as a major problem to successful clinical xenotransplantation. Previous reports suggested that consumptive coagulopathy is initiated by the expression of tissue factor in the porcine graft [72-74]. In response to the binding of xenoreactive antibody and/or activation by complement, endothelial cells in the graft are activated to increase tissue factor activity and initiate intragraft thrombosis and consumptive coagulopathy.

During inflammation, type I activation of endothelial cells induces P-selectin and vascular leakiness of plasma proteins; this process takes 10-20min. Type II activation of endothelial cells is triggered by stimulation of tumor necrosis factor-α and interleukin-1, induces more effective leukocyte recruitment by synthesis of adhesion proteins, such as E-selectin and CD106 (vascular cell adhesion molecule-1, VCAM-1), and is sustained for 6-24h after cytokine-mediated activation. Type I and type II activations are believed to be associated with hyperacute rejection and AHXR, respectively. The activated endothelial cells and the generated thrombin subsequently activate platelets, leukocytes, and other inflammatory cells in the recipient, initiating a vicious cycle.

Recent *in vitro* studies by Lin *et al.* [75] have indicated that porcine aortic endothelial cells (PAECs) are able to induce human tissue factor exposure on human platelets and monocytes through an immune response-independent pathway. This problem has been investigated *in vivo* in pig-to-baboon kidney [76] or liver [71] transplantation models.

For example, the rapid development of consumptive coagulopathy in a pig-to-baboon liver xenotransplantation model has been studied [71]. Using genetically-modified pig liver transplantation into baboons, it has been observed that there is a massive loss of platelets from the circulation within minutes after reperfusion [50]. The development of thrombocytopenia was accompanied by thrombin formation.

Determination of the exact mechanism by which thrombotic microangiopathy and consumptive coagulopathy are initiated after xenotransplantation is important because it may enable further genetic modification of the pig or suggest therapy that might prevent them. The introduction of genes for human thrombomodulin, tissue factor pathway inhibitor [76, 77], or CD39 [78] have been suggested to overcome the coagulation incompatibilities between pig and primate.

RECENT ADVANCES IN KIDNEY XENOTRANSPLANTATION

Table **1** summarizes recent experiments and their outcomes in the field of kidney xenotransplantation. In 2004, Baldan *et al.* [79] reported the longest survival to date reaching 90 days in life-supporting kidney xenotransplantation. However, in Baldan *et al.*'s experiments, the median survival in different experimental groups testing different immunosuppressive regimens was not different than previous experiments in the literature (Table **1**). The introduction of GTKO pigs together with the thymokidney technology prolonged the median survival significantly [44, 80]. Although the prolonged survival of pig kidney grafts in NHPs was achieved, it has been shown that immunosuppressive regimens used in experimental setting cannot be used in clinical trials (Table **1**), such as anti-CD154mAb, cobra venom factor, and whole body irradiation of the recipient.

Table 1: Recent advances in kidney xenotransplantation (selected publications)

Author [Ref#]	Year	Pigs	Recipients	N.	Mean (Median) Survival (days)	Immunosuppression	Outcome
Azimzadeh [85]	2009	GTKO	Baboon	7	n.a	None (n=1), ATG+anti-CD154+CVF+MMF+Cs (+/- CTLA4-Ig)	Early graft failure, complement deposition
		GTKO/CRP	Baboon	5	n.a	ATG+anti-CD154+CVF+MMF+Cs (+/- CTLA4-Ig)	CRP (either CD46 or CD55), reduced early graft failure incidence, minimal complement deposition
Burdorf [86]	2009	GTKO	Baboon	3	4 (5)	ATG+anti-CD154+CVF+MMF+Cs (+/- CTLA4-Ig)	n.a.
		GTKO/CD55	Baboon	3	8 (12)	ATG+anti-CD154+CVF+MMF+Cs	n.a.
		GTKO/CD46	Baboon	2	9 (9)	ATG+anti-CD154+CVF+MMF+Cs (+/- CTLA4-Ig)	n.a.
Cozzi E [82]	2009	GTKO/CD55/CD59/CD39/HT	Cyno	6	16 (16)	CyP+CSA+MMF+Cs	Kidney failure, abdominal bleeding (n=1), AHXR
Greisemer [80]	2009	GTKO	Baboon	7	51 (49)	(a) Thymokidney+Rituximab+ATG+LoCD2b + anti-CD154+TAC+MMF (n=4), (a) - LoCD2b (n=2), (a) – TAC + WBI (n=1)	Died from drug reaction, invasive CMV infection, AMI, pleural effusion from proteinuria, ARDS,
Le Bas-Bernardet [83]	2009	GTKO/CD55/CD59/CD39/HT	Baboon	5	13 (13) (ISed)	None (n=2) or CyP+TAC+MMF+C1 inhibitor	AHXR
Salvaris [81]	2009	GTKO/CD55/CD59/HT	Baboon	6	3 (3)	None	HAR, CC
Ezzelarab [87]	2009	GTKO	Baboon	3	3 (3)	CVF only (n=1), low-dose anti-CD154+CTLA4-Ig+MMF (n=1), ATG+CVF+anti-CD154+MMF+Cs(n=1)	AHXR, CC, renal artery thrombosis
Greisemer [84]	2010	GTKO	Baboon	2	16 (16)	Splenectomy+WBI+Thymus Irridation+ ATG+LoCD2b+TAC+GTKO BM (+CVF in one case)	Renal failure, pulmonary edema, gross enlargement of the kidney, hemorrhage and thrombi
Lin [77]	2010	GTKO	Baboon	1	7	ATG+anti-CD154+CVF+MMF+Cs	CC
		GTKO/CD46	Baboon	6	9 (10)	None (n=1), ATG+anti-CD154+MMF (n=4), ATG+anti-CD154+MMF+Cs (n=1)	Fluid overload, CC

Legend: AHXR= acute humoral xenograft rejection, ATG= antithymocyte globulin, CC= consumptive coagulopathy, CRP= complement-regulatory protein, Cs= corticosteroids, CVF= cobra venom factor, HAR= hyperacute rejection, HIA= heterotopic intra-abdominal, HIT= heterotopic intra-thoracic, IS= immunosuppression, MMF= mycophenolate mofetil, n.a= not available, OHT= orthotopic, PGI2= prostacycline, RAPA= rapamaycin, TAC= tacrolimus, TM= thrombotic microangiopathy. AMI= acute myocardial infarction, ARDS= acute respiratory distress syndrome, BM= bone marrow, CMV= cytomegalovirus, CSA= cyclosporine, cyno= cynomolgus monkey, CyP= cyclophosphamide, LoCD2b= mouse anti-human CD2b antibody, WBI= whole body irradiation.

With the availability of multiple genetically-modified pigs, several groups aimed to decrease heavy immunosuppressive treatment in recipients to make regimens applicable to the clinic (Table **1**). Salvaris *et al.* showed in a non-immunosuppressed pig-to-NHP model that the combination of GTKO with expression of CD55/CD59/HT (H-transferase) improved renal xenograft survival [81]. Recently, under the Xenome Project of the European Union, pigs with multiple genetic modifications (GTKO/CD55/CD39/HT) were transplanted into NHPs. Cozzi *et al.* [82] and Le Bas-Bernardet *et al.* [83] reported similar outcomes using different clinically-applicable immunosuppressive regimens (Table **1**).

Greisemer *et al.* [84], with the goal of inducing transplantation tolerance, performed GTKO pig-to-baboon renal xenotransplants using an extensive immunosuppressive regimen combined with GTKO pig bone marrow administration. Unfortunately, their results were not good enough to compare with previous experiments (Table **1**).

With the knowledge of the importance of coagulation dysregulation and thrombocytopenia limiting the extended survival in xenotransplantation, Lin *et al.* studied the role of tissue factor expression on circulating platelets and peripheral blood mononuclear cells (PBMCs) following either GTKO or GTKO/CD46 pig kidney transplantation in baboons [77]. They showed that tissue factor was detectable on platelets on post-transplant day 1, but was not detectable on PBMCs until consumptive coagulopathy was beginning to develop. Graft histopathology showed fibrin deposition and platelet aggregation. Therefore, we believe that prevention of recipient platelet activation will be critical for successful pig kidney transplantation.

IMMUNOLOGICAL TOLERANCE

The induction of immunological tolerance to the graft is the ultimate and ideal goal for xenotransplantation (and allotransplantation). Considerable efforts have been made to achieve this goal either by pig bone marrow transplantation (to induce mixed chimerism) (reviewed by Tseng [88]) or by pig thymus transplantation in the host [89]. After kidney allotransplantation, the induction of mixed chimerism, even if only transient, has been associated with the induction of tolerance to the graft in both nonhuman primate [90] and clinical models [91]. To date, however, neither of these approaches has been convincingly successful in models of xenotransplantation.

There is increasing interest in the potential role of T regulatory cells (reviewed in [92]) and/or mesenchymal stem cells to induce a state of tolerance to a xenograft, but to date there has been very little exploratory work reported. The possibility of inducing B-cell tolerance in neonates, as has been achieved in ABO-incompatible allografts [93, 94], is also intriguing [95]. However, there are obviously a number of other barriers, such as thrombotic microangiopathy and consumptive coagulopathy, that need to be overcome before tolerance is likely to be induced.

PIG ORGAN FUNCTION IN PRIMATES

Even if the immunologic and coagulation barriers can be overcome, the question has been asked as whether a pig organ will function satisfactorily in the primate bodily environment. Will the organ carry out all of the functions required of it, *i.e.* all of the functions of a native primate organ? The physiological aspects of xenotransplantation have been relatively recently reviewed [96].

In summary, current evidence is that pig hearts function well in primates. Successful orthotopic life-supporting pig heart transplantation in baboons has been followed by satisfactory function for periods of up to 53 days [97, 98]. The pig heart has been demonstrated to recover from an initial ischemic injury occurring during the transplant operative procedure [98].

Pig kidneys function adequately with one or two possible exceptions, *e.g.*, handling of phosphate [99]. However, one major problem following pig kidney transplantation in nonhuman primates is the development of proteinuria that can be considerable. This results in low albuminemia with its accompanying complications, such as peripheral edema. Although this can be prevented or corrected by the continuous intravenous infusion of human albumin, this would clearly not be a realistic long-term therapeutic option in a patient with a pig kidney graft. Whether the proteinuria is related to the immune response, or is simply a physiologic incompatibility remains uncertain.

CROSS-SPECIES INFECTIOUS TRANSMISSION (XENOZOONOSIS)

The potential for the development of a xenozoonosis in the recipient of a pig graft, *i.e.* the potential for a porcine microorganism to cause infection in the recipient, has been of concern for a number of years [100-102]. These potential risks, particularly with regard to porcine endogenous retroviruses (PERV), are now considered to be much less significant than they were a few years ago [101-104], and a clinical trial would be deemed justified if there were a realistic possibility that the graft would be life-saving for the patient. Furthermore, activation of PERV could now be prevented by siRNA technology [105, 106], although this is unlikely to be necessary. Nevertheless, largely because of the possibility of the transfer of a porcine infectious microorganism, xenotransplantation will be highly-regulated by national regulatory authorities, such as the Food and Drug Administration in the USA. The likely regulatory requirements have recently been reviewed by Schuurman [107].

CLINICAL PERSPECTIVE

There are clearly problems that remain to be overcome before pig organs can be used in clinical transplantation. As truly long-term survival of pig organ grafts may be limited for some time by the early onset of graft atherosclerosis or other forms of chronic rejection (until this problem can be resolved), initial clinical trials may involve 'bridging' a patient in end-stage organ failure, particularly of the liver [108] or heart [109], until a suitable allograft becomes available. This would not only be life-saving – and therefore ethically justified - but would also enable valuable experience to be gained of pig organ function in humans as opposed to nonhuman primates.

However, 'bridging' would not be a clinical option if sensitization to pig antigens, *e.g.*, swine leukocyte antigens (SLA), resulted in an increase in panel-reactive antibodies, *i.e.* antibodies to human leukocyte antigens (HLA), which might either preclude subsequent allotransplantation or be detrimental to the outcome of such a procedure. Fortunately, though limited, current evidence is that antibodies that develop after exposure to a pig xenograft (if immunosuppressive therapy has been unsuccessful in preventing sensitization) are not cross-reactive against HLA, and so would not be detrimental to a subsequent allograft (reviewed in [110]). In contrast, patients with a high level of HLA-reactive antibodies may be at greater risk of rejecting a pig xenograft, though again the evidence for this remains limited (reviewed in [110]).

The potential therapeutic possibilities offered by xenotransplantation are so considerable that it is an area of research that should be pursued vigorously until the barriers have been overcome. The number of patients who might benefit from xenotransplantation may therefore run into the hundreds of thousands or even millions if it can achieve its potential.

The increasing availability of genetically-modified pigs is steadily drawing clinical xenotransplantation closer. Treated 'non-viable' tissues from WT pigs, such as dermis scaffolds and small intestinal stroma (SIS), are already being used on a large scale in clinical surgery, and steps are underway to improve outcomes by using GTKO pigs for these purposes. There is evidence to indicate that tissues from GTKO pigs will generate a weaker inflammatory response in the recipient.

The encouraging results of pig islet transplantation in diabetic monkeys [85, 86], particularly when islets from genetically-engineered pigs are transplanted, suggest that clinical islet xenotransplantation is almost certain to be initiated within a few years. Pig organ transplantation in patients with end-stage organ failure is likely to follow, initially as a bridge to allotransplantation.

In summary, therefore, further genetic engineering of pigs is required to protect the organs and islets from the primate immune response, particularly from the innate immune system. Recent advances and therapeutic alternatives in vascularized organ xenotransplantation have been recently reviewed [111]. Most important, genetically-engineered pigs are required whose organs and cells are protected from the coagulation dysregulation that occurs. In particular, modifications are required to prevent (i) tissue factor activity on the graft and (ii) activation of recipient platelets to express tissue factor and initiate consumptive coagulopathy. An immunosuppressive regimen is required to prevent cellular rejection and a T cell-dependent elicited antibody response, and this regimen must be one that is clinically-applicable and not associated with a high incidence of complications, such as infection or malignant disease. In this respect, an alternative is to express the immunosuppressive agent in the graft. Recently developed genetically-engineered pigs have been discussed according to their potential contribution to clinical xenotransplantation [111]. The need of further experimental studies to understand the impact of new genes is obvious.

ABBREVIATIONS

AHXR	=	acute humoral xenograft rejection
Gal	=	Galα1,3Gal
GTKO	=	α1,3-galactosyltransferase gene-knockout
NeuGc	=	N-glycolylneuraminic acid

REFERENCES

[1] UNOS - United Network for Organ Sharing (UNOS) http://www.unos.org (accessed July 10th, 2009).

[2] Taniguchi S, Cooper DKC. Clinical xenotransplantation - past, present and future. Ann R Coll Surg Engl 1997; 79: 13-19.

[3] Cooper DKC, Lanza RP. Xeno - The Promise of Transplanting Animal Organs into Humans. Oxford University Press, New York, 2000, pp. 1-274.

[4] Cooper DKC, Gollackner B, Sachs DH. Will the pig solve the transplantation backlog? Annu Rev Med 2002; 53: 133-147.

[5] Cooper DKC, Ye Y, Rolf LL, Zuhdi N. The pig as potential organ donor for man. In Cooper DKC, Kemp E, Reemtsma K, White DJG (eds). Xenotransplantation. Springer, Heidelberg, 1991, pp. 481-500.

[6] Cooper DKC, Dorling A, Pierson RN III, *et al.* α1,3-galactosyltransferase gene-knockout pigs for xenotransplantation: where do we go from here? Transplantation 2007;84:1-7.

[7] Princeteau M. Greffe renale. Journal of Medicine de Bordeaux 1905; 26: 549-555.

[8] Reemtsma K. Renal heterotransplantation from nonhuman primates to man. Ann NY Acad Scie 1969; 162: 412-418

[9] Bailey LL, Nehlsen-Cannarella SL, Concepcion W, *et al.* Baboon-to-human cardiac xenotransplantation in a neonate. JAMA 1985; 254: 3321-3329.

[10] Starzl TE, Fung J, Tzakis, A, Todo S, *et al.* Baboon-to-human liver transplantation. Lancet 1993; 341: 65-71

[11] Lexer G, Cooper DKC, Rose AG, *et al.* Hyperacute rejection in a discordant (pig to baboon) cardiac xenograft model. J Heart Transplant 1986;5:411–418.

[12] Rose AG, Cooper DKC. Venular thrombosis is the key event in the pathogenesis of antibody-mediated cardiac rejection. Xenotransplantation 2000;7:31-41.

[13] Watts A, Foley A, Awwad M, *et al.* Plasma perfusion by apheresis through a Gal immunoaffinity column successfully depletes anti-Gal antibody: experience with 320 aphereses in baboons. Xenotransplantation 2000;7:181-185.

[14] Buhler L, Yamada K, Kitamura H, *et al.* Pig kidney transplantation in baboons: anti-Galα1-3Gal IgM alone is associated with acute humoral xenograft rejection and disseminated intravascular coagulation. Transplantation 2001;72:1743–1752.

[15] Chen G, Sun H, Yang H, *et al.* The role of anti-non-Gal antibodies in the development of acute humoral xenograft rejection of hDAF transgenic porcine kidneys in baboons receiving anti-Gal antibody neutralization therapy. Transplantation 2006;81:273-283.

[16] Gollackner B, Goh S-K, Qawi I, *et al.* Acute vascular rejection of xenografts: roles of natural and elicited xenoreactive antibodies in activation of vascular endothelial cells and induction of procoagulant activity. Transplantation 2004;77:1735-1741.

[17] Inverardi L, Clissi B, Stolzer AL, *et al.* Human natural killer lymphocytes directly recognize evolutionarily conserved oligosaccharide ligands expressed by xenogeneic tissues. Transplantation 1997;63:1318-1330.

[18] Baumann BC, Forte P, Hawley RJ, Rieben R, Schneider MK, Seebach JD. Lack of galactose-α1,3-galactose expression on porcine endothelial cells prevents complement-induced lysis but not direct xenogeneic NK cytotoxicity. J Immunol 2004;172:6460-6467.

[19] Rieben R, Seebach JD. Xenograft rejection: IgG1, complement and NK cells team up to activate and destroy the endothelium. Trends Immunol 2005;26:2-5.

[20] Fox A, Mountford J, Braakhuis A, *et al.* Innate and adaptive immune responses to nonvascualr xenografts: evidence that macrophages are direct effectors of xenograft rejection. J Immunol 2001;166:2133-2140.

[21] Yamada K, Sachs DH, DerSimonian H. Human anti-porcine xenogeneic T cell response. Evidence for allelic specificity of mixed leukocyte reaction and for both direct and indirect pathways of recognition. J Immunol 1995;155:5249-2556.

[22] Dorling A, Lechler RI. T cell-mediated xenograft rejection: specific tolerance is probably required for long term xenograft survival. Xenotransplantation 1998;5:234-245.

[23] McCurry KR, Parker W, Cotterell AH, *et al.* Humoral responses to pig-to-baboon cardiac transplantation: implications for the pathogenesis and treatment of acute vascular rejection and for accommodation. Hum Immunol. 1997;58:91-105.

[24] Cozzi E, Bhatti F, Schmoeckel M, *et al.* Long-term survival of non-human primates receiving life-supporting transgenic porcine kidney xenografts. Transplantation 2000;70:15-21.

[25] Cozzi E, Vial C, Ostlie D, *et al.* Maintenance triple immunosuppression with cyclosporin A, mycophenolate sodium and steroids allows prolonged survival of primate recipients of hDAF porcine renal xenografts. Xenotransplantation 2003;10:300-310.

[26] Byrne GW, Davies WR, Oi K, *et al.* Increased immunosuppression, not anticoagulation, extends cardiac xenograft survival. Transplantation. 2006;82:1787-1791.

[27] Buhler L, Awwad M, Basker M, *et al.* High-dose porcine hematopoietic cell transplantation combined with CD40 ligand blockade in baboons prevents an induced anti-pig humoral response. Transplantation 2000;69:2296-2304.

[28] Dalmasso AP, Vercellotti GM, Platt JL, Bach FH. Inhibition of complement-mediated endothelial cell cytotoxicity be decay accelerating factor. Potential for prevention of xenograft hyperacute rejection. Transplantation 1991;52:530–533.

[29] Oglesby TJ, White D, Tedja I, *et al.* Protection of mammalian cells from complement-mediated lysis by transfection of human membrane cofactor protein and decay-accelerating factor. Trans Assoc Am Phys 1991;104:164–172.

[30] Cozzi E, White DJ. The generation of transgenic pigs as potential organ donors for humans. Nat Med 1995;1:964–966.

[31] Byrne GW, McCurry KR, Martin MJ, McClellan SM, Platt JL, Logan JS. Transgenic pigs expressing human CD59 and decay-accelerating factor produce an intrinsic barrier to complement-mediated damage. Transplantation 1997;63:149-155.

[32] Loveland BE, Milland J, Kyriakou P, *et al.* Characterization of a CD46 transgenic pig and protection of transgenic kidneys against hyperacute rejection in non-immunosuppressed baboons. Xenotransplantation 2004;11:171-183.

[33] Cooper DKC, Good AH, Koren E, *et al.* Identification of α-galactosyl and other carbohydrate epitopes that are bound by human anti-pig antibodies: relevance to discordant xenografting in man. Transpl Immunol 1993;1:198-205.

[34] Cooper DKC, Koren E, Oriol R. Genetically engineered pigs. Lancet 1993;342:682-683.

[35] Phelps CJ, Koike C, Vaught TD, *et al.* Production of α1,3-galactosyltransferase-deficient pigs. Science 2003;299:411-414.

[36] Kolber-Simonds D, Lai L, Watt SR, *et al.* α1,3-galactosyltransferase null pigs *via* nuclear transfer with fibroblasts bearing loss of heterozygosity mutations. Proc Natl Acad Sci USA 2004;19:7335-7340.

[37] Morgan BP, Berg CW, Harris CL. "Homologous restriction" in complement lysis: roles of membrane complement regulators. Xenotransplantation 2005;12:258-265.

[38] Galili U, Shohet SB, Kobrin E, Stults CL, Macher BA. Man, apes, and Old World monkeys differ from other mammals in the expression of alpha-galactosyl epitopes on nucleated cells. J Biol Chem 1988;263:17755–17762.

[39] Oriol R, Ye Y, Koren E, Cooper DKC. Carbohydrate antigens of pig tissues reacting with human natural antibodies as potential targets for hyperacute vascular rejection in pig-to-man organ xenotransplantation. Transplantation 1993;56:1433-1442.

[40] Good AH, Cooper DKC, Malcolm AJ, *et al.* Identification of carbohydrate structures that bind human antiporcine antibodies: implications for discordant xenografting in man. Transplant Proc 1992;24:559-562.

[41] Kobayashi T, Cooper DKC. Anti-Gal, α-Gal epitopes, and xenotransplantation. In: *αGal and Anti-Gal: α-1,3-Galactosyltransferase, α-Gal Epitopes, and the Natural Anti-Gal Antibody.* Galili U, Avila JL (eds). Kluwer Academic/Plenum, New York, London. (Subcellular Biochemistry Series, volume 32). 1999. pp.229-257.

[42] Kuwaki K, Tseng YL, Dor FJMF, *et al.* Heart transplantation in baboons using α1,3-galactosyltransferase gene-knockout pigs as donors: initial experience. Nat Med 2005;11:29-31.

[43] Tseng Y-L, Kuwaki K, Dor FJMF, *et al.* α1,3-galactosyltransferase gene-knockout pig heart transplantation in baboons with survival approaching six months. Transplantation 2005;80:1493-1500.

[44] Yamada K, Yazawa K, Shimizu A, *et al.* Marked prolongation of porcine renal xenograft survival in baboons through the use of α1,3-galactosyltransferase gene-knockout donors and the cotransplantation of vascularized thymic tissue. Nat Med 2005;11:32-34.

[45] Hara H, Long C, Lin YJ, Tai HC, Ezzelarab M, Ayares D, Cooper DKC. *In vitro* investigation of pig cells for resistance to human antibody-mediated rejection. Transpl Int. 2008;21:1163-1174. .

[46] Bhatti FN, Schmoeckel M, Zaidi A, *et al.* Three-month survival of hDAF transgenic pig hearts transplanted into primates. Transplant Proc. 1999;31:958.

[47] McGregor CG, Davies WR, Oi K, *et al.* Cardiac xenotransplantation: recent preclinical progress with 3-month median survival. J Thorac Cardiovasc Surg. 2005; 130(3):844-851.

[48] Zaidi A, Schmoeckel M, Bhatti F, *et al.* Life-supporting pig-to-primate renal xenotransplantation using genetically modified donors. Transplantation 1998;65:1584-1590.

[49] Ramirez P, Chavez R, Majado M, *et al.* Life-supporting human complement regulator decay accelerating factor transgenic pig liver xenograft maintains the metabolic function and coagulation in the nonhuman primate for up to 8 days. Transplantation 2000;70:989-998.

[50] Ekser B, Long C, Echeverri GJ, *et al.* Impact of thrombocytopenia in survival of baboons after pig liver transplants: clinical relevance. Am J Transplant 2009, in press.

[51] Hara H, Gridelli B, Lin YJ, Marcos A, Cooper DKC. Liver xenografts for the treatment of acute liver failure: clinical and experimental experience and remaining immunologic barriers. Liver Transplant 2008;14:425-434.

[52] Nguyen BH, Zwets E, Schroeder C, Pierson RN 3rd, Azimzadeh AM. Beyond antibody-mediated rejection: hyperacute lung rejection as a paradigm for dysregulated inflammation. Curr Drug Targets Cardiovasc Haematol Disord. 2005;5:255-269.

[53] Nguyen BN, Azimzadeh AM, Zhang T, *et al.* Life-supporting function of genetically modified swine lungs in baboons. J Thorac Cardiovasc Surg 2007;133:1354-1363.

[54] Zhu X, Dor FJMF, Cooper DKC. Pig-to-non-human primate heart transplantation: immunologic progress over 20 years. J Heart Lung Transplant 2007; 26: 210-218.

[55] Baumann BC, Stussi G, Huggel K, *et al.* Reactivity of human natural antibodies to endothelial cells from Galalpha(1,3)Gal-deficient pigs. Transplantation 2007;83:193-201.

[56] Hara H, Ezzelarab M, Rood PPM, *et al.* Allosensitized humans are at no greater risk of humoral rejection of GT-KO pig organs than other humans. Xenotransplantation 2006;13:357-365.

[57] Cooper DKC. Xenoantigens and xenoantibodies. Xenotransplantation 1998;5:6-17.

[58] Ezzelarab M, Ayares D, Cooper DKC. Carbohydrates in xenotransplantation. Immunol Cell Biol 2005;83:396-404. .

[59] Bouhours D, Pourcel C, Bouhours JE. Simultaneous expression by porcine aorta endothelial cells of glycosphinogolipids bearing the major epitope for human xenoreactive antibodies (Galα1-3Gal), blood group H determinant and N-glycolylneuraminic acid. Glycoconj J 1996;13:947-953.

[60] Varki A. Loss of N-glycolylneuraminic acid in humans: mechanisms, consequences, and implications for hominid evolution. Am J Phys Anthropol 2001;(Suppl 33):54-69.

[61] Seebach JD, Comrack C, Germana S, LeGuern C, Sachs DH, DerSimonian H. HLA-Cw3 expression on porcine endothelial cells protects against xenogeneic cytotoxicity mediated by a subset of human NK cells. J Immunol 1997;159:3655-3661.

[62] Dorling A, Monk NJ, Lechler RI. HLA-G inhibits the transendothelial migration of human NK cells. Eur J Immunol 2000;30;586-593.

[63] Forte P, Baumann BC, Weiss EH, Seebach JD. HLA-E expression on porcine cells: protection from human NK cytotoxicity depends on peptide loading. Am J Transplant 2005;5:2085-2093.

[64] Ide K, Ohdan H, Kobayashi T, Hara H, Ishiyama K, Asahara T. Antibody- and complement-independent phagocytotic and cytolytic activities of human macrophages toward porcine cells. Xenotransplantation 2005;12:181-188.

[65] Burlak C, Twining LM, Rees MA. Terminal sialic acid residues on human glycophorin A are recognized by porcine Kupffer cells. Transplantation 2005;80:344-352. .

[66] Rees MA, Butler AJ, Brons IG, *et al.* Evidence of macrophage receptors capable of direct recognition of xenogeneic epitopes without opsonization. Xenotransplantation 2005;12:13-19. .

[67] Kuwaki K, Knosalla C, Dor FJMF, *et al.* Suppression of natural and elicited antibodies in pig-to-baboon heart transplantation using a human anti-CD154 monoclonal antibody-based regimen. Am J Transplant 2004;4:363-372.

[68] Shimizu A, Yamada K, Yamamoto S, *et al.* Thrombotic microangiopathic glomerulopathy in human decay accelerating factor-transgenic swine-to-baboon kidney xenograts. J Am Soc Nephrol 2005;16:2732-2745.

[69] Gaca JG, Lesher A, Aksoy O, *et al.* Disseminated intravascular coagulation in association with pig-to-primate pulmonary xenotransplantation. Transplantation 2002;73:1717-1723.

[70] Buhler LH, Basker M, Alwayn IPJ, *et al.* Coagulation and thrombotic disorders associated with pig organ and hematopoietic cell transplantation in nonhuman primates. Transplantation 2000;70:1323-1331.

[71] Lin CC, Ekser B, Long C, *et al.* Consumptive coagulopathy is not associated with a humoral immune response after genetically-modified pig liver transplantation in baboons Submitted for publication.2009.

[72] Dorling A, Lechler RI. Disordered thromboregulation after xenografting. Curr Opin Organ Transplant 2001;6:36-41.

[73] Cowan PJ, Aminian A, Barlow H, *et al.* Protective effects of recombinant human antithrombin III in pig-to-primate renal xenotransplantation. Am J Transplant 2002;2:520-525.

[74] Cowan PJ, d'Apice AJF. The coagulation barrier in xenotransplantation: incompatibilities and astrategies to overcome them. Curr Opin Organ Transplant 2008;13:178-183.

[75] Lin CC, Cooper DK, Dorling A. Coagulation dysregulation as a barrier to xenotransplantation in the primate. Transpl Immunol 2009;21:75-80.

[76] Lin CC, Chen D, McVey JH, Cooper DKC, Dorling A. Expression of tissue factor and initiation of clotting by human platelets and monocytes after incubation with porcine endothelial cells. Transplantation. 2008;86:702-709. .

[77] Lin CC, Ezzelarab M, Shapiro R, *et al.* Tissue factor expression on recipient platelets initiates consumptive coagulopathy in pig-to-primate kidney xenotransplantation. Am J Transplant 2010; 10: 1556-68.

[78] Dwyer KM, Robson SC, Nandurkar HH, *et al.* Thromboregulatory manifestations in human CD39 transgenic mice and the implications for thrombotic disease and transplantation. J Clin Invest 2004:113:1440-1446.

[79] Baldan N, Rigotti P, Calabrese F, *et al.* Ureteral stenosis in HDAF pig-to-primate renal xenotransplantation: a phenomenon related to immunological events? Am J Transplant 2004; 4: 475-481.

[80] Griesemer AD, Hirakata A, Shimizu A, *et al.* Results of Gal-knockout porcine thymokidney xenografts. Am J Transplant 2009; 9: 2669-2678.

[81] Salvaris E, Hawthorne WJ, Peirce S, *et al.* Improved survival of GalT KO/hCD55-hCD59 pig renal xenografts in non-immunosuppressed baboons. (Abstract IXA-O-2.9). Xenotransplantation 2009; 16: 358.

[82] Cozzi E, Simioni P, Nottle MB, *et al.* Preliminary study in a life supporting pig to primate xenotransplantation model using GAL KO pigs transgenic for human CD39, CD55, CD59 and fucosyltransferase (Abstract LB IXA O-4). Xenotransplantation 2009; 16:544.

[83] Le Bas-Bernardet S, Tillou X, Poirier N, *et al.* First xenotransplantations of GAL KO, CD55, CD59, CD39, HT transgenic pig kidneys in baboons. (Abstract LB IXA O-3). Xenotransplantation 2009; 16:543.

[84] Griesemer AD, Liang F, Hirataka A, *et al.* Occurrence of specific humoral non-responsiveness to swine antigens following administration of GalT-KO bone marrow to baboons. Xenotransplantation 2010; 17: 300-312.

[85] Azimzadeh AM, Kelishadi SS, Ezzelarab M, *et al.* Early graft failure of GTKO pig organs in baboons is reduced by hCPRP expression. (Abstract IXA-O-2.2). Xenotransplantation 2009; 16: 356.

[86] Burdorf L, Stoddard T, Zhang T, *et al.* Does addition of CTLA4Ig to an anti-CD154-based regimen prevent anti-non-Gal antibody production after GalTKO or GalTKO/hCRP pig organ xenografting? (Abstract IXA-O-5.6). Xenotransplantation 2009; 16: 368.

[87] Ezzelarab M, Garcia B, Azimzadeh A, *et al.* The innate immune response and activation of coagulation in α1,3-galactosyltransferase gene-knockout xenograft recipients. Transplantation 2009; 87: 805-812.

[88] Tseng Y-L, Sachs DH, Cooper DKC. Porcine hematopoietic progenitor cell transplantation in nonhuman primates: a review of progress. Transplantation 2005;79:1-9. .

[89] Barth RN, Yamamoto S, LaMattina JC, *et al.* Xenogeneic thymokidney and thymic tissue transplantation in a pig-to-baboon model: I. Evidence for pig-specific T-cell unresponsiveness. Transplantation 2003;75:1615-1624.

[90] Kawai T, Cosmi B, Colvin RB, *et al.* Mixed allogeneic chimerism and renal allograft tolerance in cynomologus monkeys. Transplantation 1995; 59: 256-262.

[91] Spitzer TR, Delmonico F, Tolkoff-Rubin N, *et al.* Combined histocompatibility leukocyte antigen-matched donor bone marrow and renal transplantation for multiple myeloma with end stage renal disease: the induction of allograft tolerance through mixed lymphohematopoietic chimerism. Transplantation 1999;68:480-484. .

[92] Muller YD, Golshayan D, Ehirchiou D, Wekerle T, Seebach JD, Buhler LH. T regulatory cells in xenotransplantation. Xenotransplantation. 2009;16:121-128.

[93] West LJ, Pollock-Barziv SM, Dipchand AI, *et al.* ABO-incompatible heart transplantation in infants. N Engl J Med 2001;344:793-800.

[94] Fan X, Ang A, Pollock-Barziv SM, *et al.* Donor-specific B-cell tolerance after ABO-incompatible infant heart transplantation. Nat Med 2004;10:1227-1233.

[95] Rood PPM, Tai H-C, Hara H, *et al.* Late onset of development of natural anti-nonGal antibodies in infant humans and baboons: implications for xenotransplantation in infants. Transplant Int 2007;20:1050-1058.

[96] Ibrahim Z, Busch J, Awwad M, Wagner R, Wells K, Cooper DKC. Selected physiologic compatibilities and incompatibilities between human and porcine organ systems. Xenotransplantation 2006;13:488-499. .

[97] Vial CM, Ostlie DJ, Bhatti FN, *et al.* Life supporting function for over one month of a transgenic porcine heart in a baboon. J Heart Lung Transplant 2000;19:224-229.
[98] McGregor CGA, Davies WR, Oi K, *et al.* Recovery of cardiac function after pig-to-primate orthotopic heart transplant (Abstract). Am J Transplant 2008; 8(suppl 2): 205.
[99] Soin B, Smith KG, Zaidi A, *et al.* Physiological aspects of pig-to-primate renal xenotransplantation. Kidney Int 2001;60:1592-1597.
[100] Onions D, Cooper DKC, Alexander TJL, *et al.* An assessment of the risk of xenozoonotic disease in pig-to-human xenotransplantation. Xenotransplantation 2000;7:143-155.
[101] Fishman JA, Patience C. Xenotransplantation: infectious risk revisited. Am J Transplant 2004;4:1383-1390.
[102] Patience C, Patton GS, Takeuchi Y, *et al.* No evidence of pig DNA or retroviral infection in patients with short-term extracorporeal connection to pig kidneys. Lancet 1998;352:699-701.
[103] Paradis K, Langford G, Long Z, *et al.* Search for cross-species transmission of porcine endogenous retrovirus in patients with living pig tissue. The XEN 111 Study Group. Science 1999;285:1236-1241.
[104] Fishman JA. Xenosis and xenotransplantation: current concepts and challenges (Abstract PL5:2). Xenotransplantation. 2005;12:370.
[105] Dieckhoff B, Petersen B, Kues WA, Kurth R, Niemann H, Denner J. Knockdown of porcine endogenous retrovirus (PERV) expression by PERV-specific siRNA in transgenic pigs. Xenotransplantation. 2008;15:36-45.
[106] Ramsoondar J, Vaught T, Ball S, *et al.* Production of transgenic pigs that express porcine endogenous retrovirus small interfering RNAs. Xenotransplantation. 2009;16:164-180.
[107] Schuurman HJ. Regulatory aspects of pig-to-human islet transplantation. Xenotransplantation. 2008; 15:116-120.
[108] Ekser B, Gridelli B, Tector AJ, Cooper DKC. Pig liver xenotransplantation as a bridge to allotransplantation: which patients might benefit? Transplantation. 2009;88:1041-9.
[109] Ibrahim Z, Ezzelarab M, Kormos R, Cooper DKC. Which patients first? Planning the first clinical trial of xenotransplantation: a case for cardiac bridging. Xenotransplantation 2005;12:168-172. .
[110] Cooper DKC, Tseng Y-L, Saidman SL. Allo- and xeno-antibody cross-reactivity in transplantation. Transplantation 2004;77:1-5.
[111] Ekser B, Kumar G, Veroux M, Cooper DKC. Therapeutic issues in the treatment of vascularized xenotransplants using gal-knockout donors in nonhuman primates. Curr Opin Organ Transplant 2011; 16: 222-30.

Index

A

C

D

E

F

G

H

I

K

Massimiliano Veroux and Pierfrancesco Veroux (Eds)

L

N

P

Q

R

S

T

W

Made in the USA
Las Vegas, NV
03 November 2026

57424114R00240